Psychosocial Occupational Therapy
A Holistic Approach

Psychosocial Occupational Therapy
A Holistic Approach

Second Edition

Franklin Stein, Ph. D., OTR/L, FAOTA
University of South Dakota
Department of Occupational Therapy
Vermillion, South Dakota

Susan K. Cutler, Ph.D., NCSP
Morningside College
Sioux City, Iowa

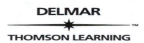

DELMAR
™
THOMSON LEARNING

Australia Canada Mexico Singapore Spain United Kingdom United States

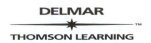

DELMAR

THOMSON LEARNING

Psychosocial Occupational Therapy-A Holistic Approach, 2nd Edition
by Franklin Stein
Susan K. Cutler

Health Care Publishing Director:
William Brottmiller

Editorial Assistant:
Maria D'Angelico

Production Editor:
Mary Colleen Liburdi

Executive Editor:
Cathy L. Esperti

Executive Marketing Manager:
Dawn F. Gerrain

Illustrator:
SoundLightMind

Acquisitions Editor:
Candice Janco

Channel Manager:
Jennifer McAvey

Cover Design:
The Drawing Board

www.thomsonrights.com
Library of Congress Cataloging-in-Publication Data applied for and on file.

NOTICE TO THE READER

Contents

Preface to the Second Edition ix

Preface to the First Edition with Revision...xi

Disablement Theory from World Health Organization (WHO) xiii

Acknowledgments...xix

1 Introduction to the Holistic Approach in Psychosocial Practice 1

2 A Short History of the Treatment of Individuals with Mental Illness
   and the Emergence of Occupational Therapy...27

3 The Community Care Model and the Roles of the Occupational Therapist
   and Certified Occupational Therapy Assistant (COTA): 1960–2000 65

4 Theoretical Models Underlying the Clinical Practice of
   Psychosocial Occupational Therapy 109

5 The Occupational Therapy Treatment Process: The Basis for
   Achieving Positive Mental Health Goals 187

6 Evaluation and Assessment of the Individual with Psychosocial Dysfunction 241

7 Medications Related to Psychosocial Issues 301

8 Applying the Group Process to Psychosocial Occupational Therapy
   by Beverlea Tallant, Ph.D., OT(C) 359

9 Vocational Exploration and Employment and Psychosocial Disabilities
   by Joyce Tryssenaar, M. Ed., OT(C)...391

10 Stress Management, Biofeedback, and Relaxation Techniques 417

11 Leisure-Time Occupations, Self-Care, and Social Skills Training............................463

12 Exercise, Nutrition, and Alternative Treatment Techniques...................................497

13 Creative and Expressive Arts and Their Application to Psychosocial Treatment.......................539

14 Quality Assurance, Continuous Quality Improvement,
    Reimbursement, and Documentation
    by Rita Chang, MS, OTR 559

15 Evaluating and Designing Clinical Research Studies..591

    Epilogue...611

    Glossary 613

    Appendix A: Diagnosis of Mental Disorders...639

    Appendix B: Severity of Psychosocial Stressors and Level of Functioning 645

    Appendix C: Role Delineation of COTA 647

    Appendix D: Useful Internet Sites 653

    Appendix E: Calories Expended per Hour for Typical Activities.................................655

    Index 657

Contributors

Rita Chang, M.S., OTR
St. Michael's Hospital
Stevens Point, Wisconsin

Beverlea Tallant, Ph.D., OT(C)
School of Occupational and Physical Therapy
McGill University
Montreal, Quebec, Canada

Joyce Tryssenaar, M. Ed., OT(C)
McMaster University
Hamilton, Ontario, Canada

Preface

Preface to the Second Edition

The health care system in the United States is undergoing dramatic changes, with managed care under attack and plans for changes in Medicare, especially with coverage for medications. Americans are using alternative medicine in increasing numbers. It has been estimated that almost 40 percent of the population uses some type of alternative medicine, whether it be herbal remedies, acupuncture, or yoga. There is concern also by the medical community that herbal medicines do interact with prescriptive medications and may cause adverse effects. However, alternative or complementary medicine will continue to be widely used because consumers believe they are effective and easily attainable. Occupational therapy is directly affected by the political decisions made in health care and the consumers' perceptions of what quality care is. Heart disease, stroke, and cancer are still the leading causes of death in the United States. However, psychosocial disabilities are an enormous problem at the beginning of the 21st century, coinciding with the rapid pace of living and rising expectations in one's standard of living. Anxiety disorders and depression are widespread and of epidemic proportions. There are also increased diagnoses of attention deficit hyperactivity disorders among schoolchildren. Violence in the schools and an increase in the use of tobacco, drugs, and alcohol among youth are of extreme concern for parents and educators. How can occupational therapists contribute their expertise and knowledge in the field of psychosocial practice?

In the second edition of this text, the authors have

▶ included material on the role of the COTA in psychosocial practice, with review of this section by Gwen Hawley, Director of the COTA program at Lake Area Tech in Watertown, SD

▶ included the World Health Organization's newest definition of disablement

▶ reviewed carefully the chapter on medications with the help from Dr. Steven Waller, Associate Dean, University of South Dakota Medical School and Professor of Physiology and Pharmacology

▶ updated references and included recent references on mental illness and homelessness, forensic psychiatry, object relations, and borderline personality

▶ added an appendix with useful Internet sites for occupational therapists working in psychosocial areas

The chapters on group occupational therapy, vocational exploration, and quality assurance have been edited and revised by the guest authors.

In the fall of 1999 Frank spent a sabbatical at the University of Uppsala in Sweden. He had the opportunity to visit a number of mental health centers and to discuss occupational therapy with clinicians. He would like to thank publicly the support from the Swedish occupational therapists, Ingrid Söderback and Helena Lindstedt from Uppsala, Ann-Britt Ivarsson from Orebro, and Mona Eklund from Lund; and Sisko Salo-Chydenius from Helskinki, Finland who interacted with him and widened his perspectives in the role of occupational therapy in psychosocial practice.

Frank Stein, Vermillion, SD
Susan K. Cutler, Sioux City, IA
July 6, 2000

Preface to the First Edition with Revision

Occupational therapists have always considered that treatment, if it is to be successful, should consider the totality of a patient or client's life. A holistic approach implies that the clinician considers both the organic and functional aspects of an individual's illness and applies treatment methods that take mind-body relationships into consideration. The holistic practitioner emphasizes the biopsychosocial aspects of both etiology and treatment. The holistic approach is congruent with the wellness model for clients. Swarbrick (1997) defines wellness from an occupational therapy perspective: "Wellness is a lifestyle that incorporates a good balance of health habits, such as adequate sleep and rest, productivity, exercise, supportive thought processes and social resources. This balance influences social roles and associated activities" (p. 1). The concept of mind, body, and spirit is essential in understanding the individual's illness. On the other hand, a nonholistic approach is one dimensional, for example, treating patients singly with medication, surgery, or ascribing to one theory of psychosocial treatment. The holistic practitioner is not tied to a "Procrustual Bed" whether it be a specific drug, treatment method, or theory. The holistic practitioner seeks the most effective treatment method by considering the total needs of the individual while empowering the client to take an active role in the treatment process. Clinical research is incorporated into practice by basing clinical judgment on research evidence. In a holistic approach, it is essential that the clinical practitioner maintain good interdisciplinary relationships with other team members. In working with the individual who is mentally ill, a holistic practitioner uses language that is acceptable top all health care professionals. For example, in diagnosing individuals with mental illness, the DSM-IV (APA, 1994) is accepted by psychiatrists, psychologists, nurses, counselors, school psychologists, special educators, and occupational therapists as a practical guide. Common criteria are used in evaluating outcome.

Etiology of mental illness is of interest to all mental health practitioners. Theories underlying the basis of treatment are shared by the mental health team. Although the team shares a common language in diagnosing mental illness, an understanding of etiology and the criteria for successful outcome, there are differences in the specific role functions of mental health practitioners. For example, psychiatrists are primarily responsible for diagnosing the patient's illness, for prescribing medication and in some cases, carrying out psychotherapy. Psychologists use projective and objective tests in evaluating psychodynamic aspects of a patient's illness and also engage in psychotherapy. Occupational therapists emphasize the functional aspects of an individual's life, which include the ability to work, engage in leisure activities, be independent in self-care, and have adequate social relationships. In holistic treatment, the members of the mental health team combine their expertise and efforts in helping the patient.

Effective psychiatric rehabilitation includes (a) reducing symptoms, such as anxiety, phobias, depression, hallucinations, delusions, and thinking disorders; (b) enabling the patient to work at a job that gives him or her satisfaction; (c) discovering leisure activities that are fulfilling; (d) restoring or developing independent living and interpersonal skills; and (e) helping the patient develop a sense of meaning in life by fulfilling spiritual needs.

In this book, the authors bring together a holistic approach by using historical references, current occupational therapy practice, and research evidence. Traditional as well as alternative or complimentary treatment techniques are described and evaluated. Occupational therapy's link to its historical roots, as well as the emerging trends in community mental health care, is emphasized. At a time of expanding roles in occupational therapy, the past, present, and future of occupational therapy in mental health are considered.

Proposed Definition of Occupational Therapy

In this book, the authors define occupational therapy as an applied science and rehabilitation profession concerned with enabling individuals with disabilities to reach their maximum potential in performing functions in daily living, employment, and leisure, through the use of purposeful activities. The occupational therapist's treatment goals are to maintain, restore, and develop physical and psychological functions. The occupational therapist works with clients throughout the life span to prevent and treat disabilities and to restore or develop function. The outcome of treatment will depend on the competence of the therapist, the scientific basis of the activity prescribed, the environment in which the activity takes place, and the motivation and will of the patient to improve. This definition is compatible with the *Uniform Terminology for Occupational Therapy* (3rd ed., 1994).

A purposeful activity occurs within the context of work, self-care, play and leisure, has meaning to the patient, and is related to the patient's goal of maximum independence (AOTA, 1993; Hong & Yates, 1995). Examples of purposeful activities are simulated work activities, creative expression, relaxation exercise, animal-facilitated therapy, arts and crafts, horticulture, sports, table games, and self-care exercises. Activities that are not purposeful and repetitious and monotonous, for example, putting pegs in a board, cone stacking, watching televi-

sion obsessively, compulsive gambling, and other tasks without value to the individual that are used to fill time.

Assumptions underlying the definition of occupational therapy are:

▶ Development is sequential and hierarchical and dependent on critical stages of learning (Gesell, 1928; Lorenz, 1981; Piaget, 1926).

▶ Human life includes a process of continuous adaptation to the home, work, and leisure environments and promotes self-survival and self-actualization (Maslow, 1968; Rogers, 1951).

▶ An important component of occupational therapy is to help clients self-actualize their life goals realistically [by reaching their maximum potential in performing ADL, work, and leisure activities] (Reilly, 1974).

▶ Biological, psychological, and environmental factors may interrupt the adaptation process any time throughout the life cycle (Erikson, 1963).

▶ The inability to adapt to a change such as a disability increases the degrees of handicap in ADL, work, and leisure activities (Rusk, 1971).

▶ Purposeful activity facilitates the adaptive process, and relates to the areas of ADL, work, and leisure (AOTA, 1994).

▶ Intrinsic motivation and compliance are important influences on the patient's rehabilitation and recovery (Kielhofner, 1997).

▶ Clinical research enables the occupational therapist to objectively evaluate the effectiveness of a specific treatment method (Stein & Cutler, 1996, 2000).

Within the definition of occupational therapy, it is vital that psychosocial occupational therapists differentiate between impairment, disability, and handicap as consistent with the definition from the World Health Organization (World Health Organization, 1980):

▶ Impairment is any loss or abnormality of physiological, psychological, or anatomical structure or function such as blindness, deafness, astereognosis, mental retardation, or lack of pain sensation. For example, a psychiatric impairment is a delusion, hallucination, severe anxiety, phobia, depression, or any other symptom that interferes with carrying out normal human activities.

▶ Disability is any restriction or lack of ability (resulting from an impairment) to perform an activity in the manner or within the range considered normal for a human being. These human activities include walking, running, speaking, writing, dressing, feeding oneself, or listening. A psychiatric disability results from the symptoms of an illness such as delusions that prevent an individual from engaging normally in human interactions. The symptoms of depression can cause an individual to become disabled in performing the activities of daily living.

▶ Handicap is a disadvantage imposed on a given individual, resulting from an impairment or a disability that limits or prevents the fulfillment of a role that is normal (depending on age, sex, and social and cultural factors) for that individual. A psychiatric handicap is the inability to perform normal role functions as a student, worker, husband, wife, father, or mother or to engage in leisure activities, or be independent in self-care or social functioning. The handicap can also be aggravated by environmental factors such as a stigma, which produces a negative attitude toward individuals with mental illness and thereby prevents individuals with mental illness

from obtaining employment. These differences are depicted in Figure P–1.

Disablement Theory from World Health Organization (WHO)

In 1997, the World Health Organization reconceptualized the International Classification of Impairments, Disabilities and Handicaps (ICIDH). The new model (International Classification of Impairments, Activities and Participation [ICIDH–2]) changed the focus from the disease and disability to the consequences of the impairment. One reason for the change was the inadequacy of the diagnosis by itself to predict (a) health care intervention, (b) need for and time spent in health care, (c) intensity of care needed, (d) effectiveness of hospitalization, (e) receipt of disability benefits, (f) ability to work, and (g) social integration into the community (WHO, 2000). In this model, the ability to predict outcome is based on the diagnosis and the disability (e.g., function and disablement). Function includes the ability to (a) learn and apply knowledge, (b) communicate and understand knowledge, (c) manipulate objects, (d) move about, (e) perform self-care and domestic activities, (f) engage in major life activities such as work and school, and (g) partake in interpersonal and social relationships. Figure P–2 depicts the conceptualization.

Examples cited by WHO using this model include attention deficit disorder and panic disorder. In attention deficit disorder, the impairment includes poor attention, problems in concentration, and increased arousal. Activity limitations include difficulty with completion of homework assignments and taking turns. Participation restrictions include exclusion from everyday class activities. In panic disorder, the impairment is described as severe and uncontrolled anxiety. The activity limitation

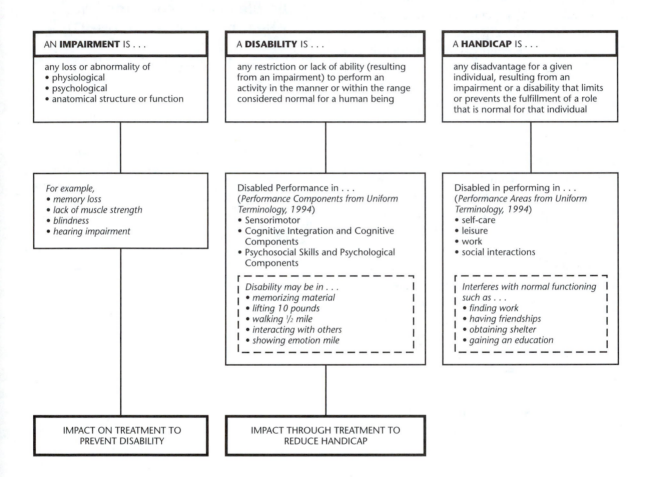

Figure P–1. This figure shows the differences between impairment, disability, and handicap as defined by the World Health Organization in 1980. Although there is a relationship, each term denotes a different type of loss. The impairment can lead to either a disability or handicap. Treatment for the impairment is designed to prevent a disability, while treatment for the disability is designed to reduce the handicap. Occupational therapists should evaluate the client to determine the effect of the impairment on either a disability or handicap, and then provide treatment to alleviate the condition. (Adapted from *Handbook of Psychiatric Rehabilitation* [p. 5], by R. P. Libermann [Ed.], 1992; Boston: Allyn and Bacon; and the *International Classification of Impairments, Disabilities, and Handicaps [ICIDH]* (pp. 27–29), by World Health Organization [WHO], 1980, Geneva, Switzerland: Author.)

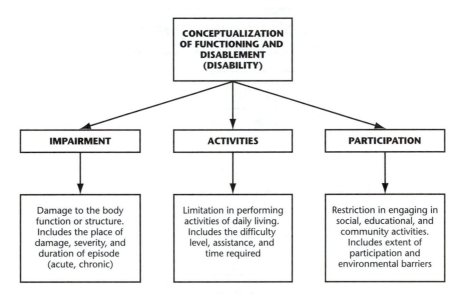

Figure P-2. The new conceptionalization of ICIDH (WHO, 1999). Disability is conceptualized as including both functioning and disablement. Impairment, activity, and participation are integral concepts, which then determine the functioning and disablement of the disability.

includes the inability to go out alone, while the participation restriction involves lack of social interactions. The concepts are seen as dynamic and impacting on the individual's ability to function independently in social and community contexts (see Figure P–3). In Figure P–4, the model is applied to an individual with schizophrenia.

In this book, we use the words *patient, member, client, individual,* and *person* interchangeably. We are aware of the connotations of these words. It seems to us that the word "patient," which is defined as an individual awaiting or under medical treatment, connotes an individual with an abnormal condition. The very use of this term may imply a pejorative meaning. This is especially true when the terms "patient with a psychiatric illness," "patient with an emotional disturbance," "patient with mental illness," "patient with schizophrenia," or "patient who is paranoid" are used. In actuality, occupational therapists work with people who have impairments that cause them to be disabled. Throughout history and in different culture individuals who have been unable to care for themselves or unable to regulate their feelings have been cared for at both extremes of cruelty and humanism. We have tried to convey in this book the attitudes toward the individual with mental illness that are reflected historically and that are practiced in the moral holistic tradition of occupational therapy.

REFERENCES

American Occupational Therapy Association (AOTA). (1993). Position paper: Purposeful activity. *American Journal of Occupational Therapy, 47,* 1081–1082.

American Occupational Therapy Association (AOTA). (1993). *Uniform terminology for occupational therapy: Application to practice* (3rd ed.). Rockville, MD: Author.

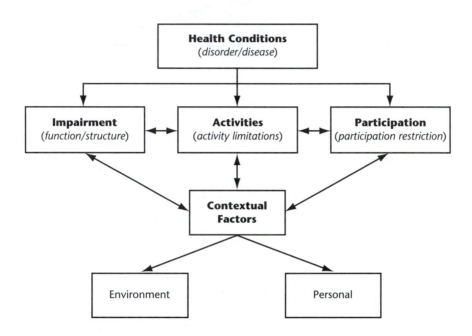

Figure P-3. The concepts included in the functioning and disablement are seen as dynamic and impact on the individual's ability to function independently in social and community contexts.

American Psychiatric Association. (1994). *Diagnostic and statistical manual of mental disorders* (4th ed.). Washington, DC: Author.

Erikson, E. (1963). *Childhood and society* (2nd ed.). New York: W. W. Norton.

Gesell, A. (1928). *Infancy and human growth.* New York: McGraw Hill.

Hong, C. S. , & Yates, P. (1995). Purposeful activities? What are they? *British Journal of Occupational Therapy, 58,* 75–76.

Kielhofner, G. (1997). *Conceptual foundations of occupational therapy* (2nd ed.). Philadelphia: F. A. Davis.

Liberman, R. P. (Ed.). (1992). *Handbook of psychiatric rehabilitation.* Boston: Allyn and Bacon.

Lorenz, K. Z. (1981). *The foundation of ethnology.* New York: Springer-Verlag.

Maslow, A. (1968). *Toward a psychology of being* (2nd ed.). New York: Van Nostrand Reinhold.

Piaget, J. (1926). *The language and thought of the child* (M. Gabain & R. Gabain, Trans.). London: K. Paul, Trench, Trubner.

Reilly, M. (1974). *Play as exploratory learning.* Beverly Hills, CA: Sage.

Rogers, C. (1951). *Client-centered therapy.* Boston: Houghton-Mifflin.

Rusk, H. (1971). *Rehabilitation medicine* (4th ed.). St. Louis, MO: C. V. Mosby.

Stein, F., & Cutler, S. K. (1996). *Clinical research in allied health and special education* (3rd ed.). San Diego, CA: Singular Publishing Group.

Stein, F., & Cutler, S. K. (2000). *Clinical research in occupational therapy* (4th ed.). San Diego, CA: Singular Publishing Group.

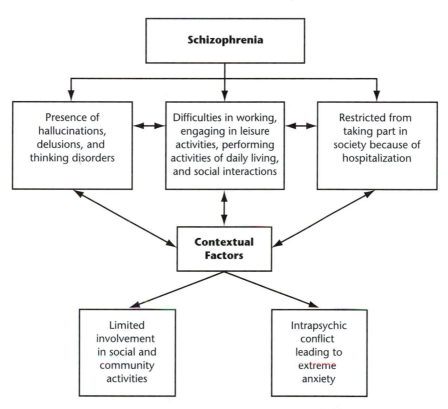

EXAMPLE OF THE INTERACTION OF FUNCTIONING AND DISABLEMENT CONCEPTS

Figure P-4. The functioning and disablement of schizophrenia are presented as an example of the ICIDH–2 model.

Swarbrick, P. (1997). Wellness model for clients. *Mental Health Special Interest Section Quarterly, 20*(1), 1–4.

World health Organization (WHO). (1980). *International classification of impairments, disabilities, and handicaps (ICIDH).* Geneva, Switzerland: Author.

World Health Organization (WHO). (2000, December). *ICIDH-2: International Classification of functioning, disability and health.* Prefinal draft, full revision. Geneva, Switzerland: Author. Retrieved January 23, 2001 from the World Wide Web: http://www.who.int/icidh/ICIDH-2PFDec-2000.pdf.

Acknowledgments

Writing a book and putting one's thoughts on paper is a retrospective journey through time. One's ideas, concepts, philosophy, and theories are shaped by experiences in life, and the people encountered. My ideas about psychology and mental illness were initially learned from professors at Brooklyn College (Evelyn Raskin, Wayne Dennis, Ivan London, Harold Proskansky, Martin Lean) and from friends (Stanley Berger, Larry Posner, Gerald Schecter, Leon Miller). At the Brooklyn Day Center I met Jennie Stiffler, an occupational therapy intern who later became my wife, and Bill Roach and Jane Foley, psychosocial occupational therapists. Virginia Scullin, director of Occupational Therapy for the New York State Department of Mental Hygiene, encouraged me to continue my education by offering me a scholarship to complete my studies at New York University.

▶ *To the professors at New York University:* Freida Behlen, Hugh Banks, Sophie Chiotelis, George Deaver, Claire Glasser, Claude Grant, Robert Hoppock, Bernard Katz, Edith Lawton, Isabel Robinault, Howard Rusk, Muriel Zimmerman

▶ *To the colleagues at New York State Psychiatric Institute:* Gail Fidler, Susan Babbit Fine, Alice Trei, and psychiatric residents Ronald Fieve, Robert Spitzer

▶ *To colleagues at Brooklyn After Care Clinic:* Ed Busby, Donald Carmichael, Floyd Carneal, Elizabeth Robinson, George Serban, Jane Tucker, Doreen Weinstein

▶ *To colleagues at the counseling psychology department at Queens College*

▶ *To fellow doctoral students in psychology at New York University:* Larry Randolph, Frank Di Bernardo

▶ *To colleagues and students at Boston University:* Abby Abildness, Irene Allard, Olga Baloueff, Evelyn Bloch, Tina Brollier, Beverly Bullen, Sharon Cermak, Judy Chiswell, Linda Duncombe, Wimberly Edwards, Carroll English, Maureen Fleming, Bob Gilbert, Carmella Gonnella, Anne Henderson, Ruth Jacobson, Jerry Johnson, Moya Kinnealey, Matt Luzzi, Dottie Marsh, Patti Maurer, Lucy Miller, Rosalie Miller, Ellie Nystrom, Frances Palmer, Whitney Powers, Stan Rosenzweig, Richard Schwartz, Sharan Schwartzberg, Alice Schaefer, Roger Soule, Shirley Stockmeyer, Barbara Sussenberger, Nancy Talbot, Catherine Trombly, Nancy Watts, Hilda Versluys

▶ *To colleagues and students at University of Wisconsin—Milwaukee:* Martin Blackwell, Karen Conrad, Fred Cox, Tina Dale, Joyce Engel, Rene Gratz, Michael Hauer, Barbara Jacobsen, Lisette Kautzmann, Byong Kim, Rosemary Kwako, Ted and Phyllis King, Elizabeth Larson, Carol Leonardelli, John

Lynch, Virgil Mathiowetz, Jim McPherson, Susan Nikolic, Sharon Pape, Fred Pairent, Cindy Schoenleber, Sandy Spaulding, Virginia Stoffel, Mary Taugher, Ronald Tikofsky, Ruth Zemke

▶ *To colleagues and students at University of Manitoba*

▶ *To colleagues and students at University of South Dakota:* Dorothy Anne Elsberry, Marie Axtmann, Rosemary Bartowski, Bob Bing, Barbara Brockevelt, Frank Gainer, Diane Hawkins, Linda Kamp, Barbara and Bernie Kleinman, Jo Moore, Barbara Papik, Deb Picasso, Marianne Ross, Denise Rotert, Evelyn Schlenker, Peggy Stoddard, Cliff Summers

▶ *To colleagues in AOTA and the Occupational Therapy community:* Bea Abreu, Claudia Allen, Linda Baldwin, Carolyn Baum, Marie Louise Blount, Estelle Breines, Sharon Brintnell, Chick Christiansen, David Clark, Florence Clark, Barbara Cooper, Florence Cromwell, Rosemary Crouch, Elizabeth Devereaux, Karen Diasio-Serrett, Mary Donohue, Winnie Dunn, Paul Elsworth, David Etheridge, Ann Fisher, Diane Gibson, Ellie Gilfoyle, Grace Gilkeson, Nedra Gillette, Kay Grant, Ruth Hansen, Diane Harlowe, Barbara Hemphill, Jim Hinojosa, Helen Hopkins, Margot Howe, Sat Izutsu, Jacie Jurkowski, Gary Keilhofner, Jean Kiernat, Lorna Jean King, Marge Kirchman, Valerie Knotts, Ellen Kolodner, Ruth Levine, Lela Llorens, William Mann, David Nelson, Anne Opzoomer, Ken Ottenbacher, Paul Petersen, Barbara Posthuma, Kitty Reed, Rhona Reiss-Zukas, Patricia Reynolds, Barbara Rider, Charlotte Royeen, Phil

Shannon, Jane Slaymaker, Roger Smith, Anne Spencer, Karen Stone, Bev Tallant, Julia Van Deusen, Pat Wilbarger, Joane Wyrick

▶ *To past friends:* Jean Ayres, Doris Beasley, Joe Chase, Mary Fiorentino, Alice Jantzen, Ruth Robinson, Wilma West

▶ *To my colleagues on the Editorial Board of Occupational Therapy:* Diana Bailey, Evelien Bongers, Marjorie E. Concha, Susan Esdaile, Joyce Engel-Knowles, Suzanne L. Floyd, Rita Goble, Angela Harth, Clare Hocking, Chia Swee Hong, Clephane Hume, Noomi Katz, Indira Ramesh Kenkre, Deborah Labovitz, Gwynnyth Llewellyn, Lilian Vieira Magalhaes, Ana Maria Montes Palma, Julie Piergrossi, Helene Polataijko, Sisko Salo-Chydenius, Tsuyoshi Sato, Maria Schwarz, Mei-Jin Chen Sea, Kathleen Sinclair, Ingrid Soderback, Sylvie Tétreault, Rhoda Weiss-Lambrou, Elizabeth Yerxa

▶ *Clerical help:* Cheryl Hovorka, Rene Bilka, and Cherity Lindgren.

▶ And to all the other friends, colleagues, and students who have shared with me their knowledge and experiences

▶ And to my family: Jennie, David, Sharon, Jacqueline, Natalie, Barbara, Craig, Jessie, and Chris.

▶ Sue Cutler and I owe a special thanks to Candice Janco and Sandy Doyle of Singular Publishing Group for the editorial assistance and help that any writer needs in making a book come to fruition.

Frank Stein
January 20, 1998

CHAPTER

Introduction to the Holistic Approach in Psychosocial Practice

> *The whole of human organization has its shape in a kind of rhythm. It is not enough that our hearts should beat in a useful rhythm, always kept up to a standard at which it can meet rest as well as wholesome strain without upset. There are many other rhythms which we must be attuned to: the larger rhythms of night and day, of sleep and waking hours, of hunger and its gratification, and finally the big four—work and play and rest and sleep, which our organism must be able to balance even under difficulty. The only way to attain balance in all this is actual doing, actual practice, a program of wholesome living as the basis of wholesome feeling and thinking and fancy and interests.*
>
> —A. Meyer, (1922/1977), The Philosophy of Occupational Therapy,
> *Archives of Occupational Therapy, 1*, p. 641.

Operational Learning Objectives

By the end of this chapter, the learner will:

1. Examine common attitudes and major issues related to mental illness.

2. Examine his or her own attitudes toward mental illness.

3. Define, compare, and contrast mental illness and mental health.

4. Comprehend and discuss the most current definition of mental illness as defined in DSM–IV (APA, 1994).

5. Use "People First" language.

6. Identify the five key issues affecting the practice of psychosocial occupational therapy.

7. Identify how the family's reaction can affect the individual with mental illness by analyzing biographical material from contemporary literature.

Key Questions for Occupational Therapy Students Studying Psychosocial Dysfunction

What are some key questions that occupational therapy students and clinicians should consider in studying psychosocial dysfunction?

▶ What is mental illness? What is normality?

▶ How does mental illness differ from mental retardation?

▶ How is mental illness diagnosed?

▶ What are typical attitudes toward mental illness?

▶ What is the history of the treatment of individuals with mental illness?

▶ What current controversies surround the care and treatment of individuals with mental illness?

▶ Are the homeless mentally ill?

▶ What is the role of self-help groups in the treatment of individuals with mental illness?

▶ Is mental illness inherited?

▶ What is the role of the environment in the onset of mental illness?

▶ What is the role of stress in the onset of mental illness?

▶ How do people recover from mental illness?

▶ What does current research on mental illness suggest in the treatment of mental illness?

▶ What are the current theories regarding the multiple causes of mental illness?

▶ How is the DSM–IV (APA, 1994) used in the diagnosis of mental illness?

▶ What are the ethical considerations in treating mental illness?

▶ What are the differential roles of professionals in evaluating and treating those individuals with mental illness?

▶ What are the major theories and frames of references guiding treatment?

▶ What common evaluation instruments are used by occupational therapists?

▶ What treatment techniques are used by psychosocial occupational therapists?

An outline of the process of psychosocial dysfunction showing the relationship between the factors causing mental illness, the symptoms that occur, and the comprehensive evaluation, treatment, and rehabilitation is found in Figure 1–1. The authors have proposed a model for understanding how individuals develop mental illness and then are diagnosed through evaluations, treated, and rehabilitated. Throughout the book the reader is encouraged to refer to this model as the process of mental illness is discussed.

ATTITUDES TOWARD MENTAL ILLNESS

Attitudes are formed by knowledge, experience, personal values, and beliefs. These attitudes affect how each of us interacts with our environment. Attitudes can be changed if one is willing. Attitudes toward mental illness affect how the therapist treats the patient or client. The attitude scale in Table 1–1 lists some of the controversial issues attached to mental illness. At this time, the reader should take the *Attitudes Toward Mental Illness Scale* to assess his or her personal attitudes.

After taking the scale, consider the following controversial questions as a basis for understanding one's own attitudes. Each individual should explore his or her own attitudes to see

Process of Social Dysfunction

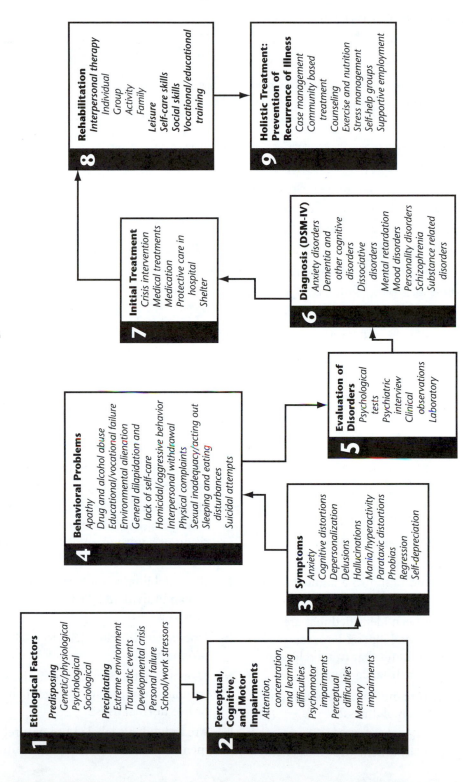

Figure 1–1. Outline of the process of psychosocial dysfunction. The process is sequential, beginning with etiological factors. Dysfunctional aspects, problems, and symptoms are considered in the evaluation and diagnosis, and these components occur before treatment can begin. The treatment approach is holistic and is aimed toward rehabilitation and prevention of recurrence.

Table 1–1. Attitudes Toward Mental Illness Scale

Circle Y or N to show your attitude.	Yes	No
1. Mental illness is inherited.	Y	N
2. Individuals with mental illness are not as intelligent as normal people.	Y	N
3. Mental illness is due to faulty parenting.	Y	N
4. Most homeless people are mentally ill.	Y	N
5. People with mental illness who are convicted of crimes should be put in prison.	Y	N
6. People should be hospitalized for mental illness if they are diagnosed with schizophrenia.	Y	N
7. Individuals diagnosed with depression are generally malingerers.	Y	N
8. People who abuse alcohol and drugs are mentally ill.	Y	N
9. People should not be forced to have treatment if they are mentally ill.	Y	N
10. Electroconvulsive therapy is the treatment of choice for those with severe depression.	Y	N
11. People with dementia should be in mental hospitals.	Y	N
12. Community treatment is better than hospital care for those with mental illness.	Y	N
13. Tough-love is a positive way to treat adolescents who are acting out.	Y	N
14. Parents should not use physical punishment to discipline children.	Y	N
15. Prozac® should be used often with patients who are depressed.	Y	N
16. Neuroleptics treat symptoms rather than cure people.	Y	N
17. The best indication of normality is the ability to work.	Y	N

Source: © F. Stein, 1994.

how they affect interactions with individuals with mental illness. References that explore the issues, either pro or con, are included with each section as resources for the reader.

Mental illness is inherited. (Tsuang, Kendler, & Lyons, 1991)

▶ Have genetic studies shown a familial relationship?

▶ Have any genes been identified that are implicated in mental illness? For example, have genes been found that cause schizophrenia, bipolar, substance abuse?

▶ What is the nature–nurture relationship in the etiology of mental illness?

▶ What is the relationship between the interaction of the environment with the genetic predisposition and the individual's temperament in causing mental illness?

▶ Have studies of identical twins shown a convincing evidence for a genetic predisposition or environmental cause in mental illness?

▶ If mental illness is inherited, what actions can an individual take to prevent the onset of illness?

▶ Does a genetic cause lead to a self-fulfilling prophecy?

▶ Does a genetic cause mean individuals with mental illness cannot change their behavior or live normal lives?

▶ Are individuals labeled prematurely with mental illness because family members may be seeking an explanation for the aberrant behavior?

Individuals with mental illness are not as intelligent as normal people. (Sternberg & Grigorenko, 1997)

▶ How does mental illness differ from mental retardation?

▶ What is the distribution of intelligence in people with mental illness?

▶ Why do evaluators sometimes obtain low intelligence scores in individuals with mental illness?

▶ What is the effect of low motivation, distraction, poor attention or inattentiveness, anxiety, inaccurate perceptions, and the presence of psychotic behavior on test results?

Mental illness is due to faulty parenting. (Bisbee, 1991)

▶ Why do counselors and psychologists blame parents for mental illness in their children?

▶ Is Parent Effectiveness Training (Gordon, 1976) important in the child's psychological development?

▶ Can a child develop mental illness regardless of the parent's effectiveness?

▶ Does mental illness occur because of the interactions between the genetic predisposition for the illness and environmental factors such as dysfunctional family, poor parenting, stress, poverty, homelessness, school failure, peer pressure, and lack of support or encouragement in developing a positive self-image?

▶ Can effective parenting with children who are mentally ill help them make a good adjustment in school, work, personal relations, self-care, and leisure activities?

Most homeless people are mentally ill. (Snow & Anderson, 1993)

▶ What percentage of homeless people are mentally ill?

▶ Why do people become homeless?

▶ How does homelessness affect one's mental health?

▶ Should people who are homeless be treated for mental illness without their consent?

▶ Should occupational therapists reach out to homeless individuals in the community?

▶ What are the conditions for hospitalization for those people who are homeless who have mental illness?

People with mental illness who are convicted of crimes should be put in prison. (Szasz, 1963)

▶ Should every individual be responsible for his or her behavior regardless of whether he or she is mentally healthy or mentally ill?

▶ Should society encourage responsibility in every individual?

▶ If individuals with mental illness are imprisoned, should they be in rehabilitation programs and receive psychiatric treatment?

▶ If an individual pleads insanity, should he or she be punished for the crime?

People should be hospitalized for mental illness if they are diagnosed with schizophrenia. (Pasamanick, Scarpitti, & Dinitz, 1967)

▶ Should people be hospitalized even if they are not harmful to themselves or others but show signs of schizophrenia?

▶ Can individuals with schizophrenia function adequately in mainstream society, such as in work, leisure, school, and self-care activities?

▶ How can short-term hospitalization help an individual with schizophrenia reduce the positive symptoms of delusions, hallucinations, and thinking disorders?

▶ Why does long-term hospitalization cause regression in individuals with schizophrenia?

▶ Are there instances of individuals with schizophrenia making adequate adjustments in society?

▶ Is community care better than hospitalization in helping individuals to overcome dysfunction or symptoms?

▶ How do alternatives to hospitalization, such as halfway houses, supported employment, foster care, support groups, and day treatment centers help individuals with schizophrenia improve their functioning?

Individuals with depression are generally malingerers. (Montgomery & Rouillon, 1992)

▶ Why do people malinger?

▶ Why are individuals with depression overly fatigued?

▶ What is the relationship between depression and vegetative signs (e.g., sleeping, eating, and sexual dysfunction)?

▶ Why do people with depression have difficulties with work, school, personal relationships, leisure activities, and self-care?

▶ Why do individuals with depression feel they have no control over their behavior?

▶ What types of therapy are effective in mobilizing individuals with depression?

▶ Why is stress a factor in precipitating symptoms?

People who abuse alcohol and drugs are mentally ill. (Wekesser, 1994)

▶ Is alcoholism inherited?

▶ Are most individuals with alcoholism depressed?

▶ Why do people become alcoholics or substance abusers?

▶ Why is Alcoholic Anonymous (12–Step Program) effective with certain individuals who abuse alcohol or chemical substances?

▶ Is there an alcoholic personality?

▶ What are the best treatment methods for people who are alcohol or substance abusers?

People should not be forced to have treatment if they are mentally ill. (Szasz, 1974)

▶ Should people who are harmful to themselves or others be forced to have treatment?

▶ When are symptoms of mental illness not a danger to self or others?

▶ Should we restrict the freedom of people who are mentally ill by hospitalization or imprisonment?

Electroconvulsive Treatment (ECT) is the treatment of choice for those with severe depression. (Abrams, 1997; American Psychiatric Association, 1978; Breggin, 1979)

▶ Are there clinical research studies to show that ECT is effective with individuals who are severely depressed?

▶ How frequently is ECT used with individuals with severe depression?

▶ Are there effective alternatives to ECT to reduce symptoms of depression?

▶ What is the neurophysiological explanation for how ECT relieves depression?

▶ Does excessive use of ECT cause brain damage?

▶ What is the relationship between ECT and loss of memory?

People with dementia should be in mental hospitals or long-term facilities. (Binstock, Post, & Whitehouse, 1992)

▶ When are the symptoms of dementia a danger to the individual or to others?

▶ What individual freedoms should a person with dementia have?

▶ What are the alternatives to hospitalization or nursing facilities when treating individuals with dementia?

▶ How should the therapist consider the severity of dementia in deciding on hospitalization?

▶ Can individuals with severe dementia live successfully with supportive services at home or in the community?

▶ How can we help family caregivers reduce their stress when caring for family members with dementia?

Community treatment is better than hospital care for those with mental illness. (Prior, 1993)

▶ Why is community care treatment better than hospitalization for some individuals with mental illness?

▶ What can individuals learn in a community mental health center that will help them be more functional?

▶ Does long-term hospitalization cause individuals with mental illness to lose skills in self-care, leisure, work, and interpersonal relationships?

▶ Are there aspects of hospital care that are beneficial to individuals with mental illness?

▶ When is hospitalization effective for individuals with mental illness?

Tough-love is a positive way to treat adolescents who are acting out. (Dobson, 1983; York & York, 1980)

▶ Why does Tough-love work with certain adolescents?

▶ How can a parent be compassionate and yet impose firm limits on an adolescent?

▶ When is Tough-love perceived as rejection by the adolescent?

▶ When is Tough-love counterproductive, resulting in the adolescent acting out to a greater degree?

Parents should not use physical punishment to discipline children. (Walsh, 1991)

▶ Does physical punishment help children develop ethical behavior?

▶ What is the relationship between punishment and discipline?

▶ When is punishment considered abusive?

▶ Should punishment ever be used with children?

▶ What are the alternatives to punishment when teaching children ethical behavior?

▶ Why is punishment sometimes used excessively in dysfunctional families?

▶ What happens to children who have been excessively punished?

▶ Do children who are punished have a greater probability of becoming mentally ill than those who are not punished?

Prozac® should be used often with patients who are depressed. (Kramer, 1993; Murray, 1996)

▶ What is the neurophysiological explanation for how Prozac® works?

▶ Does Prozac® cause dependency?

▶ What are the common side effects of Prozac®?

▶ What are the alternatives to Prozac® or other medications?

▶ Are there long-term detrimental effects in taking Prozac®?

▶ What is the clinical research evidence for the effectiveness of Prozac®?

Neuroleptics treat symptoms rather than cure people. (Bernstein, 1995)

▶ What is the neurophysiological explanation for how a neuroleptic works?

▶ Can neuroleptics become addictive?

▶ What is the relationship between neuroleptics and detrimental symptoms such as tardive dyskinesia?

▶ Should neuroleptics be used in conjunction with other treatments (e.g., psychotherapy and occupational therapy)?

▶ What major psychiatric symptoms do neuroleptics reduce most effectively?

The best indication of normality is the ability to work. (Offer & Sabshin, 1991)

▶ What is normality?

▶ Can an individual who is mentally ill work?

▶ Does the ability to work always indicate normality?

▶ What is the relationship between unemployment and depression?

▶ What is the relationship between job dissatisfaction, anxiety, and depression?

▶ Does job satisfaction increase self-esteem and mental health?

WHAT IS MENTAL HEALTH AND WHAT IS MENTAL ILLNESS?

An understanding of normality and mental health and abnormality and mental illness is important if one is to work effectively with individuals with a psychosocial dysfunction. Jantzen (1969) stated:

In devising our roles as occupational therapists we need to be aware of the types of problems that may be called mental illness if we are to determine how we may help deal with such problems. We need to know what is considered healthy behavior if we elect to promote health. (p. 252)

Berger (1977) provided us with a good discussion of these issues.

People considered normal or healthy in one society or group might be considered abnormal, unhealthy or deviant in another society. There is no one definition of a "normal person" applicable to all people, at all times, in all situations.

It is a mistake to equate the "normal" person with the ideal or idealized one. People who function within the designation "healthy" are also imperfect, make mistakes, have "crazy thoughts" at times, have inner conflicts, and are not *absolutely* aware, honest, reliable, or responsible *all* the time.

Upon deep reflection I am compelled to state unequivocally that the idea of a *totally normal person* is not grounded in reality. From a realistic viewpoint, the concept of a healthy or normal person covers a wide area of human functioning and adaptation. The healthier a person, the greater is his adaptive capacity to integrate and react rationally or appropriately to unexpected, changing, or stressful events in his environment. Normality is to be strived for, although never absolutely achieved. We only know people who are *more-or-less* normal. (pp. 18–19)

According to Berger (1977), some of the characteristics for being normal or mentally healthy are:

▶ realistic acceptance of oneself and capacities

▶ ability to accept responsibility for one's behavior

▶ ability to work effectively with others

▶ sense of humor and a capacity for play

▶ ability to perceive reality without distortion

▶ recognition of one's feelings

▶ ability to learn and not to deny criticism and rejection

▶ ability to stand by one's convictions

▶ involvement in life or *joie de vivre*

▶ capacity to be flexible and deal adequately with unexpected events and situations

▶ ability to self-regulate stress

Another definition of mental health is provided by the Canadian National Health and Welfare (Health and Welfare Canada, 1988):

> Mental health is the capacity of the individual, the group and the environment to interact with one another in ways that promote subjective well-being, the optimal development and use of mental abilities (cognitive, affective and relational), the achievement of individual and collective goals consistent with justice and the attainment and preservation of conditions of fundamental equality. (p. 7)

A more systematic discussion of mental health as proposed by Jahoda (1958) is found in Chapter 5 of this book.

What is a mental disorder? Before answering this, one must distinguish between a mental disorder and a mental health problem.

> A *mental disorder* may be defined as a recognized, medically diagnosable illness that results in the significant impairment of an individual's cognitive, affective or relational abilities. Mental disorders result from biological, developmental and/or psychosocial factors, and can—in principle, at least—be managed using approaches comparable to those applied to physical disease (that is, prevention, diagnosis, treatment and rehabilitation).
>
> A *mental health problem*, on the other hand, is a disruption in the interactions between the individual, the group and the environment. Such a disruption may result from factors within the individual, including physical or mental illness, or inadequate coping skills. It may also spring from external causes, such as

the existence of harsh environmental conditions, unjust social structures, or tensions within the family or community. An effective response to mental health problems must therefore address a broader range of factors. (Health and Welfare Canada, 1988, p. 8, italics added)

The difference between a mental disorder and mental health is further depicted in Figure 1–2. In this figure, mental health and mental disorder are described as a continuum along which any individual can lie.

A mental disorder is defined in DSM–IV (APA, 1994) as a "behavioral, psychological, or biological dysfunction in the individual" (pp. xxi–xxii). It is important to note that in the DSM–IV a distinction is made between classifying people and classifying the disorders people have. For example, the terms " a schizophrenic" or "an alcoholic" are avoided because they classify people instead of the disorder. Instead, "an individual with schizophrenia" or "a person who abuses alcohol" are used to emphasize People First language. Throughout this book, we have attempted to follow the same distinction.

FIVE KEY ISSUES AFFECTING THE PRACTICE OF PSYCHOSOCIAL OCCUPATIONAL THERAPY

Occupational therapy as a profession began comparatively late in the history of medicine. There were no occupational therapists during the Middle Ages in Europe, in Colonial America, or even up until the 1900s. Although there were no occupational therapists, enlightened health practitioners throughout history have recommended activities as beneficial for individuals with mental illness. In the following chapters we have sought to bring together the research and theories that underlie practice and the clinical techniques of occupational therapy practiced in clinics, mental hospitals, and community mental health centers that have evolved progressively during the last 200 years.

Humanism as a philosophical value assumes the dignity and worth of mankind and the capacity of each individual for self-realization (Rogers, 1961). Occupational therapists within a humanistic tradition work directly with individuals in activities to prevent illness, treat symptoms, and restore function. For example, in prevention, occupational therapists work with children who are learning disabled in public school to prevent academic failure (Parham, 1998), treat individuals with depression by reducing

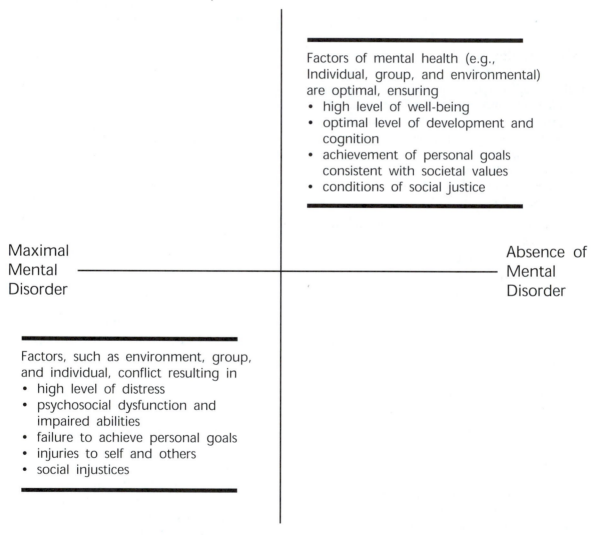

Optimal Mental Health

Factors of mental health (e.g., Individual, group, and environmental) are optimal, ensuring
- high level of well-being
- optimal level of development and cognition
- achievement of personal goals consistent with societal values
- conditions of social justice

Maximal Mental Disorder

Absence of Mental Disorder

Factors, such as environment, group, and individual, conflict resulting in
- high level of distress
- psychosocial dysfunction and impaired abilities
- failure to achieve personal goals
- injuries to self and others
- social injustices

Minimal Mental Health

Figure 1–2. Optimal and minimal mental health. (Adapted from *Mental Health for Canadians: Striking a Balance by Health and Welfare Canada,* 1988, p. 9)

anxiety through cognitive behavioral therapies (CBT) (Stein & Smith, 1989), and rehabilitate individuals with mental illness by enabling them to return to work (Brollier & Shepherd, 1990). In a holistic approach to occupational therapy, prevention, treatment, and rehabilitation are interrelated (Figure 1–3).

The growth and development of the occupational therapy profession can be viewed in perspective as analogous to the growth of scientific medicine. Only since the beginning of the 20th century has there been progress in medicine that has positively affected the treatment and rehabilitation of the patient with a chronic illness.

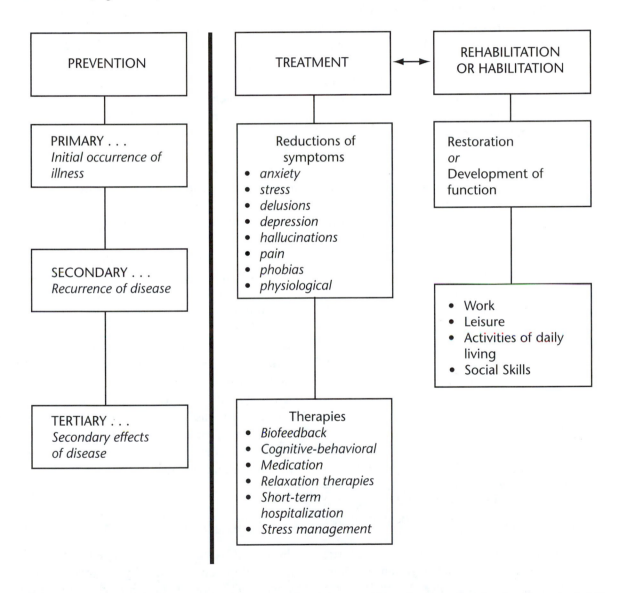

Figure 1–3. Model for a holistic approach in occupational therapy. Although prevention, treatment, and rehabilitation are separate entities, they are interrelated. Treatment leads to rehabilitation, which may lead to further treatment.

For example, antiseptic surgery was developed by Lister in the late 1800s (Truax, 1944), penicillin and other antibiotic therapies have been commercially available only since World War II, and chlorpromazine was first introduced in the late 1950s as the "miracle drug" for mental illness (Solomon, 1966). Before 1900 physicians could offer little hope when treating infection, communicable disease, or chronic illness. The concepts of primary, secondary, and tertiary prevention were introduced during the 1950s (Caplan, 1961), and the investigation of chronic diseases produced some advances only about 40 years ago when researchers were able, through computer analysis, to identify multiple risk factors such as smoking, obesity, hypertension, cholesterol, and lack of exercise that, along with the genetic predisposition, lead to heart disease and stroke (U.S. Department of Health, Education, and Welfare, 1968). The same approach is now being applied to other causes of diseases and disabilities.

The future of psychosocial occupational therapy is tied to the same major issues that confront all health care workers when treating patients. Currently, there are many philosophical, social, and ethical issues in the health care system that directly affect the occupational therapist as well as provide a glimpse of future problems.

Humanistic Caring

The *first* issue involves the availability of caring professionals who will respond to patient needs by first establishing rapport and a therapeutic relationship. This kind of treatment contrasts sharply with depersonalized health care where the patient is viewed anonymously and the health care worker dispenses treatment indifferently. If we are to help resolve this problem we must work toward individualizing treatment in

psychosocial occupational therapy by carefully evaluating patients and determining what approach or technique is most effective for each individual. We should avoid a "Procrustean bed" where the treatment is applied to all patients. We should explore a wide range of treatment modalities (e.g., biofeedback, relaxation therapy, exercise, sensory and cognitive stimulation, group dynamics, prevocational programming, and creative expression) to determine their efficacy with specific patients. We should provide caring treatment to patients with chronic disabilities, those who have been left in nursing homes or geriatric wards of psychiatric hospitals with little activity. Even if other health care workers have given up on certain patients, we should maintain an optimism and respect for these patients. We must incorporate activities into treatment on a personal level with the main objective of occupational therapy to help the individual to cope with the everyday demands of life.

As health care workers, we need to recognize the meaning of illness to the one who is disabled and to the caregivers who must live beside the patient. Serious mental illness represents a loss to both the patient and to the family. We need to tell ourselves, as we work with our patients and clients, that they are not routine cases, that they are persons who may feel helpless, and that many times they have families who feel pain and sorrow. We must not let ourselves fall into institutional traps where patients become part of a bureaucracy and are treated without individual care.

Self-Regulation

The *second* issue concerns the need to advocate the development of healthy lifestyles in our patients. The present health system frequently causes patients to be dependent for their well-being on medications alone. We need to develop public mental health programs in schools and local communities so that we may share with the lay public our knowledge of the use of holistic activities in fostering health. Likewise, children should be as familiar with their own anatomy, physiology, and psychological identity as they are with reading and writing. We can facilitate the learning of basic cognitive skills, as well as the healthy psychological expression of feelings through art, music, literature, drama, and dance. We have much to contribute to Health Maintenance Organizations that try to prevent mental illness. We have the potential to be helpful in prenatal and child care programs to help parents select toys and activities that foster social, physical, cognitive, and emotional development. We can assist in geriatric centers in fostering active participation and social engagement. By joining with other health care workers such as psychologists, recreational therapists, dietitians, nurses, counselors, and psychiatrists, we can help patients through educational programs to raise their level of knowledge about emotional and social growth and self-regulation of health through exercise and good nutrition. No longer should we treat our clients with mental illnesses as passive consumers. In these ways, we can prevent people from turning to faith healers, palmists, cultists, and others on the fringes of medicine who promise instant improvement and miraculous cures.

We are presently in the throes of a health consumer revolution in which citizens are demanding more information about medications, surgery, vitamins, herbs, exercise, and alternative treatments. As occupational therapists, we can take an active part in this movement by becoming knowledgeable about these treatments and working cooperatively with self-help groups in the community, such as the National Alliance for the Mentally Ill (NAMI; http://www.nami.org).

Equality of Mental Health Care

The *third* issue is in the distribution of psychiatric care. Presently, there is a gap between psychiatric care that is afforded to the middle class as opposed to care afforded to the poor (Carling, 1995). For example, there is a great discrepancy between psychiatric treatment provided in community mental health centers attracting the best trained professionals as compared with health care provided in the emergency rooms of local hospitals where many times poor individuals with psychiatric emergencies are treated mainly with drugs. Over the past 35 years the gap has continued to widen as the poor are left in the downtown areas of the cities, while middle-class families have moved to the suburbs. In the central core of many large cities live the poor, the minorities, the aged, and the homeless who are under continual stress and are most vulnerable to crime, family disorganization, and mental illness (Conrad, Matters, & Hanrahan, 1999). As occupational therapists we must advocate health care for all as a right, not as a privilege, with a particular concern for those in our society who are the most disadvantaged and at risk for mental illness.

A system of health care that emphasizes prevention of mental illness for populations at risk (e.g., dysfunctional families, children who have been abused, and families with alcohol and substance addictions) must evolve. Occupational therapists must be certain that their voices are heard when health care plans are presented. Our experience as clinicians working with individuals with severe disabilities is essential in providing input in designing comprehensive mental health programs that emphasize prevention and holistic treatment.

Preventative Approaches

The *fourth* issue is the problem of health abuse that is directly related to lifestyles that contribute to illness. There is a need to advocate health programs that counteract the effects of self-abuse caused by poor nutrition, drug abuse, lack of exercise, malaise, smoking, and alcoholism. Rather than treating the costly consequences of self-abuse, we should focus society's attention on community programs that promote physical and mental health.

The present effort in reducing premature heart disease is a good example that can be applied to preventative psychiatry. The annual economic costs in the United States resulting from cardiovascular disease in 2000 have been estimated by the American Heart Association (AHA) to be 326.6 billion dollars (AHA, 1999). From 1970 to 1995 there was a decrease in the death rate among males of working age between 40 and 65 (Blair et al., 1995). This decrease has been attributed to an increased awareness of the effects of a low-fat diet, reduced smoking, and increased physical fitness in our society. A reduction in the amount of fat consumed plus exercise programs that encourage aerobic activities, such as jogging, bicycling, tennis, and brisk walking, have led to these favorable results.

Schizophrenia, a problem of enormous proportions in our country, is an example of a chronic psychiatric illness that has not been systematically approached from a preventative perspective. Approximately 1 percent of the population of industrialized countries is diagnosed as schizophrenic. There are approximately 200,000 patients who are institutionalized in hospitals and nursing homes in the United States with a diagnosis of schizophrenia (U.S. Department of Health and Human Services, 1999; Regier et al., 1993). Another 400,000 individuals with schizophrenia are in the community, living lives of "quiet desperation." Many of these people are disabled as the result of insufficient or faulty treatment during hospitalization, lack of special educational programs, poor social skills, inadequate vocational preparation, and a host of other factors (Liberman, 1992). Individuals with schizophrenia many times give up on life, have difficulty competing in society, and are forced to escape to an institutional environment that fosters dependency. Other individuals with a diagnosis of schizophrenia are able to live normal lives in the community.

Estimates of the incidence and prevalence of mental illness indicate the enormity of the problem (Table 1–2). According to the Surgeon General (U.S. Department of Health and Human Services, 1999), approximately 5 million American adults suffer from the most severe mental illnesses (e.g., schizophrenia, manic-depressive, major depression, panic disorder, and obsessive-compulsive disorder), while approximately 10 percent of the population experience a mental illness during any given year (U.S. Department of Health and Human Services, 1999). Key areas of research within NIMH (2000) include:

► basic behavioral and neuroscience research, designed to examine the interaction of cognition, emotions, and interpersonal relationships;

► schizophrenia, the most chronic and disabling of the severe mental disorders, which affects more than 2 million Americans;

► mood disorders, including depression and manic-depressive illness (bipolar disorder), that debilitate 19 million Americans each year;

► ADHD, which affects 3 to 5 percent of school-aged children;

► anxiety disorders, including phobias, panic disorder, posttraumatic stress disorder, and obsessive-compulsive disorder, that together affect 19 million people in the United States;

▶ autism, a severe pervasive developmental disorder that affects 1 to 2 children out of every 1000, and that commonly arises before a child's 3rd birthday;

▶ rural mental health, serving almost 60 million people;

▶ child and adolescent violence, including risk factors, prevention, and intervention;

▶ eating disorders, including anorexia nervosa, bulimia, and binge eating disorder;

▶ Alzheimer's disease and other brain and mental disorders that rob 12 percent of older Americans of full and satisfying lives.

Most individuals reported to have a mental illness are in the community; however, an estimated 121,000 are hospitalized because of the illness (U.S. Department of Commerce, Bureau of the Census, 1996).

Mental health programs should move toward preventing mental illness among the most vulnerable individuals, such as those who are under continual stress, because of poverty, minority status, or severe occupational demands. The occupational therapist can be an integral part of the mental health team in the schools, along with the psychiatrist, psychologist, social worker, special educator, and speech–language pathologist. Through the skillful use of activity, the occupational therapist can aid in building independence, self-esteem, and a feeling of competence in children who are emotionally disturbed.

Holistic Medicine

The *fifth* issue in the health care system in this country is the need for generalists or primary health care workers who can treat the patient as a whole person in contrast to specialists, who divide the patient and treat his or her parts separately. Holistic medicine, which is concerned with an individual's psychological, social, physical, and spiritual dimensions (e.g., health status, lifestyle change, management of stress, and diet and exercise), offers an excellent framework for treatment and rehabilitation. For example, many times the failure of a patient to comply with treatment is related to orthotic devices and prostheses that remain unused because the therapist did not spend the time with the patient to explain the purpose of wearing or using a device. Diets that are not in accord with the patient's cultural traditions may not be adhered to. Exercise programs that are indicated for individuals with depression are not adhered to because a compliance program was not considered. Hearing aids, eyeglasses, and back braces may be unacceptable to adolescents because they are not cosmetically attractive. The main purpose of the holistic approach is to try to integrate every aspect of treatment to prevent splintering effects such as those described earlier. Problems and discontinuities in treatment frequently occur when the total needs of the patient are not considered.

In occupational therapy there is a growing trend toward specialty certification, such as in hand therapy, neurodevelopmental therapy, sensory integration, and work evaluation. The rise of these specialty sections has given impetus to specialization in the field of occupational therapy. There is no doubt that specialization has positive benefits in that it creates experts and generates knowledge in defined areas. The danger of specialization is that it may create narrowly educated health care professionals who focus on single aspects of illness or treatment techniques rather than taking a broadly based view of occupation. The abuse of specialization

Disorder	Description	Statistics	Etiology	Age/Gender
	characterized by delusions, hallucinations, thinking disorder, and disorganized behavior that is present for at least 6 months (APA, 1994)	▲ (NIMH, 1999) ▲ Approximately 2 million out of a population of 240 million are affected each year (NIMH, 2000)	in neurophysiological changes ▲ Environmental factors exacerbate condition (Jablensky, 1995)	early adulthood ■ No gender differer common in lower 1996)
Mood disorders (Affective disorders)	Disorder that includes the two clinical syndromes of major depressive disorder (MDD) and manic-depressive (bipolar disorder) (APA, 1994)	▲ 10 million adults in U.S. ▲ MDD: 1.1% of adult population in U.S. ▲ Manic-depressive: 1.0% of adult population in U.S. (NIMH, 2000)	▲ Genetic disposition to both (Burvill, 1995) ▲ Stress and environmental factors (Boyer & Nemerhoff, 1996)	■ MDD: F:M::2:1; av onset is mid 20s, (APA, 1994) ■ Bipolar: average a teens, 20s, or 30s difference (Boyer 1996)
Anxiety disorders	Set of disorders that includes obsessive-compulsive disorder (OCD), phobias, panic disorder, and post-traumatic stress disorder (PTSD) (Ninan, 1996)	▲ OCD: 1.5 to 2.1% (Ninan, 1996) ▲ Social phobia: 2% (Ninan, 1996) ▲ Panic disorder: 1.5 to 3.5% (Ninan, 1996) ▲ PTSD: 3.5% of civilians, 20% of Vietnam veterans (Ninan 1996)	▲ Familial, genetic, and environmental factors (Ninan, 1996) ▲ Traumatic environment event (Ninan, 1996)	■ OCD: median age 23; gender onset i equal (Ninan, 199 ■ Phobias: F:M::2:1; of onset is 13 (Nin ■ Panic: median age F:M::3.5:1 (Ninan, ■ PTSD: no gender c variable age of on 1996)
Substance-related disorders	"Disorders related to the taking of a drug of abuse (including alcohol), to the side effects of a medication, and to toxin exposure" (APA, 1994, p. 175)	▲ 18 million individuals with alcoholism in U.S. (McMicken, 1996) ▲ 1 million individuals with cocaine addictions ▲ 600,000 individuals with heroin addictions (Schnoll, 1996)	▲ Genetic or biochemical predisposition ▲ Implication of personality traits (McMicken, 1996)	■ M:F::4:1; variable (McMicken, 1996; 1996)
Eating disorders	Disturbances of attitudes and behavior such as anorexia nervosa and bulimia	▲ 1 to 5% of population (Dell, 1996) ▲ 0.5 to 1% of general population are anorexic (APA, 1994) ▲ 1 to 3% of general population are bulimic (APA, 1994)	▲ Genetic predisposition ▲ Variety of biological, environmental, and family factors contribute (Dell, 1996)	■ 90 to 95% are fem middle or upper S 1996) ■ mean age of onse old (Dell, 1996)

comes through in medicine when those trained in highly technical procedures limit themselves to the use of specific treatment methods, placing the patient into a "Procrustean bed" where the patient is fitted to the treatment technique rather than selecting the most effective treatment technique available for the individual. It is more efficacious to evaluate the patient and then to select the treatment method based on both individual factors and knowledge of a broad spectrum of treatment techniques than to treat on a one-dimensional approach. An alternative to specialization is an eclectic approach in which the therapist is receptive to applying a wide range of treatment procedures while conferring with the individual patient. We should use any or all of the following treatment methods: cognitive-behavioral treatment, sensory motor integration, creative arts, psychoeducational approaches, psychodynamic therapies, relaxation therapy, biofeedback, or any treatment method for scientific reasons because it is appropriate to the individual case and not because of an emotional or biased attachment to a specific method. There is a dilemma in that, if we educate occupational therapists to be generalists, they may remain superficial, and if we educate therapists to become specialists, they may become too narrow in their roles. However, there is a compromise solution to this dilemma. That is, we can educate therapists in clinical reasoning and problem-solving skills and in a variety of treatment techniques so that they will be able to evaluate and implement treatment methods that are effective with specific individuals. The question is not whether one treatment method is more effective than another but whether one individual can benefit from one method as opposed to another. Skill in applying different methods of treatment based on the individual needs of the patient is the important factor. A holistic approach to psychosocial treatment is consistent with the occupational therapy philosophy of considering the total needs of the patient in the context of the cultural and social environment.

Other current issues in the health care system also affect the occupational therapist as a humanistic treatment agent. One of these is the excessive use of drugs in solving emotional problems. Patients now equate treatment with taking a pill. Sometimes, however, the side effects of drug treatment are more detrimental than no treatment. Because of this, a new group of treatment-induced illnesses has resulted and are known as clinical iatrogenesis. We must educate and empower our patients to use naturalistic approaches to health, such as good nutrition, exercise, relaxation methods, use of leisure time activities, and self-regulation. We must change the opinion of some health care workers who perceive occupational therapy as a luxury, not a necessary part of treatment. We must change this perception because it is false. The mere fact that we do not dispense drugs or perform surgery does not necessarily make occupational therapy more or less powerful. The effectiveness of occupational therapy should be validated through clinical research.

We have introduced the concept of occupational therapy as a humanistic approach to health care. The historical origins of occupational therapy are based on the moral treatment begun in hospitals in the 1800s in which the respect and the sanctity of the individual were integrated into patient care. We should not lose this perspective even during a period of specialization of function, depersonalization of treatment, rising costs of health care, and an age of computerization. Occupational therapists can serve their patients more effectively if they take the time to get to know the people they treat as individuals and to work in a client-centered manner. The following chapters present objectively the evolution of treatment models in caring for individuals with mental illness. The holistic humanistic framework that is advocated is consistent with the core of occupational therapy and with the pioneers of moral treatment.

A parallel theme in this book is the importance of the patient's or client's role in the treatment process. How the client views therapy in his or her role in treatment is a vital factor. In the following excerpts, in which clients describe their experiences in occupational therapy, we can gain insights into the patient's thinking.

FAMILIES AND MENTAL ILLNESS

Autobiographical Accounts of Mental Illness and Occupational Therapy

How does the patient or family perceive occupational therapy? To fully understand the impact of occupational therapy on the individual with emotional illness, we have selected excerpts from two contemporary autobiographies in which the authors describe their personal experiences in occupational therapy. In the first excerpt, from the book, *I'm Dancing as Fast as I Can* (1979), Barbara Gordon portrays her emotional collapse from abusing drugs that were initially used to control her stress. The second excerpt is from John Neary's (1975) book, *Whom the Gods Destroy: An Account of a Journey Through Madness.* The next two excerpts are from the perspective of how mental illness affects family dynamics. Louise Wilson (1968), in the book, *This Stranger, My Son: A Mother's Story,* and *Wasted: The Story of My Son's Drug Addiction* by William Chapin (1972), strongly express the impact of mental illness on the family.

I'm Dancing as Fast as I Can

Barbara Gordon (1979), described her experiences in occupational therapy in an autobiographical novel after being hospitalized for mental illness:

I had been in the hospital about a month when I decided one morning to go to the occupational therapy building. Julie had been urging me to go, but I told her I knew I would never regain my sense of self playing with clay or weaving a basket. Now I wanted to get away, at least for awhile, from the sickness and squalor of the hall. Was that progress? I didn't think so, I was just curious to see what the other crazies were doing.

Once I arrived in the large, airy O.T. building, I found myself strolling from room to room, just looking. People of all ages were deeply involved in working with clay, weaving cloth, making potholders, doing needlepoint. I forced myself to sit down and try to do something. But I only had to glance at the man on my left or the woman on my right to feel hopelessly inept. As I tried to make something out of the lifeless gray clay I held in my hand, somewhere deep inside me I heard a voice saying, "It's eleven o'clock on a Tuesday morning and you're sitting here modeling clay for your health. Barbara Gordon, you are in occupational therapy, next thing you know you'll be weaving baskets" and I gave up in despair and wandered into another room filled with even more people purposefully engaged in the process of making of something. But in the art therapy room, I saw gobs and gobs of bright acrylic paint, and the brilliance of the colors knocked me out. I took a brush and began literally throwing the paint on a canvas. If I couldn't tell Julie, I could show her the anguish I felt. So I decided to draw the color of the fire blazing in my head—an orange, yellow, red jungle of a fire. Then I painted the gray fog that seemed to surround my brain like a shroud. And that afternoon I brought the childish primitives to her office so she could see what I no longer had the words to describe. Like a five-year old home from kindergarten with her finger paintings, I rushed in the door saying "See, Julie, this is how it hurts. This is how I feel. This is how I look. I'm a monster. See my monster."

She looked at the paintings and smiled. "A gentle monster Barbara." So the painting began: faces with white, empty eyes, monsters, ogres, coffins, dead men, gray, black, brown, umber. It would be a long time before I would look outside and paint flowers. (pp. 181–182)

For Barbara Gordon, the experience in occupational therapy gave her the opportunity to express her feelings. "See Julie, this is how it hurts." She painted her anguish and shared her emotion. This is one of the important goals for the therapist, that is, to help the patient paint out his or her feelings.

Whom the Gods Destroy: An Account of a Journey Through Madness

John Neary, a journalist, in writing of his mental illness in *Whom the Gods Destroy: An Account of a Journey Through Madness* (1975), gives an account of his initial encounter with the occupational therapist.

He gained nothing in his bargaining session with the occupational therapist. Flatly, he told her that he would have no part of occupational therapy. The only therapy he needed was getting out of the hospital, he insisted; the only occupation he knew was reporting and writing—how did woodwork, pottery, pounding tin, relate to him? Insistently, the slight, fine-boned woman in the brown cardigan talked to him, not arguing with him, simply maintaining her hope that he would come to her O.T. group.

His initial resistance to occupational therapy ended and he began a woodworking project. When he did go to O.T., it reminded him of woodshop or art class in high school, a time-wasting period for goofing off then—and now too, obviously, for some of the patients on 5-E.

McCabe felt he was under close scrutiny, and set out to prove to whoever might be watching that he was all there. He found a saw, hammer, nails, a square, in a rack of tools, and some scraps of pine and made a tiny wall box for Carrie, assembling it and painting it green in one work period, his hands trembling so badly he could scarcely hammer the pin-sized finishing nails.

This first experience in occupational therapy was a challenge to him. He wanted to prove through a non-verbal activity that he wasn't completely hopeless. The activity was completed which gave him apparent feelings of self-esteem. His severe anxiety (his trembling) did not diminish his desire to complete the project.

The next O.T. period, he asked for a soldering iron and, to his surprise, the therapist sent an aide off to find one. When it appeared, he got coat hangers from his locker, cut them into four-inch lengths and began scraping the black enamel from the tips of the short rods.

When the therapist asked him what he was up to, he told her, without thinking, "a tesserac . . . a model of X to the fourth power." It suddenly occurred to him how nonsensical he must sound, no doubt as though he were making the whole thing up, or telling her he was undertaking a model of some hallucination. "It's kind of model we used to make in high school math." He remembered the math teacher he and his friends called Wild Bill, one of the few teachers he had ever had who set no ground rules inside his subject; any way you got it was okay with the grizzled, grumpy, rumpled, wrinkled former submarine skipper who somehow had wound up teaching mathematics to a bunch of kids most of whom were bound for the mills or an apartment kitchen. McCabe had never tried a tesserac for Bill, fearing then his own ineptitude as compared to those metal shop wizards who brought in flawless gems of the solder-er's and tinsmith's art. He would now essay a tesserac, constructing here in the fifth-floor O.T. room of the Illinois State Psychiatric Institute a model of X^4.

He had no brace for the soldering iron, no clamps with which to hold the little rods together, no previous experience whatever at soldering and, it seemed to McCabe, Pompadour was slamming his clay down on the work table to eliminate the air bubbles with more that adequate vigor.

"This is a model of the fourth dimension, Mr. McCabe?" The O.T. teacher had made the rounds of the class and had returned to look on. "No," he said. "Each little rod stands for X, you see. One rod is X. Move X through a plane its own length and you have X squared, so this rectangle is a model of that. Now move the plane through space, you have a model of X to the fourth power. Not really, but a model, you know, of the idea." His voice shook.

He tried to solder as he spoke, heating the coil with the red tip of the rod, dropping huge blobs of the stuff onto the joint. Instead of the neatly soldered joints he remembered from solid geometry class, his model looked as though it had been dipped in chewing gum. His fingertips were badly scorched. The shaky table was part of the reason. He felt he was under scrutiny not only by the O.T. teacher, but by the others in the class as well. Some teased him—suggested he was really building a radio. It made him feel under enormous pressure as he touched the cherry top of the iron to the solder and, coupled with the rising feeling of that electrical surge, he could barely control his hands. Shaking like a Bowery drunk, he assembled the cube, then affixed the struts in what he hoped were parallel angles. If he was off, they would have to be melted free—probably undoing the cube in the process.

As McCabe worked, Ernest, sitting next to him, quietly pieced together tiny chips of turquoise-colored stone into the pattern of an Indian head complete with war bonnet, gluing them down with untranquilized watch-maker-ly precision onto the lid of a jewelry box he had made. At a table by the window, the chubby girl who had chalked the inspirational message on the blackboard tapped at an old Royal standard typewriter, working on her journal of her hos-pital stay in faded pica. Pompadour pinched his ashtray, a big platter-sized affair made to look like a lopsided Salvador Daliesque face, Richard Speck in two dimensions—or Pompadour himself. Not bad, McCabe noted to himself—do-it-yourself Rorschach, the switch being that the O.T. lady no doubt did the interpretations. What did his tesserac say about him?

He said yes when the O.T. lady asked if she could enter his tesserac in the hospital art fair. (pp. 235–237)

In this occupational therapy session the patient selected an abstract project where he was given the freedom to express himself without being judged or evaluated. The freedom to design creatively an original project gave him a sense of identity. This was confirmed by the occupational therapist who asked him to enter his tesserac (a kind of mathematical model) in the hospital art fair. The activity served as a link to his childhood. ("It's a kind of model we used to make in high school math.")

This Stranger, My Son, a Mother's Story

Louise Wilson (1968) described the anguish and life crises of her son with mental illness as he struggled toward maturity. It is the chronicle of an adolescent boy who was diagnosed with paranoid schizophrenia. The mother tells a story that is representative of many families in which one member is emotionally ill, while other children are normal. Tony, the adolescent with mental illness, was a first child in a family with three other healthy siblings. The father was a successful surgeon and the mother was a free-lance artist. Tony was born during World War II while the father was a surgical resident in the Navy. Tony was a fitful infant, unable to sleep and extremely sensitive to extraneous noises. He cried very often and would only stop if he was picked up or rocked in his mother's arms.

Pediatricians found no physical ailments and he was tentatively diagnosed as a hyperactive baby. Tony's cognitive development was accelerated, speaking in complete sentences at an early age, and showing strong sensitivity and interest in nature. During his childhood years, Tony became very attached to his mother and he could not emotionally tolerate being apart from her or of being alone. Tony had a severe emotional reaction when his mother had to leave home for two weeks when her father died. Another traumatic event in Tony's early life that was extremely anxiety provoking was the birth of his sister. Tony expressed hostility toward his new sister and toward his mother for giving birth to another child. As Tony became older, he demanded more and more of his mother's time, and pleaded more intensely for her attention. Tony was unable to play with other children and he appeared fearful in his relationships. He was outwardly belligerent to his sister. Tony's mother reacted inconsistently to him, using either punishment or reason. Neither one worked and Tony failed to respond positively. Tony was fearful when initiating conversation with strangers. During his grade school years, he was shy and seclusive, clinging to his mother or homeroom teacher. Tony, however, excelled in his academic studies. His day-to-day life in the family was filled with temper tantrums, hostility toward his siblings, negativism, and the type of acting out behavior that is annoying and disruptive to family and friends. On the other hand, his mother noted that he had a "tremendous intellectual curiosity."

The mother felt that Tony was difficult so she sought help from pediatricians, family practitioners, and psychiatrists. She was told frequently that Tony's acting out behavior was due to psychological and parental problems. Tony seemed to the mother to be two children, one a talented academic student and the other, a child who was emotionally disturbed and withdrawn. He would not establish relationships with his peers and he acted out his feelings without control in the home. He was seen as the disturbing force in the household. He was a continual problem in a family where the other three children were growing up normally. Tony created a climate of terror and anxiety in the home. He threatened, antagonized, and battled. He was unhappy, isolated, and at war with others and himself. As he grew older, the parents had more difficulty in tolerating his behavior and they desperately sought help that would prevent him from being institutionalized. He underwent personal counseling and psychotherapy in a continual pattern of initial optimism and then acknowledged failure. The underlying fears of the family were that he would permanently harm one of the family members or he would commit suicide. Eventually, their only solution was for Tony to be placed in a modified halfway house with six other adolescents. A psychoanalytic psychiatrist and his wife were the caretakers in this home. This was seen by the family as the last hope for Tony. The mother ends the story of Tony with a quiet desperation and ambivalence so typical of the parent with a child with mental illness. This example occurred when the parents were visiting Tony while he was being treated in a residential program:

> "Please take me home," he whispered. "Please. You say you love me; then take me home. I think of my home, it's so beautiful; maybe I've never told you how beautiful it is. I think of the view out over the garden in back; the birds coming to the feeder, and keep seeing that print of the covered wagon over my desk."
>
> The mother responds: "Tony, you will be home. That's all we want. Please help us; please help yourself." (p. 150)

Why did treatment fail for Tony? What did the parents expect from Tony? In retrospect, what would have been the best treatment environment for Tony? What were the healthy parts of Tony that could have been mobilized by the therapist? In what ways could the family be more integrated into the long-term treatment goals? These questions challenge the very nature of psychiatric treatment. They must be answered if patients like Tony are to be helped.

Wasted: The Story of My Son's Drug Addiction

In another excerpt, William Chapin (1972) portrays, with compassion and frustration, the story of an adolescent with drug addiction. The author describes how the family becomes intertwined in the drug addict's life. The addict's roller coaster emotional life with the promises and regrets are meshed with the family's hopes and disappointments.

The father, a journalist, describes his son's (Mark) early infant development, childhood, and troubled adolescence. Mark was a second child, born under natural childbirth to middle-class, educated parents. He accomplished his developmental landmarks within the normal expectations; for example, he walked at 11 months and spoke at the appropriate time. He was an active child, experiencing temper tantrums occasionally as well as expressing laughter. The father, in retrospect, characterized Mark's childhood as normal. Mark attended nursery school and actively participated in games and childhood play. The parents were sometimes inconsistent in their discipline and expressed guilt in the way they handled him. Moreover, the father was a heavy drinker and occasionally lost control of his actions in disciplining the child. Throughout Mark's life his mother felt that she was unable to establish a mature relationship with him and she felt inept and "heartbroken" in not being able to control his drug addiction. The family moved frequent-

ly during Mark's childhood and the father, in reaction to the stress of moving and change, frequently increased his drinking. At one point the drinking became so uncontrollable that the father consulted a psychiatrist.

In public school in the San Francisco area, Mark seemed initially to be a good academic achiever. However, the family did not seem able to establish firm roots in any community and there continued to be frequent changes in Mark's life. Consequently, Mark did not sustain any long-lasting friendships during his childhood. The family moved to Japan when an opportunity arose for the father. Mark, at 9 years old, had a traumatic experience with an illness during this period, that was first diagnosed as appendicitis. Because of language difficulties, Mark was not properly treated.

In preadolescence, Mark developed an interest in poetry and music, and continued to achieve normally in elementary school. The father confessed that he spent little time with his son while his drinking increased and he withdrew further from family responsibilities. After living in Japan for a number of years, the family returned to the San Francisco area where Mark was enrolled as a freshman in a large public high school. Mark's beginning as a drug addict started with his accessibility to marijuana and later experimentation with LSD while in high school. This was during the 1960s, a time of adolescent protest and a general malaise among the youth that was related to the Vietnam War. Why did Mark become vulnerable to drugs while other adolescents did not experiment? From the parents' perspective, Mark did not have a strong bond with them and they seemed unable to provide him with the consistent values and models that he needed. Another hypothesis to explain Mark's attraction to drugs was that with his fragile ego and withdrawn lifestyle, he was unprepared to cope with stress. Consequently, as an escape from his failures in interpersonal relationships, he created a drug fantasy for himself that denied reality. Whatever the explanation, Mark progressively became a heavy user of drugs, which eventually caused brain damage and an inability to care for his most basic needs.

As a result, his ability to learn was severely affected and his whole existence centered around obtaining drugs and experimenting with his emotions. The family was unable to influence Mark or to affect his behavior. They referred Mark for psychotherapy but it was unsuccessful. "Fights, quarrels, recriminations and resentments prevailed in the . . . household . . . and most of the trouble centered on Mark. One day he would be a victim, the next day the catalyst" (p. 62).

Mark's life was in continual crisis with failure in school, fights with his parents, inability to care for his personal hygiene, police arrests, and progressively heavier drug use. His only positive involvement was in music. However, it was intermittent and not sustained. He regressed rapidly.

> His memory suffered lapses. His handwriting became crabbed and shaky. He would laugh when there was nothing to laugh at. He would turn on the gas stove to heat water for tea; ten seconds later he would leave the house. He began to leave cigarettes burning on the edges of tables and bookcases . . ." (pp. 91–92)

Mark was unable to complete high school. Mark's years from 18 to 21 were the most difficult for him and the family. Now that he was no longer in school, had no job, was unable to care for himself, and was heavily addicted to amphetamines, the family searched for psychiatric treatment facilities. Mark went from psychiatrists, to the state hospital, to psychologists, to alternative living environments, to Synanon (a specialized treatment center for addicts), all with the same poor result. Mark was unable to benefit from individual psychotherapy, medication, and group living arrangements. Mark eventually became institutionalized and dependent on others. He was unable to live by himself or to maintain a job. At 21 years old the drug addiction had worn Mark down so completely that his only prospect was to live the rest of his life in a state institution. His life, as far as his father was concerned, was wasted.

Why did psychiatric treatment fail with Mark? How could the family have been more involved in treatment? How could Mark's positive interests in poetry and music be used constructively? When was the best time to intervene therapeutically in Mark's drug abuse? What activities would have been helpful in treatment?

The therapist must be prepared to answer these and similar questions as part of the treatment process. Unfortunately, the very nature of psychiatric treatment demands unique solutions that cannot be generalized in practice. For each individual, the occupational therapist formulates short- and long-term goals, considering the psychiatric diagnosis, developmental landmarks, and the potential impact of the family on the course of treatment.

REFERENCES

Abrams, R. (1997). *Electroconvulsive therapy* (3rd ed.). New York: Oxford University Press.

Alfred, D. C. (1996). Schizophrenia. In J. W. Hurst (Ed.), *Medicine for the practicing physician* (4th ed., pp. 15–19). Stamford, CT: Appleton & Lange.

American Heart Association (AHA). (1999). *Economic cost of cardiovascular diseases.* Retrieved May 24, 2000, from the World Wide Web: *http://www.americanheart.org/statistics/10econom.html.*

American Psychiatric Association. (1978). *Task force report electroconvulsive therapy.* Washington, DC: Author.

American Psychiatric Association. (1994). *Diagnostic and statistical manual of mental disorders* (4th ed.). Washington, DC: Author.

Berger, M. M. (1977). *Working with people called patients.* New York: Brunner/Mazel.

Bernstein, J. G. (1995). *Handbook of drug therapy in psychiatry* (3rd ed.). St. Louis: C. V. Mosby.

Binstock, R. H., Post, S. G., & Whitehouse, P. J. (1992). *Dementia and aging: Ethics, values, and policy choices.* Baltimore: Johns Hopkins University Press.

Bisbee, C. C. (1991). *Educating patients and families about mental illness: A practical guide.* Gaithersburg, MD: Aspen.

Blair, S. N., Kohl, H. W., Barlow, C. E., Paffenbarger, R. S., Gibbons, L. W., & Macera, C. A. (1995). Changes in physical fitness and all-cause mortality: A prospective study of healthy and unhealthy men. *Journal of the American Medical Association, 273,* 1093–1098.

Boyer, W., & Nemerhoff, C. B. (1996). Mood disorders: Depression and mania. In J. W. Hurst (Ed.), *Medicine for the practicing physician* (4th ed., pp. 22–27). Stamford, CT: Appleton & Lange.

Breggin, P. R. (1979). *Electroshock: Its brain-disabling effects.* New York: Springer.

Brollier, C., & Shepherd, J. T. (1990). Developmental disabilities and long-term mental illness: New work programs. *Work: A Journal of Prevention, Assessment & Rehabilitation, 1,* 45–54.

Burvill, P. W. (1995). Recent progress in the epidemiology of major depression. *Epidemiology Review, 17*(1), 21–31.

Caplan, G. (Ed.). (1961). *Prevention of mental disorders in children: Initial explorations.* New York: Basic Books.

Carling, P. J. (1995). *Return to community: Building support systems for people with psychiatric disabilities.* New York: Guilford.

Chapin, W. (1972). *Wasted: The story of my son's drug addiction* (1st ed.). New York: McGraw–Hill.

Conrad, K. J., Matters, M. D., & Hanrahan, P. (1999). *Homelssness prevention in treatment of substance abuse and mental illness: Logic models and implementation of eight American projects.* Binghamton, NY: Haworth.

Dell, M. L. (1996). Eating disorders. In J. W. Hurst (Ed.), *Medicine for the practicing physician* (4th ed., pp. 40–44). Stamford, CT: Appleton & Lange.

Dobson, J. C. (1983). *Love must be tough: New hope for families in crisis.* Waco, TX: Word Books.

Gordon, B. (1979). *I'm dancing as fast as I can.* New York: Harper & Row.

Gordon, T. (1976). *P.E.T. Parent Effectiveness Training: The tested new way to raise responsible children.* New York: New American Library.

Health and Welfare Canada. (1988). *Mental health for Canadians: Striking a balance.* Ottawa: Ministry of Supply and Services.

Jablensky, A. (1995). Schizophrenia: Recent epidemiologic issues. *Epidemiologic Reviews, 17*(1), 10–20.

Jahoda, M. (1958). *Current concepts of positive mental health.* New York: Basic Books.

Jantzen, A. C. (1969). Definitions of mental health and mental illness. *American Journal of Occupational Therapy, 23,* 249–253.

Kramer, P. D. (1993). *Listening to Prozac.* New York: Penguin Books.

Liberman, R. (1992). *Handbook of psychiatric rehabilitation.* Boston: Allyn & Bacon.

McMicken, D. B. (1996). Alcohol: Tolerance, addiction, and withdrawal. In J. W. Hurst (Ed.), *Medicine for the practicing physician* (4th ed., pp. 1975–1983). Stamford, CT: Appleton & Lange.

Meyer, A. (1977). The philosophy of occupational therapy. *Archives of Occupational Therapy, 1,* 1–10. Reprinted in *American Journal of Occupational Therapy, 31,* 639–642. (Original work published 1922)

Montgomery, S. A., & Rouillon, F. (1992). *Long-term treatment of depression.* New York: John Wiley.

Murray, M. T. (1996). *Natural alternatives to Prozac.* New York: William Morrow.

National Institute of Mental Health. (NIMH) (2000). *Facts about the National Institute of Mental Health (NIMH).* Retrieved January 1, 2001, from the World Wide Web: *http://www.nimh.nih.gov/about/factsabout.cfm.*

Neary, J. (1975). *Whom the gods destroy: An account of a journey through madness.* New York: Atheneum.

Ninan, P. T. (1996). Anxiety disorders. In J. W. Hurst (Ed.), *Medicine for the practicing physician* (4th ed., pp. 28–33). Stamford, CT: Appleton & Lange.

Offer, D., & Sabshin, M. (Eds.). (1991). *The diversity of normal behavior: Further contributions to normatology.* New York: Basic Books.

Parham, L. D. (1998). The relationship of sensory integrative development to achievement in elementary students: Four year longitudinal patterns. *The Occupational Therapy Journal of Research, 18,* 104–127.

Pasamanick, B., Scarpitti, F. R., & Dinitz, S. (with Albini, J., & Lefton, M.). (1967). *Schizophrenics in the community: An experimental study in the prevention of hospitalization.* New York: Appleton–Century–Crofts.

Prior, L. (1993). *The social organization of mental illness.* London: Sage.

Regier, D. A., Narrow, W. E., Rae, D. S., Manderscheid, R. W., Locke, B. Z., & Goodwin, F. K. (1993). The de facto U.S. mental and addictive disorders service system. Epidemiologic catchment area prospective 1-year prevalence rates of disorders and services. *Archives of General Psychiatry, 50,* 85–94.

Rogers, C. (1961). *On becoming a person.* Boston: Houghton–Mifflin.

Schnoll, S. H. (1996). Psychoactive substance use disorders. In J. W. Hurst (Ed.), *Medicine for the practicing physician* (4th ed., pp. 54–57). Stamford, CT: Appleton & Lange.

Snow, D. A., & Anderson, L. (1993). *Down on their luck: A study of homeless street people.* Berkeley: University of California.

Solomon, P. (Ed.). (1966). *Psychiatric drugs.* New York: Grune & Stratton.

Stein, F., & Smith, J. (1989). Short-term stress management techniques to a schizophrenic patient. *American Journal of Occupational Therapy, 43,* 162–191.

Sternberg, R. J., & Grigorenko, E. L. (Eds.). (1997). *Intelligence, heredity, and environment.* New York: Cambridge University Press.

Szasz, T. S. (1963). *Law, liberty, and psychiatry: An inquiry into the social uses of mental health practice.* New York: Macmillan.

Szasz, T. S. (1974). *The myth of mental illness: Foundations of a theory of personal conduct* (Rev. ed.). New York: Harper & Row.

Truax, R. (1944). *Joseph Lister, father of modern surgery.* Indianapolis, IN: Bobbs–Merrill.

Tsuang, M. T., Kendler, K. S., & Lyons, M. J. (Eds.). (1991). *Genetic issues in psychosocial epidemiology.* New Brunswick, NJ: Rutgers University Press.

U.S. Department of Commerce, Bureau of the Census. (1996). *Statistical abstract of the United States,* 1996 (116th ed.). Washington, DC: Government Printing Office.

U.S. Department of Health, Education, and Welfare, National Institutes of Health. (1968). *The Framingham study: An epidemiological investigation of cardiovascular disease* (DHEW Publication No. NIH 74–618) Washington, DC: Government Printing Office.

U.S. Department of Health and Human Services. (1999). *Mental health: A report of the surgeon general.* Rockville, MD: U. S. Department of Health and Human Services, Substance Abuse and Mental Health Services Administration, Center for Mental Health Services, National Instituties of Health, National Institute of Mental Health. Retrieved January 23, 2001 from the World Wide Web: *http://www.surgeongeneral.gov/library/mentalhealth/home.html.*

Walsh, K. (with Lee, J. M., & Aufderheide, J. A.). (1991). *Discipline for character development.* Birmingham, AL: R.E.P. Books.

Wekesser, C. (Ed.). (1994). *Alcoholism.* San Diego, CA: Green Haven.

Wilson, L. (1968). *This stranger, my son: A mother's story.* New York: G. P. Putnam.

York, P., & York, D. (1980). *Toughlove: A self-help manual for parents troubled by teenage behavior.* Sellersville, PA: Community Service Foundation.

CHAPTER

2

A Short History of the Treatment of Individuals with Mental Illness and the Emergence of Occupational Therapy

> *Occupational Therapy has demonstrated its value through many centuries of use in the treatment of the mentally ill. The idle patient either expends his energy in destructive violence or in preoccupation that soon reduces him to helpless regressive vegetation. Studies have shown that as occupational and recreational activities increase, destruction and violence diminish.*
>
> —*W. E. Barton, (1957),* Occupational Therapy for Psychiatric Disorders, in W. R. Dunton & S. Licht *Occupational Therapy: Principles and Practice,* p. 195

Operational Learning Objectives

By the end of this chapter, the learner will:

1. Discuss and differentiate the factors in a psychiatric treatment program that, on the one hand, can potentially facilitate improvement in the patient with mental illness and, on the other hand, cause further regression into illness.

2. Discuss the naturalistic approach to mental health.

3. Identify practices in ancient and nonindustrial societies that fostered mental health.

4. Discuss the relationships between mental health and the following variables: nutrition, extended family, continuity of daily life patterns, health perspective, realistic life goals, exercise, music, and dance.

5. Define holistic medicine and its relationship to mental health.

6. Discuss the factors that characterize the inhumane era in the care of those with mental illness during the Middle Ages in Europe.

7. Define Moral Humanistic Treatment of the 19th century and discuss its relationship to the use of activities in mental hospitals.

8. Discuss the contributions of Pinel, Reil, Tuke, Kirkbride, and Rush, who as 19th century psychiatric reformers advocated activity programs in mental hospitals.

9. Discuss the rise of the mental hygiene movement in the United States and its relationship to the emergence of the occupational therapy profession at the beginning of the 20th century.

10. Evaluate the benefits of occupational therapy in mental hospitals during the 1920s and 1930s.

11. Discuss the contributions of the pioneers in psychiatric occupational therapy (i.e., Adolph Meyer, William Rush Dunton, Jr., and Louis Haas).

12. Define dynamic treatment and the influence of psychoanalytic theory in the practice of occupational therapy in the first half of the 20th century.

13. Discuss the emergence of the Certified Occupational Therapy Assistant (COTA) during the 1950s and 1960s.

14. Critically evaluate the patient's perceptions of occupational therapy by examining autobiographical accounts.

In this chapter the authors trace the historical roots of psychosocial occupational therapy by examining two major current streams: holistic medicine and moral treatment. Holistic medicine is viewed as a logical extension of the ancient Hellenistic concept of wellness, which is based on man's harmony with nature (Heidel, 1941). The concepts of holistic medicine continue to be practiced in several nonindustrial societies in the world and have recently received credibility in traditional medical care in Western nations by the emphasis of diet, exercise, and relaxation therapies (Workshop on Alternative Medicine, 1994). The second major stream, moral treatment, emerged as a counterbalance to the inhumane care of those with mental illness that had engulfed most of Western Europe from the Middle Ages up until the 19th century (Mora, 1985). Humanistic care emphasized the rights of those with mental illness to treatment based on the use of activities toward the goal of helping the individual achieve mental restoration (Barton, 1957). The original writings of the early pioneers in psychiatry, occupational therapy, and the mental hygiene movement are cited in this context. From a historical perspective, the practice of psychosocial occupational therapy is consistent with the traditions of holistic medicine, humanistic care, and moral treatment. The landmarks in 20th century psychiatry are outlined in Table 2–1.

OVERALL GOALS OF PSYCHIATRY

In examining the literature on the history of psychiatry, one realizes that one way to measure the degree of civilization of a society is to determine how individuals with mental illness are treated. Individuals with mental illness have been punished (Ackerknecht, 1968), locked in dungeons and abused (Pinel 1801/1947), exterminated by the Nazis during World War II (Annas & Grodin, 1992), and, in the 1990s, left homeless, neglected, and untreated (Federal Task Force on Homelessness and Severe Mental Illness, 1992). The search for immediate solutions and instant changes in the behavior of individuals with mental illness led to radical methods in the 1930s through the 1960s in which individuals were literally shocked, cajoled, drugged, threatened, and surgically experimented on (Valenstein, 1986). On the other hand, there were many instances in agrarian societies and early civilizations that had provided humane care for individuals with mental illness (Alexander & Selesnick, 1966; Heidel, 1941; Leon & Rosselli, 1975; Veith, 1975).

Table 2–1. Landmarks in 20th Century Psychiatry

1900–1910	• Dynamic psychotherapy (Freud, 1938)
	• Mental Hygiene Movement (Beers, 1908)
1920s	• Rapid growth in large psychiatric hospitals
1930–1940s	*Biological treatments*
	• Prefrontal surgery (Moniz, 1936; Freeman & Watts, 1942)
	• Insulin shock (Sakel, 1938)
	• Metrazol shock (Meduna, 1936)
	• Electroconvulsive (Kalinowsky, 1959)
1950s	• Introduction of neuroleptics (Delay, Deniker, & Harl, 1952; Malitz & Hoch, 1966)
	• Large number of patients discharged from hospitals (Regier & Burke, 1985)
	• Therapeutic community, group therapy (Jones, 1953)
1960s	• Community Mental Health Center Act (P.L. 88–164, 1963) (Bachrach, 1976)
	• Deinstitutionalization (Goffman, 1961)
	• Antipsychiatry movement (Laing, 1965; Szasz, 1965)
1970s	• The rise of homeless populations in cities (Cohen & Thompson, 1992)
	• Legal protections: Rights of those with mental illness to treatment (Slovenko, 1985)
1980s	• Insurance coverage for mental illness (Trachtenberg, 1993)
	• Growth of self-help and family support groups
	• Increased research in biological factors in the etiology of mental illness
	• Psychophysiological approaches to treatment unifying bio/psych/sociological perspectives
1990s	• Identification of genetic markers—vulnerability hypothesis
	• Health promotion
	• Health Maintenance Organizations and mental health (Christianson & Osher, 1994; Stroul, Pires, Armstrong, & Meyers, 1998)

Occupational therapy, in the tradition of humanistic care, is conservative in nature, and the occupational therapist uses activities creatively to produce positive changes in the patient's behavior. If we make the assumption that mental illness, although biological in nature, is also a functional disorder in everyday living (Albee, 1982), then we act on the basis that the main treatment approach should be to enable the individual with mental illness to become functional in his or her life and to mas-ter the environment. In this approach drug treatment and other biochemical interventions are ancillary to occupational therapy. For example, an individual who is having difficulty with stress on the job may receive transient relief of symptoms of anxiety through a tranquilizer drug. However, the basic problem of work adjustment obviously cannot be cured by a drug. The more complex therapeutic method of working directly with the patient in creative problem solving to find new approaches in dealing with job satisfaction and reduction of stress takes more time and effort on the therapist's part than the mere administration of a drug.

If a group of specialists in the field of mental health today were to formulate an ideal treatment environment for individuals with mental illness they would probably arrive at the following conclusions:

▶ The length of initial treatment or acute care is as short as possible, so as to not disrupt the family or to threaten the individual's ability to resume working (Katz, 1985).

▶ An extensive evaluation of the individual should include an in-depth personal history, a neurological examination, and a complete physical examination.

▶ The treatment environment is as normalizing as possible with a respect for privacy, providing opportunities for self-improvement in a well-maintained housing unit (Carling, 1995).

▶ Individualized treatment is based on scientific findings, administered by mental health practitioners such as psychiatrists, psychiatric nurses, occupational therapists, psychologists, social workers, rehabilitation counselors, and psychiatric aides.

▶ The goals of psychosocial rehabilitation are linked to a holistic follow-up plan that includes medication management, readjustment in the community, a vocational goal, family involvement, suitable housing, opportunities for socialization, enrichment of leisure time, self-regulation of stress, and a community support system to prevent reccurence of symptoms (Anthony, Cohen, & Cohen, 1984; Liberman, 1992).

▶ The treatment approach is humanistic with caring attitude toward the patient and a respect for the sanctity of the individual (Rogers, Gerdlin, Kiesler, & Trevax, 1967).

In a theoretical study, Anthony, Cohen, and Farkas (1982) presented 10 essential ingredients in psychiatric rehabilitation that can serve as a model for operationally developing a comprehensive treatment program. These are listed in Table 2–2. These essential ingredients define quality assurance in a psychiatric rehabilitation program.

On the other hand, we consider the following factors to increase the chances of regression into illness and generally create a poor prognosis:

▶ A lengthy hospitalization that is primarily custodial

▶ No attempt to understand the dynamics and present history of the individual's life

▶ Incarceration in a locked facility that is poorly maintained and where the individual's basic needs in self-care, nutrition, exercise, and personal decision-making are not adequately met

▶ Treatment is routinized with an emphasis on medication and somatic therapies and there is no attempt to utilize a team approach. The patient spends most of the time idle (e.g., watching television or being inactive) without planned activities or rational treatment or is overprogrammed so there is no time for individual problem-solving

▶ The institutional approach is essentially psychologically or physically punitive to the patient without respect for individual differences

▶ The patient is discharged without any follow-up plan for maximum community adjustment, continuity of care, or prevention of recurrence of symptoms

Throughout the history of the treatment of those with mental illness, there are instances when society fostered a stigma attached to mental illness. This attitude has prevailed for many

Table 2-2. The Essential Ingredients of a Psychiatric Rehabilitation Program

Ingredient	*Example of How Observed*
1. Functional assessment of client skills in relation to environmental demands	1. Client records show a listing of client skills and deficits in relation to environmental demands; strengths and deficits are behaviorally defined and indicate client's present and needed level of functioning.
2. Client involvement in the rehabilitation assessment and intervention phases	2. Record forms have places for sign-off and comments; percentage of clients who actually sign off; sample of audiotapes of client interviews indicate client understanding of *what* a program is doing and *why.*
3. Systematic individual client rehabilitation plans	3. Written or taped examples of objective, behavioral, step-by-step client plans; a central "bank" of available rehabilitation curricula; client records specify on which plans client is working.
4. Direct teaching of skills to clients	4. Practitioners can identify the skills they are capable of teaching, describe the teaching process, and demonstrate their teaching techniques. Program's daily calendar reflects blocks of time devoted to skill training.
5. Environmental assessment and modification	5. Practitioners can describe characteristics of client's environment to which client is being rehabilitated and how the environment may be modified to support the client's skills level. Functional assessment should have assessed unique environmental demands.
6. Follow-up of clients in their real-life environments	6. Client records indicate a monitoring plan and description of practitioner and client feedback sessions; record-keeping forms provide spaces for changes in the intervention plan. Percentage of clients whose plans have changed; number of appointments for "follow-along" services.
7. A rehabilitation team approach	7. Team members can verbally describe each client's observable goals and the responsibilities of each team member in relation to those goals (may refer to client's records for this information).
8. A rehabilitation referral process	8. Client responses indicate requesting specific outcomes by specific dates; telephone referrals demonstrate the same rehabilitation referral ingredients.
9. Evaluation of observable outcomes and utilization of evaluation results	9. Agency records show the pooled outcome dates for all clients; agency directors can verbally describe their most significant client outcomes in the settings.
10. Consumer involvement in policies and planning	10. Administrators can list the number of joint meetings with consumers; consumer ratings of satisfaction with the environment to which client is being rehabilitated and rehabilitation program.

Source: Taken from "A Psychiatric Rehabilitation Treatment Program: Can I Recognize One If I See One?" by W. Anthony, M. Cohen, & M. Farkas (1982), *Community Mental Health Journal, 18*(2), p. 95. Reprinted by permission.

centuries in the care of individuals who were segregated away from society because they were thought to be either suffering from an incurable illness or possessed by a demonic force (Zilboorg, 1935). There are also examples of individuals like Philippe Pinel, a French physician, who in 1793 in the "lunatic asylum" of the Becetre in Paris ordered the removal of chains from patients to be replaced by a humane treatment (Pinel, 1801/1947).

In the section that follows, the roots of occupational therapy have been traced from the enormous amount of literature on the history of psychiatry. It is difficult to attribute concepts of etiology and treatment to specific time periods. There have been historical instances throughout the world of false causes of mental illness, such as demonology and possession. Instances of barbaric care also have been reported in the 1990s. For the student interested in the history of psychiatry, we recommend investigation of the primary sources listed in the references to gain insight into how the present practice of psychiatry evolved and to understand occupational therapy's place in this process.

NATURALISTIC APPROACH TO MENTAL HEALTH

Many of the early civilizations used natural remedies in treating diseases and disabilities (Alexander & Selesnick, 1966; Basham, 1976). Exercise, music, dance, and drama were recommended by Greek physicians for individuals suffering from mental illness. Asclepiades, a Greek physician who died approximately 100 B.C., prescribed bathing, exercise, and massages in light and airy rooms for the mentally ill (Alexander & Selesnick, 1966). The concept of a healthy mind in a healthy body influenced the Greeks in their approach to mental illness. They believed that illness was caused by man's lack of harmony with nature and that treatment should be used to balance the forces within the individual. Hippocrates (460–377 B.C.) advocated the idea that it is nature that heals the patient, and the doctor's role is to assist the patient to reach harmony with the natural forces within himself or herself (Heidel, 1941).

Soranus (98–138 A.D.), a Roman physician, believed that patients should be treated in pleasant surroundings with activities that relieve mental anguish. He stressed the importance of the healer working directly with the patient through discussions of the patient's occupation (Alexander & Selesnick, 1966).

The concept of medicine in ancient India stressed the importance of preventative actions in diet, physical exercise, and a good mental attitude as staving off illness (Basham, 1976). The ancient Peruvians used collective confessions, which are described as a type of group catharsis where the priests listened to individuals expressing their sorrows and guilt feelings. Afterward the priests lightly stroked the backs of the individuals with illness with straw and finally "priest and penitents spat on a handful of grass which was thrown into a river" (p. 481). This might have been a symbolic way of washing away the sins (Leon & Rosselli, 1975).

Other ritualistic methods of dealing with mental illness are prevalent in African societies where the Shaman (healer) uses incantations and the power of words to ward off the illness. Music, dance, and drama are also incorporated into the ritual of working out the illness (Lambo, 1975). In dynamic psychiatry, this process can be interpreted as a form of motor abreaction, which is defined as the living-out of an unconscious impulse through motor expression (Hinsie & Campbell, 1960).

In understanding the ancient tradition of treating mental illness in China, one must understand the concepts of yin and yang, which are considered to be the two primary forces in man. The two forces oppose each other and represent the female and male characteristics in each person. The Chinese believed strongly that man should live in harmony with nature and with the two forces in his or her body. They concluded that disease affects the entire human being. In Chinese medicine, the health of the individual is built up to prevent illness; in contrast, in Western medicine the emphasis is on treating the disease. Disease can be interpreted in this view as faulty living and not adhering to the prescribed "way" of carrying out life's task according to the right framework of Confucian ethics. Treatment, therefore, was achieved by having the individual alter one's lifestyle by conforming to the accepted precepts. In addition, the closely knit family system of Chinese society created a secure environment where the individual could be cared for by family members and protected from the secondary effects of illness. There are published data that have implied that there is less incidence of mental illness in China because of the nature of its society and the primary involvement of the family (Veith, 1975).

There are also contemporary examples of agrarian societies that are in the tradition of naturalistic medicine that have developed life patterns and self-regulating mechanisms that encourage holistic health and, therefore, minimize mental illness. Sula Benet (1976), an anthropologist, described the lifestyle patterns of the long-living people of the Caucasus located in the former Soviet Union. Factors were identified in their lifestyles that contributed to their healthy existences. These guidelines for healthful living were probably developed over a long period of time and were shaped by human experience in dealing with physical and mental illness. They are linked to ancient practices of natural healing.

Nutritional Factors in Mental Health

The dietary pattern of individuals who live long lives includes a high intake of natural vitamins from fresh vegetables, fruits, and milk products. There is a dietary rhythm in their everyday lives that includes a consistent atmosphere associated with a pleasurable and relaxed environment. Food preparation and selection are given high priority in their social interactions. Because this is an agrarian society, natural foods are abundant and include spices, beans, herbs, nuts, and honey. Packaged foods and processed meats are hardly used because they are not available. Spring water is available and fresh meat is usually boiled and roasted. The diet is high in bulk and low in fatty acids such as cholesterol. It has been known for centuries that diet has a direct relationship to physiological changes and plays a

prominent role in the overall health of the individual (Lankford, 1994).

There are some health practitioners (Miller, 1996) who propose that mental illness may be linked to dietary deficiencies. They advocate that individuals with mental illness, such as those diagnosed with schizophrenia, may benefit from large doses of vitamins (megavitamins). This field, orthomolecular psychiatry (Osmond & Hoffer, 1962), is based on the premise that certain individuals with mental illness can benefit from vitamins, such as B-complex and C. Although the field of orthomolecular psychiatry is not widely accepted by traditional psychiatrists, it remains a fertile area of investigation (Hoffer, 1973; Pauling, 1968). Other researchers have found little evidence to support the use of vitamin supplementation in the treatment of mental illness (Kleijnen & Knipschild, 1991; Lipton, et al., 1973).

However, it is known that some diseases of the nervous system are caused by vitamin deficiencies (McArdle, Katch, & Katch, 1994). For example, abnormal brain wave patterns and convulsions may result from deficiencies of vitamin B_6, B_{12}, and degeneration of peripheral nerves is related to deficiencies in vitamin B_{12} (Mahan & Escott–Stump, 1996). It has also been found that a ketogenic diet, composed of fatty acids and amino acids of protein may be helpful in controlling seizures, especially in children (Chapman & Giles, 1997).

Another example of the possible relationship between nutrition and mental health is in the area of hyperactivity. Feingold (1975) found that some children with hyperactivity have allergic reactions to salicylates, artificial food coloring, and artificial food flavoring. Based on his clinical observations, he devised a diet that eliminates artificial ingredients. However, a recent review of the research on Feingold's diet (Krummel, Seligson, & Guthrie, 1996) found no positive effects of reducing sugar and artificial food colors from diets on attention-deficit hyperactivity disorder. The researchers recommend that "the goal of diet treatment is to ensure a balanced diet with adequate energy and nutrients for optimal success" (p. 31). It is a probable conclusion based on research evidence and clinical observations that good nutrition and eating habits contribute to the mental health of the individual, while poor nutrition and inadequate diets negatively affect the overall health and can lead to chronic diseases (President's Council on Physical Fitness and Sports, 1996).

Extended Family and Mental Health

The social structure of the family in many agrarian societies is organized around generations of families living together in the same household and providing security and support for each member. Family loyalty and commitment are emphasized and aged members of the family are venerated. This type of structure creates a secure bond between family members and reduces the stress that accompanies individual striving and new learning. For example, in this structure the grandparents educate the younger generations based on long histories of experiential learning. The new parent does not have to learn through trial and error, but can benefit from the experiences of the elders.

How can this experience be compared with Western societies' family patterns? In the United States most families are centered around the nuclear family that is the result of a mobile and transient society where families change residences rapidly and seek independence from their parents. The nuclear parents are dependent on their own limited experiences and education and on the widely published self-help manuals and books that explain how to raise children, develop a relationship, assert their feelings, and cope with any and every problem that can possibly arise in developing social relationships and raising children. In industrial countries support groups and community organizations have taken the place of the extended family. Because stressful experiences have a definite role in the precipitation of emotional and physical disorders (Pelletier, 1977; Selye, 1976; Stein & Miller, 1993), the extended family, or as a substitute, community support groups, can provide a source of comfort and solace to the individual at times when stress and trauma arise. For the nuclear family and individuals living alone, support networks such as social action groups (e.g., Alliance for the Mentally Ill [AMI]) and self-help groups (i.e., Recovery Incorporated and Alcoholics Anonymous) have replaced the extended family that traditionally has been needed by the individual during emotional crises.

Continuity of Daily Life Patterns

"A rhythmic regularity characterizes Caucasian life and is probably a major source of its healthfulness" (Benet, 1976, p. 159). Continuity in an individual's life refers to the daily patterns of everyday existence that the individual maintains regarding sleep, work, diet, sex, exercise, leisure, relaxation, and personal interactions. The individual may establish a daily pattern of living that is conducive to good physical and emotional health. For the individual, the rhythm of life affects the ability to combat stress and disease. Investigators studying sleep found a direct relationship between sleep deprivation and reduction of natural immune responses (Hartman, 1973; Irwin et al., 1996). The pattern of occupational adjustment and stress-related factors attached to work have also been documented by researchers (Holt, 1993). The disturbing effects of changes in occupational and work tasks have been implicated as precipitating causes of emotional illness. In Western society it is important for the individual to establish a daily pattern of life that is congruent to health. For most individuals the body reacts favorably to a familiar and stable environment that creates a psychological climate of trust and security. On the other hand, discontinuities in daily life such as inadequate amounts of sleep, alterations in the work–sleep pattern where the individual alternately works at night and sleeps during the day, frequent changes in food habits, and lack of routines in exercise and leisure activities reduce the individual's ability to cope with stress and, therefore, make one vulnerable to mental illness. The accumulation of evidence in research studies has resulted in the identification of mechanisms by which stress reactions can dampen the immune system and therefore make the individual susceptible to illness (Ader, Felten, & Cohen, 1991; Valdimarsdottir & Stone, 1997). Researchers using the model of psychoneuroimmunology have generated studies examining the relationships between stress and the variables of AIDS and cancer.

Health Perspective

The active desire to be physically and emotionally healthy is an important factor. Holistic health practitioners and researchers (Edlin & Golanty, 1992; Mattson, 1982) have emphasized the importance of individuals taking more responsibility for their own health.

For the people living in the Caucasus, good health is a primary goal of life that is related to the individual's attitude and lifestyle. Physical and mental health are active states of mind to which people aspire. On the one hand the individual advocating a natural approach to health strives to develop a lifestyle that facilitates health

and increases one's ability to cope with stress. On the other hand, a negative attitude toward health and a lack of insight into how to master the environment contribute to inadequate adjustment and vulnerability to mental illness.

Realistic Life Goals

Benet (1976) found that,

Clearly defined behavior patterns and achievable life goals reduce emotional tensions. The Caucasians live in a stable culture whose expectations do not overreach the possibilities of attainment and whose competition, if found at all, is in nonvital activities such as sports, dancing, and music. (pp. 160–161)

Researchers and theorists (Coker, Osgood, & Clouse, 1995; Holland, 1973) have found that vocational satisfaction and work adjustment depend on the congruence of the individual's personality with cognitive traits. Mental health, therefore, would be affected by the matching of an individual's personality, interests, intelligence, education, and experiences to realistic life goals. The inability to realize one's potentials and strive toward unrealistic goals affect vocational satisfaction and, as a result, mental and physical health (Bogg & Cooper, 1995). Continual patterns of failure in highly competitive areas of life can produce symptoms such as feelings of inadequacy, low self-esteem, anxiety, and depression, all of which are cardinal signs of mental illness.

Exercise and Mental Health

The role of exercise in health has been well substantiated. Regular, systematic exercise has a positive effect on the cardiovascular, respiratory, and muscular systems. Its beneficial effects on the heart, blood vessels, oxygen supply, digestion, and muscles of the body have been documented by investigators throughout the world during the last 45 years (Eckstein 1957; Ekert & Montoye, 1984; Morris & Crawford, 1958; Simonson, 1972; Towner & Blumenthal, 1993). Sula Benet (1976) found in her study that many Russian physicians believe that regular exercise helps develop resistance to diseases and is a major factor in longevity. There is also increasing evidence that moderate, regular exercise is related to a positive sense of well-being (International Society of Sports Psychology, 1992; Morgan & Goldstein, 1987).

Folkins and Sime (1981), in an extensive review of the relationship between physical fitness training and mental health, concluded that exercise led to improved mood, positive self-concept, and good work behavior. To support this conclusion they cited the following studies. Kavanagh, Shepard, Tuck, and Quereshi (1977) found marked improvement in reducing depression for a group of severely depressed male patients with cardiac problems after 4 years of exercise-oriented rehabilitation. Scott (1960) reported an improved sense of well-being associated with fitness. Morris and Husman (1970) found a sense of improved "life quality" resulting from a fitness training program for college students. Greist et al. (1979), while investigating the effect of running on reducing depression reported a positive relationship. The literature also contains evidence of the positive effects of exercise on inhibiting phobic reactions (Orwin, 1974), reducing anxiety (Martinsen, 1993), and improving mood (Steptoe, Edwards, Moses, & Matthews, 1989). In general there is enough evidence to conclude that regular, moderate physical exercise has a positive effect on the emotional state of the individual.

Music and Mental Health

From the time of recorded history, music has played an important role generally in medicine and particularly in relieving the suffering of individuals with mental illness (Pavlicevic, 1999; Tame, 1984; Wrangsjo & Korlin, 1995). Music is present in all societies and is incorporated into almost every aspect of our lives, such as listening for relaxation, creating a relaxing mood for work and leisure, expressing patriotism and pride, visualizing pleasurable scenes, and reminiscing about joyful past experiences. Podolsky (1954) described case studies in which music produced curative effects. He concluded that the potential value of music as a resocializing agent in treating individuals with mental illness is immeasurable:

> Music is capable of changing mood; it overcomes depressed feelings and calms over-active patients. It can change a dissatisfied and destructive mood to a satisfied and constructive one. Since music has this power it is being used quite widely on mental patients to bring them out of seclusion, relieve tensions and afford contact with reality by relaxation and the creation of an emotional outlet. (p. 19)

Music has been shown to produce physiological and psychological effects as well as having social, educational, and aesthetic attributes (Darrow, Gibbons, & Heller, 1985). Girard (1954), in reviewing the literature, made the following conclusions:

1. Music has the property of producing various moods, and by means of appropriate music, an anxious mood may be dispelled by a hopeful mood induced by music.

2. Music has the property of facilitating self-expression and by expressing the tension that gives rise to anxieties, the latter are quite often eliminated.

3. The associative response whereby music stimulates the process of thought, and of both memory and fantasy formation, makes it evident that such stimulation may facilitate the expression of repressed or unconscious

mental elements which gives rise to anxiety. Thus the anxiety is eliminated. (p. 106)

Juliette Alvin (1978) presented detailed case histories of using music as therapy with children with autism. These children were unable to develop normal relationships and they lived in isolated worlds closed off from communication with others. Their behavior seems irrational, bizarre, and difficult to understand. The author used music to "help the child to discover his innate creativity, express himself through any kind of sound, beautiful, violent, rough or timid, that would be helpful to encourage him to come out of his loneliness through a world of music" (p. viii). Gradually, through music, the children were able to appreciate their own ability to express themselves by experimenting with such musical instruments as a cymbal, chime bars, xylophone, drums, piano, and cello. The musical experiences for these children were positive and therapeutic and are examples of a natural approach to mental health that is significant in a holistic framework. Other researchers have reported using music therapy effectively with individuals who are elderly (Bernard, 1992), have dementia (Casby & Holm, 1994; Koger & Brontons, 1999), are depressed (Lai, 1999), and have had a stroke to improve hand grasp and functional performance (Cofrancesco, 1985).

Benet (1976) noted that the Caucasians used music to relieve pain as well as a tranquilizer. She found that specific songs were used for different illnesses. Group singing was also used to distract the patient from his pain and also to persuade "God" to cure him. The effect of music on ß-endorphins has been explored recently by researchers demonstrating the effect of music in reducing pain (McKinney, Tims, Kumar, & Kumar, 1997).

Dance and Mental Health

Among aboriginal people, dance is incorporated into the daily life patterns to celebrate important occasions (e.g., births), to influence nature (e.g., rain dances), to stir up passions (e.g., war dances), to relate tribal stories, and to create sexual excitement (Meerloo, 1960). Dance is an action-oriented art form that serves as a strong outlet for emotional expressions and is especially appropriate for individuals with mental illness (Levy, 1988; Nagpal & Ruta, 1997).

Spontaneous dance is an overflow of strong emotions that are expressed at a time of joy. For example, the jump of joy in hearing unexpected good news and the celebration after a sports victory are examples of unrehearsed expressions of happiness. Spontaneous dance can be interpreted as an extension of human movement. The emotional expressions of the body in the way we stand, walk, and use our limbs can be interpreted as expressions of body language. Individuals walking slowly with their heads down as compared to strident walkers holding their chins up are examples of expressing feelings through bodily movement.

In the society in the Caucasus, dance was highly ritualized and regulated and was an integral part of courtship. It provided the individual an opportunity to share as an active participant in the society. It encouraged a sense of belongingness to the community (Benet, 1976). Palo-Bengtsson, Winblad, and Ekman (1998) found that social dancing, when used with individuals with dementia, was a positive influence on feelings, communication, and behavior.

Dance, like art, music, poetry, drama, and literature, is an excellent activity for expressing one's feelings. It is part of the culture of every society whether it be in the form of folk dancing, ballet, modern dance, ballroom dancing, or tribal dancing. It is a universal expression that arises from our deepest emotions and bodily feelings.

Summary

In summary, the naturalistic approach to mental health that was first advanced by the ancient Greeks (Hippocratic medicine) and later practiced in part by agrarian civilizations and non-industrial societies is the basic foundation for the holistic health movement. This philosophical perspective on health incorporates a wide variety of diverse approaches to preventing illness, maintaining health, and healing disease. The lifestyle of the individual, as it encompasses nutrition, exercise, music, social and family relationships, everyday activities of daily living, and attitudes toward health and life goals, affects the overall health of the individual. These multiple factors are considered by practitioners of a naturalistic or holistic health approach to be essential in designing a program for preventing or treating mental illness. Consistent with this approach is the concept that the patient should take a major responsibility in his or her treatment. It is interesting to note that the specific treatment methods related to the holistic health model place a heavy emphasis on stress reduction, for example, progressive relaxation (Jacobson, 1958; Lehrer & Woolfolk, 1993), autogenic training (Luthe & Schultz, 1969), biofeedback training (Brown, 1977; Schwartz & Associates, 1995), rolfing (Rolf, 1977), and bioenergetics (Lowen, 1976).

For the occupational therapist, the natural holistic approach to mental health provides an excellent model that can be incorporated into a comprehensive activity treatment program for the individual with mental illness. In parallel to holistic health, the moral humanistic tradition in health care was a direct result of the reaction against the inhumane care toward individuals with mental illness during the Middle Ages.

THE INHUMANE ERA IN THE CARE OF THOSE WITH MENTAL ILLNESS

Zilboorg (1941) summarized the general attitude toward individuals with mental illness during the Middle Ages in Western Europe in the following quote:

> The whole field of mental diseases was thus torn away from medicine. Medicine at first did not seem to relinquish this territory unwillingly. Medical psychology as a legitimate branch of the healing art practically ceased to exist. It was recaptured by the priest and incorporated into his theurgic system. Seven hundred years of effort seemed for a long while to have spent themselves in vain. The ardent voice one hears in Hippocrates' discourse on the *Sacred Diseases* was lost in the wilderness; it was silent for nearly twelve centuries. (p. 103)

During this period, individuals with mental illness were considered to be possessed by demons (Alexander & Selesnick, 1966). The clergy rather than the medical profession was responsible for caring for individuals with mental illness. Exorcism was practiced by the clergy as a way of ejecting the "insane" influence of the demon from the body of the individual with mental disturbance. Although physical illness was recognized as a natural phenomenon, mental illness was seen as a supernatural and religious problem. If exorcism did not cure the individual of his insanity, the person could be chained in a dungeon or tortured until he repented and freed himself of his demonic influence. Individuals with mental illness were also rejected by their families and left to live in the streets or to wander from village to village, becoming like "untouchables" who were feared rather than pitied. As the clergy became more and more frustrated by the inability to "cast out the demons" from the insane, the theory of witchcraft was proposed as an explanation for deviant and heretical behavior that threatened the very order of the society.

The book that influenced the public's attitudes toward the persecution of witches or those possessed by demons was the *Malleus Maleficarum* written by two Dominican clergymen and published in 1486 (Alexander & Selesnick, 1966). This book was a handbook of sorts that identified individuals who were deviant, namely, those with mental illness. In this book the causes of witchcraft were linked to sexual lust and cohabitation with demons. The witches, after conviction, were burned at the stake. The witchcraft theory dominated the attitudes toward individuals with mental illness for over 400 years from approximately the middle of the 15th century, during the Salem witch trials in Massachusetts in the 17th century, and even up to the 18th century. It is incredible to note that the number of people who were persecuted as witches during this time was in the millions (Michelet, 1939).

Although the Middle Ages are generally associated with the inhumane care of the "insane," it also should be noted that there were instances of rational methods of treatment based on the Greek ideal of natural medicine and compassion. Alexander and Selesnick (1966) found in reviewing Medieval literature that Bethlehem Hospital in London, established in 1247, was originally a place of comfort and shelter for individuals with mental illness. When patients were able to leave Bethlehem Hospital "in the care of their relatives, they were given arm badges to wear so that they could be returned to the hospital if their symptoms should reoccur" (p. 53). Unfortunately, Bethlehem Hospital became the infamous "Bedlam" hundreds of years after its founding. Another instance of humane care during the Middle Ages was the development of a form of foster family care for the "insane" in Geel, Belgium. "From the second half of the 14th century, Geel gradually became a place of pilgrimage specifically for mental

patients. The custom originated to lodge the insane in the houses of the local population" (Pierloot, 1975, pp. 139–140). This practice of providing halfway houses was the first recorded example of a community providing care for individuals with mental illness, and it indirectly is the precursor to the community mental health concept fostered in Great Britain and in the United States during the 1960s.

The Renaissance did not change the inhumane course of treatment for individuals with mental illness. The 300 years between the rebirth of classical learning and the 19th century were characterized as "the great confinement" by Michael Foucault (1965) in his essay, *Madness and Civilization: A History of Insanity in the Age of Reason*. For example, during the 17th century, one out of every hundred inhabitants of the city of Paris was confined in a general hospital, prison, or workhouse. The "insane" were found mingled with the unemployed, the idle, vagabonds, and criminals. Those confined were many times forced to work because idleness was perceived as a destructive element and a threat to the order of the society.

The confinement of the "insane" also produced the phenomenon of displaying them for entertainment purposes. "One went to see the keeper display the madmen the way the trainer . . . put the monkeys through their tricks" (Foucault, 1965, p. 68). Many hospital administrators charged admission to see the "lunatics." They were confined to dungeons, chained to the walls and beds, put on leashes, and kept like vicious animals with minimal care to keep them alive. "There was no need to protect them; they had no need to be covered or warmed" (p. 68).

Various methods of curing or controlling individuals with mental illness were tried: dunking them into water, "stone cutting," which involved making an incision in the skin on the forehead and removing an imaginary stone, bloodletting, using magical charms and amulets, laying on of hands, rotating chairs, castrating males, starving patients, using various drugs such as camphor and digitalis, inducing high fever, removing teeth, engaging in numerous other inhumane practices in the hope of finding a magical cure. By the end of the 18th century in Western Europe, there was a growing moral indignation to the brutal treatment of those with mental illness.

MORAL TREATMENT AND THE USE OF OCCUPATION DURING THE 19th CENTURY

During the 19th century the physicians who were responsible for the care of individuals with mental illness came to recognize the importance of activity in mental hospital care. The quote below from Pinel (1801/1947), the first psychiatrist to advance moral treatment, links activity to recovery. This was one of the key concepts that laid the foundation for the profession of occupational therapy.

> Prescribed physical exercises and manual occupations should be employed in all mental hospitals. There is no longer any question about the desirability of such practices since the continuous and unanimous experience in all public asylums such as prisons and hospitals has demonstrated its effectiveness in maintaining health. Rigorously executed manual labor is the best method of securing good morale and discipline. This fact is especially true in relation to hospitals for the alienated and I am firmly convinced that such institutions must be conducted in that manner if they are to be of lasting usefulness. I have conclusively shown that very few of these patients should be denied active occupation even while they are in a state of marked agitation. What a distressing sight it is, to see in all our national establishments, numbers of mental patients in a continuous

and purposeless state of excitement, or what is worse, plunged into inertia and stupor! What better method is there of prolonging the excitement, fits of passion, and delirious flights of the imagination than indolence? Continuous work, on the other hand, interrupts the chain of morbid thoughts, fixes the attention of more pleasant subjects and by means of exercise maintains order in any group of patients and at the same time permits the rejection of many detailed and often useless regulations for the maintenance of internal discipline. The return of convalescent patients to their previous interests, to the practice of their profession; to industriousness and perseverance have always been for me the best omen of a final recovery. (p. 63)

For Pinel occupation meant farming, manual work, music, and practical activities directly related to an individual's former work and avocational interests. Pinel's concept of curative activity is directly related to the definition of occupation used by contemporary occupational therapists. *Occupation* is defined as integral groups of activity within the context of a culture, for example, fishing, cooking, playing, or working. These activities are considered to be self-initiated, purposeful, and socially sanctioned (Pendleton, 1996).

Pinel recognized that this approach in the use of occupation was revolutionary in the care of individuals with mental illness. It was to replace the harsh treatment that existed during the Middle Ages and that unfortunately exists in some institutions even up to the present time. Pinel's (1801/1947) statement below called for an end to cruelty to patients within the mental hospital, a theme that has been repeated for the last 200 years.

> To place the agitated mental patients in continuous isolation and restraint, to surrender them without protection to the brutality of attendants under the pretext of dangers inherent to their health, to rule them, in a word, with an iron rod, so as to hasten the end of an existence

considered deplorable, is undoubtedly a very convenient method of management but at the same time is a reversion to the barbarous dark ages. It is not only contrary to the established fact that this type of insanity is curable in a great many patients who are permitted limited liberty within the hospital, but it is also proven that harmless activity or at least diminished restraints and the observance of other rules and intelligent treatment make this condition amenable to improvement. Nothing is better established than the beneficial influence which the chief of a mental hospital exerts than when he brings to it dignity and the most enlightened principles of humanity. (p. 67)

It is ironic to note that an article excerpted from *Le Monde* in September (1980) entitled "Psychiatric Hospitals: Excellence and Squalor," raised the issue of cruel and inhumane treatment for individuals with mental illness in the country where Pinel unlocked the chains 200 years ago.

Looking into psychiatric hospitals means stepping onto the shoes of a host of administrators, ministry inspectors, humanists and doctors who have for over two centuries been tirelessly castigating but without getting anywhere, the practice of shutting away the individuals with mental illness. It means entering a universe of fear and suffering, fear of the violence inherent to asylums and fear of the outside world (very frequently we had to resort to subterfuge to penetrate this tightly closed environment) the suffering present in the world of asylums, which are rejected wholesale by society in a reaction that is both primitive and continuing; and the suffering caused by the disrepute into which these institutions have very often fallen. A total of 105,000 patients live in France's psychiatric hospitals. (Brisset, September 4, 1980, p. 12)

The moral movement in the early 19th century engulfed many parts of Europe and America. Johann Christian Reil (1759–1813), a German physician, also believed that physical work should be part of the everyday routine for the patient. He felt that, as the patient improved, assigned work should proceed from physical and mechanical work to art and mental work. This concept of sequencing activities into higher levels of abstraction has been the basis of many present-day occupational therapy activity programs that start patients on simple routine activities and work upward to more creative and challenging activities relating to the individual patient's ability to concentrate and conceptualize. The quote below from Reil (1803/1947) illustrates the range of activities he advocated in the treatment of individuals with mental illness:

Even so, some variety must be used to prevent the indifference to which monotony may lead. Building blocks and the assembly of picture cut-outs should be used as well as swimming, dancing, balancing, drill, vaulting, quoits, jumping rope, and other gymnastic exercises, since they strengthen both the mind and body. In fact this subject deserves special consideration, and a gymnasium designed especially for the needs of the insane would be most useful. It is a pity that insane patients cannot have the same use of them as is made in the education of children.

Patients should be instructed in drawing, painting, singing, music and other arts in which they exhibit talent. A concert, in particular would enable them to concentrate on one subject. Still another thought deserves mention. Could not plays especially adapted for performance in insane asylums be prepared? Those patients who most nearly approximate normal could produce them while the others would look on. Such a performance would demand the closest attention. Through the proper assignment of roles other advantages could be gained, such as ridiculing the follies of each patient. The patients should imitate, memorize and correct errors in speech. At the beginning they should read aloud mechanically, later with expression and finally relate from memory the content of what they have read. In conversion they should be taught to give defin-itive answers. They should be urged to portray scenes of their former life by narrative or by acting them out. Later they should be given more complicated tests of attention such as the discussion of abstract things in confusing cir-cumstances. They should be required to keep a diary of all events which they witness and in order to test their observation some incidents would be invented without their knowledge. All these and other exercises of attention and thought must be adapted to the strength of the patient so as not to fatigue him. Other methods of general body care such as baths, motion and massage with oil should also be employed. (pp. 343–344)

Reil's concepts, in a way, are precursors to the contemporary uses of exercise, psychodrama, creative arts in therapy, bibliotherapy, journal-ing, and massage. These activities are the basis for treatment in many programs.

In another part of Europe, in England, Samuel Tuke (1784–1857) advocated moral treatment for individuals with mental illness. Moral treatment, as conceived by Tuke, was associated with exercise, recreation, manual work, and crafts. Tuke also prescribed that patients work alongside the hospital staff in the everyday maintenance of the institution. The quotation below from Tuke (1813/1947) emphasizes the importance of activity in a humane treatment environment for individuals with mental illness:

Every means is taken to seduce the mind from its favorite but unhappy musing, by bodily exercise, walks, conversations, reading, and other innocent recreations, the good effect of exercise, . . . has been very striking in several instances at this institution.

Some years ago, a patient much afflicted with melancholic and hypochondriacal symp-toms, was admitted by his own request. He had walked from home, a distance of 200 miles, in company with a friend, and on his arrival, found much less inclination to converse on the absurd and melancholy views of his own state, than he had previously felt.

This patient was by trade a gardener, and the superintendent immediately perceived, from the affect of his journey, the propriety of keeping him employed. He led him into the garden, and conversed with him on the subject of horticulture; and soon found that the patient possessed a very superior knowledge of pruning, and of the other departments of his art. He proposed several improvements in the management of the garden, which were adopt-ed, and the gardener was desired to furnish him with full employment. . . .

The female patients in the Retreat, are employed, as much as possible, in sewing, knit-ting or domestic affairs; and several of the con-valescents assist the attendants. Of all the modes by which the patients may be induced to restrain themselves, regular employment is perhaps the most generally efficacious; and those kinds of employment and doubtless to be preferred, both on a moral and physical account, which are accompanied by consider-able bodily action; that are most agreeable to the patient, and which are most opposite to the illusions of his disease. (pp. 255–257)

Thomas Kirkbride (1809–1883), one of the founders of the American Psychiatric Association, had a far reaching influence on the practice of hospital psychiatry. In the quote below from his major work, *On the Construction, Organization, and General Arrangement of Hospitals for the Insane* (1854/1948), Kirkbride gave practical advice on the day-to-day activities for the "insane." He favored a highly structured regimen where the patient is involved in pleasur-able social and educational activities that range from the time he is awakened in the morning until he goes to bed at night. He believed strong-ly in a consistent activity program that involved regular exercise, lectures, music, arts and crafts, and entertainment. Kirkbride was strongly against the use of restraint, physical abuse, and seclusion in patient management.

ARRANGEMENTS OF HOSPITALS
FOR THE "INSANE"

The hospital day begins at five o'clock in the morning, at which hour the attendants and those engaged in the domestic departments, are expected to rise and prepare for their morning duties. By six, it is intended the patients should be getting ready for breakfast, which meal, during the whole year, is taken at half past six o'clock, and previous to which, medicine is given to those for whom it may be deemed desirable in the different wards, by persons specially deputed for the purpose. Before this, too, the Supervisors are expected to ascertain the general condition of the patients, and the mode in which those employed are performing their duties. The officers resident in the hospital take all their meals half an hour after the patients, so that those to whom the duty is specially delegated can have a personal supervision of the dining rooms, and the general serving of food. Immediately after breakfast, the rooms and wards are put in order, preparatory to examination by the medical officers at their morning visit, which they begin a few minutes after eight o'clock, accompanied by the supervisors, and during which the condition and wants of every patient are carefully ascertained, and every room is inspected. Previous to the commencement of this visit, the cards form the watch-clocks are examined, written reports are received from the supervisors and companions of the patients, detailing their observation of the previous day and evening, and verbal reports are made of the state of the patients in the early morning. Before this visit, or immediately after, arrangements are made for driving, walking, visiting interesting places, and for the special occupations and amusements of the patients during the day, as well as for whatever requires attention in the city. At eight o'clock in summer, and at nine in winter, the patients start out driving in the large carriages which go into Philadelphia and the adjacent country, and in the pony and donkey phaetons, the German town wagons, etc., all of which, but the first, are often driven by the patients, being used only inside of the enclosures, the roads within which at each department are nearly two miles in extent. About the same time, the patients from all the wards, accompanied by a portion of their attendants, pass into the grounds to walk, and in good weather they are expected thus to spend at least a couple of hours every morning out of the house. Before returning, or afterwards, they have an opportunity to visit the museums and reading rooms, the greenhouse, gymnastics hall, various summer houses, the calisthenium or ten-pin alley, amusement hall, etc., and to engage in the various games there provided, or in those more specially calculated for the open air. In addition, the male patients have the use of the carpenter and other workshops, and of the gardens and grounds, in working in which, many take much interest. The female patients also resort to their workrooms. Many too, of both sexes, walk outside of the enclosures, visiting objects of interest in the vicinity, and often extending their excursions to a considerable distance.

After the out-door exercise, the usual indoor resources are at command—reading, writing, conversation, games of nearly every kind, and whatever work is likely to be interesting to individual patients. During all this period, as well as in the afternoon and evening, the supervisors and companions to the patients pass among them in the different wards, the latter especially giving their attention wherever deemed most important, and taking care that there is no falling off in the amount of exercise, in the amusements, or occupations in which the inmates are engaged. At all these periods, the medical and other officers, too, give what time they are able to spare to professional visits at irregular hours, and to the exercise of such personal influence as they can bestow, which is often of great value in the cases under care.

At noon, medicine is again administered to those who are taking it regularly, and preparations are made for dinner, which is on the table at half past twelve. Early in the afternoon, the hour depending somewhat on the season, all are expected to be again in the open air, and securing, as much as possible, the advantages which result from it, sunshine, exercise, and whatever else can be combined with these valuable agents for preserving as well as restoring health. The same places of resort for occupation and amusement are open, as in the morning and as many as can be accommodated are again out driving.

Tea is ready at six o'clock in winter, and half past six in summer; after which, except in very warm weather, few go outside of the yards connected with the wards. Then begin the special arrangements for making the evenings pass pleasantly. Preparations are made for the lectures and other entertainments in the lecture rooms, or gymnastic halls, or for the officers' tea parties; one of these entertainments takes place regularly every evening of the week for nine months at each department, commencing at half past seven o'clock, and lasting about one hour—the character of these exercises being greatly varied, as has been before detailed. After leaving the lecture rooms, the patients frequently accessible in the parlors, and have music, games, and other diversions, filling up the time to half past nine, between which and ten o'clock, all persons are expected to retire for the night. The only difference when there is no lecture-room entertainment, is, that much more music, more reading aloud, and all the games that are popular, while small tea parties now and then make a pleasant variety. The evening visit of the physicians is made soon after tea, or immediately after lecture, when particular directions are given for the night.

At half past nine P.M., the regular night-watcher calls at the physician's office for instructions in regard to special duties. The night-watch consists of those regularly employed for the purpose of passing through the wards, to see to the safety of the buildings, the condition of the patients, and to attend to their wants, etc., and of those who may be appointed to be with the very sick. Every ward is visited at stated periods, and when passed

through, the night-watcher, by touching a pull connected with the watch-clocks, makes a mark on the revolving card, which shows that the duty has been performed, and also the exact time at which it was done. This pull can be made only at one point in each ward, and the card itself is accessible only to the officer having it in charge. The night-watch remains of duty till the attendants are up, and have taken the custody of the wards in the morning, so that at no time, day or night, are the wards left without someone directly responsible for their care. (pp. 77–79)

Benjamin Rush (1745–1813), the father of American psychiatry, listed remedies for hypochondriasis in his work entitled *Medical Inquiries and Observations Upon the Diseases of the Mind* (1812/1947).

OF THE REMEDIES FOR HYPOCHONDRIASIS

Exercise, especially upon horseback. *Labor* is still more useful, particularly in the open air.

Employment, or business of some kind. Man was made to be active. Even in paradise he was employed in the health and pleasant exercises of cultivating a garden. Happiness, consisting in folded arms, and in pensive contemplation beneath rural shades, and by the side of purling brooks, never had any existence, except in the brains of ad poets, and love-sick girls and boys. Hypochondriac derangement has always kept pace with the inactivity of body and mind which follows wealth and independence in all countries. It is frequently induced by this cause in those citizens, who retire, after a busy life, into the country, without carrying with them a relish for agriculture, gardening, books or literary society.

Building, commerce, a public employment, an executorship to a will; above all, agriculture, have often cured this disease. The last, that is agriculture, by agitating the passions by alternate hope, fear, and enjoyment, and by rendering bodily exercise or labour necessary, is calculated to produce the greatest benefit. Great care should however be taken never to advise retirement to a part of the county where good society can not be enjoyed upon easy terms.

In those cases in which the body can not be employed, the mind should be kept constantly busy. Mr. Cowper often relieved his melancholy by reading novels. Hence he has well said,

"*Absence* of occupation is not rest,
A mind quite *vacant* is a mind *distrest*."

I knew a lady in whom this disease was brought on by a disappointment in love, who cured herself by translating Telemachus into English verse. The remedy here was, chiefly constant employment.

Dr. Burton, in his Anatomy of Melancholy, delivers the following direction for its cure: "Be not idle, be not solitary." Dr. Johnson has improved this advice by the following commentary upon it. "When you are idle, be not solitary; and when you are solitary, be not idle." The illustrious Spinola, upon hearing of the death of a friend inquired of what disease he died? "Of having nothing to do," said the person who mentioned it. "Enough," said Spinola, "to kill a general." Not only the want of employment, but the want of care, often increases, as well as brings on this disease. This was exemplified in the two instances formerly mentioned, of suicide being induced by situations in which the heart wished and cared for nothing.

Concerts, evening parties, and the society of the ladies to gentlemen affected with this disease, have been useful. Of the efficacy of the last, Mr. Green has happily said,

"With speech so sweet, so sweet a mien,
They excommunicate the spleen."

Certain amusements. Those should be preferred, by which, while they interest the mind, afford exercise to the body. This chase, shooting, playing at quoits, are all useful for this purpose. The words of the poet, Mr. Green, upon this subject, deserve to be committed to memory by all physicians:

"To cure the mind's wrong bias, spleen,
Some recommended the bowling green;

Some hilly walks—all exercise,
Fling but a stone—the giant dies."

Chess, checkers, cards, and even push-pin, should be preferred to idleness, when the weather forbids exercise in the open air. The theater has often been resorted to, to remove fits of low spirits; and it is a singular fact, that a tragedy oftener dissipates them than a comedy. The remedy, though distressing to persons with healthy minds, is like the temperature of cold water to persons benumbed with frost; it is exactly proportioned to the excitability of their minds, and it not only abstracts their attention from themselves, but even revives their spirits.

A female patient of mine, in whom this disease had several times been excited by family afflictions, lost a favorite child in November 1811, which produced many of its symptoms. Soon afterwards her husband became sick. The lighter and dissimilar distress occasioned by this event, suddenly removed her disease, and she regained with the recovery of her husband, her usual health and spirits. Mirth, or even cheerfulness, when employed as remedies in low spirits, are like hot water to a frozen limb. They are disproportioned to the excitability of the mind, and, instead of elevating, never fail to increase its depression or to irritate. Mr. Cowper could not bear to hear his humorous story of John Gilpin read to him in his paroxysms of this disease. It was to his "heavy heart" what Solomon happily compares to the conflict produced by pouring vinegar upon nitre, or in other works, upon an alkaline salt. (pp. 177–178)

The additional excerpts from Esquirol (1838/1948) and Leuret (1840/1948), who were French psychiatrists in the forefront of moral treatment during the 19th century, illustrate the importance of activity in the context of humanistic care.

Corporal exercises, riding on horseback, the game of tennis, fencing, swimming and traveling, especially in melancholy, should be employed, in aid of other means of treatment.

The culture of the earth, with a certain class of the insane, may be advantageously substituted for all other exercises. We know the result to which a Scotch farmer arrived by the use of labor. He rendered himself celebrated by the cure of certain insane persons, whom he obliged to labor in his fields. (Esquirol, 1948, p. 59)

Among the alienated, intelligence and emotion cannot be restored to their previous condition without the use of moral treatment; and that is the only kind of treatment which has a direct influence on the symptoms of insanity.

To prevent the effects of idleness and boredom, all psychiatrists recommend diversions and work. The diversions available in a hospital or convalescent home are very limited in number, and those physicians who prescribe them admit that they are not as effective as work. In a German hospital at Halle I have seen work for patients organized as systematically as it is in industry. (Leuret, 1840/1948, p. 27)

Moral treatment for those with mental illness during the 19th century was an important impetus to the emergence of occupational therapy. For example, in Worcester State Lunatic Hospital in Massachusetts, which was established in 1833, a philosophy of humanitarianism was applied by the superintendent, Dr. Samuel B. Woodward, a distinguished physician. "The thrust of Woodward's moral treatment focused on regular routines, individualized care, occupational therapy and religious training. . . . He emphasized the utility of occupational therapy to keep inmates active, he assigned varied tasks and constructive leisure activities, such as reading in the hospital library and attendance at religious services" (Bell, 1980, p. 17). The therapeutic program established by Woodward was judged at that time to have produced a significant recovery rate among the middle-class inmates.

No discussion of the history of psychiatry is complete without citing the work of Dorothea Dix (1802–1887) who worked diligently to improve the care of those with mental illness. She devoted her adult life to visiting the jails, poorhouses, and private homes where they were confined (Colman, 1992). She documented the physical abuse and neglect that had reduced them to pitiful creatures. She petitioned legislators to consider the public financing of mental institutions where individuals could receive adequate humanistic caring. The asylum that Dorothea Dix projected was one where individuals with mental illness would be given the opportunity to participate actively in a wide variety of therapeutic activities in an atmosphere of respect and tranquility (Colman, 1992). Unfortunately, what later emerged was the building of asylums that offered merely custodial, depersonalized care.

THE EMERGENCE OF THE PROFESSION OF OCCUPATIONAL THERAPY AND THE MENTAL HYGIENE MOVEMENT: 1900–1950

The 19th century psychiatric reformers such as Pinel in France, Tuke in England, Reil in Germany, and Rush in the United States changed the course of caring for individuals with mental illness from a perspective of custodial neglect to a model of humanistic concern. Although the care of these individuals was in the hands of the medical community, still no systematic, acceptable treatment procedures were practiced in mental hospitals. Occupational therapy and other mental health professions came into existence after the turn of this century.

American psychiatry, as previously noted, was greatly influenced by Benjamin Rush, who played an important role in developing a psychiatric treatment program at Pennsylvania Hospital in Philadelphia. Rush, however, based his recommended treatment practices on a somatic approach to mental illness that involved bloodletting, emetics, a meager diet, and two therapeutic mechanisms, the tranquilizer chair and the gyrator. "The former was a chair with straps that bound the patient's wrist and feet. A box like wooden hat that lowered onto the head and attached to the chair back prevented head movement. . . . Rush reasoned that the rapid rotation helped to flow blood toward the head, thereby restoring the blood vessels to normalcy. Both instruments evoke images of Inquisition Chambers" (Bell, 1980, p. 7). In retrospect we can conclude that Rush introduced a medical model in the field of psychiatry in place of a demonic model. However, the medical model did have remnants of a prescientific era in the history of psychiatry.

Tuke's influence on American psychiatry led to the founding of four private mental hospitals that were patterned after the religious-humanistic structure of William Tuke's Retreat at York, England. These were the Friend's Asylum at Frankfurt, Pennsylvania; Bloomingdale Asylum in New York City; the McLean Asylum in Massachusetts; and the Hartford Retreat in Connecticut. In all of these institutions with a moral-humanistic philosophy, the concept of occupational therapy was strengthened. In the Bloomingdale Asylum during the early 1900s, the first systematic occupational therapy program was developed by Louis Haas, one of the early leaders in the American Occupational Therapy Association.

Some of the most important factors that changed the course of psychiatry from 1900 to 1950 were psychoanalysis and the related schools of psychotherapy; the common sense eclectic approach of the psychiatrist Adolph Meyer; the rapid rise of mental hospital care, the application of biological treatments such as Electric Convulsive Therapy, Metrazol, and insulin shock, psychosurgery, and chemothera-

py; and the Mental Hygiene Movement. The practice of occupational therapy was affected by all of these factors. However, the biological approach to treatment relegated occupational therapy to a secondary or adjunctive role. In this approach the occupational therapist was used by the psychiatrist as a type of "weather vane" to record the patient's behavior and to describe the effects of the biological treatment.

Occupational Therapy in Mental Hospitals

With the rapid growth in the building of mental hospitals during the 1920s and 1930s, occupational therapy was increasingly prescribed. For example, in 1922 only 4.8 percent of the patients in New York's 13 state mental hospitals received occupational therapy; and 5 years later the percentage rose to 31.9 percent (Bell, 1980). Occupational therapy programs at that time were organized around "step systems," in which patients started on simple, repetitive activities and advanced to more complicated, creative tasks. Progress in behavior brought the patient along until it was felt that recovery had occurred and the patient could be discharged. However, the chances for discharge from a mental hospital during the first half of the 20th century were not very good (Strauss, Schatzman, Bucher, Ehrlich, & Sabshin, 1964). The rise in the number of hospital beds in psychiatric institutions and the occupancy rates continued until the later part of the 1950s when a combination of factors, mainly the community mental health movement and the increased use of tranquilizer drugs, reversed the trend of long-term custodial care (Weinberg, 1967).

During this period, which can be designated "the custodial-repressive era" in American psychiatry, occupational therapy was perceived as a humane intervention that kept patients active in producing arts and crafts and in physical tasks while they were institutionalized. In addition to arts and crafts, puppetry was used in occupational therapy programs. Phillips (1996), in a historical review of drama and puppetry, noted that drama was used for "insight–oriented therapy" (p. 229) in Sheppard and Enoch Pratt Hospitals. "Drama was recognized by some occupational therapists as a natural socializing agent as well as an occupation that supported a wide variety of interests" (p. 232). Phillips believed that drama would be a beneficial tool for an occupational therapist "to promote competence, enhance self-concept, and improve socialization" (p. 229).

Bell (1980), in the quote below, summarized the functions of occupational therapy in mental hospitals:

> Mental health authorities acclaimed the efficacy of occupational therapy. The *American Journal of Psychiatry* documented its beneficial results, asserting that it had "unquestionable" value. Dr. C. S. Miller of Jackson State Hospital in Louisiana referred to it as "one of the greatest helps we have in handling mental cases." Dr. Henry Frost of Boston State Hospital in Massachusetts, claimed that it helped some of his more difficult patients return to normal life. Horatio Pollock of the New York State Department of Mental Hygiene stated that occupational therapy was the "best available method of treating the vast majority of chronic mental patients" and, if introduced on a large scale, it would transform any hospital into an active therapeutic center.
>
> Pollock and other advocates of occupational therapy believed that it struck at the root of all evil in mental institutions, the problem of enforced idleness. Patients condemned to a monotonous existence devoid of activities or diversions exhibited bad temper and developed untidy and destructive habits. Occupational therapy countered this torporous condition by giving the patients' energy outlets ranging from such simple endeavors as sorting colors

or sandpapering parts of wooden toys to projects of stimulating technical exactitude. Calisthenics and games complemented work therapy. Varied physical education and recreation included tug-of-war, horse-shoe pitching, shuffleboard, handball, tennis, basketball, soccer, and baseball. Some persons, especially severe cases of paranoia or schizophrenia, could not be reached through an activities program. Nevertheless, those chronic inmates who engaged in work and recreation seemed to deteriorate less rapidly, and the acutely disordered had a faster convalescence. Occupational therapy simply enabled many patients to forget their troubles, lose their delusions and hallucinations, and concentrate on a concrete task.

> Hospital administrators recognized the economic value of occupational therapy, a potent factor accounting for their enthusiastic and wide acceptance of it. Employed patients had little time for mischief, and in economic terms this translated into fewer broken chairs, tables, lamps and windows. A ward of patients on a regimen of definite duties also reduced the cost of supervision. The smaller staff maintained discipline and worked in an atmosphere free from the need for constant vigilance over restless patients lost in aimless activities. Occupational therapy contributed to the economical administration of a hospital by justifying the employment of patients in every area of institutional life. This source of cheap labor was eagerly exploited by economy-minded administrators who directed patients to the tasks necessary for maintaining the hospital.

> At many institutions patients, under the guise of occupational therapy classes, did the general plumbing, carpentry, and electrical repair work. They replaced downspouts, plastered walls, painted rooms, reupholstered chairs and couches, and fixed the damaged tables and broken lamps. They performed other basic services. A typical example occurred at Colorado Psychopathic Hospital, where patients did laundry, baking and sewing. Kalamazoo State Hospital in Michigan operated on a policy of reclamation, allowing nothing

to be thrown out that could be used again; patients cut old clothes into rags that were woven into rugs. This was a general practice at other institutions, here inmates made the hospital's furniture, clothing and linens. At Watertown State Hospital in Illinois, patients made window shades, screens, bedsprings, baskets, chairs, tables, brooms, brushes, coat hangers, pillows, pillow-cases, sheets, quilts, bath towels, table napkins, curtains, dresses, overalls, trousers, suits, scarves and mittens. (pp. 120–121)

Adolph Meyer

One of the most influential psychiatrists at the turn of the century to advocate the use of occupational therapy in the treatment of the "insane" was Adolph Meyer (1866–1950). In 1933, William Alanson White (Lief, 1948), the noted American psychiatrist, wrote in his memoirs:

In many respects, Dr. Meyer has been the outstanding influence in the development of psychiatry in this country, for about forty years and practically no major enterprise has been projected in the field of psychiatry which he has not influenced in some way. (p. viii)

Adolph Meyer made an important contribution to the field of psychiatry in general and to occupational therapy in particular. Meyer (1895/1948) wrote a report to the governor of Illinois: "Occupation is, with good right, called the most essential side of hygienic treatment of most insane patients, and the last thirty years have brought great and practical investigation in this field" (p. 59).

Meyer (1895/1948) also believed strongly in an individual approach to the patient that did not rely on drugs. For example, he stated:

any method merits such praise if it does not do any harm, either directly or in making the attendants and physicians believe that a drug can do away with more time-taking care. There is always some danger that the patient may get

tonics instead of good desirable food, sedatives instead of administering a simple bath, etc. It is especially dangerous to keep standing formulas for sedative and hypnotic purposes, because the attendants or even the physicians may be tempted to use what is ready, without going into the trouble of individualizing. (p. 57)

Meyer believed that patients living in an asylum should have an environment that simulates the family. He felt that the attendants and personnel should share with the patients in the everyday life activities (Meyer, 1922/1977). This idea was later incorporated during the 1950s in the therapeutic community. He also believed in a natural, humanistic approach to the treatment of the patient with psychiatric illness. In his most quoted book *Psychobiology*, published posthumously in 1957, Meyer advocated a therapeutic approach in which the patient's individual assets are used in countering pathology. Meyer believed that the therapist should first obtain an in-depth history of the patient's past experiences and a basis for formulating treatment goals:

From the data thus obtained we build a definite plan for the therapeutic procedure and formulate the outlook for the case, sizing up the time and influences needed for readjustment of a state of balance. From this point on, pathology and therapy—study and service—become, even more than with the first contact, an unavoidable and continuous blend. (p. 161)

Meyer's approach to mental illness is consistent with a holistic materialistic philosophy. He believed the therapist should be concerned with the patient's total life, including sleep habits, nutrition, daily routine, and personal adjustment. "It is the therapist's goal to bring about in the patient a 'modus vivendi,' a way of seeking, creating and finding a line of behavior that will best help him adapt to himself and his environment" (Meyer, 1957, p. 169).

Meyer considered progress to be judged on the basis of examining the individual's ability to work, rest, play, socialize, and express himself or herself. He considered occupational therapy as a social laboratory to help the patient develop the adaptive skills that are necessary to overcome his or her illness. Meyer considered his approach to be based on common sense and not on sterile theory. He believed that the most important task of the mental health worker is to help the patient to help himself or herself. He advocated a mental health model that did not emphasize drugs, custodial care, incarceration, or psychosurgery. Meyer's theory, consistent with contemporary occupational therapy, placed great emphasis on individualizing treatment by utilizing the assets and positive strengths of the patient. Occupation in the broadest sense was an important component of Meyer's theory of psychobiology.

Clifford Beers and the Mental Hygiene Movement

The National Committee for Mental Hygiene was founded in 1909 by Clifford Beers who wrote the book, *A Mind That Found Itself* (1908). In this book Beers described his mental illness, which led to his being hospitalized in three mental institutions. His book is acknowledged in the history of psychiatry as an important impetus to the mental hygiene movement in the United States. This movement was a grass roots effort to bring to the American consciousness the pitiful conditions in mental hospitals and the need for progressive change in the care of those with mental illness. The mental hygiene movement also fostered preventable psychiatry and child-guidance clinics.

Beer's book was instantly popular throughout the world and went through numerous reprints during his lifetime. He gained worldwide recognition for his courage to publish his autobiography and for his efforts to establish a national and later international organization to promote mental health and to prevent mental illness.

In *A Mind That Found Itself*, Beers chronicles his emotional breakdown and eventual recovery. After graduation from Yale University in 1897, Beers worked as a clerk in an insurance firm in New York City. Beers had been worried about an older brother who had recently died of a brain tumor. The emotional stress precipitated a depression. He was unable to work and to care for his most basic needs. He became actively suicidal and delusional, which led to his initial hospitalization. During this time Beers experienced the abuse by untrained and poorly paid attendants who frequently used physical force and restraints. He found firsthand that mental hospitals were frequently controlled by uncaring administrators who made enormous profits at the expense of those who were mentally ill.

His road to recovery occurred when he developed interests in drawing and writing, activities that reinforced his ability to regain his self-esteem.

> I usually spent part of the night drawing . . . while I was at the height of my wave of self-centered confidence, that I decided that I was destined to become a writer of books—or at least one book; and now I thought I might as well be an artist, too, and illustrate my own works. (p. 115)

However, his interest in drawing and writing were actually discouraged by his physician and attendants, and he consequently regressed to the point where he was forcibly placed in a straight-jacket and held in seclusion in a padded cell. His sufferings intensified when he was placed in a violent ward that was cold, foul smelling, and without the minimal humane care given to an animal in captivity. He was beaten, half-starved, confined, insulted, and deprived of his human rights.

> Thus day after day, I was repressed in a manner which probably would have driven many a

sane man to violence . . . Deprived of my clothes, of sufficient food, or warmth, of all sane companionship and of my liberty I told those in authority that so long as they should continue to treat me as the vilest of criminals, I should do my best to complete the illusion. (pp. 178–179)

Beers was describing a typical experience of patients with psychiatric illness who fulfill the worst expectations (e.g., self-fulfilling prophesy) of the attendants and psychiatrists. The patient was behaving as prophesied by the "keepers."

Beers describes his improvement as coinciding with the betterment of conditions in the ward:

I was no longer subjected to physical abuse, . . . I was no longer cold and hungry. I was allowed a fair amount of outdoor exercise . . . But above all, I was again given an adequate supply of stationery and drawing materials, which became as tinder under the focused rays of my artistic eagerness . . . Art and literature again held sway. (p. 182)

Finally, after 2 1/2 years of hospitalization, Beers was discharged. He then decided to dedicate his life to improving the care of those with mental illness, a project that led to the publication of his book, which received encouragement from the current leaders in the field of psychiatry and psychology, such as Adolph Meyer, William James, Macfie Campbell, and William Welch. Clifford Beers was instrumental in bringing psychiatry under the scrutiny of community groups eager to bring about progressive reform. Psychiatric care was no longer the absolute domain of isolated mental hospital administrators who were not responsive to the mental health movement.

William Rush Dunton, Jr.

William Rush Dunton, Jr. (1868–1966) had a principal role in establishing occupational ther-

apy as a profession. He was the founder and editor of *Occupational Therapy and Rehabilitation* and the author of numerous articles and books on occupational therapy, including *Reconstruction Therapy* (1919) and *Prescribing Occupational Therapy* (1957a). Dunton, a psychiatrist, advocated the use of occupational therapy early in his career in 1895 while working in Sheppard and Enoch Pratt Asylum and later at Johns Hopkins Medical School.

Dunton (1957a) established the ethical principle of occupational therapy as a medical modality prescribed by the physician. The prescription to the psychiatric occupational therapist should include basic information regarding the patient's background, the medical reason for referring the patient, and such treatment objectives as "to diminish excitement" or "to increase attention." The specific activity used in treatment was selected by the occupational therapist.

Dunton believed that occupational therapy provided an excellent opportunity for the patient to develop a hobby that encouraged healthy interests. He gave examples of appropriate hobbies such as collecting objects, playing a musical instrument, collecting postage stamps (philately), reading inspirational books (bibliotherapy), and engaging in arts and crafts. Dunton (1957b) in *Occupational Therapy: Principles and Practice* stated that:

It has been said that the individual who has an indoor and outdoor hobby is doubly insured against mental breakdown when emotional upsets occur. They may serve as safety values and interest can be directed toward one or the other with a lessening of tension. (p. 34)

Dunton (1957b) also formulated principles guiding the selection of activities that have become an accepted part of the occupational therapy treatment philosophy:

1. That work should be carried out with cure as the main object.

2. The work must be interesting.

3. The patient should be carefully studied.

4. That one form of occupation should not be carried to the point of fatigue.

5. That it should have some useful end.

6. That it preferably should lead to an increase in the patient's knowledge.

7. That it should be carried on with others.

8. That all possible encouragement should be given the worker.

9. That work resulting in poor or useless product is better than idleness. (pp. 47–48)

Louis Haas

Louis Haas was one of the pioneers in the field of psychiatric occupational therapy who, as director of the Men's Therapeutic Occupations in Bloomingdale Hospital in White Plains, New York during the early 1900s, used crafts specifically to meet the individual needs of the patient.

Haas (1925) wrote the textbook, *Occupational Therapy for the Mentally and Nervously Ill*, which set forth his philosophy of treatment, as well as described in detail the major crafts that can be used effectively in occupational therapy. Haas used his considerable background in industrial arts in developing a model for practice in psychiatric occupational therapy. His philosophy of treatment was based on the belief that "occupation can create a real work world in which the man can live and engage in activities to the extent that he is conscious of the satisfaction of having done an interesting day's work, that occupation can help him gain control of himself" (Haas, 1925, p. 23).

Haas categorized patients into the following groups, which served as the basis for selecting appropriate therapeutic crafts:

1. "The individual who seems to live in a world apart from his surroundings and gives little evidence of being aware of anything that goes on about him" (p. 23). Haas felt that occupational therapy's main purpose with this individual was to bring him back to reality.

2. "Another type of individual is dissatisfied with everything and everyone including himself" (p. 23). Haas prescribed activities for this type of individual that provided continuity and did not allow him or her to constantly change when he or she was dissatisfied. According to Haas, the occupational therapist has to be firm with this type of patient.

Haas described other patient types as overactive, fearful, and confused. For these patients specific crafts were also prescribed.

As an occupational therapist, Haas (1925) reacted against diversionary crafts. He believed that activities should be purposeful and suited to the individual needs of the patient, as for example in the following quote:

It is, therefore, readily seen that occupation for mental and nervous patients must consist of much more than the mere doing of something diversional: *being busy is not necessarily therapeutic.* Experience has taught us that certain crafts meet a large percentage of occupational needs, while other crafts meet just certain needs. Certain modifications must be made to make them available for the treatment of some patients, and finally certain equipment must be gathered together and arranged within properly constructed shops to make the efficient presentation of the occupational treatment possible. All this presupposes that the worker has a sure foundation in the crafts and a full supply of ingenuity, and a deep insight into the patient's needs, acquired by experience and nourished by sympathetic supervision, and cooperation of the physicians. (p. 25)

The environment of the occupational therapy department was an important component for a successful program according to Haas. The environment should stimulate "a normal atmosphere in which the man may spend a certain part of his time" (p. 51). Haas felt that, ideally, the occupational therapy department in a psychiatric hospital should be located in a detached building specifically designed for activity programs. Haas recommended that the occupational therapy building should be U-shaped with a central court used for an exhibition area displaying examples of patients' completed projects. The rooms in the occupational therapy department building were separated into the major crafts employed. These included 12 major therapeutic crafts. The list of crafts in Table 2–3 are ranked, according to Haas, in consideration of the relative importance of the craft as a therapeutic modality for men.

Haas placed considerable emphasis on the physical plant of an occupational therapy department. Equipment such as workbenches, tables, stands, looms, tool racks, and cupboards for the tools should be carefully selected by the occupational therapist in designing a treatment program.

He also set forth what the progress note in occupational therapy should contain. He recommended that each week the occupational therapist should note the actual pieces of work completed, the patient's attitudes toward work, and the results obtained. The craft product was used as a measure of the patient's progress, although Haas recognized that the craft activity was only a means to help the patient improve. Haas presented the following motto as a summary of what the craft should mean in occupational therapy: "The very best that is possible is but good enough" (p. 132). Haas (1925) elaborated on this by stating:

> It does mean that the instructor and the director of occupational therapy, with the patient's welfare ever in mind, will continually examine the crafts used, the methods of presentation, and the processes of construction employed; the materials used; and finally that the designs and even the sources of inspiration for these designs should be studied in effort to make possible the best results. (p. 132)

Haas played an important part in the development of psychosocial occupational therapy. His philosophy and practical recommendations were used as models for occupational therapy departments throughout the 1920s, 1930s, and even into the 1950s.

During the 1930s the emphasis of occupational therapists working with those with mental illness was placed on the quality of the craft completed in the mental hospital. For example, in a brief report by Scullin (1930), a description of an annual visitation for occupational therapists included display of articles produced by patients. The articles included wall hangings of stitchery, appliqué, block printing, weaving,

Table 2–3. Relative Importance of Crafts as Therapeutic Modality

Craft	Relative Importance
Basketry	1
Brushes and Chair Caning	2
Carpentry	3
Art Metal	4
Printing	5
Jewelry	6 (tied)
Concrete Work	6 (tied)
Blacksmithing	8 (tied)
Bookbinding	8 (tied)
Weaving	10 (tied)
Tennis Racket Restringing	10 (tied)

Source: Adapted from *Practical Occupational Therapy* by L. Haas, 1944, Milwaukee, WI: Bruce.

hooked rugs, chair seats, copper bookends, linoleum block prints, and other artwork. The author includes a comment regarding the value of the articles:

> The articles were thoughtfully planned and well executed. They represented the keen interest of the individual patient in doing the work and proved to what degree of pleasure and perfection the aide can guide a patient who has been aroused and interested by a special project. One could indeed visualize in studying these articles the pride and pleasure of the ones who executed them. When a piece of work has been well done and admired by all, often a new trend of thought is established and confidence and concentration restored. (Scullin, 1930, p. 240)

DEVELOPMENT OF DYNAMIC TREATMENT (1950–1960)

Barton (1957), a superintendent at Boston State Hospital in Massachusetts, was one of the first psychiatrists to identify the use of occupational therapy as a dynamic factor in treating the psychiatric patient. During the years from 1940 to 1950 occupational therapy in psychiatry was considered to be an adjutant modality, secondary to the physician who was the prime treatment agent using psychotherapy, electroconvulsive treatment, insulin shock, Metrazol, or barbiturates. Occupational therapy was used mainly as a diversional or relaxing activity that the physician or nurse prescribed in managing the patient's behavior. Barton, within a psychoanalytic framework, perceived occupational therapy as a primary, dynamic modality. For example, he proposed the following:

> The work at hand may provide sublimation for symptoms of disease. Hostile feelings and aggressive impulses can be dissolved, and so can feelings of guilt, in the stream of activity. It is possible to work out one's needs for creative-

ness and in one's productive activities there is room for expression of fantasy. The principal goals of therapy, then, are to provide motivation along the pathway to recovery, to relieve personal anxiety, and to substitute creative activities for destructive fantasy. When a patient is acutely ill, he needs the help of the persons best trained and equipped to evaluate his potentialities and to apply the known dynamic principles to work or recreational activities. The point of departure may well be the occupational therapy class on the ward. Here the psychiatric nurse, under the stimulation and guidance of the occupational therapist, helps the patient take the first faltering steps toward the world outside his troubled self. After progress has been made in the simple activities suitable for use on the ward, he may next graduate to the group in the occupational therapy clinic. As the patient continues improving, it soon becomes possible to assign him to useful work around the hospital. Eventually, when he has demonstrated his capacity to carry responsibility and a full day's work, it is but a step to a job in the community. Patients under treatment with an acute mental illness do not always require intensive group work of personal, individualized attention by a therapist. There are those who can be assigned at once to hospital industry. (Barton, 1957, p. 180)

Barton also differentiated the application of occupational therapy with various psychiatric diagnostic groups. Table 2–4 summarizes Barton's recommendations.

Dynamic treatment is based on psychoanalytic theory and it emphasizes the relationship between the patient and the therapist, that is, transference. With the introduction of dynamic treatment, the focus changed from mainly maintenance care to an active involvement with the patient, and a new optimism was generated that mental illness can be reversible (Linn, Weinroth, & Shamah, 1962). The occupational therapist became part of a psychiatric treatment

Table 2–4. Occupational Therapy Activity Related to Psychiatric Diagnosis

Diagnostic Group	Principal Symptoms	Examples of O.T. Activities
Psychoneurosis	Anxiety	Carpentry
• phobic	• fear	
• conversion-hysteria	• physical disturbance	
• obsessive-compulsive	• repetitious behavior	
Psychotic disorders	Loss of contact with reality	Clerical
• manic-depressive	• emotional lability	• practical everyday tasks
• schizophrenia	• isolate-break with reality	• group activities
• paranoia	• delusionary processes	• individual responsibility
Senility	Chronic brain impairment	Motivation in everyday events
Mental deficiency	Intellectual deficits	Activity mastery
Epilepsy	Seizures	Positions of responsibility

Source: Adapted from "Occupational Therapy for Psychiatric Disorders" by W. Barton, 1957. In *Occupational Therapy Principles and Practice* (pp. 177–196) by W. R. Dunton & S. Licht, Eds., 2nd ed., Springfield, IL: Charles C. Thomas.

team of specialists, who increasingly emphasized the psychotherapeutic relationship. Meyer's theory of psychobiology was eclipsed by Freudian psychoanalysis (Serrett, 1985). Activity became a means to help the patient work through psychological conflicts. This is illustrated in the following quote by Semrad and Day (1959): "The general objective in the augmentation of psychotherapy or any therapeutic effort . . . is to afford the patient a therapeutic experience by providing opportunities for the expression of sublimation of emotional needs and drives" (p. 1). This model, typical of American psychiatry in the late 1950s, emphasized the symbolic nature of activities in meeting psychotherapeutic goals.

Semrad and Day defined three specific roles of activity programs (numbers added by authors):

1. Activity and therapy activities serve as anxiety–relieving mechanisms.

2. An activity serves on a trial and error basis as a procedure for developing ego skills which contribute to the individual's total capacity to negotiate interpersonal relationships with due regard to himself and to those he cathexes [Expresses feelings].

3. Each therapeutic worker must appreciate himself as a tool, as an available object whom the patient can recathexis as he progresses from his narcissistic state back to using his old capacity. Furthermore, the patient can increasingly add to his skills by his relationship with this therapeutic person. (p. 6)

Semrad and Day used the terminology of psychoanalysis such as catharsis, sublimation, ego, and cathexis. The last term, *cathexis*, a term Freud (1938) introduced, expresses the idea of psychical energy that is directed at people or objects. To the psychoanalytic occupational therapist, activity provided the opportunity for the individual to enhance personality growth (O'Kane, 1968). Although activity was perceived as a principal method to achieve therapeutic change in patients, psychoanalysts emphasized the importance of the occupational therapist as a treatment agent in the interactive encounter with the patient. The use of self was introduced as an important component in the occupational therapy process (West, 1959).

Use of Self as Treatment Agent

The use of "self as a therapeutic tool" is a term that was first introduced by the psychiatrist Jerome Frank (1958). In an article in the *American Journal of Occupational Therapy*, "The Therapeutic Use of Self," Frank placed the psychiatric occupational therapist into the role of psychotherapist, as exemplified in the following quotes:

> All forms of psychotherapy, including the psychotherapeutic aspect of occupational therapy, try to reinforce the health aspects of the patient's self and help him to modify its flaws. They do this by trying to engage him in new and different interpersonal transactions which will confirm his health expectancies and disappoint his pathological ones. The main therapeutic tool for this purpose is the self of the therapist. . . .
>
> Occupational therapists, like psychiatrists, are practitioners of a healing art who perceive themselves as help givers; that is persons able to relieve suffering and to improve the effectiveness of others. . . .
>
> The therapeutic role of the occupational therapist is confined to trying to bring about modifications in the acting self of the patient . . . . He tries to help the patient modify his expectancies in a limited area of his functioning—the task he is doing—in the hope that the self–confidence thus gained will generalize to other areas of the patient's life. . . .
>
> To use himself effectively the therapist must also have a clear realization of his own abilities and limitations. (pp. 222–223)

The advocacy by Frank of the occupational therapist's dynamic role in the treatment of those with mental illness was part of the evolu-

tionary process in the history of psychiatry. This movement toward the humane care of those individuals, which began in the 18th century, was linked to an activity framework. Reformers understood the need for activities in mental hospitals as a means to promote mental and physical health. The dynamic approach in psychiatry, influenced by psychoanalytic theory, emphasized the patient-therapist relationship as a key component in treatment. The humanistic use of activities with patients with mental illness became combined with psychotherapy to form the current philosophy underlying the practice of psychosocial occupational therapy. The treatment environment, activity selected, the therapeutic relationship, and the motivation of the patient to improve are the key components in the effectiveness of occupational therapy (Stein, 1969).

EMERGENCE OF THE CERTIFIED OCCUPATIONAL THERAPY ASSISTANT (COTA)[1]

As a result of the rapid growth of the occupational therapy profession during the 1950s and 1960s, the profession began to explore the development of an assistant-level person trained through a specific educational course of study. This person was meant to assist the occupational therapist and provide for the lack of manpower in the field (AOTA, 1958).

Standards were initially developed for the training and recognition of the assistant-level person in the field of psychiatry and were adopted by the American Occupational Therapy Association in October 1958. Initially, the assistant was to be trained in a 3-month hospital-

---

[1] The material contained in this section was originally written by Susanne Floyd who was the former director of Occupational Therapy at Concordia Lutheran College in Mequon, WI.

based program only for a specialty area. These training programs were developed in state and county psychiatric institutions for current occupational therapy aides who were paid their salaries while attending the course work. A majority of these graduates returned to their base hospitals for practical application. The curriculum was divided into hour units on topics such as personality development, the use of activity, and the development and application of recreational and craft skills.

In 1960, standards for training occupational therapy assistants for general practice were approved and implemented (Crampton, 1967). Some of these programs were developed specifically for preparing occupational therapy assistants to work with geriatric patients who had chronic disabilities. It was planned that the Certified Occupational Therapy Assistant would be utilized as an activity director to help develop effective activity programs in nursing homes and other long-term care facilities under the supervision and evaluation of occupational therapy consultants. The length of these educational programs was between 12 and 18 weeks. AOTA has continually revised the guidelines for training and supervision of the COTA. This information is contained in *Essentials*, published by the American Occupational Therapy Association (AOTA, 1995).

One such typical program was sponsored by the Wisconsin State Board of Health and was supported by federal funds (Wisconsin State Board of Health, 1968). This course ran for 4 months with the academic part being given during the first 3 months and a full-time practical experience during the fourth month. Such topics as personality development (43 hours), physical development (57 hours), use of activity with geriatric patients (50 hours), arts and crafts skills (171 hours), organization skills (25 hours) were covered.

During the middle to late 1960s, AOTA Committee on Occupational Therapy Assistants began to explore a combination of community college-based learning coupled with a fieldwork or practice component. Initially, some programs were developed to be 6 months in length, gradually developing to 1-year certificate programs.

As the scope of the occupational therapy profession grew, the demand for increased skill of the assistant also grew. The majority of occupational therapy assistant programs in the year 2000 are currently in junior, community, or technical colleges, and are generalist programs not aimed at one area of the profession. Of the 178 assistant programs now available, almost all of the programs offer 2-year associate degrees.

A resolution was adopted by the American Occupational Therapy Association Representative Assembly in 1981 that required "all educational programs for training as the Certified Occupational Therapy Assistant be required to offer an associate degree (by 1985) (AOTA, 1981).

The broader-based background provided by the academic institution has helped to develop the much needed oral and written language, communication, and basic science skills required to maintain medical records and to converse, learn, and work with other health care paraprofessionals and professionals. This unified educational level approach for the assistants allowed a clear delineation of their role and enabled COTAs to be more competitive in the job market.

The specific roles of the COTA in psychosocial practice are discussed in Chapter 5. Additional information about the role delineation of the COTA is in Appendix C.

SUMMARY

Bing (1981), in an historical review of the legacy of occupational therapy, identifies two individuals, Thomas Kidner (1866–1932) and Eleanor Clark Slagle (1876–1942), who summarize the early philosophy that has framed the practice of occupational therapy:

> May we, therefore, look at occupational therapy—with increased faith as the years go by—as a natural means of aiding in the restoration of the sick and disabled to health and working capacity (which means happiness) because it appeals to all our human attributes. (Kidner, 1931, p. 11)

> The story of the profession of occupational therapy will never be fully told, nor will that of the patients who have so abundantly appreciated the opportunities of the service. There has been no fanciful crusading "for the cause"; it has meant that a few have perhaps borne many burdens, but in the slow process that make permanent things of great value, it can be said that there is a fine body of professional workers, experienced and well trained, coming forward and being welcomed to a really great human service, that of helping to show the way to the person with large disabilities to make the best of his incomplete self. (Slagle, 1938, p. 382)

The history of psychosocial occupational therapy can be seen as a mosaic with various historical pieces having important influences. The naturalistic philosophy of the Greeks first proposed in the Hippocratic writings in the 6th century B.C. and developed through the experiences of agrarian societies throughout the world has found a renewed interest in Western countries. The naturalistic philosophy has been incorporated in the current worldwide holistic health movement (Collinge, 1996; Edlin & Golanty, 1992; Hastings, Fadiman, & Gordon, 1981; Long, 1990; Mattson, 1982; Pelletier, 1979; Peters & Woodham, 2000) that emphasizes nutrition, exercise, reduction of stress, self-actu-alization, spirituality, and a rhythmic continuity of life. This tradition has been an important thread in the history of occupational therapy. The next important influence was the moral-humanitarianism of the 19th century. This movement was a reaction to the inhumane care of those with mental illness during the Middle Ages and later periods that linked mental illness to demonic possession and witchcraft. Occupational therapy as a mental health profession emerged after the turn of the 20th century at a time when psychotherapy was initiated, and the mental hygiene movement was founded.

In the next chapter we discuss the occupational therapist's role in community mental health. This change in role from working primarily in an institutionalized setting to community settings is still in the process of transformation in the 21st century.

BIBLIOGRAPHY FOR ADDITIONAL READING

Altschule, M. (1965). *Roots of modern psychiatry: Essays in the history of psychiatry* (2nd ed.). New York: Grune and Stratton.

Bromberg, W. (1954). *The mind of man: A history of psychotherapy and psychoanalysis.* Philadelphia: Lippincott.

Deutsch, A. (1949). *The mentally ill in America: A history of their care and treatment from colonial times* (2nd ed.). New York: Oxford University Press.

Galdston, I. (Ed.). (1976). *Historic derivations of modern psychiatry.* New York: McGraw-Hill.

Kraepelin, E. (1962). *One hundred years of psychiatry* (W. Baskin, Trans.). New York: Philosophical Library.

Roback, A. (1961). *History of psychology and psychiatry.* New York: Philosophical Library.

Shorter, E. (1998). *A history of psychiatry: From the era of the asylum to the age of prozac.* New York: J. Wiley.

Szasz, T. (Ed.). (1973). *The age of madness.* Garden City, NJ: Anchor.

REFERENCES

Ackerknecht, E. (1968). *A short history of psychiatry.* New York: Hafner.

Ader, R., Felten, D. L., & Cohen, N. (1991). *Psychoneuroimmunology* (2nd ed.). San Diego: Academic.

Albee, G. (1982). Preventing psychopathology and promoting human potential. *American Psychologist, 37,* 1043–1050.

Alexander, F. G., & Selesnick, S. T. (1966). *The history of psychiatry: An evaluation of psychiatric thought and practice from prehistoric times to the practice.* New York: Harper and Row.

Alvin, J. (1978). *Music therapy for the autistic child.* London: Oxford University.

American Occupational Therapy Association. (1958). Project committee on recognition of occupational therapy assistants, final report. *American Journal of Occupational Therapy, 13,* 269.

American Occupational Therapy Association. (1981). Guide for supervision of occupational therapy personnel, official position paper, adopted March 1981 by the Representative Assembly of AOTA. *American Journal of Occupation Therapy, 35,* 815–816.

American Occupational Therapy Association. (1995). *COTA information packet (a guide for supervision).* Rockville, MD: Author.

Annas, G. J., & Grodin, M. A. (1992). *The Nazi doctors and the Nuremberg Code: Human rights in human experimentation.* New York: Oxford.

Anthony, W. A., Cohen, M. R., & Cohen, B. (1984). Psychiatric rehabilitation. In J. Talbott (Ed.), *The chronic mental patient: Five years later* (pp. 213–252). New York: Grune & Stratton.

Anthony, W., Cohen, M., & Farkas, M. (1982). A psychiatric rehabilitation treatment program: Can I recognize one if I see one? *Community Mental Health Journal,18*(2), 83–96.

Bachrach, L. L. (1976). *Deinstitutionalization: An analytic review and sociological perspective* (DHEW Publication No. [AMD] 76–351). Washington, DC: Government Printing Office.

Barton, W. E. (1957). Occupational therapy for psychiatric disorders. In W. Dunton & S. Licht (Eds.), *Occupational therapy principles and practice* (2nd ed., pp. 177–196). Springfield, IL: Charles C. Thomas.

Basham, A. L. (1976). The practice of medicine in ancient and medieval India. In C. Leslie (Ed.), *Asian medical systems: A comparative study* (pp. 18–43). Berkeley: University of California.

Beers, C. A. (1908). *A mind that found itself.* New York: Doubleday.

Bell, L. (1980). *Treating the mentally ill: From colonial times to the present.* New York: Praeger.

Benet, S. (1976). *How to live to be 100: The life style of the people of the Caucasus.* New York: Dial.

Bernard, A. (1992). The use of music as a purposeful activity: A preliminary investigation. *Physical and Occupational Therapy in Geriatrics, 10*(3), 35–45.

Bing, R. (1981). Occupational therapy revisited: A paraphrasic journey. *American Journal of Occupational Therapy, 35,* 499–518.

Bogg, J., & Cooper, C. (1995). Job satisfaction, mental health, and occupational stress among senior civil servants. *Human Relations, 48,* 327–341.

Brisset, C. (1980, September 4). Psychiatric hospitals excellence and squalor. *Le Monde* (Paris), p. 12.

Brown, B. (1974). *Stress and the art of biofeedback.* New York: Harper and Row.

Carling, P. J. (1995). *Return to community: Building support systems for people with psychiatric disabilities.* New York: Guilford.

Casby, J. A., & Holm, M. B. (1994). The effect of music on repetitive disruptive vocalization of persons with dementia. *American Journal of Occupational Therapy, 48,* 883–889.

Chapman, D. P., & Giles, W. H. (1997). Pharmacologic and dietary therapies in epilepsy: Conventional treatments and recent advances. *Southern Medical Journal, 90,* 471–480.

Christianson, J. B., & Osher, F. C. (1994). Health maintenance organizations, health care reform, and persons with serious mental illness. *Hospital and Community Psychiatry, 45,* 898–905.

Cofrancesco, E. M. (1985). The effect of music therapy on hand grips strength and functional task performance in stroke patients. *Journal of Music Therapy, 22*(3), 129–145.

Cohen, C. I., & Thompson, K. S. (1992). Homeless mentally ill or mentally ill homeless? *American Journal of Psychiatry, 6,* 816–822.

Coker, C. C., Osgood, K., & Clouse, K. R. (1995). *A comparison of job satisfaction and economic benefits of four different employment models for persons with disabilities.* Menomonie, WI: Rehabilitation Research and Training Center on Improving Community-Based Rehabilitation Programs, University of Wisconsin–Stout.

Collinge, W. (1996). *The American Holistic Health Association complete guide to alternative medicine.* New York: Warner.

Colman, P. (1992). *Breaking the chains: The crusade of Dorothea Lynde Dix.* White Hall, VA: Shoe Tree.

Crampton, M. W. (1967). Educational upheaval for occupational therapy assistants. *American Journal of Occupational Therapy, 21,* 317–318.

Darrow, A. A., Gibbons, A. C., & Heller, G. N. (1985, September-October). Music therapy past, present, and future. *The American Music Teacher, 35*(1), 18–20.

Delay, J., Deniker, P., & Harl, J. M. (1952). Utilization en thérapeutique psychiatrique d'une phenothiazine d'action centrale élective [Use of phenothiazine in psychiatry]. *Annales medico psychologiques* (Paris), *110,* 112.

Dunton, W. R. (1919). *Reconstruction therapy.* Philadelphia: W. B. Saunders.

Dunton, W. R. (1957a). *Prescribing occupational therapy.* Springfield, IL: Charles C. Thomas.

Dunton, W. R. (1957b). The prescription. In W. R. Dunton & S. Licht (Eds.), *Occupational therapy: Principles and practice* (pp. 29–52). Springfield, IL: Charles C. Thomas.

Eckstein, R.W. (1957). Effects of exercise and coronary artery narrowing on coronary collateral circulation. *Circulation Research, 5,* 230.

Edlin, G., & Golanty, E. (1992). *Health and wellness: A holistic approach* (4th ed.). Boston: Jones and Bartlett.

Ekert, H. M., & Montoye, H. J. (Eds.). (1984). *Exercises and health.* Champaign, IL: Human Kinetics.

Esquirol, J. (1948). *Mental maladies* (E. K. Hunt, Trans.). Reprinted in S. Licht (Ed.), *Occupational therapy source book* (pp. 57–59). Philadelphia: Williams and Wilkins. (Original work published 1838)

Feingold, B. (1974). *Why your child is hyperactive.* New York: Random House.

Federal Task Force on Homelessness and Severe Mental Illness. (1992). *Outcasts on Main Street: Report of the Federal Task Force on Homelessness and Severe Mental Illness.* (DHHS Publication No. ADM 92–1904). Washington, DC: U.S. Department of Health and Human Services.

Folkins, C., & Sime, W. (1981). Physical fitness and mental health. *American Psychologist, 36,* 373–389.

Foucault, M. (1965). *Madness and civilization: A history of insanity in the age of reason* (R. Howard, Trans.). New York: Random House.

Frank, J. (1958). The therapeutic use of self. *American Journal of Occupational Therapy, 12,* 215–225.

Freeman, W., & Watts, J. (1942). *Psychosurgery.* London: Baillere, Tindall and Cox.

Freud, S. (1938). *The basic writings of Sigmund Freud* (A. A. Brill, Trans.). New York: Modern Library.

Girard, J. (1954). Music therapy in the anxiety states. In E. Podolsky (Ed.), *Music therapy* (pp. 101–106). New York: Philosophical Library.

Goffman, E. (1961). *Asylums: Essays on the social situation of mental patients and other inmates.* New York: Doubleday/Anchor.

Greist, J. H., Klein, M. H., Eischens, R. R., Fairs, J., Gurman, A. S., & Morgan, W. P. (1979). Running as treatment for depression. *Comprehensive Psychiatry, 20*(1), 41–54.

Haas, L. (1925). *Occupational therapy for the mentally and nervously ill.* Milwaukee, WI: Bruce.

Haas, L. (1944). *Practical occupational therapy.* Milwaukee, WI: Bruce.

Hartmann, E. (1973). *The functions of sleep.* New Haven, CT: Yale University.

Hastings, A. C., Fadi man, J., & Gordon, J. S. (Eds.). (1981). *Health for the whole person: The complete guide to holistic medicine.* Toronto: Bantam.

Heidel, W. (1941). *Hippocratic medicine.* New York: Columbia University.

Hinsie, L., & Campbell, R. (1960). *Psychiatric dictionary* (3rd ed.). New York: Oxford.

Hoffer, A. (1973). Orthomolecular treatment of schizophrenia. *Canadian Journal of Psychiatric Nursing, 14*, 11–14.

Holland, J. (1973). *Making vocational choices: A theory of careers.* Englewood Cliffs, NJ: Prentice-Hall.

Holt, R. R. (1993). Occupational stress. In L. Goldberger & S. Breznitz (Eds.), *Handbook of stress: Theoretical and clinical aspects* (2nd ed., pp. 342–367). New York: Free Press.

Howells, J. G. (Ed.). (1975). *World history of psychiatry.* New York: Brunner/Mazel.

International Society of Sports Psychology. (1992). Physical activity and psychological benefits: A position statement from the International Society of Sports Psychology. *Journal of Applied Sport Psychology, 4*(1), 94–99.

Irwin, M., McClintick, J., Costlow, C., Fortner, M., White, J., & Gillin, J. C. (1996). Partial night sleep deprivation reduces natural killer and cellular immune responses in humans. *FASEB Journal, 10*, 643–653.

Jacobson, E. (1958). *Progressive relaxation.* Chicago: University of Chicago.

Jones, M. (1953). *The therapeutic community.* New York: Basic Books.

Kalinowsky, L. B. (1959). Convulsive shock treatment. In S. Arieti (Ed.), *American handbook of psychiatry* (Vol. 2, pp. 1499–1520). New York: Basic Books.

Katz, S. E. (1985). Psychiatric hospitalization. In H. I. Kaplan & B. J. Sadock (Eds.), *Comprehensive textbook of psychiatry* (4th ed., pp. 1576–1591). Baltimore: Williams and Williams.

Kavanagh, T., Shepard, R. J., Tuck, J. A., & Quereshi, S. (1977). Depression following myocardial infarction: The effect of distance running. *Annals of the New York Academy of Sciences, 301*, 1029–1038.

Kidner, T. (1931). Occupational therapy, its development, scope and possibilities. *Occupational Therapy and Rehabilitation, 10*, 11.

Kirkbride, T. S. (1948). *On the construction, organization and general arrangements of hospitals for the insane.* Philadelphia: Lindsay & Blakiston. Excerpts reprinted in S. Licht (Ed.), *Occupational therapy sourcebook* (pp. 77–79). Philadelphia: Williams and Wilkins. (Original work published 1854)

Kleijnen, J., & Knipschild, P. (1991). Niacin and vitamin B_6 in mental functioning: A review of controlled trials in humans. *Biological Psychiatry, 29*, 931–941.

Koger, S. M. & Brontons, M. (1999). Music therapy for dementia symptoms. [CD-ROM]. *The Cochran Library (Oxford), 4.*

Krummel, D. A., Seligson, F. H., & Guthrie, H. A. (1996). Hyperactivity: Is candy causal? *Critical Review of Food, Science, and Nutrition, 36*, 35–47.

Lai, Y. (1999). Effects of music listening on depressed women in Taiwan. *Issues in Mental Health Nursing, 20*, 229–246.

Laing, R. D. (1965). *The divided self: An existential study in sanity and madness.* Middlesex: Penguin Books.

Lambo, T. A. (1975). Mid and West Africa. In J. G. Howells (Ed.), *World history of psychiatry* (pp. 579–599). New York: Brunner/Mazel.

Lankford, T. R. (1994). *Foundations of normal and therapeutic nutrition.* Albany, NY: Delmar.

Lehrer, P. M., & Woolfolk, R. L. (1993). *Principles and practice of stress management* (2nd ed.). New York: Guilford.

Leon, C., & Rosselli, H. (1975). Latin America. In J. G. Howells (Ed.), *World history of psychiatry* (pp. 476–506). New York: Brunner/Mazel.

Leuret, F. (1948). *Du traitement moral de la folie* [On the moral treatment of insanity]. Paris: J. B. Bailliere. In S. Licht (Ed.), *Occupational therapy source book* (p. 63). Philadelphia: Williams and Wilkins. (Original work published 1840)

Levy, F. J. (1988). *Dance/movement therapy: A healing art.* Reston, VA: American Alliance for Health, Physical Education, Recreation, and Dance.

Liberman, R. P. (Ed.). (1992). *Handbook of psychiatric rehabilitation.* Boston: Allyn & Bacon.

Licht, S. (Ed.). (1948). *Occupational therapy sourcebook.* Philadelphia: Williams and Wilkins.

Lief, A. (Ed.). (1948). *The commonsense psychiatry of Dr. Adolf Meyer: Fifty-two selected papers.* New York: McGraw-Hill.

Linn, L., Weinroth, L. A., & Shamah, R. (1962). *Occupational therapy in dynamic psychiatry: An introduction to the four-phase concept in hospital psychiatry.* Washington, DC: American Psychiatric Association.

Lipton, M. A., Ban, T. A., Kane, F. J., Levine, J., Mosher, L. R., & Wittenborn, R. (1973). *Megavitamin and orthomolecular therapy in psychiatry.* Washington, DC: American Psychiatric Association.

Long, S. (1990). *Holistic health and biomedical medicine: A countersystem analysis.* Albany: State University of New York.

Lowen, A. (1976). *Bioenergetics.* London: Coventure.

Luthe, W., & Schultz, J. (1969). *Auogenic therapy: Vol II. Medical applications.* New York: Grune and Stratton.

Mahan, L. K., & Escott-Stump, S. (1996). Vitamins. In L. K. Mahan & S. Escott-Stump (Eds.), *Krause's food, nutrition, & diet therapy* (9th ed., pp. 77–122). Philadelphia: W. B. Saunders.

Malitz, S., & Hoch, P. H. (1966). Drug therapy: Neuroleptics and tranquilizers. In S. Arieti (Ed.), *American handbook of psychiatry* (Vol. 3, pp. 458–476). New York: Basic Books.

Martinsen, E. W. (1993). Therapeutic implications of exercise of clinically anxious and depressed patients. *International Journal of Sports Psychology, 24*(2), 185–199.

Mattson, P. (1982). *Holistic health in perspective.* Palo Alto, CA: Mayfield.

McArdle, W. D., Katch, F. I., & Katch, V. L. (1994). *Exercise physiology: Energy, nutrition and human performance* (4rd ed.). Baltimore: Williams & Wilkins.

McKinney, C. H., Tims, R. C., Kumar, A. M., & Kumar, M. (1997). The effect of selected classical music and spontaneous imagery on plasma b-endorphin. *Journal of Behavioral Medicine, 20,* 85–99.

Meduna, L. J. (1936). *Die Konvulsionstherapie de Schizophrenie* [Convulsive therapy for schizophrenia]. Halle: Marhold.

Meerloo, J. A. M. (1960). *The dance: From ritual to rock and roll—ballet to ballroom.* Philadelphia: Chilton.

Meyer, A. (1948). Action in Kanakee. In A. Lief (Ed.), *The commonsense psychiatriatry of Dr. Adolf Meyer; Fifty-two selected papers edited, with biographical narrative* (pp. 43–76). New York: McGraw-Hill. (Original work published 1895)

Meyer, A. (1957). *Psychobiology* (E. Winters & A. Bowers, Comp. & Ed.). Springfield, IL: Charles C. Thomas.

Meyer, A. (1977). The philosophy of occupational therapy. *Archives of Occupational Therapy, 1,* 1–10. Reprinted in *American Journal of Occupational Therapy, 31,* 639–642. (Original work published 1922)

Michelet, J. (1939). *Satanism and witchcraft: A study in medieval superstition.* New York: The Citadel Press.

Miller, M. (1996). Diet and psychological health. *Alternative Therapies in Health Medicine, 2*(5), 40–48.

Moniz, E. (1936). *Tentatives opératoires dans le traitement de certaines psychoses* [Surgical techniques in the treatment of certain psychoses]. Paris: Masson.

Mora, G. (1985). History of psychiatry. In H. I. Kaplan & B. J. Sadock (Eds.), *Comprehensive textbook of psychiatry* (4th ed., pp. 2034–2054). Baltimore: Williams and Williams.

Morgan, W. P., & Goldstein, S. E. (Eds.). (1987). *Exercise and mental health.* New York: Hemisphere.

Morris, A., & Husman, B. (1970). Life quality changes following an endurance conditioning program. *American Corrective Therapy Journal, 32,* 3–6.

Morris, J., & Crawford, M. (1958). Coronary heart disease and physical activities of work: Evidence of a national necropsy study. *British Medical Journal, 2,* 1458.

Nagpal, M. & Ruta, A. M. (1997). Joy in schizophrenia: Through dance/movement therapy. *Journal of the California Alliance for the Mentally Ill, 8,* 53–55.

O'Kane, C. P. (1968). *The development of a projective technique for use in psychiatric occupational therapy.* Buffalo: State University of New York.

Orwin, A. (1974). Treatment of a situational phobia. *British Journal of Psychiatry, 125,* 95–98.

Osmond, H., & Hoffer, A. (1962). Massive niacin treatment in schizophrenia: Review of nine year study. *Lancet, 1*, 316.

Palo-Bengstsson, L, Winblad, B., & Ekman, S. (1998). Social dancing: A way to support intellectual, emotional and motor functions in persons with dementia. *Journal of Psychiatric & Mental Health Nursing, 5*, 545–554.

Pavlicevic, M. (1999). *Music therapy; Intimate notes.* London: Jessica Kingsley.

Pauling, L. (1968). Orthomolecular psychiatry. *Science, 160*, 265–271.

Pelletier, K. (1977). *Mind as healer, mind as slayer: A holistic approach to preventing stress disorders.* New York: Delta.

Pelletier, K. (1979). *Holistic medicine: From stress to optimum health.* New York: Delacorte.

Pendelton, H. M. (1996). The occupation of needlework. In R. Zemke & F. Clark (Eds.), *Occupational science: The evolving discipline* (pp. 287–296). Philadelphia: F. A. Davis.

Peters, D. & Woodham, A. (2000). *Complete guide to integrative medicine: Combining the best of natural and conventional care.* London: DK Publishing, Inc.

Phillips, M. E. (1996). The use of drama and puppetry in occupational therapy during the 1920s and 1930s. *American Journal of Occupational Therapy, 50*, 229–233.

Pierloot, R. (1975). Belgium. In J. G. Howells (Ed.), *World history of psychiatry* (pp. 136–149). New York: Brunner/Mazel.

Pinel, P. (1947). *Traite medico-philosophique sur l'alienation mentale, ou la manie* [Medical philosophical treaties on mental alienation]. Paris: Chez Richard, Caille et Ravier. Excerpts reprinted in *Occupational Therapy and Rehabilitation, 26*, 63–68. (Original work published 1801)

Podolsky, E. (Ed.). (1954). *Music therapy.* New York: Philosophical Library.

President's Council on Physical Fitness and Sports. (1996). *Physical activity and health: A report of the surgeon general.* Pittsburgh, PA: U.S. Department of Health and Human Services, Centers for Disease Control and Prevention, National Center for Chronic Disease Prevention and Health Promotion.

Regier, D. A., & Burke, J. D. (1985). Quantitative and experimental methods in psychiatry. In H. I. Kaplan & B. J. Sadock (Eds.), *Comprehensive textbook of psychiatry* (4th ed., pp. 295–311). Baltimore: Williams and Williams.

Reil, J. C. (1947). *Rapsodieen uber die Anwendung der psychichen Curmethode auf Geisteszerruttugen* [Rhapsodies on the psychic treatment of the insane]. Halle, Germany: In der Curtschen Buchhandlung. Excerpts reprinted in *Occupational Therapy and Rehabilitation, 26*, 342–345. (Original work published 1803)

Rogers, C. R., Gerdlin, E. T., Kiesler, D. J., & Trevax C. B. (1967). *The therapeutic relationship and its impact: A study of psychotherapy with schizophrenics.* Madison: University of Wisconsin Press.

Rolf, I. (1977). *Rolfing.* Santa Monica, CA: Dennis Landman.

Rush, B. (1947). *Medical inquiries and observations, upon the diseases of the mind.* Philadelphia: Kimber & Richardson. Excerpts reprinted in *Occupational Therapy and Rehabilitation, 26*, 177–180. (Original work published 1812)

Sakel, M. (1938). The pharmacological shock treatment of schizophrenia. *Nervous and Mental Disease* (Monograph, No. 62). New York: Nervous and Mental Disease Publication.

Schwartz, M. S. and Associates. (1995). *Biofeedback: A practitioner's guide* (2nd ed.). New York: Guilford.

Scott, M. (1960). The contribution of physical activities to psychological development. *Research Quarterly, 31*, 307–320.

Scullin, V. (1930). Report on institute exhibit. *Occupational Therapy and Rehabilitation, 9*, 239–240.

Selye, H. (1976). *The stress of life* (Rev. ed.) New York: McGraw-Hill.

Semrad, E. V., & Day, M. (1959). Techniques and procedures used in the treatment and activity program for psychiatric patients. In W. L. West (Ed.), *Changing concepts and practices in psychiatric occupational therapy: Proceedings of the Allenberry Workshop Conference on the Function and Preparation of the Psychiatric Occupational Therapist* (pp. 1–22). New York: American Association of Occupational Therapy.

Serrett, K. D. (1985). Another look at occupational therapy's history: Paradigm or pair-of-hands. *Occupational Therapy in Mental Health, 5*(3), 1–26. [Special issue: Philosophical and historical roots of occupational therapy]

Simonson, E. (1972). Evaluation of cardiac performance in exercise. *American Journal of Cardiology, 30,* 722.

Slagle, E. (1938). Occupational therapy. *Trained Nurse Hospital Review, 100,* 382.

Slovenko, R. (1985). Law and psychiatry. In H. I. Kaplan & B. J. Sadock (Eds.), *Comprehensive textbook of psychiatry* (4th ed., pp. 1960–1990). Baltimore: Williams and Williams.

Stein, F. (1969). Three facets of psychiatric occupational therapy: Models for research. *American Journal of Occupational Therapy, 23*(6), 491–494.

Stein, M., & Miller, A. H. (1993). Stress, the immune system, and health and illness. In L. Goldberger & S. Breznitz, (Eds.), *Handbook of stress: Theoretical and clinical aspects* (2nd ed., pp. 127–141). New York: The Free Press.

Steptoe, A., Edwards, S., Moses, J., & Matthews, A. (1989). The effects of exercise training on mood and perceived coping ability in anxious adults from the general population. *Journal of Psychosomatic Research, 33,* 537–547.

Strauss, A., Schatzman, L., Bucher, R., Ehrlich, D., & Sabshin, M. (1964). *Psychiatric ideologies and institutions.* London: Collier-Macmillan.

Stroul, B. A., Pires, S. A., Armstrong, M. I., Meyers, J. C. (1998). The impact of managed care on mental health services for children and their families. *Future of children, 8,* 119–133.

Szasz, T. S. (1965). *Psychiatric justice.* New York: Macmillan.

Tame, D. (1984). *The secret power of music: The transformation of self and society through musical energy.* Rochester, VT: Destiny Books.

Towner, E. A., & Blumenthal, J. A. (1993). The efficacy of exercise in the management of hypertension. *Homeostatis, 34,* 338–345.

Trachtenberg, R. L. (1993). Comprehensive mental health benefits: A sound investment. *Journal of American Health Policy, 3*(5), 15–21.

Tuke, S. (1947). *Description of the Retreat, an institution near York, for insane persons of the Society of Friends: Containing an account of its origin and progress, the modes of treatment, and a statement of cases.* Philadelphia: Isaac Pierce. Excerpts reprinted in *Occupational Therapy and Rehabilitation, 26,* 248–263. (Original work published 1813)

Valdimarsdottir, H. B., & Stone, A. A. (1997). Psychosocial factors and secretory immunoglobulin A. *Critical Reviews in Oral Biology & Medicine, 8,* 461–474.

Valenstein, E. S. (1986). *Great and desperate cures: The rise and decline of psychosurgery and other radical treatments for mental illness.* New York: Basic Books.

Veith, I. (1975). The Far East. In J. G. Howells (Ed.), *World history of psychiatry* (pp. 662–704). New York: Brunner/Mazel.

Weinberg, S. K. (Ed.). (1967). *The sociology of mental disorders: Analyses and readings in psychiatric sociology.* Chicago: Aline.

West, W. L. (1959). *Changing concepts and practices in psychiatric occupational therapy. Proceedings of the Allenberry Workshop conference on the Function and Preparation of the Psychiatric Occupational Therapist.* Allenberry Inn, Boiling Springs, PA, November 13–19, 1956. New York: American Occupational Therapy Association.

Wisconsin State Board of Health. (1968). *An occupational therapy assistants program: A demonstration project.* Washington, DC: Department of Health Educational and Welfare. (PHS Grant #3CH 53-4)

Workshop on Alternative Medicine. (1994). *Alternative medicine: Expanding medical horizons* (NIH Publication No. 94–066). Washington, DC: Government Printing Office.

Wrangsjo, B., & Korlin, D. (1995). Guided imagery and music as a psychotherapeutic method in psychiatry. *Journal of Association of Music Imagery, 4,* 79–92.

Zilboorg, G. (1935). *The medical man and the witch during the renaissance.* Baltimore: Johns Hopkins.

Zilboorg, G. (1941). *A history of medical psychology.* New York: W. W. Norton.

CHAPTER

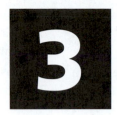

The Community Care Model and the Roles of the Occupational Therapist: 1960–2000

> We must strengthen and improve the programs and facilities serving the mentally ill and the mentally retarded. The emphasis should be upon timely and intensive diagnosis, treatment, training and rehabilitation so that the mentally afflicted can be cured and their functions restored to the extent possible. Services to both the mentally ill and the mentally retarded must be community based and provide a range of services to meet community needs.
>
> —President John F. Kennedy, Mental Illness and Mental Retardation Message to the Congress of the United States, February 5, 1963.

Operational Learning Objectives

By the end of this chapter, the learner will:

1. Discuss the negative effects of institutionalization on the patient with mental illness.

2. Discuss the social and psychological factors that led to the Community Mental Health Movement.

3. List the essential components of a community support system for those with chronic mental illness.

4. Describe alternative community models for treating those with mental illness.

5. Describe the goals and functions of a Community Mental Health Center.

6. Discuss the role of occupational therapy in a community mental health program.

7. Differentiate the treatment objectives for patients with acute illness and chronic illness who are attending an outpatient program.

8. Discuss the purposes of vocationally oriented activities in a Community Mental Health
   Center.

9. Describe the role of occupational therapy in
   a community residential treatment program
   for youth who are at risk for delinquency or
   incarceration.

10. Apply criteria for evaluating the effective-
    ness of a community mental health treat-
    ment program.

THE EMERGENCE OF THE COMMUNITY CARE MODEL IN PSYCHIATRY

Why and how did comprehensive community
mental health centers (CMHC) replace mental
hospitals as the primary focal point of treatment for those with mental illness? The concept
of a mental hospital in the early 19th century
was proposed as a humane alternative to the
harsh treatment provided to those with mental
illness, who frequently were imprisoned or left
to wander in city or rural areas. The mental
hospital was first planned as a place of refuge to
protect those with mental illness from being
exploited and maltreated. Ironically, a century
later the mental hospital was the target of attack
as being an environment that fostered individuals to regress further into their illness and as a
result to lose their capacity to live independently (Goffman, 1959). The negative effects of
institutionalization intensified as state mental
hospitals became huge human warehouses that
created artificial microcosms of false security
(Wales, 1960).

From 1920 to 1957, the number of individuals admitted to mental hospitals increased dramatically, resulting in overcrowded facilities and
burgeoning state and federal costs. For example,
in 1920 there were approximately 220,000
patients in mental hospitals in the United States
out of a total population of 106 million. In 1956
the number of patients in mental hospitals
increased to 632,804 in a total population of 168
million. The proportion of those with mental
illness who were hospitalized in 1920 was 207
per 100,000; in 1956 it was 377 per 100,000
(Weinberg, 1967). A shift away from increased
hospitalization occurred in 1957 and continued
into the 1990s (Stein, 1992).

The community mental health movement
emerged during the 1960s amidst a climate of
political, social, and cultural changes (Ellek,
1991). There was a general reaction against the
forced isolation of individuals with disabilities
and minorities from the mainstream of society.
Political changes were sought to reverse the
trends toward incarcerating delinquents, segre-
gating blacks, and institutionalizing those with
developmental disabilities and mental illness.
The description below of a ward in a mental
hospital by Beckenstein (1964), a director of the
Brooklyn State Mental Hospital, was a common
reaction by many mental health professionals:

THE NEGATIVE EFFECTS OF INSTITUTIONALIZATION

Typically, the walls were bare, heavy chairs and
benches were pushed in line against the walls,
there were no curtains or draperies at the windows—only prison-like guards. The few parlor
wards in which an effort was made to create a
less depressing atmosphere were decorated
with large ferns in flower pots which were
placed inside large brass containers. These containers were kept highly polished and, like the
custodian's keys, became a symbol of the mental health institution. In the dining room, only
spoons were provided, for fear the patients
might harm themselves or each other if they
were given the usual eating utensils. Disturbed
patients were seldom taken outdoors unless an
enclosure, called a "bull-pen," was available.
The reading matter on hand consisted mostly

of out-dated magazines and discarded children's books.

The patients themselves, particularly those in the regressed and disturbed wards, were as unattractive in appearance as were their surroundings. Their clothes were ill-fitting, trousers were held up by a piece of string, hair was uncombed. Apathetic patients simply sat around all day, propped against the wall, or on the floor in attitudes of hopelessness and despair. Others, shouting and yelling, were kept in restraint. To prevent suicide, all furniture and accessories which might have made the atmosphere of the ward less discouraging were removed. Yet, even when such precautions had not been taken, the incidence of suicide in the hospital was extremely low.

Generally, the personnel were neatly uniformed, but many had large bunches of keys attached to their belts by long cords, for penalties were imposed if a door were left unlocked. Moreover, as might be expected, their attitude toward the patients reflected the penal approach of the institution. The therapeutic program was limited. There was some occupational therapy, some recreation, some supportive therapy, but this was frequently reserved for newly admitted patients. The hospitals were hampered by inadequate funds, ill-trained personnel and overcrowded facilities.

These abuses were perpetuated by a public attitude which viewed the mental patients as hopeless, and which embraced the belief that they be isolated from the community, and cared for with minimum financial burden to the outside world. Many progressive hospital directors and their staffs tried valiantly to counteract these attitudes. They recognized and stressed the need for therapy, and for community clinics which might provide both prophylactic and posthospital care. Many tried to make the public aware of the dangers of "desocialization" and regression which were the concomitants of institutional practice. (pp 178–179)

Reforms and Shifts in the Mental Health System in the United States

The movement away from institutionalization had political support in the United States. (See Table 3–1 for legislative chronology.) For example in 1963, the United States Congress, with the support of President Kennedy, authorized funds for the construction of comprehensive CMHCs. Further legislation provided for a full range of mental health services that included, in addition to 24-hour-a-day hospital care, outpatient individual and group psychotherapy, crisis intervention, part-time hospitalization, preventive mental health consultations in schools and community agencies, vocational rehabilitation, and support for halfway houses that enabled individuals to live in supportive community residences (Karno & Schwartz, 1974).

In 1970 the total number of residents in all mental health facilities was reduced to 345,050, or 170 per 100,000 population (Gruenberg & Turns, 1975). Since 1970, the proportion of individuals in mental hospitals has continued to decrease, while short-term acute care hospitalization and outpatient and community care have increased. In 2000, there were approximately 200,000 individuals hospitalized in mental health facilities in the United States, including state and county, private, general, and VA hospitals (U.S. Substance Abuse and Mental Health Services Administration, Center for Mental Health Services, 1999) (Figure 3–1.)

There are a number of explanations for the decrease in the hospitalization rates for the mentally ill. The first was the introduction of tranquilizer drugs on a wide scale, which reduced the intensity of symptoms (Starr, 1982). The second was the availability of community care facilities for those with chronic mental illness (Koran, 1977; Mechanic, 1969; Stein, 1992). Community programs, such as Day Treatment Centers and Outpatient Clinics made accessible

Table 3-1. National Institutes of Mental Health Legislative Chronology

1946:	P.L. 79-487, the National Mental Health Act, authorized the surgeon general to improve the mental health of U.S. citizens through research into the causes, diagnosis, and treatment of psychiatric disorders.
1949:	The National Institute of Mental Health (NIMH) was established on April 15th.
1953:	Reorganization Plan No. 1 assigned Public Health Service to the newly created Department of Health, Education, and Welfare.
1955:	P.L. 84-182, the Mental Health Study Act, authorized NIMH to study and make recommendations on mental health and mental illness in the United States. The act also authorized the creation of the Joint Commission on Mental Illness and Health.
1963:	P.L. 88-164, the Mental Retardation Facilities and Community Mental Health Centers Construction Act, provided for grants for assistance in the construction of community mental health centers nationwide.
1965:	P.L. 89-105, amendments to P.L. 88-164, provided for grants for the staffing of community mental health centers.
1966:	P.L. 89-793, Narcotic Addict Rehabilitation Act of 1966, launched a national program for long-term treatment and rehabilitation of narcotic addicts.
1968:	NIMH became a component of the newly created Health Services and Mental Health Administration.
1968:	P.L. 90-574, Alcoholic and Narcotic Rehabilitation Amendments of 1968, authorized funds for the construction and staffing of new facilities for the prevention of alcoholism and the treatment and rehabilitation of alcoholics.
1973:	NIMH became a component of the newly created Alcohol Drug Abuse and Mental Health Administration (ADAMHA).
1984:	P.L. 98-509, Alcohol Abuse, Drug Abuse, and Mental Health Amendments, authorized funding for block grants for fiscal years 1985 through 1987, as well as extending the authorizations for federal activities in the areas of alcohol and drug abuse research, information dissemination, and development of new treatment methods.
1992:	P.L. 102-321, the ADAMHA Reorganization Act, abolished ADAMHA, created the Substance Abuse and Mental Health Services Administration, and transferred NIMH research activities to NIH.
1996:	P.L. 104-204, the Mental Health Parity Act, implemented on January 1, 1998, provided annual and lifetime dollar limits for mental heath benefits to be the same as that of other physical illnesses for large-size employers. Substance abuse and chemical dependency are excluded.

to patients, have become the models for treating those with mental illness (Herz, Endicott, & Spitzer, 1971). The major purpose of these community programs is to help the individual who had been hospitalized for a psychiatric disorder to relearn the skills necessary for living independently in the community.

Carling (1995) states that deinstitutionalization led to a paradigm shift in the field of mental health.

> We have moved from an era of institutional and facility–based thinking in which these people were seen exclusively as their illnesses (i.e., as patients), through a "transitional" period in which these individuals were seen princi-

pally in terms of their disabilities (i.e., as service recipients needing a comprehensive community support system) (Turner & TenHoor, 1979), to a world view in which these people are seen principally as citizens who happen to have disabilities, but share with all citizens the potential for, and right to, full community participation and integration. (p. 31)

A third explanation for the decrease in hospitalization rates for those with mental illness is the increase in the number of individuals with mental illness who are incarcerated in prisons or who are homeless. The number of individuals with mental illness has not been reduced in the last 40 years in spite of political reforms. What

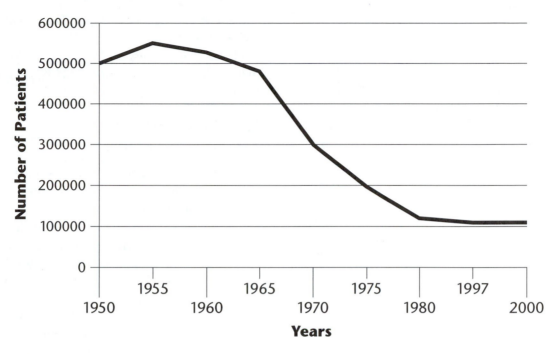

Figure 3–1. Number of patients in mental hospitals. (Adapted from "Quantitative and Experimental Methods in Psychiatry" by D. A. Regier and J. D. Burke, 1985. In H. I. Kaplan & B. J. Sadock, *Comprehensive Textbook of Psychiatry* (4th ed.), Baltimore: Williams & Wilkins.) Latest statistics available from *Hospital Statistics 2001 Edition*, by the Health Forum — An American Hospital Association.

has occurred is a shift in where those with mental illness can be found. In any given day there are approximately 200,000 individuals who are hospitalized for mental illness, 283,800 who are mentally ill and incarcerated, and 500,000 homeless who are mentally ill.

Homelessness, Incarceration, and Mental Illness

Based on a number of research studies, the National Coalition for the Homeless (1999a) has estimated that 12 million adult residents in the United States have been homeless at some point in their lives. Approximately one-fourth of this population are considered to be mentally ill (Koegel, 1996).

Vast increases in homelessness did not occur until the 1980s, when incomes and housing options for those living on the margins began to diminish rapidly.... However, a new wave of deinstitutionalization and the denial of services or premature and unplanned discharge brought about by managed care arrangements may be contributing to the continued presence of seriously mentally ill persons within the homeless population.

Mental disorders prevent people from carrying out essential aspects of daily life, such as self-care, household management and interpersonal relationships. Homeless people with mental disorders remain homeless for longer periods of time and have less contact with family and friends. They encounter more barriers to employment, tend to be in poorer physical health, and have more contact with the legal system than homeless people who do not suffer from mental disorders. (National Coalition for the Homeless, 1999b, p. 1)

According to the United States Office of Justice (1999), an estimated 283,800 offenders were diagnosed with mental illness. In addition, 547,800 individuals on probation were mentally ill. Family dysfunction seems to be contributing to the incarceration of individuals with mental illness. Many in this population were physically or sexually abused by their parents. Almost 50 percent of their parents had problems with alcohol or substance abuse. Parents and siblings were incarcerated to a large degree. It is important to note that 40 percent of this population were unemployed prior to their incarceration.

Forensic Psychiatry

Forensic psychiatry, a relatively new area for health professionals, deals with individuals who are incarcerated because of aggressive, dangerous, and socially unacceptable behavior, and who, in addition, have a mental illness (Lloyd, 1995). The most common diagnoses found in the forensic population include schizophrenia, substance abuse, organic disorders, personality disorders, and mood disorders (Farnsworth, Morgan, & Fernando, 1987)

Occupational therapists play an important role in the rehabilitation and habilitation of patients in forensic psychiatry units and prisons (Dorwart & Hendricks, 2000). Lloyd (1995) advocated that patients who have been in criminal institutions should be prepared to return to the community with positive personal assets and adaptive skills so that they can integrate into the community. Occupational therapy treatment goals in forensic units include stress management, improvement of social skills and daily living skills, reduction of psychiatric symptoms, vocational rehabilitation, and improvement in

problem-solving abilities (Best, 1996; Crawford & Mee, 1994; Dressler & Snively, 1998; Dorwart & Hendricks, 2000; Farnsworth et al., 1987; Lloyd & Guerra, 1988; MacKain & Streveler, 1990; Penner, 1978).

Goals for Community Mental Health Programs

All people with mental disorders, including those who are homeless, require ongoing access to a full range of treatment and rehabilitation services to lessen the impairment and disruption produced by their condition. However, most people with mental disorder do not need hospitalization, and even fewer require long-term institutional care. According to the Federal Task Force on Homelessness and Severe Mental Illness, only 5 to 7 percent of homeless persons with mental illness need to be institutionalized; most can live in the community with the appropriate supportive housing options (Federal Task Force on Homelessness and Severe Mental Illness, 1992). Unfortunately, there are not enough community-based treatment services, nor enough appropriate, affordable housing, to accommodate the number of people disabled by mental disorders in the United States.

> Federal demonstration programs have produced a large body of knowledge on the service and treatment needs of homeless individuals with serious mental illnesses. Findings indicate that homeless persons with mental disorders are willing to use services that are easy to enter and that meet their perceived needs. . . . Findings also reveal that persons with mental disorder and persons with addictive disorders share many of the same treatment needs, including carefully designed client engagement and case management, housing options, and long-term follow-up and support services. Studies also emphasize the importance of service integration, outreach and engagement; the use of case management to negotiate care sys-

tems; the need for a range of supportive housing and treatment options that are responsive to consumer preferences; and the importance of meaningful daily activity. When combined with supportive services, meaningful daily activity in the community (including work), and access to therapy, appropriate housing can provide the framework necessary to end homelessness for many individuals. . . .

Finally, the commitment to making deinstitutionalization work as it was intended must be renewed. People with mental illness must be able to live as independently as possible with the help of expanded comprehensive, community-based mental health services and other supports. It is crucial that polices be proactive rather than reactive. Services such as crisis intervention, landlord-tenant intervention, continuous treatment teams and appropriate discharge planning in jails and inpatient facilities must be made available in all communities. (National Coalition for the Homeless, 1999b, pp. 1–2)

In 1980, the Community Support Program was incorporated into the Mental Health Systems Act (Turner & TenHoor, 1979; National Institute of Mental Health [NIMH], 1987). This legislation outlined guidelines for a community support system funded by federal grants for those with chronic mental illness. Legislation mandated that an adequate community program provide staff and resources to perform the following functions. These goal functions were proposed as recognition that those with chronic mental illness are vulnerable to the everyday stressors in life and that they need community services to prevent rehospitalization. The following is taken from the goals as reported in Tessler and Goldman (1982):

▶ identification of the target population, whether in hospitals or in the community, and outreach to offer appropriate services to those willing to participate

▶ assistance in applying for entitlements (Medicare and Medicaid)

▶ crisis stabilization services in the least restrictive setting possible, with hospitalization available when other options are insufficient

▶ psychosocial rehabilitation services, including but not limited to:

   ▶ goal-oriented rehabilitation evaluation

   ▶ training in community living skills, in the natural setting wherever possible

   ▶ opportunities to improve employability

   ▶ appropriate living arrangements in an atmosphere that encourages improvements in functioning

   ▶ opportunities to develop social skills, interests, and leisure-time activities to provide a sense of participation and worth

▶ supportive services of indefinite duration, including supportive living and working arrangements, and other such services for as long as they are needed

▶ medical and mental health care

▶ backup support to families, friends, and community members

▶ involvement of concerned community members in planning and offering housing or working opportunities

▶ protection of client rights, both in hospitals and in the community

▶ case management, to ensure continuous availability of appropriate forms of assistance. (p. 16)

Bachrach (1992) defines psychosocial rehabilitation in terms of eight fundamental concepts:

▶ enabling an individual with long-term mental illness to develop to the fullest extent his or her capacities

▶ emphasis on the environmental factors such as housing, employment, social skills, and family relations that require changes in the environment to meet the needs of the individual while also helping the individual to adapt to the environment

▶ enlarging on the positive strengths of the individual and improving the competencies in terms of the healthy part of the person

▶ restoring hope to the individual and a will to improve that is "future oriented"

▶ creating optimism in the individual that he or she will be able to engage in work activities. It is a premise that work gives the individual a sense of personal achievement and mastery. The concept of work also includes supported employment, creative activities, hobbies, and volunteer opportunities

▶ engaging the individual with long-term mental illness in social and recreational activities such as social clubs, resocialization programs, educational opportunities, drop-in centers, and family education

▶ involving the individual in every aspect of his or her treatment with the therapist taking into account the individual's values, experiences, feelings, ideas, and goals. In effect this is treating the individual as a consumer who is actively involved in the treatment process

▶ psychosocial rehabilitation is an ongoing process firmly committed to the concept of continuity of care

Stein (1990) developed a treatment model based on this plan. This treatment model was presented to the Winnipeg Mental Health Association and is reproduced in Table 3–2.

Dowell and Ciarlo (1989) identified nine program goals for CMHCs:

to increase the range and quality of services of public mental health services, to make services equally available and accessible to all, to provide services in relation to the existing needs, to decrease state hospital admissions and residents, to maximize citizen participation in community programs, to prevent development of mental disorders, to coordinate mental health-related services in the catchment area, to provide services which reduce suffering and increase personal functioning. (p. 196)

Currently, CMHCs provide five essential mental health functions in 1,500 service areas in the United States: (a) inpatient hospitalization, (b) outpatient services, (c) partial hospitalization, (d) emergency and crisis intervention, and (e) consultation and education. Of these, approximately 86 percent of all mental health care is outpatient, 5 percent is inpatient or emergency hospitalization, and 9 percent is partial hospitalization (e.g., night hospital) (U.S. Department of Health and Human Services, 1996).

Readjustment of the Patients to Community Living

An individual discharged from a mental hospital during the 1960s faced major psychological, social, vocational, and financial problems (Stein, 1962). Adjustment to community living meant relearning the social patterns of behavior that are different from institutional life. In the psychiatric hospital, the patient adapted to hospital norms and regulations that were equated with compliance to authority and order. The ward attendant usually set the social expectations for the patient. Passive dependency was rewarded, while assertive behavior was considered negative. The patient with an acute illness who acted out required constant surveillance and became the focal point of the staff's attention and supervision until the symptoms became stabilized and the patient's behavior was controlled. This is the point where the patient was judged to be socialized to the hospital environment. Frequently, the patient was discharged with a residual handicap in interpersonal relationships, a lowered self-esteem, and a social stigma for being a "former mental patient." The need for

Table 3–2. Individualized Treatment Plan (ITP) *(developed upon patient's discharge from hospital, and approved by case manager, patient, and family or surrogate family)*

Assumptions Underlying the ITP

- There are biopsychosocial vulnerabilities to mental illness that include genetic-developmental and environmental factors. (Predisposing causes)

- Stress can trigger mental illness in an already vulnerable individual. (Precipitating causes)

- Successful treatment helps the individual to resist stress and develop hardiness. (Secondary prevention)

- Mental illness is episodic in nature—treatment helps individual over the "rough periods."

Content of Interventions	Rationale	Potential Risks	Methods or Operational Plan
Medication	To relieve symptoms	• Side effects may be uncontrolled • Too little or too much medication may cause adverse effects	• Dosage • Amount of dosage and how long the medication should be taken can affect results
Housing • Family • Halfway house • Boarding • Temporary shelter	To provide safe and supportive habitat	Unsafe neighborhood may create additional stress if neighborhood is in slum area with drugs, crime, and poverty	• Specific housing environment • Goal is for individual to feel safe and secure in environment
Vocational or Educational • Specialized placement • Supportive employment • Temporary employment • Transitional employment • School • Day treatment	To assist in gaining employment	Possible job failure if plan is unrealistic and gives false hopes to individual, the chance for success is diminished	Designated vocational plan that is • relevant • understandable • measurable • behavioral • achievable
Support Group	To provide ongoing support for self-care, leisure, and social activities	Group may be overly critical	Individual is introduced to support group before discharge from hospital
Counseling or Psychotherapy • Individual • Group	To provide outpatient counseling as needed	Process may foster dependency	Individual is transitioned into treatment while in hospital
Case Manager Follow-up (Hospital to outpatient to community)	To provide outreach to vulnerable individual in the community	Individual may feel loss of privacy	Every individual is provided case manager in hospital: mental health professional, psychiatrist, psychologist, nurse, social worker, or occupational therapist

Copyright © F. Stein, 1990.

transitional services that prevented the patient from being readmitted to a mental hospital generated alternative treatment models in community mental health.

Gage, Cook, and Fryday-Field (1997), in an exploratory study of the client's transition from an acute care setting to their homes in the community, concluded that the occupational therapist has an important role to play in pre- and postdischarge planning. Data were collected through telephone interviews from 27 discharged clients. Resources for successful adjustment to the community depend on intra- and interpersonal resources, adaptive devices and techniques, and the importance of occupation (Greene & Cruz, 1981).

MODELS FOR COMMUNITY MENTAL HEALTH

Joshua Bierer (1964), one of the early advocates of community psychiatry as an alternative to the mental hospital, listed four issues underlying effective treatment in the community.

1. The successful treatment of mental illness requires a change in societal attitudes; that is, elimination of the social stigma attached to mental illness.

2. The treatment of mental illness should be an interdisciplinary approach.

3. The recognition that the patient's active participation, motivation, and will to recovery are the most potent and valuable dimensions in treatment.

4. The very nature of community care of those with mental illness implies that patients work together with staff in political decisions affecting the very existence of community treatment programs.

Early experiments in community psychiatry led to alternative models such as therapeutic social clubs, night hospitals or partial hospitalization, halfway houses, aftercare clinics, crisis intervention or crisis service teams, case management, mental health consultation, support groups, and day treatment centers.

Therapeutic Social Clubs

Therapeutic social clubs include self-governing groups where patients can socialize and take part in recreational and educational activities in an informal atmosphere. Therapeutic social clubs are initiated in the hospital for patients who are ready for discharge into the community or as an aftercare support group for individuals newly adjusting to the community. Activities include cooking, table games, painting, lectures, films, concerts, role playing, and other group projects suggested by the patients (Jones, 1953). Fountain House in New York City was a model for social clubs that incorporated psychological rehabilitation methods into an informal atmosphere (Beard, Propst, & Malamud, 1982).

Night Hospital or Partial Hospitalization

The American Partial Hospitalization Association (AAPH) has defined partial hospitalization as "a time-limited, ambulatory treatment program that offers intensive, coordinated, and structured clinical services within a stable therapeutic milieu" (AAPH, 1991, p. 1). This includes day, evening, night, and weekend day treatment programs (Ettlinger, Beigl, & Feder, 1972). The major purpose of a night hospital is to prevent rehospitalization of individuals who can work during the day, yet need a supportive environment during their free time. According to Linn, Caffey, Klett, Hogarty, and Lamb (1979), partial hospitalization is at least as effective as inpatient units in the treatment of patients with psychosis or schizophrenia.

Halfway House

A halfway house is a supportive group residence where patients live together in the community.

The total organization and maintenance of the halfway house is carried out by the patients under supervision from house parents or mental health staff. This transitional environment encourages the patient to become independent and responsible in the activities of daily living (Friedlob, Janis, & Deets-Aron, 1986).

Aftercare Clinic

As an outpatient setting, an aftercare clinic provides a continuity of services for discharged patients that includes individual and group therapy, supervision of medication, and family and vocational counseling. Periodic appointments are arranged by the social worker to provide follow-up care (Wilberding, 1991).

Crisis Response Services

The crisis response service is directed at helping the client and family to cope with emergencies by providing 24-hour standby assistance. A home intervention team is available to visit the client in the home and to arrange for short-term and partial hospitalization, temporary placement in a halfway house, or family counseling (Biss & Curtis, 1993; Carling, 1995).

Case Management

Case management is an important aspect for the client who has returned to the community, the homeless, and individuals living in shelters. The role of the case manager is intensive and ongoing, providing a continuity of care (Moeller, 1991). The case manager works with the patient in a "client-directed and client-empowering" manner.

Specific functions should include identifying clients who need and desire case management services; working with each client to develop a comprehensive service plan based on the client's needs and goals; providing information to help the client make an informed choice about opportunities and services; assisting the client, on request, to obtain needed services, supports, and entitlements; being available during and after regular working hours; and advocating at the systems level for needed systems improvement. Close contact between client and case manager during hospitalizations is essential, as are a variety of mechanisms to closely coordinate hospital and community services. (Carling, 1995, p. 55)

Berthaume, Bailey, Horowitz, and McCrory (1994) examined the role of the case manager in referral of clients for medication, to outpatient counseling, or to social clubs. In a survey of 70 case managers, they found that the clients who were the most impaired were referred most often to day treatment programs with fewer additional support services recommended, while clients with the least impairment were referred to clubhouse or supported employment programs as well as to many other support services.

Scaletti (1999), in discussing a role for occupational therapists in community mental health, lists five steps that an occupational therapist can use in working with children, adolescents, and their families. These five steps include developmental casework, mutual support, coalitions of mutual interest, proactive community participation, and social movements.

Mental Health Consultation

One of the most important concerns of community mental health practitioners has been in the area of preventative psychiatry. Mental health consultancies to schools, places of employment, and community organizations are a direct outgrowth of the community mental health movement (Haylett & Rapoport, 1964).

In general, the consultant's role is to help community organizations assess the need for mental health services in the development of systematic programs of prevention (Watanabe & Watson, 1987). "As a consultant, an occupational therapist gives expert advice or information on organizational, program development, supervisory, or clinical issues or any combination of these to persons seeking this service" (Richert & Gibson, 1993, p. 550).

Community Support Groups

Self-help groups of former patients and their families operate as social action groups in offering support networks and community referral sources. These groups include local mental health associations, Alliance for the Mentally Ill, Recovery, Inc., Alcoholics Anonymous, Emotions Anonymous, Compassionate Friends, and Women's Crisis Line. Specific purposes of these groups are to advocate positive changes in the care and treatment of those with mental illness, remove the stigma of mental illness, protect the rights of those with mental illness, and sponsor educational programs and forums that increase the public awareness of mental health concerns (Carling, 1995).

Rural Mental Health

Providing mental health services to rural areas is another issue that is complicated by cultural and geographic factors (Murray & Keller, 1986). Bartels and Hogan (1986), in a survey of mental health problems in rural areas in North Dakota, found that the following mental health problems predominated (p. 43):

► alcoholism

► drug abuse

► depression/loneliness

► marital problems

► adolescent adjustment

► stress

► problems with parenting

► adjustment to aging

► psychiatric problems

► lack of recreation

Bartels and Hogan (1986) discussed 10 community developmental activities that have been successful in linking the rural community and the mental health system. These innovative activities included:

► rural stress workshops, dealing with stress management, stressors, and identifying copers

► commitment law seminars, discussing involuntary commitment to mental hospitals

► substance abuse education

► press relations, having a casual discussion with local news editors about mental health and available programs

► training for citizen participation on community mental boards

► organizing advisory boards for mental health programs

► conducting county commission reports regarding mental health services

► establishing a food pantry

► assisting in employment conflicts

► advocating for mental health services for those in need

DAY TREATMENT CENTER: THE GOALS AND FUNCTIONS

The guiding philosophy of the day treatment center is that the individual with mental illness treated in the community can develop the interpersonal and daily living skills to be independent. The general treatment goals for members attending a day treatment center include the following (Meltzoff & Blumenthal, 1966; Woodside, 1985):

General Treatment Goals of a Day Treatment Center

▶ Cultivate interpersonal relations with others through socialization groups and friendships.

▶ Adjust to family living and actively participate in household activities.

▶ Make use of community facilities through social and recreation groups. Develop avocational interests and leisure time pursuits.

▶ Foster self-confidence, feelings of personal worth, and a high self-regard for one's own abilities and characteristics.

▶ Formulate realistic life plans that include obtaining a job and achieving personal goals.

▶ Develop tolerance for frustration and stress without suppressing or internalizing feelings; be able to delay gratification and impulsive behavior.

▶ Demonstrate ability to modulate feelings and to have a stable level of happiness, cheerfulness, and optimism without severe mood swings of depression or mania.

▶ Accept responsibility for one's personal appearance, behavior, day-to-day decisions, and personal needs. Self-regulate behavior independently and at times be able to help others.

The Structure of a Day Treatment Center

A therapeutic milieu is created in a day treatment center that typically has an average daily attendance of between 20 and 60 individuals. On admission, the former patient is referred to as a consumer, client, or "member" of the community. The professional staff includes psychiatrists, psychologists, social workers, nurses, vocational counselors, recreational therapists, and occupational therapists. Support staff includes secretaries, maintenance workers, and aides. Volunteers direct various interest groups related to adult education, photography, computer operation, and leisure activities that can enrich a therapeutic program. The staff, members, and volunteers interact informally to create a climate of mutual understanding and trust. This climate helps to break down the artificial barriers of communication between patients and therapists. Day treatment centers are usually located in a central area that is easily accessible and away from the stigma of being associated with a mental hospital. Members are expected to arrive and leave at specified times in the morning and evening. This experience helps the member to develop independent living skills that are necessary in preparation for competitive employment in the community (Lang & Cara, 1989; Stein, 1984).

Activity Program and Treatment Methods

Although the emotional climate of the day treatment center is permissive, there is structure and goal direction in the activity program (Schecter, 1974). Activities are frequently structured around creative arts and recreational activities, such as swimming, bowling, volleyball; field trips to museums, parks, movies, factories, restaurants; activities of daily living such as budgeting, shopping, and cooking; prevocational preparation; task groups; and therapeutic groups such as art and music therapy, psychodrama, and role playing. Opportunities for the members' self-government are encouraged in group decisions involving everyday problems of maintenance, plans for social events, fundraising, and legislative lobbying. Periodic community meetings are held where staff, members, and their families are invited to discuss mutual problems. These meetings are helpful in communicating to the members' families the therapeutic purposes of the day treatment center.

COMMUNITY MENTAL HEALTH CENTERS

Occupational Therapist's Role

Because readjustment in the community depends to a great extent on a person's ability to be independent, a major role in psychosocial rehabilitation falls within the occupational therapy area. Jaffe (1980) developed a model for the role of occupational therapy as a community consultant in prevention, with indirect or nontreatment roles. Occupational therapists became involved in a pilot project aimed at the educational and cultural needs of children in a small community in southeastern Michigan. The therapist served as program consultant and assisted in orienting, training, and educating other occupational therapists in "community organization, expanded professional roles, and in preventative health goals of a community" (p. 50). A discussion of objectives for field training in community mental health, community experience during the field training, and supervisory and communication networks in the program

were the parts of the model utilizing the role of the occupational therapist as a community consultant.

In examining the challenges of occupational therapy to changes in the mental health system, Fidler (1991) proposed that occupational therapists address four very basic questions in assessment and rehabilitation: (a) What are the patient performance skills? (b) What are the strengths, abilities, and interests of the patient and what are the external resources? (c) What are the internal and external factors that interfere with the patient's ability to achieve his or her goals? and (d) What interventions and remedial activities must be used to help the patient fulfill his or her lifestyle performance expectations?

The occupational therapist works in alliance with the client or member to plan a goal-directed program. During the initial interview, the occupational therapist discusses the general goals of occupational therapy with the member and establishes rapport and the basis for building a therapeutic relationship. One of the overall goals of treatment is to help the member prepare for employment. The problems of work are discussed in terms of evaluating work potential, establishing work habits, and managing occupational stress. The occupational therapist uses groups to discuss such practical information as initiating a job search, preparing for a job interview, filling out an application form, taking personnel tests, and handling feedback and criticism on the job. The occupational therapist recommends individuals who show potential for further education or training in a specific occupation to the State Division of Vocational Rehabilitation counselor. The timing of the member's referral is extremely important. A premature referral or a prolonged delay in referral can frequently dampen the member's motivation to do work.

In general, the occupational therapist plays a key role in helping individuals to mobilize their potential assets toward a work-related goal. Table 3–3 describes the hierarchical experiences and skills that underlie a member's progress toward full-time employment in the community.

Teske (1986) described the development of a community program in Ypsilanti, Michigan, in which occupational therapists served as advocates for former patients with mental illness. Deinstitutionalization had increased the number of discharged patients, and the Full Circle Community Center was developed to provide support services. Instead of direct treatment for those who needed adjustment to community life, occupational therapists were involved in indirect service delivery, such as creating task forces, meeting health needs, and providing volunteer work.

Adams (1990) identified three important functions of occupational therapists working at CMHCs: "Program planning, evaluation, and implementation; collaboration with other community-based professionals; and interfacing with other service providers, with relatives, and with the public" (pp. 1–2). In a discussion of these roles, Adams stated that the functions of program planning and evaluation were completed by occupational therapists in the hospital; however, "service provision in community mental health, especially in work readiness training and independent living skills training, requires skills the occupational therapist may not have gained in an academic setting" (p. 1). Occupational therapists must work with other professionals in the community. Adams concludes by defining the role of the occupational therapist in community mental health as a "'boundary spanner'—one who interfaces with others to bridge gaps in service provision" (p. 2).

Learnard and Deveraux (1992) developed the conceptual model of occupational therapy in an independent practice in rural Maine. The clients served had a diagnosis of severe mental illness. The conceptual model consisted of planning, environmental structure, and skill building. Planning was defined as an activity that "required a clear understanding of the client's goals and of the resources that were available for them" (p. 869). Environmental structure aided

Table 3–3. Hierarchical Steps Toward Full-time Employment in the Community

1. Evaluation of skills and aptitudes	Process of identifying occupational strengths and aptitudes through work samples and objective tests
2. Occupational information group	Exploration of educational requirements and tasks involved in specific jobs (e.g., through *Dictionary of Occupational Titles)*
3. Individual counseling	Formulation of short- and long-term vocational goals
4. Vocational training	Formal training or education to prepare the client for a specific job
5. Pre-employment counseling	Group discussion of factors related to securing a job and work adjustment
6. Transitional volunteer work	Placement in a nonpaying position that promotes the client's ability to meet the demands of a job
7. Supportive employment	Placement in a noncompetitive work environment where the client works in a transitional setting within the community
8. Transitional tryout work	Transitional job in the community in which the client receives job coaching
9. Special placement	A concerted effort to place the client in a job that matches his or her abilities and interests

clients in learning and allowed them to gain the greatest level of functioning in an activity. The environment structure facilitated the client's cognitive, sensorimotor, and psychosocial development. Finally, for the skill-building component, the focus was the functional skills of the clients. In this phase, the therapist completed a review of the client's abilities and deficits in work, activities of daily living, and leisure and used direct or indirect services to assist the person in developing skills and/or compensatory strategies. Plans for a client were changed to suit the client's current needs, and with different disciplines, yielding a variety of perspectives in the design of an intervention plan. The importance of occupational therapy in the intervention was explained as follows:

> Occupational therapy's holistic approach to service provision, its long-standing emphasis on rehabilitation outcomes, the variety of activities it can offer, and its ability to assess clients' function in an environmental context and adapt physical and social environments all provide a strong base for community practice. (Learnard & Deveraux, 1992, p. 871)

In an interview with Robnett (1997), Learnard stated that the occupational therapist working in community mental health should help create circles of support that will facilitate a functional environment for the person with mental illness. To Learnard, the environment is adjusted to fit each person's self-determined needs by utilizing the community, such as friends, family, and neighbors, as well as the occupational therapist and other team members. Learnard views the scope of community practice as truly holistic with concern for the environment, the individual skills of the client, and the future plans as envisioned by the client.

Occupational Therapy Facilities

In 1969, Ozarin described the physical facilities for occupational therapy in a CMHC:

> The physical facilities for OT programs in a community mental health center should reflect the center's treatment philosophy and the role of OT in the program, the types of patients served, and the availability of community resources. . . . Activity areas in community mental health centers should be flexible and multipurpose. . . . Adequate office space should be provided for the occupational therapist, preferably next to the activity area. . . . A program that serves a large number of chronic patients may have to establish its own sheltered workshop, particularly if there are no suitable ones in the community. (p. 48)

Occupational therapy facilities in a day treatment center in the 1960s were usually divided into three areas: homemaking/kitchen, clerical office, and industrial work-shop (Stein, 1962).

▶ *Homemaking/Kitchen:* A homemaking/ kitchen area was available in most day treatment centers to help individuals learn independent living skills in a socially supportive environment. In this area the member practiced budgeting, cooking, laundering, cleaning, and other household skills. Members were encouraged to plan and complete activities that enhance self-esteem and renew concern for appearance. Sometimes relatives of members tended to shield them from taking part in household responsibilities, which, many times, was a way of fostering dependency and diminishing self-worth. Members in the day treatment center could tangibly demonstrate to their relatives their skills and by so doing take a more active part in the family household.

The member's performance in the homemaking area could also be used for evaluating potential for independent living and work. Simulated work tasks were analyzed into component skills required for adequate performance. A member's performance in simulated work tasks could be evaluated to determine if the member has aptitude or ability. Subsequently, members having ability in this area could be referred to the State Division of Vocational Rehabilitation for training and eventual placement. Those demonstrating entry-level vocational skills could be referred directly to the State Employment Service or other specialized placement agencies for those with disabilities.

▶ *Clerical Office:* The clerical office was another major area in a day treatment center where an individual had the opportunity to test his or her abilities and interests in office tasks. Members who had worked in a clerical position before hospitalization could regain office skills and self-confidence while practicing on various business machines. Clerical tests were used to evaluate the level of performance compared with the minimum requirements for clerical workers. These tests included business arithmetic, spelling, typing, use of shorthand, use of calculator, filing systems, use of copy machines, and typing from a transcriber.

The member who was ready for employment gained skills by practicing. Skills such as filling out an application form, filing, transcribing material, and typing were tested. Attention was given to anticipating any difficulty that a person might encounter when he or she applied for a job. Frequently, the member was concerned with personal acceptance by a prospective employer. Discussions and practice job interviews were held to rehearse any anticipated problems.

▶ *Industrial Workshop:* Members preparing for industrial or assembly line work many times needed to organize their work habits and learn to follow written or verbal instructions. Machine woodworking involving the use of drill press, band saw, circular saw, and wood lathe could be used in the evaluation of manual capacities. Attention span, the ability to concentrate, initiative, and independent work habits were factors used in determining a member's employability for industrial and assembly line work. The member could also be evaluated for potential in small assembly work, electronics, and related job tasks. The *Dictionary of Occupational Titles* (a periodic publication available through the Department of Labor) was used by the occupational therapist to explore related occupations with the client. The most recent edition was published in 1999 (Schaerfl, 1999).

The Support Network, Madison, Wisconsin (Prototype of Day Treatment Center)

An example of a day treatment center using a comprehensive rehabilitation model is the Support Network located in Madison, Wisconsin. This treatment program is organized in a flexible pattern, adapting to the individual needs of the members and to the resources available in the local community.

The Support Network Day Treatment Program was established in 1976. It was the first community psychosocial rehabilitation program in Wisconsin (Stein & Test, 1985) to work specifically with individuals with mental illness. The majority of the clients served through the Support Network are diagnosed with chronic schizophrenia. They have found that the most common problems identified with the individuals with chronic schizophrenia discharged from mental hospitals are a high vulnerability to deal with stress; difficulties in coping with everyday problems and basic living skills; extreme dependency on others; inability to find and hold jobs; and severe difficulties in interpersonal relationships.

To help the individual with chronic schizophrenia to overcome these problems, the staff formulated three basic treatment objectives:

1. Improve the member's ability to function independently in the community.

2. Reduce the member's dependency on the state hospital and subsequently to reduce rehospitalization.

3. Improve the member's quality of life in the community.

To accomplish these objectives, the professional staff, composed of psychiatrists, psychologists, social workers, counselors, nurses, and occupational therapists, provide a supportive milieu and a wide range of individual and group therapies. The program is centrally located in a downtown area in a renovated house. Initially, it was open five afternoons and four evenings a week. When it was first conceptualized, the program was organized around eight structured components. This model has been replicated in various forms throughout the world. It continues to serve as a classical model for community mental health. The eight components are described below.

▶ *Prevocational:* This part of the program includes a food service where members prepare and serve meals; a communication/clerical unit where members send out mailings, make community posters, and perform other clerical activities; and the "outreach" unit where members visit, telephone, and write other members who

become ill and who are unable to attend the day treatment center.

▶ *Educational Classes:* Small classes (six to eight people) are offered in cooking, budgeting, housekeeping, transportation, academic subjects, and mental health. New classes are organized around members' interests.

▶ *Social and Recreation:* Activities in sports, arts and crafts, yoga, field trips to community events, picnics, parties, and social outings are organized to promote friendships and leisure time interests.

▶ *Members' Self-governance:* Weekly meeting of staff and members are held to discuss program policy issues and to recommend new activities or discontinue groups.

▶ *Medical Coverage:* A majority of the members attending the day treatment center are on some type of psychotropic medication, for example, antipsychotic agents, Lithium, minor tranquilizers, antidepression drugs, sleeping pills; and antiparkinsonian drugs. (An outline of the main functions and side effects of psychotropic drugs are listed in Chapter 7.) The psychiatrists and nurses are responsible for monitoring the effects of the drugs and making changes when needed.

▶ *Counseling:* Ongoing personal counseling is provided either from the Support Network staff or consulting psychotherapists in the community. Stress management and relaxation are taught by the occupational therapist and psychologist. Each member has a case manager to help integrate the program components of housing, medication, support groups, work, and leisure.

▶ *Outreach:* The members and professional staff emphasize the importance of crisis intervention and the teaching of adaptive skills in coping with unforeseen emergencies such as housing eviction, death of a relative, or the loss of a job. The outreach program provides members with a continual link to the Support Network.

▶ *Community Referral:* Community agencies are interconnected with the Support Network. They include the State Division of Vocational Rehabilitation, Goodwill Industries, sheltered workshop, Alliance for the Mentally Ill and other community support groups, Visiting Nurses Association, housing agencies and authorities, job placement centers, and crisis intervention when needed.

Two short case histories, one of an individual with acute mental illness and another of an individual with chronic mental illness, are personal examples of the successful use of a day treatment center in psychosocial rehabilitation (Stein, 1962).[1]

INDIVIDUAL WITH ACUTE MENTAL ILLNESS

S. K., a 44-year-old attractive woman, with a history of several short-term hospitalizations, was referred to a day treatment center as an emergency admission after one month of convalescent care in her home. S. K. was suffering a severe depression that prevented her from meeting the minimal requirements for independent living. The sister with whom she was living contacted the social worker and the psychiatrist in the after-care clinic that she was attending asking for assistance. A return to the state hospital was considered as an option. However, S. K. refused to voluntarily return to the state hospital. Referral to the day treatment center as an alternative to rehospitalization was made in order to increase her skills for independent living, to prevent regression, and to encourage socialization. Medication was to be supplied and supervised by the psychiatrist and nurse in the day treatment center. S. K. attended the Day Treatment Center for six months during which time she was initially pessimistic and expressed doubt about her ability to improve. However, after considerable support and reassurance from the total staff, S. K. was eventually able to mobilize herself to seek employment. She obtained a clerical position shortly afterward and continued to make a good adjustment one year after discharge from the day treatment center.

In the day treatment center, the occupational therapist used a variety of activities with S. K. during the first three months. S. K. did hand sewing initially, where she was involved in a socialization group with eight other members. The other members accepted her into the group, which was helpful, since she tended to depreciate herself. S. K. also participated in an art group where she enjoyed painting. However at the end of the session, the finished art product was promptly deposited in the waste can. The socializing environment and permissive approach allowed S. K. to express herself spontaneously. After the first planning conference, the staff felt that definite improvement had occurred in her self-esteem and lessening of depression. A change in her activity program toward a vocationally oriented goal was recommended. S. K. was placed in the clerical area for a work evaluation and was referred to the employment counseling group by the psychiatrist. She had the necessary skills to work in an office. However, she still seemed to lack self-confidence and she sought reassurance constantly. She was given this reassurance and was encouraged toward seeking employment by other members in group therapy, and by the occupational therapist. A second planning conference was held with S. K. in which the staff took a direct approach and emphasized the importance of seeking work at this time. S. K. took the staff's advice and was successful in finding employment as a clerical worker in a credit office. This woman,

---

[1] Minor editing changes were made from original article for inclusion in this book.

depressed, acutely-ill, and temporarily non-productive, after six months of treatment in the day treatment center with emphasis upon work adjustment, creative expression, and socialization was able to mobilize her abilities toward obtaining employment in the community. (p. 33)

PATIENT WITH CHRONIC MENTAL ILLNESS

L. M., an individual with chronic schizophrenia who had spent 18 years in a state mental hospital during the prime of his life, was referred to a day treatment center at the age of 42. Prior to hospitalization he had attended an art school where he earned a certificate in advertising art. He had worked for only a few months before the onset of his illness.

In the state hospital L. M. was in a locked ward where he remained in a catatonic stupor intermittently for ten years, at times being fed intravenously. He regressed in the state hospital to the point where he was incontinent of urine and feces and completely out of contact with his immediate surroundings. L. M.'s symptoms gradually receded in the last six years of hospitalization and he was finally placed on convalescent care. His treatment in the hospital during the 18 years included electro-shock, insulin shock, sodium amytal injections and thorazine. An excerpt from the last note in the state hospital written by the psychiatrist is as follows: "patient is a chronic schizophrenic who has made an excellent hospital adjustment . . . goes to art classes and does excellent work. . . apparently hallucinating but doesn't act anti-socially to these. He expresses interest in getting a job as an illustrator with some advertising company but **it is doubtful whether he can maintain sufficient drive and interest to hold a position for long."** [bold added]

L. M. was referred to the day treatment center for readjustment to the community and stimulation toward employment after one month of convalescence at home. The program in the day treatment center was mainly organized toward preparing L. M. for employment.

The occupational therapist organized L. M.'s activity program around the preparation of an art portfolio for a prospective employer. Techniques in advertising art were practiced by L. M. with the support of the occupational therapist. Contacts with commercial artists in the community were made, to determine what should go into an art portfolio and the level of quality expected in getting an entry level job.

During this time L. M. was attending college at night taking commercial art courses. He had been sponsored at the college through the Division of Vocational Rehabilitation. L. M. gained self-esteem and confidence, from other members at the day center who recognized his artistic abilities. He gained additional self-confidence when he was requested to do a poster, or design a birthday card for a member or for one of the professional staff. This made him feel useful and productive, important in his reintegration of self, after spending most of his life in a passive-dependent state. L. M. assisted other members engaging in art activities in the occupational therapy program. L. M. felt that the day treatment center was truly a therapeutic community and he showed a sense of pride and responsibility in actively participating in patient government.

After one year in the day treatment center, L. M. felt he was ready for employment. He was also encouraged and motivated by the staff. He was referred to various employment agencies and he presented his art portfolio to many employers. He showed remarkable resiliency and refused to be discouraged even after repeated rejections. After awhile he found a position as a delivery man in a small advertising firm through the state employment agency specializing in placements for individuals with physical and mental disabilities. In spite of his advanced training and skill in art he accepted this position because it put him in contact with the field of commercial art. This initial job eventually led him to a full-time commercial art position.

After discharge from the Day Treatment Center, L. M. has been successful in his job and social interactions. He lived with his older parents, while working full time, attending art school at night and doing free-lance art work in his spare time. Over the years he has continued to keep in contact with the members and staff of the Day Treatment Center trying to be of help to other people like himself who had been severely ill for long periods of time. Remarkably, after 20 years of non-productivity, L. M. had been able to return to the community through the transitional experience of a day treatment center. (pp. 33–34)

Supported Competitive Employment

A successful psychosocial rehabilitation agency in Chicago, Thresholds, was awarded a 3-year grant from the Robert Wood Johnson Foundation to "provide community employment and ongoing support to persons with a wide range of psychiatric impairments and diversity of career goals" (Cook & Razzo, 1992, p. 23). Although approximately 50 percent of the clients had been employed during their participation in the program, a survey taken during the 1987/1988 fiscal year revealed that many of these clients were no longer employed 6 months after discharge from the program. "It appeared that clients were unable to maintain the vocational gains they had made, with agency support, after leaving the agency. Moreover, there was evidence that clients benefited from *longer* rather than *shorter* periods of employment support" (p. 24). As a result, the agency designed a program that would (a) provide maximal flexibility allowing for individualization of services based on the needs of the client and (b) provide training at the workplace so that maximum generalization of task and support could be provided. Thirdly, services were to be provided outside of the agency setting to reduce stigma of the client.

The program, called the Thresholds' Supported Competitive Employment (SCE) Program consisted of three components: (a) a day program in which members of an interdisciplinary team assisted the client in achieving such goals in employment, self-care, independent living, education, socialization, and coping skills to prevent rehospitalization; (b) a placement program for those completing goals from (a) and who needed continued vocational support to ensure retention of present jobs; and (c) a long-term program for clients who "often had been unsuccessful in finding or maintaining employment . . . [but who] desired some sort of structured programming" (p. 32). Clients in the latter component focused on independent living skills and social skills necessary for community employment.

Success in the program has been attributed to a number of factors. First, because clients have different needs, no one program will meet everyone's needs. By providing a number of different types and amounts of employment support, clients and team members reported a high level of satisfaction and success. Second, telephone calls, as well as face-to-face meetings, were found to be an effective type of support. The telephone provided convenient check-ins for both employers and clients and allowed for contact in a "non-stigmatizing context" (p. 38). Third, recognition that vocational support is not effective unless therapists consider social and interpersonal needs and developmental issues, along with skills training and vocational support. By emphasizing a holistic approach to rehabilitation, using a multidimensional outcome model (Anthony & Farkas, 1982), therapy can be structured to meet the needs of individual clients, rather than structuring the client to meet the needs of the program. Cook and Razzo (1992) suggest, however, that this may not occur unless we rethink two basic assumptions of funding: "first, that clients need support for a time-limited period, after which they should be 'closed'; and second, that support needs 'fade' in a simple linear fashion over time on the job" (p. 40).

COMMUNITY CARE MODEL APPLIED TO YOUTH AT RISK

In addition to the growth of CMHC, attempts have been made to find alternatives to the institutional care among those involved in criminal activity, antisocial behavior, or substance abuse. Reforms have been introduced to change the environment from penal institutions and mental hospitals to community care facilities. This model is within the tradition of humanistic caring and moral treatment. Reformers raised the questions: Is institutional care self-defeating, demoralizing to the individual, and a factor in increasing antisocial attitudes? Are there community rehabilitation models that are effective alternatives to institutionalization? These questions threaten the very existence of locked institutions that do not prepare the individual adequately for independent living in the community.

Therapeutic Goals for Youth at Risk

The residential treatment center (RTC) in the community provides an opportunity to intervene in the youth at risk's life to prevent delinquency and to increase the avenues for achieving success. The RTC is organized to provide therapeutic services in three essential areas: cognitive and educational development, vocational identity, and social value systems.

These three areas are critical in effecting change in a youth's life. In the cognitive-educational area we find that, characteristically, children who are socially disadvantaged are not prepared for a traditional middle-class curriculum when they enter the primary grades. Riessman (1967) in a study, *The Culturally Deprived Child*, presented a composite of disadvantaged youths

who, typically, have skills in externally oriented physical activities. These youths, according to Reissman, are content-centered and are concrete and inductive in analyzing information.

Minorities underutilize CMHCs, often because the philosophy of the CMHCs does not reflect their beliefs and values. One culturally specific model of community mental health was developed by Camphinha-Bacote (1991) for African-American clients with a dual diagnosis of substance abuse and mental illness. In another case, Yau (1997) developed a program for Southeast Asian adolescents and young adult refugees. He advocated that occupational therapists can help clients by "developing occupational therapy services that are appropriate and culturally relevant" (p. 1). This can be done by providing opportunities to "(1) practice appropriate human occupations and establish more satisfying relationships; (2) facilitate release and sublimation of emotional drives; (3) enhance smooth transition and adaptation to the new environment; and (4) assist in the adoption of appropriate occupational roles" (p. 1).

Likewise, Native American youth, forced to accept values and beliefs contrary to their cultural heritage, are at risk for emotional and behavioral disorders (Barlow & Walkup, 1998). Although there is a need for more systematic data collection regarding the prevalence and incidence of mental illness in the Native American population, reports from mental health agencies and therapists suggest widespread concern about the numbers of Native American youth who are depressed and have attempted suicide or who have a conduct disorder. A survey of council members on a North Dakota Indian Reservation completed by Tyler, Clark, and Cohen (1986) cited the following problems (p. 134):

▶ parent/child relationships, home environments (53%)

▶ inhalant abuse (44%)

▶ school problems, absenteeism, dropping out of school (37%)

▶ abuse of alcohol or other drugs (32%)

▶ lack of employment opportunities (26%)

▶ lack of recreational activities (21%)

▶ low self-esteem (16%)

A wide range of stressors such as family issues (e.g., poverty, unemployment, alcoholism), interpersonal conflict, social disintegration, acculturation, and school issues appear to contribute to mental health needs. Although proposals for mental health services for Native Americans are similar to those for mainstream populations (e.g., hospitalization, outpatient care, halfway houses, therapeutic group homes, home-based interventions), the unavailability of resources, therapists, or treatment centers results in a lack of effective mental health services. Additionally, inattention to the cultural differences in healing between traditional Native American and Western mental health practices may hinder rehabilitation (U.S. Congress, 1990). In working with Native American youth, psychosocial occupational therapists who are sensitive to the cultural needs of the individual and the traditional healing practices may be more successful in helping these patients improve.

Specialized educational programs such as Head Start, compensatory education, work-study modified curriculum, Outward Bound, New Careers, Comprehensive Employment Training (CETA), and Job Corps have been used successfully in the past to meet the cognitive and educational needs of youth at risk (Altschuler & Armstrong, 1994; Ewert, 1982; Frost & Rowland, 1971; Levine, 1971; U.S. Department of Justice, Office of Justice programs, Office of Juvenile Justice and Delinquency Prevention, 1995).

In the second area (i.e., vocational identity), programs have been applied to help disadvan-taged youth develop occupational aspirations and vocational careers. Studies have shown that by the time a child is 10 years of age, he or she has already developed a self-identity that influences his or her attitudes toward classroom learning. In Erikson's terms, the child had internalized feelings of industry and activity competence (Erikson, 1963). Many educators, including Jonathan Kozol (1967) in *Death at an Early Age* and John Holt in *How Children Fail* (1964), have described the process of how the child gives up and tunes out the classroom teacher. By 10, the disadvantaged child is often in a special education program where progress may be slow and materials may not be appropriate to the child's interest or educational needs. When the student is moved to high school, work-study programs are often implemented to the detriment of academic progress. The inevitable path from early school failure to the lack of occupational preparation is thus perpetuated.

The third area for therapeutic intervention is related to social value systems. Here we are concerned with the lifestyle of the disadvantaged youth. The question faced by many professionals is, should we impose our middle-class or societal values as goals for therapy? Robert Coles (1968), a psychiatrist, in an article, "The Poor Don't Want to be Middle Class," confronted this issue directly:

> What we will continue to have is the presence of people who are still largely outside our middle-class world, with its widespread emphasis on competition, innovation, individual achievement, and constantly increasing consumption. Many of the poor have never found such goals, as well as the cautions and restraints of suburban living, possible or rewarding. They have learned to be open and direct with one another, painfully so to many of us, but from another point of view, honestly so. (p. 197)

Previous studies (Kvaraceus & Miller; 1959; Miller, 1968; Riessman, Cohen, & Pearl, 1964) comparing the social-value systems of the disadvantaged youth with middle-class youth identified the following differences:

▶ Youth at risk are fatalistic. They tend to feel that they have very little control over their own lives. Because of an external locus of control, they take less responsibility for their own behavior while blaming things that occur on external events.

▶ Youths who come from disorganized family environments tend not to see cause-and-effect relationships in the same way as youths reared in a consistent, stable, family setting. In many instances, low-income children substitute magical thinking for deductive logic. Impulsive behavior results in an inability to recognize the long-term consequences of their actions.

▶ Immediate gratification in comparison to longitudinal planning and anticipation is characteristic of disadvantaged youths who have few opportunities for systematically engaging in activities with delayed reward. They tend not to set up long-term goals for themselves and sometimes fail to see the relationship between an investment in education and the ultimate rewards.

▶ In addition, youth at risk have not developed the introspective inner life that emerges from an environment where there are opportunities for privacy and concern for the sanctity of the individual. Rather than impose the middle-class American value system on the poor, we need to separate the positive cultural and ethnic aspects of the poor from the self-defeating behavior that leads to dependence, alienation, and feelings of hopelessness.

In addition to these three areas for therapeutic intervention (cognitive, vocational, and social), Stroul and Friedman (1986) have suggested an integrated system of care:

> A system of care is a comprehensive spectrum of mental health and other necessary services which are organized into a coordinated network to meet the multiple and changing needs of severely emotionally disturbed children and adolescents. (p. iv)

The continuum proposed by Stroul and Friedman (1986) and adapted by the Children and Adolescent Service System Program (CASSP) has led to a comprehensive, nonlinear, integrated program organized around the following service dimensions: mental health, social, educational, health, vocational, recreational, and operational/case management (Nelson & Pearson, 1991). CASSP, a national program developed in 1984 and funded by NIMH, provides grants to states enabling them to develop integrated services for youth with emotional and behavioral disorders. The vision of CASSP has been to provide a comprehensive program of child-centered, community-based services in such areas as mental health, education, social skills, vocational training, and recreation (Stroul & Friedman, 1986). The purpose of CASSP is to develop interagency models of care within each state. CASSP projects provide comprehensive, collaborative statewide mental health services for children and adolescents and ensure that individuals receive all services needed to meet their individual needs. Occupational therapists can further contribute to the rehabilitation of individuals who are socially disadvantaged in the following areas: design of therapeutic curriculums, coordination of prevocational and work-study programs, and implementation of activity group therapy experiences that foster social learning and social values.

Community Residential Treatment Center: An Organizational Case Study

A community treatment model for youth at risk that replaced the traditional reform school in Massachusetts is a model that can be adapted and applied to a wide range of social disabilities (Stein, 1972). The Charles Hayden Goodwill Inn School for Boys in Dorchester, Massachusetts was a model in the 1970s of an effective community residential treatment center for youth at risk. The Hayden Inn School, a treatment facility located in a working-class neighborhood, serviced disadvantaged youths who came from the metropolitan Boston area. Hayden Goodwill Inn was first established in 1932 in conjunction with the Traveler's Aid Society as a temporary shelter for homeless boys. Through the years it developed an educational program, summer camp in a rural setting, individual counseling, and group activities in response to the needs of the youth. As a relatively small facility, individualized treatment planning was recognized as essential to the total rehabilitation.

The residential school program was divided into four basic parts: clinical treatment services, education-vocational programming, child-care counseling, and organizational and administrative functions. The basic professional staff included a rehabilitation administrator, psychiatric social worker, special education teacher, rehabilitation counselor, child-care worker, and occupational therapy consultant. Additional consultants in the medical, psychological, and educational areas were available. Outside community agencies were relied on for placement decisions and supplementary resources. Many of the youths attended public schools so that there was a continual liaison with the Boston Public School System. Neighborhood youth corps, work-study programs, youth opportunity centers, and the Massachusetts Rehabilitation Commission were used as referral sources, especially when a youth was motivated to work in the community. Family service workers were also invited to participate in decision-making conferences when appropriate. Hayden, as a residential treatment program, tried to utilize all of the appropriate resources that were available in the community for youth at risk.

The boys living in Hayden came from the most severe environmental deprivations in urban areas characterized by social disorganization, environmental blight, and family neglect. This combination of factors made the group very vulnerable to involvement in activities that led to criminal offenses, social deviance, alcoholism, drug addiction, and emotional disturbance. This population represented a chronically neglected group of children rejected by society and who, without intervention, would eventually fill those institutions that are isolated from the community: the reformatories, state institutions for individuals with mental disturbance or developmental disabilities, and county or state penal institutions.

In trying to counteract the negative effects of the environment, Hayden school offered opportunities for self-instruction and action-oriented media, such as active learning, programmed learning materials, field trips, and motion picture productions. Because these youths had difficulty with interpersonal learning and verbal communication, individual psychotherapy, especially of the introspective of psychoanalytic kind, was not stressed. Reality therapy (Glasser, 1965), where the therapist confronts the youth with immediate issues and works through specific individual problems, was more often used. Activity group therapy with opportunities for role playing and psychodrama were additional methods used to help the youth at risk develop empathy and thus become more sensitive and responsive to others.

Other Examples of Community Treatment Programs

Another prototype for treating youth at risk was Mobilization for Youth in New York City, a community rehabilitation program that was in existence during the 1960s (Grosser, 1969). The target area for the program was New York City's Lower East Side, an urban slum with a high proportion of delinquency, public welfare, unemployment, alcoholism, drug addiction, and school dropouts. The goal of the program was to prevent delinquency by changing the social environment and create opportunities for upward mobility and avenues for success within the society at large. To institute changes in the environment a council of agencies was established, which identified potential resources of the community and the need to develop new programs. The underlying theme of Mobilization for Youth was to change the environment to prevent social deviance. The community was organized to enact changes to prevent delinquency. These areas included housing, schools, vocational training, adjudication diversion, and family issues. This community model was vulnerable to political interference because of the nature of its social activism approach, and because of this it eventually was terminated.

Another alternative to custodial care is the halfway house in the community. An example was Achievement Place in Lawrence, Kansas. In this program, a therapeutic environment was created for eight youths who stayed a maximum of 6 months. A family situation was simulated by a surrogate parent team who provided models for social learning; the child was provided the traditional services in the community such as schools, mental health centers, recreational facilities, and youth services. The primary goals of this intensive treatment setting was to modify the behavior of the child by accelerating such areas as learning, peer relationships, and self-esteem.

Frequently, children or youth with mental illness are removed from their biological families as part of the therapeutic process. Although removal may be necessary in some instances, problems arise when the individual is returned to the environment that was a factor in the dysfunction. Community-based services that use a holistic approach and treat the dysfunctional family along with the child with mental illness may be a more viable model. Integrated Resources for Family Assessment, Consultation and Education (INTERFACE) is a tertiary program in Toronto, Canada that systematically treats families while treating children with mental illness (Dydyk & O'Neill, 1993). "The philosophical perspective of INTERFACE . . . [is based on the assumption] that families are generally the healthiest places for children to be raised and that intensive input to families within their community rather than removal of their children is the preferred method of intervention" (p. 40). Seven different components of INTERFACE that provide intensive services to families include an intensive family therapy unit where whole families are admitted for an in-depth evaluation of family dynamics, in-home and in-school services that provide training and support to individual family members, and foster homes in which consistent care is provided within a family structure to children who must be removed from their biological home for a period of time. This program is unique in that the team members are committed to helping staff and families build competencies and in the belief that "what happens at one level is reflected throughout the system" (p. 39).

Girls and Boys Town was founded by Father Flanagan in Omaha, Nebraska over three-quarters of a century ago as a family style, long-term residential program to help youth who were in trouble. Since that time, the services from Girls and Boys Town have expanded from residential programs to include short-term youth shelters, a national crisis hotline, training centers for parents and teachers, and foster care programs. In addition, Boys Town has a national research hospital in Omaha, Nebraska and an inner-city alternative high school. Offices are located in at least 11 states, but through the hotline, services are provided free to anyone within the continental United States, Alaska, Hawaii, Canada, Puerto Rico, and the Virgin Islands. Approximately 800 to 1,200 calls are received daily by the organization (Boys Town, n.d.)

Girls and Boys Town provides a variety of services to children and adolescents who are homeless, neglected, abused, or emotionally disturbed. These services include food, clothing, shelter, education, spiritual, and medical care. Although anyone can call, most of the calls come from individuals 19 years old and younger. The calls are made because of home and school behavior problems, requests for counseling, family problems, drug and alcohol dependency, child abuse, suicide ideation, and running away. More information about Girls and Boys Town can be obtained by calling (402) 498–1900 or requesting information through their website (www.ffbh.boystown.org).

In the 1990s, the expanded role of the occupational therapist in CMHC includes working with the homeless. Heubner and Tryssenaar (1996), using case study methodology, described the experiences of a student occupational therapist at a homeless shelter. In this setting, the occupational therapist established a group comprised of various activities suggested by the residents. The therapist noted positive changes in communication and psychosocial functioning, even among those with lower cognitive functioning and concomitant emotional disturbance.

Implications for Occupational Therapy

The treatment of youth at risk in the perspective of a community model represents a shifting of roles for the therapist who is tied to the traditional medical model. In this new role, the occupational therapist becomes familiar with the intricacies of the criminal justice system, social and cultural aspects of poverty, adolescent behavior, and community organization. Within this model, treatment techniques, such as those used under the heading of cognitive-behavioral therapy, involve the concepts of modeling behavior, hierarchical development, positive reinforcement, development of inner controls, and the creation of structured therapeutic environments such as halfway houses.

▶ *Modeling behavior* involves discovering adult or peer models with whom the adolescent can identify and aspire to be like. These models are fostered and encouraged by the therapist by helping the adolescents, through value clarification exercises, to become more aware of their primary goals in life.

▶ *Hierarchical development* implies an evaluative-treatment model where the therapist helps the adolescent to become more aware of his or her growth potential in the social, emotional, and moral areas of development.

▶ *Development of inner controls* is a critical problem area for acting-out adolescents who have not developed self-regulating behavior and act as if they are destroying or defeating themselves. Confrontation techniques include group therapy, reality therapy, and peer interaction. Setting limits are specific techniques for developing inner control.

▶ *Positive reinforcement* implies identifying personal strengths that can be fostered in the adolescent, such as vocational competencies, abilities in sports, interpersonal relations, leadership, or artistic and creative talent. Emphasis on strengths rather than deficits is reinforced by the therapist by explicit verbal recognition or by "token" rewards.

▶ *Structured environments* are community residences such as halfway houses, drop-in centers, group homes, and foster-care boarding homes. The importance of a therapeutic milieu as part of these living arrangements is essential if these environments are to become more than a "bed" for the adolescent.

▶ *Activity groups* are client-centered and heterogeneous (mixed levels of aggressiveness and passivity) groups where the therapist fosters interpersonal growth and self-regulating behavior. These groups usually have between 8 and 12 members and meet regularly for a specified period of time. The major goals of activity groups are to provide opportunities for self-expression and self-awareness.

EVALUATING THE EFFECTIVENESS OF COMMUNITY MENTAL HEALTH PROGRAMS

Although community mental health models appear to be humane approaches in treating individuals with mental illness or social disadvantages, the efficacy of these programs is still being examined. What criteria and measurement tools can be used in evaluating the effectiveness of a community mental health program (Cheah, Parker, Hadzi-Pavlovic, Gladstone, & Eyers, 1998; Eppel, Fuyarchuk, Phelps, & Phelan, 1991; Tyler, Ozcan, & Wogen, 1995; Williams & Ozarin, 1968)? The effectiveness of occupation-

al therapy in a community mental health program can be evaluated using the following questions. More extensive and detailed evaluation is possible through the use of the evaluation tool at the end of the chapter (Stein, 1986).

1. Are the goals of occupational therapy appropriate to the needs of individuals with mental illness so that they are being prepared to deal effectively with other people in work settings and to have the basic personal and leisure skills for everyday living? Are the goals *r*elevant, *u*nderstandable, *m*easurable, *b*ehavioral, and *a*chievable (RUMBA)?

2. Does the occupational therapist use specific tests, ADL scales, or client self-evaluation to continually assess functional levels of outcome?

3. What are the potential factors (e.g., stress, family, self-esteem) that interfere with the client's ability to be independent?

4. Does the occupational therapist use SOAP (subjective, objective, assessment, plan) notes in documenting progress of the client?

5. Is there a discharge plan that incorporates a holistic approach to treatment and includes continuity of care? A model for a discharge plan is the Individualized Treatment Plan presented in Table 3–2.

In a follow-up study, Test and Stein (1975) presented data that evaluated the effectiveness of a community living program as an alternative to psychiatric hospitalization. The program was staffed by a psychiatrist, psychologist, social worker, nurses, psychiatric aides, and occupational therapists. In this innovative treatment program, the staff worked primarily in the community with the patients in their homes, with family members, and with community support agencies. The primary goals of the program were to teach individual coping skills to the patient, structure a full schedule of daily living activities in the community, and prescribe chemotherapy where appropriate. Independent living skills such as laundering, shopping, cooking, eating out, grooming, budgeting, and use of transportation were emphasized with patients in their own homes and community. The staff also worked intensively with the patients in vocational activities, such as in job placement, sheltered work, job satisfaction, and work adjustment. Other areas of staff effort included helping patients develop leisure-time activities and improve social interactions.

In discussing their results, the authors concluded that a community living model is an effective alternative to hospitalization when working with clients with mental illness. In addition they found that community living increased clients' quality of life, level of adjustment, self-esteem, and personal satisfaction. This study demonstrated that a community mental health program can be an effective preventative alternative to hospitalization.

In a related study, Linn et al. (1979) used an experimental design to evaluate the effectiveness of day treatment centers in combination with psychotropic drugs in the aftercare of patients with schizophrenia. The study took place at 10 Veteran's Administration day treatment centers located in California, Texas, Illinois, Florida, Iowa, Minnesota, and Tennessee. The three major overall goals of these day treatment centers were "(1) to improve or maintain abilities to interact successfully with family and others; (2) to provide patients a place to socialize, engage in productive activities and thereby increase their psychological and social well-being; and (3) to provide a sheltered environment that sustains patients sufficiently so that they can live outside an institutional setting" (p. 1057). The study took a total of 4 years to complete. During that time the investigators evaluated and tested patients at 6-, 12-, 18-, and 24-month intervals

on social functions, symptoms, and attitudes. The results demonstrated that there were significant differences in the effectiveness of treating patients with chronic schizophrenia. They noted that "more professional staff hours, group therapy and a high patient turnover treatment philosophy were associated with poor-result centers. More *occupational therapy* [italics added] and a sustained nonthreatening environment were more characteristic of successful outcome centers" (p. 1055). This study reinforced the conclusions based on clinical observations that the Day Treatment Center with a strong occupational therapy component is an effective model for treating patients with schizophrenia.

Another example of a community-based day treatment center (in Oakland, California) for former patients with psychiatric illness that included a transitional employment program was described by Howe, Weaver, and Dulay (1981). The program was voluntary and was open to any former patient who would like to join at any time. One day of the program was devoted to a variety of open-ended activities such as physical exercises, games, arts and crafts, lunch preparation, field trips, and special interest groups such as writing and gardening. A community meeting of the professional staff, volunteers, and members was held periodically to plan events and share experiences. The second part of the program was designed for members who were interested in formulating personal goals and redirecting their lives. Initially, this part of the program included classes on human growth and development, self-care, personal goals, and basic living skills. The program was gradually expanded to include transitional sheltered workshop experiences. This part of the program was staffed by two mental health workers, a program coordinator, two adult schoolteachers, and a full-time occupational therapist whose major responsibility was to develop a transitional employment program. The members of the work-oriented program rotated through a variety of work experiences such as recycling trash, car washing and waxing, gardening and landscaping, janitorial work, and food handling (shopping, cooking, serving, baking, and catering). The members also had the opportunity to take part in educational experiences such as independent living, clerical skill training, basic reading and math skills, women's issues, and self-awareness groups. This program demonstrated how community resources can be mobilized to rehabilitate former psychiatric patients to regain self-esteem and personal direction in their lives.

Another approach to evaluating the effectiveness of a day treatment program was described by Falloon and Talbot (1982). They reviewed the individual progress of over 200 patients who were chronically mentally ill and currently attending a day treatment program. The treatment approach was based on the self-empowerment of the patients in planning realistic goals. These goals were classified into three broad categories: (a) socialization, (b) vocational activity, and (c) treatment of behavioral disturbances. After specific goals were identified by the patient, behavioral treatment strategies were formulated to meet the individual needs of the patients. Falloon and Talbot found that "almost all patients were able to set realistic goals . . . [and] that good outcome was associated with high levels of participation of patients in defining their goals and that goals covering social and vocational functioning were achieved more frequently than intrapersonal goals" (p. 283).

Coelho, Kelley, Deatsman-Kelley, and the Clinton-Eaton-Ingham Community Mental Health Board (1993) completed an evaluation of the effectiveness of a CMHC in Michigan that provides intensive support services for individuals with the dual diagnoses of mental illness and mental retardation. The authors compared an active treatment model to a standard case management model. Forty-seven clients, all at risk for institutionalization, participated, with 24 randomly assigned to active treatment and 23 to the standard treatment. The traditional case management model consisted of counseling, advocacy, individual program development and coordination, behavior management, and placement services. These services are used and planned with an interdisciplinary team approach. In contrast, the active treatment model allowed for more contact with participants in their natural environment and involved the following individualized treatments:

> (a) intensive participation, care coordination, management and advocacy with comprehensive service planning in all areas and across disciplines; (b) individualized planning with each participant involved in the selection and planning of their own services; (c) utilization of existing community resources with facilitation and support by staff as needed; (d) training, education and support in acquisition of prosocial adaptive skills and functioning; (e) behavioral programming to reduce or eliminate maladaptive behaviors, consistent with agency policies; (f) development of measurable objectives for each participant and data–based decision making regarding progress; (g) on-site consultation, training and support for care providers in day and residential settings; (h) medication monitoring provided by the agency's psychiatrist; (i) access to 24-hour crisis intervention and support; (j) individual psychotherapy. (p. 39)

The active treatment model was found to be more effective than the standard case management model in the following ways: (a) services were provided for clients who could have fallen between the cracks in a typical structured system; (b) the mental health system was educated about the needs of those with developmental disabilities and mental illness; (c) clients in the study participated in their own services; and (d) institutionalization did not occur. Although the cost for the active treatment was high, the use of the community-based treatment was less expensive than institutionalization.

SUMMARY

During the last 30 years, the community mental health movement has drastically redefined the role of the psychosocial occupational therapist. Psychosocial treatment has become more goal directed and has generated multifaceted approaches toward helping individual clients achieve independence. The CMHC model has replaced the state mental hospital and county institution in the treatment and rehabilitation for the client with chronic mental illness. The CMHC utilizes the resources of the community and empowers clients and their families in setting therapeutic goals and implementing treatment. Therapeutic activities in a CMHC are directed at helping the client improve independent living skills, interpersonal relationships, leisure activities, and work skills through a supportive environment. A comprehensive psychosocial rehabilitation program also includes prevocational evaluation, work adjustment training, and specialized job placement in the community. Community treatment models have been expanded to the habilitation of youth and adults with social and/or developmental disabilities. Preliminary research evidence indicates that the comprehensive CMHC is a viable model replacing the state mental hospital as the primary place for treating those with mental illness or developmental disability.

REFERENCES

Adams, R. (1990). The role of occupational therapists in community mental health. *Mental Health Special Interest Section Newsletter, 13*(1), 1–2.

Altschuler, D. M., & Armstrong, T. L. (1994). *Intensive aftercare for high-risk juveniles: A community care model. Program Summary.* Washington, DC: U.S. Department of Justice, Office of Justice Programs, Office of Juvenile Justice and Delinquency Prevention.

American Association for Partial Hospitalization (AAPH). (1991). *Standards and guidelines for partial hospitalization.* (Available from American Association for Partial Hospitalization, 411 K Street NW, Suite 1000, Washington, DC 20005)

Anthony, W. A., & Farkas, M. (1982). A client outcome planning model for assessing psychiatric rehabilitation interventions. *Schizophrenia Bulletin, 8*, 13–38.

Bachrach, L. L. (1992). Psychosocial rehabilitation and psychiatry in the care of long-term patients. *American Journal of Psychiatry, 149*, 1455–1463.

Bartels, B., & Hogan, K. L. (1986). The community development specialist: A new role for rural mental health. In J. D. Murray & P. A. Keller (Eds.), *Innovations in rural community mental health* (pp. 39–53). Mansfield, PA: Rural Services Institute.

Barlow, A., & Walkup, J. T. (1998). Developing mental health services for Native American children. *Child and Adolescent Psychiatry Clinics of North America, 7*, 555–577.

Beard, J. H., Propst, R. N., & Malamud, T. J. (1982). The Fountain house model of rehabilitation. *Psychosocial Rehabilitation Journal, 5*(1), 47–53.

Beckenstein, N. (1964). The new state hospital. In L. Bellak (Ed.), *Handbook of community psychiatry and community mental health* (pp. 177–188). New York: Grune & Stratton.

Berthaume, B., Bailey, D. M., Horowitz, B., & McCrory, M. V. (1994). Cost and intensity of care in case managers' referrals to psychiatric day programs. *Hospital and Community Psychiatry, 45*, 62–65.

Best, D. (1996). The developing role of occupational therapy in psychiatric intensive care. *British Journal of Occupational Therapy, 59*, 161–164.

Bierer, J. (1964). The Marlborough experiment. In L. Bellak (Ed.), *Handbook of community psychiatry and community mental health* (pp. 221–247). New York: Grune & Stratton.

Biss, S. M., & Curtis, L. C. (1993). Crisis service systems: Beyond the emergency room. *In Community, 3*(1), 1–4.

Boys Town. (n.d.). *National hotline fact sheet.* [Brochure]. Boys Town, NE: Author.

Camphinha-Bacote, J. (1991). Community mental health services for the underserved: A culturally specific model. *Archives of Psychiatric Nursing, 5,* 229–234.

Carling, P. J. (1995). *Return to community: Building support systems for people with psychiatric disabilities.* New York: Guilford.

Cheah, Y. C., Parker, G., Hadzi-Pavlovic, D., Gladstone, G., & Eyers, K. (1998). Development of a measure profiling problems and needs of psychiatric patients in the community. *Social Psychiatry and Psychiatric Epidemiology, 33,* 337–344.

Coelho, R. J., Kelley, P. S., Deatsman-Kelley, C., & Clinton-Eaton-Ingham Community Mental Health Board. (1993). An experimental investigation of an innovative community treatment model for persons with a dual diagnosis (DD/MI). *Journal of Rehabilitation, 59*(2), 37–42.

Coles, R. (1968). The poor don't want to be middle class. In G. Natchez (Ed.), *Children with reading problems* (pp. 190–197). New York: Basic Books.

Cook, J. A., & Razzo, L. (1992). Natural vocational supports for persons with severe mental illness: Thresholds Supported Competitive Employment Program. In L. I. Stein (Ed.), *New directions for mental health services No. 52: Innovative community mental health programs* (pp. 23–41). San Francisco, Jossey-Bass.

Crawford, M., & Mee, J. (1994). The role of occupational therapy in the rehabilitation of the mentally disordered offender [Conference report]. *British Journal of Occupational Therapy, 57,* 26–28.

Dorwart, K., & Hendricks, H. (2000). *Practice trends of occupational therapy in forensic psychiatry; An organization case study with a supplemental survey of occupational therapists.* Unpublished manuscript. Available from Department of Occupational Therapy, University of South Dakota, 414 E. Clark St., Vermillion, SD 57069.

Dowell, D. A., & Ciarlo, J. A. (1989). An evaluative overview of community mental health centers program. In D. A. Rochefort (Ed.), *Handbook on mental health policy in the United States* (pp. 195–236). Westport, CT: Greenwood.

Dressler, J. & Snively, F. (1998). Occupational therapy in criminal justice system. In E. Cara & A. MacRae (Eds.), *Psychosocial occupational therapy: A clinical practice* (pp. 527–552). Albany: Delmar.

Dydyk, B., & O'Neill, I. (1993). Evolution of a service: How to stay alive and healthy in a demanding mental health world. *Journal of Child and Youth Care, 8*(4), 39–52.

Ellek, D. (1991). The evolution of fairness in mental health policy. *American Journal of Occupational Therapy, 45,* 947–951.

Eppel, A. B., Fuyarchuk, C., Phelps, D., & Phelan, A. T. (1991). A comprehensive and practical quality assurance program for community mental health services. *Canadian Journal of Psychiatry, 36,* 102–106.

Erikson, E. H. (1963). *Childhood and society.* New York: W. W. Norton.

Ettlinger, R.A., Beigl, A., & Feder, S. L. (1972). The partial hospital as a transition from inpatient treatment: A controlled follow-up study. *Mt. Sinai Journal of Medicine, 39,* 251–257.

Ewert, A. W. (1982). *A study of the effects of participation in an Outward Bound short course upon the reported self-concepts of selected participants.* Unpublished doctoral thesis, University of Oregon, Eugene.

Falloon, I., & Talbot, R. (1982). Achieving the goals of day treatment. *The Journal of Nervous and Mental Disease, 170,* 279–285.

Farnsworth, L., Morgan, S., & Fernando, B. (1987). Prison based occupational therapy. *Australian Occupational Therapy Journal, 34*(2), 40–46.

Federal Task Force on Homelessness and Severe Mental Illness. (1992). *Outcasts on Main Street: A report of the federal task force on homelessness and severe mental illness.* (DHHS Publication No.

ADM 92-1904). Washington, DC: U.S. Department of Health and Human Services.

Fidler, G. S. (1991). The challenge of change to occupational therapy practice. *Occupational Therapy in Mental Health 11*(1), 1–11.

Friedlob, S. A., Janis, G. A., & Deets-Aron, C. (1986). A hospital-connected halfway house program for individuals with long-term neuropsychiatric disabilities. *American Journal of Occupational Therapy, 40*, 271–277.

Gage, M., Cook, J. V., & Fryday-Field, K. (1997). Understanding the transition to community living after discharge from an acute care hospital: An exploratory study. *American Journal of Occupational Therapy, 51*, 96–103.

Glasser, W. (1965). *Reality therapy.* New York: Harper and Row.

Goffman, E. (1959). The moral career of the mental patient. *Psychiatry, 22*, 123–142.

Greene, L. & Cruz, A. (1981). Psychiatric day treatment as alternative to and transition from full-time hospitalization. *Community Mental Health Journal, 17*, 191–202.

Grosser, C. (1969). *Helping youth: A study of six community organization programs.* Washington, DC: Government Printing Office, Office of Juvenile Delinquency and Youth Development, HEW.

Gruenberg, E., & Turns, D. (1975). Epidemiology. In A. Freedman, H. Kaplan, & B. Sadock (Eds.), *Comprehensive textbook of psychiatry: II.* (Vol. I, 2nd ed., pp. 398–413). Baltimore: Williams & Wilkins.

Haylett, C., & Rapoport, L. (1964). Mental health consultation. In L. Bellak (Ed.), *Handbook of community psychiatry and community mental health* (pp. 319–342). New York: Grune & Stratton.

Health Forum—An American Hospital Association. (2001). *Hospital Statistics 2001 Edition.* Chicago: American Hospital Association.

Herz, M., Endicott, J., & Spitzer, R. (1971). Day vs. inpatient hospitalization: A controlled study. *American Journal of Psychiatry, 127*, 1371–1381.

Heubner, J., & Tryssenaar, J. (1996). Development of an occupational therapy practice perspective in a homeless shelter: A fieldwork experience. *Canadian Journal of Occupational Therapy, 63*, 24–32.

Holt, J. (1964). *How children fail.* New York: Pittman.

Howe, M., Weaver, C., & Dulay, J. (1981). The development of a work-oriented day center program. *American Journal of Occupational Therapy, 35*, 711–718.

Jaffe, E. (1980). The role of the occupational therapist as a community consultant: Primary prevention in mental health programming. *Occupational Therapy in Mental Health, 1*(2), 47–62.

Jones, M. (1953). *The therapeutic community.* New York: Basic Books.

Karno, M., & Schwartz, D. (1974). *Community mental health: Reflections and explorations.* Flushing, NY: Spectrum.

Kennedy, J. F. (1963). Mental illness and mental retardation. Washington, DC: *Congressional Record, 109*(Pt. 2), 1837–1842.

Koegel, P. (1996). The causes of homelessness. In J. Baumohl (Ed.), *Homelessness in America* (pp. 24–33). Phoenix, AZ: Oryx.

Koran, L. M. (1997). Mental health services. In S. Jonas (Ed.), *Health care delivery in the United States* (pp. 208–246). New York: Springer.

Kozol, J. (1967). *Death at an early age.* Boston: Houghton Mifflin.

Kvaraceus, W. C., & Miller, W. B. (1959). *Delinquent behavior, culture and the individual.* Washington, DC: National Education Association.

Lang, S. K., & Cara, E. (1989). Vocational integration for the psychiatrically disabled. *Hospital and Community Psychiatry, 40*, 890–892.

Learnard, L. T., & Deveraux, E. (1992). A model for community practice. *Hospital and Community Psychiatry, 43*, 869–871.

Levine, D. U. (Ed.). (1971). *Models for integrated education; Alternative programs of integrated education in metropolitan areas.* Worthington, OH: C. A. Jones.

Linn, M., Caffey, E. M., Klett, C. J., Hogarty, G. S., & Lamb, H. R. (1979). Day treatment and psychotropic drugs in the aftercare of schizophrenic patients: A Veterans Administration cooperation study. *Archives of General Psychiatry, 36*, 1055–1066.

Lloyd, C. (1995). Trends in forensic psychiatry. *British Journal of Occupational Therapy, 58*, 209–213.

Lloyd, C. & Guerra, F. (1988). A vocational rehabilitation programme in forensic psychiatry. *The British Journal of Occupational Therapy, 51*, 123-126.

MacKain, S. J., & Streveler, A. (1990). Social and independent living skills for psychiatric patients in a prison setting. *Behavior Modification, 14*, 490–518.

Mechanic, D. (1969). *Mental health and social policy*. Englewood Cliffs, NJ: Prentice-Hall.

Meltzoff, J., & Blumenthal, R. (1966). *The day treatment center: Principles, application and evaluation*. Springfield, IL: Charles C. Thomas.

Miller, W. B. (1968). Lower class culture as a generating milieu of gang delinquency. *Journal of Social Issues, 14*, 5–19.

Moeller, P. (1991). The occupational therapist as case manager in community mental health. *Mental Health Special Interest Section Newsletter, 14*(2), 4–5.

Murray, J. D., & Keller, P. A. (1986). *Innovations in rural community mental health*. Mansfield, PA: Rural Services Institute.

National Coalition for the Homeless. (1999a). *How many people experience homelessness? Fact Sheet # 2*. Retrieved May 29, 2000, from the World Wide Web: *http://nch.ari.net/numbers.html*.

National Coalition for the Homeless. (1999b). *Mental illness and homeless. Fact Sheet #5*. Retrieved May 29, 2000, from the World Wide Web: *http://nch.ari.net/mental.html*.

National Institute of Mental Health (NIMH). (1987). *Guidelines for comprehensive state mental health plans*: P. L. 99–990. Rockville, MD: Author.

Nelson, C. M., & Pearson, C. A. (1991). *Integrating services for children and youth with emotional and behavioral disorders*. Reston, VA: Council for Exceptional Children.

Ozarin, L. D. (1969). Occupational therapy facilities in community mental health centers. *Hospital and Community Psychiatry, 20*(9), 289–290.

Penner, D. (1978). Correctional institutions: An overview. *American Journal of Occupational Therapy, 32*, 517–524.

Regier, D. A., & Burke, J. D. (1985). Quantitative and experimental methods in psychiatry. In H. I. Kaplan & B. J. Sadock (Eds.), *Comprehensive text-*

book of psychiatry (4th ed., pp. 295–312). Baltimore: Williams & Wilkins.

Richert, G. Z., & Gibson, D. (1993). Practice settings. In H. L. Hopkins & H. D. Smith (Eds.), *Willard and Spackman's occupational therapy* (pp. 546–550). Philadelphia: Lippincott.

Riessman, F. (1967). *The culturally deprived child*. New York: Harper and Row.

Riessman, F., Cohen, J., & Pearl, A. (1964). Low income behavior and cognitive style. In F. Riessman, J. Cohen, & A. Pearl (Eds.), *Mental health of the poor* (pp. 113-118). New York: The Free Press.

Robnett, R. (1997). Paradigms of community practice. *Occupational Therapy Practice, 2*(9), 30–35.

Scaletti, R. (1999). A community development role for occupational therapists working with children, adolescents and their families: A mental health perspective. *The Australian Occupational Therapy Journal, 46*, 43–51.

Schaerfl, R. A. (1999). *Dictionary of occupational titles 1991: 2 volumes in 1* (4th Rev. ed.). Indianapolis, IN: Jist Works.

Schecter, L. (1974). Occupational therapy in a psychiatric day hospital. *American Journal of Occupational Therapy, 28*, 151–153.

Starr, P. (1982). *The social transformation of American medicine*. New York: Basic Books.

Stein, F. (1962). Work adjustment of the former psychiatric patient as a function of occupational therapy. In M. Jones & D. Kandel (Eds.), *Proceedings of the Third International Congress World Federation of Occupational Therapy, Study Course V* (pp. 30–34). Dubuque, IA: W. C. Brown.

Stein, F. (1972). Community rehabilitation of disadvantaged youth. *American Journal of Occupational Therapy, 26*, 227–283.

Stein, F. (1984). Prevocational exploration and vocational rehabilitation of the psychiatric client. *Canadian Journal of Occupational Therapy, 51*, 113–120.

Stein, F. (1986). *Descriptive evaluation of a psychosocial facility*. Unpublished tool. [Available from F. Stein, University of South Dakota, Department of Occupational Therapy, 414 E. Clark St., Vermillion, SD 57069]

Stein, F. (1990, May). I*ndividualized treatment plans.* Presentation at the Winnipeg Mental Health Association, Winnipeg, Canada. [Material available from F. Stein, University of South Dakota, School of Medicine, Department of Occupational Therapy, 414 E. Clark St., Vermillion, SD 57069]

Stein, L. I. (Ed.). (1992). *New directions for mental health services: No. 56. Innovative community mental health programs.* San Francisco: Jossey-Bass.

Stein, L. I., & Test, M. A. (Eds.). (1985). *New directions for mental health services: No. 26. The training in community living model: A decade of experience.* San Francisco: Jossey-Bass.

Stroul, B. A., & Friedman, R. M. (1986). *A system of care for severely emotionally disturbed children and youth.* Washington, DC: CASSP Technical Assistance Center.

Teske, Y. T. (1986). Occupational therapist as advocate for former mental patients in the development of a community program. *Mental Health Special Interest Section Newsletter, 9*, 1–3.

Tessler, R., & Goldman, H. (1982). *The chronically mentally ill: Assessing community support programs.* Cambridge, MA: Ballinger.

Test, M., & Stein, L. (1975, August-September). *Training in community living: Research design and results.* Presentation at the 83rd Annual Convention of the American Psychological Association, Chicago.

Turner, J. E., & TenHoor, W. J. (1979). The NIMH Community Support Program: Pilot approach to a needed social reform. *Schizophrenia Bulletin, 4*, 310–344.

Tyler, J. D., Clark, J. S., & Cohen, K. N. (1986). Community consultation in an Indian reservation setting. In J. D. Murray & P. A. Keller (Eds.), *Innovations in rural community mental health* (pp. 131–141). Mansfield, PA: Rural Services Institute.

Tyler, L. H., Ozcan, Y. A., & Wogen, S. E. (1995). Mental health case management and technical efficiency. *Journal of Medical Systems, 19*, 413–423.

U.S. Congress, Office of Technology Assessment. (1990, January). *Indian adolescent mental health.* Report No. OTA-H-446. Washington, DC: Government Printing Office.

U.S. Department of Health and Human Services, Substance Abuse and Mental Health Services Administration, Center for Mental Health Services (1996). *Community Mental Health Centers Construction Monitoring Program.* Retrieved May 29, 2000 from the World Wide Web: *http://www.mentalhealth.org/publications/allpubs/archive/ken95-0013/ken950013.html.*

U.S. Department of Justice, Office of Justice Programs, Office of Juvenile Justice and Delinquency Prevention. (1995). *Guide for implementing the comprehensive strategy for serious, violent, and chronic juvenile offenders.* Washington, DC: Author.

U.S. Office of Justice (1999). *More than a quarter million prison and jail inmates are identified as mentally ill.* Retrieved May 29, 2000, from World Wide Web: *http://www.ojp.usdoj.gov/bjs/pub/press/mhtip.pr.*

U.S. Substance Abuse and Mental Health Services Administration, Center for Mental Health Services. (1999). Unpublished data. In U.S. Department of Commerce, Bureau of the Census. *Statistical abstract of the United States, 1999* (p. 144, Table No. 221). Washington, DC: Government Printing Office. Retrieved May 25, 2000, from the World Wide Web: *http://www.census.gov/statab/www/.*

Wales, B. (1960). Rewards of illness: Observations on institutionalization by a former neuropsychiatric patient. *Mental Hygiene, 44*, 55–63.

Watanabe, D. Y., & Watson, L. T. (1987). Psychiatric consultation–liaison: Role of the occupational therapist. *Mental Health Special Interest Section Newsletter, 10*(2), 1, 6, 7.

Weinberg, S. K. (1967). T*he sociology of mental disorders: Analyses and reading in psychiatric sociology.* Chicago: Aldine.

Wilberding, D. (1991). The quarterway house: More than an alternative of care. *Occupational Therapy in Mental Health, 11*(1), 65–91.

Williams, R., & Ozarin, L. (Eds). (1968). *Community mental health: An international perspective.* San Francisco: Jossey-Bass.

Woodside, H. (1985). The day center and its role as a social network. *Hospital and Community Psychiatry, 36*, 177–180.

Yau, M. K. (1997). The impact of refugee resettle-
    ment on Southeast Asian adolescents and young
    adults: Implications for occupational therapists.
    Occupational Therapy International, 4, 1–16.

Chapter 3 Appendix
Descriptive Evaluation of Psychosocial Occupational Therapy Program
University of South Dakota - Occupational Therapy Department
Developed by F. Stein, Ph.D., OTR/L, FAOTA

I.   **Description of Facility** _____

Name of Facility: _____

Address: _____

_____

City	State	Zip Code	Telephone

E-mail address: _____

URL address: _____

1. **Facility Type (check all that apply)**	2. **Maximum Capacity**	3. **Avg. Daily Census**	4. **Avg. Length Hospital Stay**
a. ____ Community Housing	_____	_____	_____
b. ____ Community Mental Health Center	_____	_____	_____
c. ____ Forensic Psychiatric Unit	_____	_____	_____
d. ____ In-Patient Psychiatric Unit in General Hospital	_____	_____	_____
e. ____ Nursing Home	_____	_____	_____
f. ____ Psychiatric Hospital	_____	_____	_____
g. ____ Residential Treatment Center (RTC) for children and adolescents	_____	_____	_____
h. ____ Veterans Administration Hospital	_____	_____	_____
i. ____ Work Adjustment Center	_____	_____	_____
j. ____ Other	_____	_____	_____

II. **Patient Characteristics**

How was information furnished? (e.g., Hospital Administrator, Published Statistics) _____

_____

A. Demographics

5. Approximate age range of patients: ____ to ____

6. Approximate percent of adult patients who are married: ____%

7-8. Approximate distribution of gender: ____% female   ____% male

9. Approximate percent of adult patients on governmental supplemental income or social security disability: _____%

10. Approximate percent of adult patients completing high school or above: _____%

B. Diagnoses: Approximate percent of patients in following diagnostic groups from DSM-IV:

11. Anxiety Disorders, (e.g., Agoraphobia) _____%

12. Childhood Disorders (e.g., Autism, ADHD, Conduct Disorder) _____%

13. Developmental Disabilities _____%

14. Eating Disorders _____%

15. Mood Disorders, (e.g., Major Depression) _____%

16. Organic Mental Disorders, (e.g., Dementia) _____%

17. Personality Disorders (e.g., Antisocial Behavior) _____%

18. Schizophrenic Disorders _____%

19. Substance-Related Disorders, (e.g., Alcoholism, Drug Addiction) _____%

20. Other _____ _____%

TOTAL   **100%**

C. Chronicity of Illness: Approximate percent of patients:

21. New psychiatric episode, first hospitalization or treatment: _____%

22. Two or three episodes of illness: _____%

23. Numerous psychiatric hospitalizations: _____%

TOTAL   **100%**

III. Percent of Current Treatment Services Offered
Who furnished information? _____

A. Approximate percent of patients receiving:

24. Electroconvulsive treatment (ECT) _____%

25. Family therapy _____%

26. Group therapy/counseling at least once weekly _____%

27. Individual psychotherapy at least once weekly _____%

28. Neuroleptic or psychotropic drugs _____%

29. Occupational therapy _____%

B.   Approximate percent of patients receiving other therapeutic services:

    30. Art therapy   _____%

    31. Bibliotherapy   _____%

    32. Dance therapy   _____%

    33. Music therapy   _____%

    34. Play therapy   _____%

    35. Recreational therapy   _____%

    36. Other _____   _____%

    37. Other _____   _____%

IV. Specific Psychosocial Occupational Therapy Services

A. Evaluation

What standardized instruments are used by the occupational therapist? (Check all tests used. Check yes even if you use a part of the instrument.)

	YES	NO	
38.	____	____	Allen Cognitive Levels (ACL)
39.	____	____	Assessment of Motor Proficiency Scale (AMPS)
40.	____	____	Attention Deficit Disorders Evaluation Scale (ADDES)
41.	____	____	Bay Area Functional Performance Evaluation (BaFPE)
42.	____	____	Canadian Occupation Performance Measure (COPM)
43.	____	____	Comprehensive Evaluation of Basic Living Skills (CEBLS)
44.	____	____	Hare Psychopathy Checklist—Revised (PCL-R)
45.	____	____	Independent Living Skills Evaluation (ILS)
46.	____	____	Kohlman Evaluation of Living Skills (KELS)
47.	____	____	Milwaukee Evaluation of Daily Living Skills (MEDLS)
48.	____	____	Mini-Mental State (MMS)
49.	____	____	Occupational Case Analysis Interview and Rating Scale (OCAIRS)
50.	____	____	Stress Management Questionnaire (SMQ)
51.	____	____	Other* _____
52.	____	____	Other* _____

*If more than two, list on opposite side.

Do you use a custom-made unpublished evaluation tool? (Check)

        YES   NO

53. _____   _____   Clinical observations

54. _____   _____   Evaluation of work adjustment

55. _____   _____   Independent living skills or ADL skills

56. _____   _____   Interest check list

57. _____   _____   Initial interview guide

58. _____   _____   Personality characteristics (mental status examination)

59. _____   _____   Other _____

60. _____   _____   Other _____

B. Treatment Techniques and Procedures: Do you use the following treatment groups in occupational therapy? (Check all groups used). After you have checked all the treatment groups that are used in occupational therapy, rank order groups in terms of importance to overall goals of hospital or agency, with rank 1 being the most important.

        YES   NO   RANK

61. _____   _____   Assertiveness training   73._____

62. _____   _____   Cognitive training   74._____

63. _____   _____   Independent living skills (e.g., cooking,   75._____
                           transportation, grooming)

64. _____   _____   Exercise group   76._____

65. _____   _____   Expressive/creative therapies   77._____

66. _____   _____   Leisure time activities   78._____

67. _____   _____   Social skills (e.g., interpersonal communication,   79._____
                           problem-solving skills)

68. _____   _____   Stress management   80._____

69. _____   _____   Values clarification   81._____

70. _____   _____   Work Adjustment training   82._____

71. _____   _____   Other _____ 83._____

72. _____   _____   Other _____ 84._____

Treatment Modalities: Do you use the following treatment modalities or activities in occupational therapy? (Check all modalities or activities used). After you have checked all the modalities or activities used in occupational therapy, rank order the **first 10 activities** in relation to overall importance in psychosocial rehabilitation with rank 1 being the most important.

YES   NO   RANK

85. ____ ____ Adaptive equipment or assistive devices   104. ____
86. ____ ____ Appreciation (e.g., music, films)   105. ____
87. ____ ____ Arts and crafts (e.g., water color, ceramics, leather)   106. ____
88. ____ ____ Assembly tasks (e.g., models or carpentry)   107. ____
89. ____ ____ Cooking, or meal preparation   108. ____
90. ____ ____ Community field trips   109. ____
91. ____ ____ Creative arts (e.g., poetry, drama, writing)   110. ____
92. ____ ____ Educational courses (e.g., literature, arithmetic)   111. ____
93. ____ ____ Horticulture   112. ____
94. ____ ____ Independent living skills (e.g., grooming, transportation)   113. ____
95. ____ ____ Individual or competitive sports   114. ____
96. ____ ____ Microcomputers   115. ____
97. ____ ____ Prescriptive exercise   116. ____
98. ____ ____ Relaxation techniques (e.g., visualization, progressive relaxation, biofeedback)   117. ____
99. ____ ____ Role playing, behavior rehearsal or psychodrama   118. ____
100. ____ ____ Simulated prevocational tasks   119. ____
101. ____ ____ Table games (e.g., Trivial Pursuit, chess)   120. ____
102. ____ ____ Other _____   121. ____
103. ____ ____ Other _____   122. ____

Description of Occupational Therapy Personnel

123. Director/Coordinator of OT Program:

Specialization: a) PsyOT ____   b) PhysMedOT ____   c) Other ____

Director/Coordinator Psychosocial Occupational Therapy Services

124. number of years in psychosocial practice   ____

125. highest degree attained: (circle)   Diploma   Baccalaureate   Masters   Doctorate

126. approximate percent time in all administrative duties   ____%

127. approximate percent of time in direct treatment   ____%

Occupational Therapy Staff

128. number of full-time OTRs (including directors)   _____

129. number of part-time OTRs   _____

130. number of full-time COTAs (assistants)   _____

131. number of part-time COTAs (assistants)   _____

Other staff under occupational therapy. List titles and numbers.

Title (e.g., recreational therapy)   Number

132. _____   _____

133. _____   _____

134. _____   _____

Occupational Therapy Staff Roles

Approximate percent of time spent in:	OTR	COTA/OT Asst
• direct patient evaluation	135. _____%	144. _____%
• direct patient treatment	136. _____%	145. _____%
• maintenance of equipment and supplies	137. _____%	146. _____%
• planning treatment groups	138. _____%	147. _____%
• preparing progress notes and reports	139. _____%	148. _____%
• professional development	140. _____%	149. _____%
• staff or team meetings	141. _____%	150. _____%
• student education	142. _____%	151. _____%
• Other _____	143. _____%	152. _____%

Occupational Therapy Facilities

153. Does the Occupational Therapy Director have an individual office?   Yes _____   No_____

154. Do the occupational therapy staff have either shared or   Yes _____   No_____
      private office space?

Check below all the laboratories or work areas used in Occupational Therapy. After you have checked off all the laboratory and clinical space used in occupational therapy, please rank order the space most widely used with 1 being the most used area.

Treatment Labs	**Rank**
155. _____ Ceramics with Kiln	165._____
156. _____ General Activity Area	166._____
157. _____ Group Therapy Room	167._____
158. _____ Gymnasium or Exercise Room	168._____
159. _____ Kitchen	169._____
160. _____ Relaxation Therapy Room	170._____
161. _____ Weaving and Fibers with Table or Floor Looms	171._____
162. _____ Woodworking with Power Machines	172._____
163. _____ Other _____	173._____
164. _____ Other _____	174._____

V. **Overall Treatment or Rehabilitation Goals of Facility**

Respondent's Title _____

(Check all appropriate goals.)

175. _____ Ability to manage stress

176. _____ Develop problem-solving abilities (e.g., look for apartment or housing)

177. _____ Development of leisure time activities

178. _____ Improve educational skills (e.g., arithmetic, reading)

179. _____ Improvement in social skills (e.g., interpersonal relationships)

180. _____ Improvement in daily living activities (e.g., grooming)

181. _____ Increase physical well being (e.g., improve dietary habits, exercise program)

182. _____ Increase self-esteem (e.g., realistic view of self and capacities)

183. _____ Preparation for employment or return to job

184. _____ Reduce alcohol or drug dependence

185. _____ Reduce smoking

186. _____ Reduction of psychiatric symptoms (e.g., hallucinations, delusions, anxiety, depression)

187. _____ Self-expression

188. _____ Improve cognitive skills

189. _____ Other _____

190. _____ Other _____

191. _____ Other _____

After you have checked off treatment goals, please rank order the **10 most important goals** of facility with 1 being most important.

ATTACH TO THE QUESTIONNAIRE THE FOLLOWING:

1. An organizational chart of the treatment facility showing occupational therapy position in the institution

2. Unpublished or custom-designed tests used by occupational therapists

3. An example of a progress note used in occupational therapy that includes initial interview, improvement, and discharge summary

Other comments regarding program and questionnaire:

CHAPTER

Theoretical Models Underlying the Clinical Practice of Psychosocial Occupational Therapy

> *Occupational therapy has its origin in philosophy. It is from philosophy that we derive and understand our assumptions, ethics, art, and science. . . . Practice . . . generates data that may be used to gain knowledge about the effectiveness of practice or to refine the theoretical foundation of the profession.*
>
> —A. C. Mosey, 1986, Psychosocial Components of Occupational Therapy, p. 5.

Operational Learning Objectives

By the end of this chapter, the learner will:

1. Describe the characteristics of a theory.

2. Describe how theories are clustered into theoretical models.

3. Define what frames of reference means and how these frames of reference relate to clinical practice.

4. Identify the major theorists within theoretical models or frames of reference.

5. Identify the major definitions, components, and assumptions of the Psychodynamic, Cognitive-Behavioral, Developmental, and Occupational-Behavioral frames of reference.

6. Discuss the major frames of reference used by occupational therapists in psychosocial practice.

7. Identify how frames of reference generate specific assessment practices and treatment techniques.

8. Generate occupational therapy activities that relate to the psychodynamic frames of reference.

9. Describe how clients use ego defense mechanisms in everyday life.

10. Discuss the impact of psychoanalytic theory on the practice of psychosocial occupational therapy.

11. Describe the history of behaviorism and how it relates to Cognitive-Behavioral frame of reference.

12. Define the Cognitive-Behavioral frame of reference and discuss how it is used in treatment with clients with depression, schizophrenia, and alcoholism.

13. Describe Allen's (1985) Cognitive Disability frame of reference.

14. Define the developmental theoretical model and frames of reference derived from this model.

15. Define the Sensory Integration frame of reference.

16. Describe the treatment approaches that are an outgrowth of the Sensory Integration (Ayres, 1963; Fisher, Murray, & Bundy, 1991) frame of reference and the developmental theoretical model.

17. Discuss systems theory and how it relates to the Occupational-Behavioral frame of reference.

18. Describe Kielhofner's (1995, 1997) Model of Human Occupation frame of reference and explain how it applies to therapeutic intervention.

19. Describe Reilly's (1974a, 1974b) Work-Play frame of reference.

20. Describe the Canadian Occupational Performance (1997) Model frame of reference.

21. Describe the Schkade and Schultz (1993) Occupational Adaptation frame of reference.

22. Describe the Occupational Science frame of reference as defined by Zemke and Clark (1996).

THEORIES AND THEORETICAL MODELS

In this chapter, some of the major questions discussed include:

▶ What are common characteristics of each theory in a theoretical model?

▶ What are the essential components or characteristics that classify a theory into a given theoretical model?

▶ How do theoretical models relate to frames of references cited in occupational therapy literature?

▶ How do theoretical models generate specific assessment procedures and treatment techniques?

Like many of the Allied Health professions, occupational therapy has had a long past and a short history. Historically, in mental hospitals, activities were used as curative modalities centuries before occupational therapy became a profession. In the past, tradition and trial and error guided the therapists in applying activities to treating those with physical and mental illness. It was not until the formulation of scientific theories and application of research toward the end of the 19th century that the understanding of the etiology of disease emerged (Dubos, 1959). It is not a coincidence that occupational therapy became a profession after the onset of the scientific revolution in medicine at the turn of the 20th century. Theories emerged predicting that diseases were caused by microorganisms that could be prevented by vaccines or treated by biological chemicals. Theories in medicine generated research studies that became the basis for clinical medicine. The direct link between theory and practice was strengthened by the quality of the research methodology (internal validity) and universality of application (external validity). In this model, theory serves to generate research that produces results that directly impact on practice (Miller, Sieg, Ludwig, Shortridge, & Van Deusen, 1988).

A scientific theory implies that phenomena or events in the world can be explained in a logical or rational way. For example, if an individual becomes depressed, a psychological theory attempts to explain the etiology of the depression. A theory also attempts to predict events in nature. For example, the theory of genetic determinacy will predict that a child born to a parent with schizophrenia will have a greater probability of showing symptoms of schizophrenia than a child born to typical parents (Battaglia et al., 1991). A scientific theory also generates a new vocabulary and a new perspective in examining, or interpreting, natural phenomena. The theory of psychoanalysis encompassed a new language where familiar terms are given specified meanings, such as id, ego, superego, unconscious, libido, and catharsis. These terms lose their ordinary connotations and they take on the precise meanings that were defined by Freud (1933/1953–1974). Scientific theories are dynamic and change to accommodate new research findings or discoveries of natural phenomena. Darwin's (1898) theory of evolution was shaped by his observations of animal behavior and examination of fossils. He formulated a theory from years of painstaking field observations. The pieces of evidence he amassed on animal and plant evolution were like mosaics that he put together like a picture puzzle to form a comprehensive theory. His research expeditions were guided by questions that continually sought to explain the wide variations in animal behavior he observed in his natural explorations in South America.

Characteristics of a Theory

In general a theory is defined as "a set of interrelated constructs (concepts), definitions and propositions that present a systematic view of phenomena by specifying relations among variables, with the purpose of explaining and predicting the phenomena" (Kerlinger, 1973, p. 9). Scientific theories are characterized by certain assumptions:

▶ A technical vocabulary, language, or terms are generated by a theory.

▶ Natural phenomena or behavior can be explained by a theory.

▶ A theory is a tentative set of beliefs that can be verified by scientific research.

▶ A theory predicts events that can be simulated in the laboratory or observed under controlled conditions.

▶ A theory enables a researcher to interpret results and to form conclusions.

▶ A theory generates knowledge and leads to the development of further theory.

▶ A theory can be completely or partially true or completely or partially false.

Theoretical Models

Theories can be clustered into theoretical models. A theoretical model has a number of theories that have similar components and assumptions. For example, in the psychodynamic theoretical model, the theories of Freud (1933/1953-1974), Adler (1939), Jung (1961), Sullivan (1953), and Reich (1949) are all interrelated because of the similarity between their components and assumptions. However, each theorist within the theoretical model has his or her own distinguishing viewpoints. In occupational therapy, frames of references have been derived from theoretical models. For example, the analytic frame of reference was derived from the psychodynamic theoretical model.

A frame of reference is a set of interrelated, internally consistent concepts, definitions, and postulates derived from or compatible with empirical data that provide a systematic description of or prescription for particular designs of the environment for the purpose of facilitating evaluation and effecting change relative to a specified part of the profession's domain of concern. (Mosey, 1986, p. 376)

Clinical practice, evaluation and assessment, and treatment techniques are derived from specific frames of reference. For example, projective tests are derived from a psychodynamic theoretical model and frame of reference. Relaxation techniques are derived from a cognitive–behavioral frame of reference. Figure 4–1 shows the relationship among theoretical models, frames of reference, and clinical practice. In the holistic practice of psychosocial occupational therapy, humanism, a theoretical model, is a thread that permeates all frames of reference and clinical practices. Humanism is a philosophical view of the world that emphasizes respect for the dignity of the individual. In a humanistic view of psychiatry, an individual's needs are of primary importance and treatment is tailored to meet these needs. Thus, client-centered treatment, a humanistic approach, underlies psychodynamic, cognitive–behavioral, developmental, and occupation frames of reference. In clinical practice, occupational therapists consider the client's need to self-actualize, and the therapist's unconditional positive regard for the client.

In the following sections, the authors discuss the major theoretical models and the occupational therapy frames of reference derived from these models. Important contributors to the theoretical models and frames of reference, as well as the definitions of the theoretical models are found in Table 4–1.

PSYCHODYNAMIC THEORETICAL MODEL

Definition/Assumptions/Components

The psychodynamic theoretical model is derived from the theories of Freud who did most of his writings at the turn of the 20th century. This model is defined as the application of verbal and nonverbal methods to understand the personality and thoughts of individuals by analyzing their dreams, free associations, and ego defense mechanisms. The psychodynamic theoretical model led to the "talking cure," which is the basis for psychotherapy. The psychodynamic movement started from the initial theories of Freud (1933/1953–1974) and led to other related theories formulated by Adler (1933/1974; 1956), Jung (1961), Sullivan (1953), Horney (1939), Blum (1953), Reich (1949), and others (see Table 4–1). The psychodynamic theoretical model also fostered art therapy, dance therapy, and poetry therapy where the therapist uses nonverbal or literary modalities to help the client express feelings in a creative nonthreatening environment. Rogerian nondirective, client-centered psychotherapy (Rogers, 1942), Berne's (1961) transactional analysis, Erikson's (1950, 1963) theory of the eight stages of man, Perls' (1965) Gestalt therapy focusing on self-awareness, Winnicott's (1965) object-relations theory, and Maslow's (1968) theory of self-actualization, were also influenced by Freud's initial work on psychoanalysis and the psychodynamic theoretical model. What are the key assumptions of the psychodynamic theoretical model?

Assumptions

1. Adult personality is formed in early childhood through genetic influences, experiences in the family, and interactions in the environment.

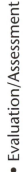

CLINICAL PRACTICE

- Evaluation/Assessment
- Treatment Techniques

MAJOR FRAMES OF REFERENCE IN PSYCHOSOCIAL OCCUPATIONAL THERAPY

HUMANISM

- Psychodynamic
- Cognitive-Behavioral
- Developmental
- Occupational Behavior

MAJOR THEORETICAL MODELS UNDERLYING PSYCHOSOCIAL PRACTICE

- Humanism
- Psychodynamic
- Behaviorism
- Developmental
- General Systems

Figure 4–1. Relationship among major theoretical models of psychosocial practice, frames of reference in occupational therapy, and clinical practice. Note that Humanism underlies all of the occupational therapy frames of reference.

Table 4-1. Relationship among Theoretical Models, Theories, and Occupational Therapy Frames of References

	Theoretical Models			
	Psychodynamic	*Behaviorism*	*Developmental*	*Systems Theory*
Theorists	S. Freud (1933)	J. Watson (1924)	A. Gesell (1928)	L. von Bertalanffy (1968)
	A. Adler (1933)	B. F. Skinner (1953)	J. Piaget (1929)	M. Reilly (1971)
	K. Horney (1939)	W. Glasser (1965)	L. S. Vygotsky (1962)	U. Bronfenbrenner (1977)
	C. Rogers (1942)	A. Ellis (1970)	K. Z. Lorenz (1965)	
	W. Reich (1949)	A. Beck (1976)	L. Kohlberg (1971)	
	H. Sullivan (1953)	A. Bandura (1977)	R. Havighurst (1972)	
	C. Jung (1961)	D. Meichenbaum (1977)		
	E. Berne (1961)			
	E. Erikson (1950, 1963)			
	F. Perls (1965)			
	D. Winnicott (1965)			

	Occupational Therapy Frame of Reference			
	Psychodynamic	*Cognitive–Behavioral*	*Developmental*	*Occupational– Behavioral*
Definition	Dynamic interpretation and analysis of personality and behavior	Application of self-regulation methods and therapeutic strategies to change thinking, behavior, and environment	A biopsychosocial model that describes the hierarchical and sequential patterns of growth as the basis for treatment	A holistic and eclectic model that focuses on the individual's daily occupations as a means to master the environment
Theorists	A. Mosey (1986)	F Stein (1982)	A. Ayres (1979)	G. Kielhofner (1995, 1997)
	G. Fidler & J. Fidler (1963)	F. Stein & S. Nikolic (1989)	B. Bobath (1978)	M. Reilly (1974b)
		F. Stein & J. Smith (1989)	L. J. King (1974)	Canadian Association of Occupational Therapists (1991)
		C. Allen (1985)	L. A. Llorens (1972)	J. Schkade & S. Schultz (1993)
				R. Zemke & F. Clark (1996)

2. Individuals can become aware of their personality strengths and problems through verbal and nonverbal activities.

3. Counseling, psychotherapy, and creative media can be used to reveal an individual's personal motives and life goals.

4. The individual's interpersonal relationships are a source of conflicts and anxiety as well as emotional support during periods of loss and stress.

5. The psychodynamic approach is based on a humanistic model of focusing on the individual and his or her capacity for personal growth. This is especially true in the theories of Rogers, Maslow, and Perls and in the theories of the existentialist psychotherapist Victor Frankl (1963).

6. The relationship between the client and the therapist is an important aspect of the psychodynamic model. Whether it is the development of transference in psychoanlaysis, an unconditional acceptance in client-centered therapy, client facilitation in Gestalt therapy, or the confrontation techniques of the existentialist therapist, the client-therapist relationship is of utmost importance.

Sigmund Freud's Contribution

Sigmund Freud (1856–1939) had a profound and revolutionary influence on the natural sciences, art, literature, anthropology, music, dance, and religion as well as psychiatry. His theories and clinical observations have been set forth in numerous books, scientific articles, and lectures that spanned a period of almost 50 years. Freud was a prolific writer who examined, in-depth, diverse areas of human behavior. Early in his career his scientific studies began with investigations into the anatomy of the nervous system; later, his interests shifted to clinical studies of hypnosis and hysteria, unconscious phenomena, transference, anxiety, ego psychology, group therapy, personality, and the structure of society. In all of his work he brought to bear a brilliant mind with an insatiable intellectual curiosity (Alexander & Selesnick, 1966; Freud, 1910/1953–1974, 1928/1953–1974). Even today, in spite of attacks by clinicians, researchers, and feminists, Freud and psychoanalysis are considered to have an important impact on society.

> Despite its flaws, Freud's work still seems to me to offer an arsenal of provocative ideas: he is brilliant about dreams, about childhood, about love, about authority, about dozens of other things. But perhaps what's most useful about Freud now is his conception of the psyche—a conception that could be of some help in reconceiving, and maybe changing the shape of, contemporary American culture. (Edmundson, 1997, p. 34)

The psychoanalytic formulations of Freud had a strong impact on the field of psychiatry in general. When Freud presented his ideas during the turn of the 19th century, psychiatrists relied primarily on a biological explanation of mental illness. The prime contribution of psychoanalysis as a therapeutic method was that it provided the psychiatrist with a psychological technique to understand the psychodynamics of the patient and the functional causes for mental illness. Psychoanalysis as a psychotherapeutic technique was a method to help the patient become aware of internal powerful forces that have the potential, if repressed, to produce painful symptoms, such as in phobias, severe anxiety, or depression. The psychiatrist searches for idiosyncratic clues in the patient's life that could account for severe anxiety or self-defeating behavior.

Freud's theories led to far-reaching changes in psychiatry during the early part of the 1900s. Psychotherapy, "the talking cure," at that time was given legitimacy as a major technique in psychiatry. After abandoning hypnosis as a technique for working with clients with mental illness, Freud's new technique, free association, encouraged the patient to consciously reveal innermost thoughts and not to censor unconscious feelings. Freud theorized that patients would be able to gain insight into the dynamics of their conflicts by working through the hidden meanings of what was revealed. In the psychoanalytic session, Freud identified the manifest content of what the patient revealed and the latent content, which is related to unconscious desires and conflicts. Dream interpretation was another technique used, and it is considered by psychoanalysts to be the "royal road to the unconscious."

Freud's theories attracted a circle of brilliant theorists and clinicians who assimilated the basic concepts of psychoanalysis in their work. Many of these early associates of Freud, such as Adler and Jung, later broke away to establish their own schools of thought. Freud had opened the path to a wide divergence in interpreting personality development, explaining emotional disorders, and discovering new treatment techniques that relied mainly on introspection. Freud led the way to the following questions: What are the primary psychological factors in development that shape an adult's personality? What are the critical developmental stages in personality development? What are the psychological factors that may contribute to the onset of neuroses and schizophrenia? What are the goals of psychotherapy and what are the associated treatment techniques?

In general, psychotherapy can be divided into two large branches: introspective therapy and behavior therapy. Psychoanalysis is the forerunner of introspective therapy, which includes under its umbrella the early theorists such as Freud (1933/1953–1974), Adler (1933/1974, 1956), Jung (1961), Sullivan (1953), Horney (1939), and Reich (1949), as well as the later theorists such as Erikson (1963), Berne (1961), Perls (Perls, Hefferline, & Goodman, 1965), and Rogers (1942). The practice of psychosocial occupational therapy has been greatly influenced by these two major streams of thought, psychoanalysis and behaviorism.

Table 4–2 outlines the major contributions of several psychodynamic theorists. These theorists are a sample of the brilliant clinicians who revised and enlarged on Freudian concepts.

It is difficult to address every major concept from the massive literature in psychoanalysis. What follows are the key concepts in psychoanalytic theory that relate to occupational therapy. Four major areas are discussed: (a) structure of the mind, (b) stages of development, (c) ego psychology, and (d) ego defense mechanisms. Examples of how these key concepts can be related to the field of occupational therapy are described.

Key Concepts in Psychoanalysis

Structure of the Mind

Freud's (1933/1953–1974) concept of the tripartite mind (id, ego, and superego) is basic to psychoanalytic thought. These three major provinces of the mind are dynamic structures that influence the total organism's adaptation and adjustment to the environment. They are not physical entities that can be seen under a microscope. The *id* represents the source of instinctual needs that are phylogenically acquired by the organism. It resides in the unconscious part of the mind, and includes all of man's physical and sexual instincts. Id impulses are revealed through dreams and through free association. Free spontaneous art activities can be used to reveal to the client unconscious feelings that are id impulses. For example, the occupational therapist can ask the client to draw a picture of a dream or fantasy. The content of the artwork can later be analyzed to help the client gain insight into unconscious thoughts or impulses that could be related to irrational behavior or anxiety. The occupational therapist, in a setting where the psychodynamic theoretical model is practiced, can help the client to work through unconscious feelings with the consultant assistance of the psychiatrist.

The *ego* emerges as the child develops and encounters the task of coping with the environment. The ego's prime function is perception of reality and accommodation in the real world. Freud believed that the ego develops in the child as the child differentiates himself or herself from the object environment. In other words, Freud conceptualized an ego structure that had the capacity to develop an autonomy of its own. This process emerged from the child's independence from his or her parents and the child's capacity to delay immediate gratification. The child's ability to learn from experience and to cope effectively with the environment are functions of the ego. The ego is like a reservoir that incorporates various tasks of the individual, such as thinking, feeling, and protection from anxiety that arise from the conflict between pri-

Table 4-2. Major Theorists in the Psychodynamic Theoretical Model

Theorists	Personality Concept	Treatment	Major References
Sigmund Freud (1856–1939) Psychoanalysis	• tripartite mind: id, ego, and superego • conscious vs. unconscious • use of defense mechanism to avoid psychic conflicts	Psychoanalyst explores with the patient traumatic events and relationships underlying psychic conflicts	Freud, S. (1933). New introductory lectures on psycho-analysis. In J. Strachey (Ed. and Trans.), *The standard edition of the complete psychological works of Sigmund Freud* (Vol. 22). London: Hogarth.
Alfred Adler (1870–1937) Individual Psychology	• lifestyle: consistent personality characteristics in reacting to social adaptation • inferiority complex	Reorganization of individual's lifestyle and creative potentialities	Adler, A. (1956). *The individual psychology of Alfred Adler: A systematic presentation in selections from his writings.* (H. L. Ansbacher & R. R. Ansbacher, Eds. and annotators). New York: Basic Books.
Carl Jung (1875–1961) Analytic Psychology	• collective unconscious: innate experiences and universal symbols carried and transmitted through generations • introversion-extroversion	Emphasis on self-realization of individual consistent with unconscious goals and personality type	Jung, C. (1961). *Memories, dreams, reflections.* New York: Vintage.
Karen Horney (1885–1952) Constructive Humanism	• the real self: inner force toward free healthy development • movement toward, away, or against others	Helping individual toward discovering real self and becoming authentic with others	Horney, K. (1939). *New ways in psychoanalysis.* New York: W. W. Norton.
Harry Stack Sullivan (1892–1949)	• self system and stages of development • consensual validation • parataxic distortions: misunderstandings in communication	Change in patient's orientation in living and interpersonal relationships	Sullivan, H. S. (1953). The interpersonal theory of psychiatry. In H. W. Perry & M. L. Gawel (Eds.), *The collected works of Harry Stack Sullivan, M.D.* (Vol. I). New York: W. W. Norton.
Fritz Perls (1893–1970) Gestalt Therapy	• individual self-regulates feelings by expressing one's needs • patient tries to counteract repression of feelings	Sensory motor exercises designed to enhance patient's awareness of physical and psychological states	Perls, F., Hefferline, R., & Goodman, P. (1965). *Gestalt therapy.* New York: Dell.

Table 4-2. Major Theorists in the Psychodynamic Theoretical Model *(continued)*

Theorists	Personality Concept	Treatment	Major References
Wilhelm Reich (1897–1957) Character Analysis	• character formation: identification of hysterical, compulsive, narcissistic, and masochistic character types	Analysis of character type and resistance to change	Reich, W. (1949). *Character analysis*. New York: Farrar Straus & Young.
Eric Erikson (1902–1994) Epigenetic Sequence	• eight stages of man	Achieve successful resolution of the conflict at each stage	Erikson, E. H. (1963). *Childhood and society* (2nd ed.). New York: Norton.
Carl Rogers (1902–1987) Client-centered Therapy	• individual has the ability to gain insight into one problems and self-actualize • unconditional positive regard	Wellness is achieved through client-therapist relationship	Rogers, C. (1942). *Counseling and psychotherapy*. Boston: Houghton Mifflin.
Eric Berne (1910–1970) Transactional Analysis	• three ego states: parent, adult, child • I'm OK, You're OK	Enable the patient to deal with adult/adult transactions	Berne, E. (1961). *Transactional analysis in psychotherapy*. New York: Grove Press.

mal feelings and superego controls. The ego's tasks are reality bound and are related to one's ability to function in a specific life role, such as a student, worker, parent, or friend. In occupational therapy, the practical tasks of life, such as work, self-care, leisure, and interpersonal relationships are ego functions.

The *superego* develops gradually and is operative when the child is around 6 years old. It represents the conscience of the individual. The superego incorporates the parents' or caretakers' ethics, values, and morals. Freud theorized that the process of the child assimilating the values of the parents or caretakers through introjection and identification occurs on an unconscious level. Personal idols of adolescents such as parents, siblings, friends, movie stars, pop singers, athletes, or teachers can influence the development of the superego as the individual incorporates the values of these individuals into his or her conscience and behavior. The individual strives for perfection based on moral standards that are derived from his or her ideals or personal idols. In occupational therapy, the individual's superego can prevent him or her from getting involved in messy activities such as working with clay, finger paints, or other media where the individual feels "dirtied." The obsessively clean individual who is fearful of making a mistake in an activity or is overly critical of the finished product is another example of a punitive superego that can prevent the individual from engaging in an activity. Perfectionistic qualities are common in individuals who are depressed, anxious, or stressful and who feel that they are unable to meet their unconscious ideals.

Psychosexual and Psychosocial Stages of Development

One of the earliest formulations by Freud (1933/1953–1974) was the psychosexual stages of child development. This was a key concept in psychoanalytic theory. Freud proposed that the early stages of life shaped the later personality of the adult. Each stage of the child's development impinged on some aspect of sexuality. For example, in the oral stage, which occurs during the first 2 years of life, the child obtains gratification from eating, sucking, and touching the mouth. It is common to observe infants putting objects in their mouths and sucking on a "pacifier." As the child matures, bodily gratification transfers to the anal area and then to the genitals. Freud theorized that as adults we can become fixated on any of these psychosexual stages. For example, the compulsive smoker still derives bodily gratification from the oral nature of the activity that maintains his or her link to childhood. The anal individual symbolically collects objects or is "stingy." Freud also theorized that as some adults become emotionally ill, they regress to an earlier psychosexual stage of development. Many times the individual going through a psychotic depression can be observed regressing toward earlier stages of development associated with oral dependency.

In contrast to Freud's theory of psychosexual stages of development is Erikson's (1963) theory of psychosocial crises. Table 4–3 compares and contrasts Freud's (1933/1953–1974) and Erikson's (1963) theories of development and provides examples of occupational therapy activities. The occupational therapy activities are hierarchical and reflect the individual's level of ego maturity and integration.

Ego Psychology

Freud's (1923/1953–1974) theory of the structure of the mind as a hypothetical construct laid the foundations for his theory concerning the development of the ego. He felt that the ego is first and foremost a bodily ego and it is ulti-

Table 4–3. Stages of Development in Psychoanalysis: Concepts of Freud and Erikson and Implications for Occupational Therapy

AGE	PSYCHOSEXUAL STAGES (FREUD, 1905)	PSYCHOSOCIAL STAGES (ERIKSON, 1963)	OCCUPATIONAL THERAPY ACTIVITY EXAMPLES
0–2	Oral Stage: *gratification in sucking and eating*	Trust vs. Mistrust: *confidence in being taken care of and protected*	Passive appreciation, such as listening to music, watching a film, appreciating nature on walks, attending sports game
2–3	Anal Stage: *gratification in controlling anal muscle tone*	Autonomy vs. Shame/Doubt: *exploration of self and body in space*	Creative exploration of media or movement, such as clay, finger paints, water color, or dance
3–5	Phallic Stage: *infantile genitality*	Initiative vs. Guilt: *development of self-identity*	Individual expression through poetry, self-portrait, and diary
5–12	Latency: *deemphasis on bodily sexual gratification*	Industry vs. Inferiority: *technical mastery of environmental tasks*	Development of skills in sports, music, dancing, building models, academics, or computer/ multimedia
12–21	Puberty, Adolescence: *development of sexual organs*	Identity vs. Identity Confusion: *self-consistency and self-awareness*	• Prevocational exploration • Social skills development • Sensory-awareness exercises
Young Adulthood	Genitality: *full mastery of sexual and reproductive capacities*	Intimacy vs. Isolation: *establishment of intimate relationships*	• Interpersonal learning through group experiences • Value clarification: love and work
Middle Adulthood		Generativity vs. Stagnation: *enriching lives of others without thought for oneself*	• Parent Effectiveness Training • Special interest groups • Support groups
Later Adulthood	Menopause	Integrity vs. Despair: *finding meaning and spirituality for one's life*	• Reminiscing • Maintaining usefulness through volunteer services • Activity continuity

mately derived from bodily sensations that are mental projections of the surface of the body. The infant at birth operates primarily on the pleasure principle which reigns unrestrictedly in the id. The pleasure principle stated that the child's id urges demand immediate gratification. The id has no temporal or spatial boundaries. The child, operating through the pleasure principle, has not developed the capacity to delay immediate pleasure for the gratification in the future. The child develops an ego as stimuli from the external world act on the organism, bombarding it with unsatisfied instinctual demands. During this phase of development,

the reality principle is substituted for the pleasure principle and aids in the development of the ego. In the ego, displeasure remains the sole means of education. The reality principle implies that the organism functions in a spatial and temporal sphere and that pleasure can be delayed.

Freud then conceived the idea that the organism deals with the external world through a prima facie conscious perception of reality. However, this conscious perception of reality is dependent on the demands of the id that influence the child's behavior. As the child develops, through reality testing, he or she is able to transform and comprise the demands of the id into ego strivings. In the process of development, the ego seeks to bring the influence of the external world on the id and its tendencies by substituting the reality principle for the pleasure principle. The ego gives the mental processes a temporal and spatial sphere and submits them to reality testing. In this context, the ego and the external world interact continuously, enabling the ego to grow through its own unique experiences. The ego also develops from the perception of the instinctual impulses of the id by controlling, obeying, or inhibiting these impulses.

This concept of ego was later elaborated by Anna Freud (1936/1963) in her work on the defense mechanisms of the ego. Theorizing within the framework of Freud's thinking, Anna Freud presented clinical data substantiating the ego's development of defense mechanisms. These methods of defense (regression, repression, reaction formation, isolation undoing, projection, introjection, turning against the self, reversal, and sublimation) enabled the ego to deal with the anxiety resulting from instinctual impulses that are blocked from direct expression. These impulses against which the ego defends itself are always the same but the particular feelings of anxiety vary according to the situation. For example, some instinctual wish may seek to enter consciousness by interplay with the superego, causing conflictual anxiety. The specific methods of dealing with anxiety define the defense mechanisms. Anna Freud emphasized the importance of economy in the mental processes demonstrated by the defense mechanisms. In short, she stressed that the organism's conflicts with its own internal impulses and the pressures of the environment influence ego development.

Another major theoretician in ego psychology was Heinz Hartmann (1939). Hartmann's approach to the ego emphasized maturational and learning processes that are crucial to ego development. His theory of ego development represented a sociological approach that elaborated on S. Freud's (1933/1953–1974) initial psychophysiological theory of ego. Hartmann presented a theory that described the organism's adaptation to an environment mainly through the cognitive functions of the ego. For instance, Hartmann assigned the ego the tasks of thinking, language, memory, productivity, and motor development, as well as perception and intention. The ego developed these tasks in response to the control of instinctual drives and the adaptation to the external world. Adaptation is also dependent on the ego's ability to deal effectively with the environment and it is a problem of both biological and sociological significance. The interplay of both heredity and environment aid in the development of the child's ego. The confrontation of problems in the child's milieu influence the growth pattern of the child's intellectual and motor development.

Erik Erikson (1963), theorizing from a maturational and sociological base, approached the problems of ego development in the context of the child's interaction with his or her immediate environment. Synthesizing Freud's conceptual framework and Hartmann's theory of ego adaptation, Erikson presented a theory of ego development that is partially based on anthropological data. His theory of ego development recognized processes of interaction that stimulate growth in the human. These processes enable the individual to master the social environment. In Erikson's theory, the ego is a process that continually develops, reacts, and interrelates the organism to its environment.

The concept of mastery of the environment was formulated by Erikson (1963) in his theory of the "Eight Stages of Man" (see Table 4–3.) He described the child's confrontation with problems in society as stages in ego development. As the child resolves one ego problem in his environment, he or she becomes prepared to confront the next phase in maturational development. Because the child is developing perceptual, motor, and learning capacities, the problem in ego development becomes increasingly more complex. As the demands of society are brought into play, the ego processes become stronger and greater demands are placed on the individual to cope with problems in society. Erikson felt that society created roles as a child develops an identity. This identity is an outgrowth of the ego's capacity to integrate and synthesize the external reality into the individual's perception of his or her unique role in society.

Implications of the Theory of Ego Psychology in the Dynamics of Schizophrenia

Although schizophrenia is a neurobiological disorder, it can also be interpreted as a disability that interferes with the individual's ability to master problems in everyday living. The presence of symptoms such as distorted perception, poor reality testing, thinking disorder, inability to concentrate, evasion of anxiety-provoking situations, and a desire to avoid making decisions result in an inadequate mastery of the environment. Psychiatric symptoms such as hallucinations (false perceptions), delusions (illogical beliefs), loss of contact with reality, schizoid or withdrawn behavior, and stylized speech are examples of the individual's retreat from reality. The ability of the individual with schizophrenia to succeed will depend on factors in the environment, such as the encouragement of family and the community, educational and vocational opportunities, support groups, creative expression, and the development of social skills. This will enable the individual to master problems in the environment. Failure to cope with life tasks

increases the individual's gradual withdrawal from active participation in society.

The following concepts are proposed as a phenomenological explanation of the individual with schizophrenia's failure in ego development (Stein, 1967).

▶ Schizophrenia is a human process of failure in environmental mastery.

▶ As a reaction to failure, the individual desires a dependent relationship to the world and a reduction of anxiety, which reduces the individual's capacity for work.

▶ The process of losing contact with reality and escaping the responsibility of "being" in the world involves the breakdown of ego functions, such as reality testing, perception, memory, thinking, attention, and judgment.

▶ These ego functions are distorted as the individual is unable to accept responsibility for self-care and work and it reinforces the individual's need for dependency and the desire to avoid anxiety and conflict.

▶ Patterns of behavior are established in the individual with schizophrenia that force him or her to enter the dependent atmosphere of an institution and thus avoid the anxiety of "being" in the world.

▶ Schizophrenia as a personal and unique reaction to the world is significant in the action and experience of the individual. Maladjustment or the inability to partake in the everyday activities of life is the prime symptom in schizophrenia, while active participation in the daily patterns of life reinforce the individual's success in mastering the environment.

The significance of the schizophrenic process lies in the incapacities of the individual. These incapacities are related to the ego defense mechanisms that have become distorted and ineffective in enabling the individual to deal with anxiety and to adjust societal demands.

Ego Defense Mechanisms

Sigmund Freud (1923/1953–1974) and later Anna Freud (1936/1963) described the development of ego defense mechanisms as dynamic characteristics in the individual. Described below are the definitions of the most common ego defense mechanisms and examples in occupational therapy of how clients use ego defense mechanisms in working with activities and in interacting with the other clients. These major defense mechanisms and other less common defense mechanisms are summarized in Table 4–4.

▶ *Introjection:* This ego defense mechanism simply means the acceptance and incorporation of others' values, attitudes, standards, and ideals as one's own. The individual in a way can accede to the normative values of others to escape punishment or to side with strength. Erich Fromm (1941), in his classical study, *Escape From Freedom*, described how the individual in a totalitarian society, such as Nazi Germany, felt helpless and insecure, and internalized the values of an all-powerful state. In this process, the individual compromises his own freedom and unique identity. The conforming individual adapts the culture and values of others. The danger of introjection is that it can lead to a "mob" psychology in which critical dissent and individualism are not tolerated. The adolescent is the most vulnerable to introjecting values of conformity without respect for the individual who stands alone. For example, adolescents who are delinquent may reject their parents' values and replace them with the values of the gang. Gullible individuals who change their

values with the times and swing with the fads of modern society have difficulty in defining their own values in life. The psychosocial occupational therapist working with adolescents who are emotionally disturbed tries to cultivate and reinforce the individual talents and interests of each person. Respect for the individual's values is emphasized when the therapist and adolescent jointly select a therapeutic activity that reflects the adolescent's interests and needs.

▶ *Isolation:* In this ego defense mechanism, the individual compartmentalizes strong experiences and separates the ideas from the feeling. Isolation is sometimes equated with intellectualization, where a person, for example, fails to express appropriate feelings in response to the death of a loved one or loss of a job and instead seems emotionally distant and unfeeling. The apathetic or indifferent client in occupational therapy has difficulty in mobilizing feelings and appears bored with activities. This reaction many times can be interpreted as an emotional insulation and fear of disclosing feelings through activities. The client is fearful of being "opened up," which may bring to the surface a flood of emotions. Instead the client presents an indifferent and overly intellectual appearance. It is important for the psychosocial occupational therapist to become aware of the client who is unable to take part in an activity that can potentially produce "emotional flooding." It is probably best to help clients with emotional difficulties and emotional constriction to gradually express themselves through activities without much therapist interpretation and to have the clients work through their feelings nonverbally.

▶ *Projection:* This is another commonly used term originally identified by psychoanalytic

Table 4–4. Major Ego Defense Mechanisms

Mechanism	Definition	Examples of Expression
Compensation	Camouflaging weaknesses by emphasizing other areas	Social skills are deliberately practiced to compensate for inadequacies in personality
Conversion	Repressed ideas or feelings used by the patient as a somatic complaint, such as a physical illness	A somatic symptom with an underlying anxiety prevents an individual from performing an activity
Denial of Reality	Refusal to believe something that is true because it's painful to accept	The finished art product reflects, symbolically or pictorially, the patient's wishes and fantasies
Displacement or Substitution	Substitution or displacement of a feeling, goal, or object that cannot be realized or is unacceptable	Angry feelings generated from others are directed at the therapist or toward the media
Idealization	Overestimating the value or an attribute of a person	Overidentification with a person, resulting in the incorporation of attributes from that person into a lifestyle
Identification	Unconsciously patterning oneself after another person	Modeling another's behavior without being aware that he/she is imitating another
Introjection	Acceptance and incorporation of others' values, attitudes, standards, and ideals as one's own	Activities and creative expression are determined by what the group is doing
Isolation	Compartmentalization of strong experiences so that the ideas are separated from the feeling or emotion	General attitude is apathetic or indifferent, regardless of the activity
Projection	Accusing others of unacceptable behavior or traits that are evident in oneself	Inability to work with others who display symptoms that are similar to the individual
Rationalization	Explaining away behavior that appears superficially to be irrational	Trying to rationalize the displaying of bizarre behavior by attributing his or her actions to outer forces
Reaction Formation	Developing characteristics or behaviors that are the opposite of tendencies we do not like in ourselves	Development of strong, rigid positions that are diametrically opposed to fears in oneself
Regression	Returning to an earlier stage of development where the needs for security and comfort were met	Creations are primitive or childlike, or client uses "free" media, such as clay, finger paint, or easel painting
Repression	Blocking from consciousness disturbing thoughts, desires, or experiences that arise in the unconscious	Sexual symbols in artistic creations are symbolically camouflaged
Reversal	Change of an instinct from an inward to an outward direction	Expression of strong feelings toward an object outwardly (e.g., clay) can be interpreted as inward expression of self-hatred
Sublimation	The process of transforming instinctual energy in a constructive or creative manner that is acceptable to society	Sexual feelings are channeled through various forms of creative expression
Turning Against the Self	Self-hatred and feelings of inferiority toward oneself are displaced by negative feelings toward others	Reliance on the therapist to make decisions reveals lack of confidence in one's ability to make decisions
Undoing	Engaging in repeated acts of ritualistic behavior to undo disapproved thought or fears	After completing a project, the patient may destroy it so as to "undo" accomplishments

theorists. It is defined as accusing others of unacceptable behavior or traits that are evident in oneself. In other words, the individual "projects" onto others characteristics that he or she dislikes in his or her own personality or behavior. The client has difficulty working cooperatively with other individuals who seem to display symptoms and behaviors similar to the client's own behaviors that are personally unacceptable on an unconscious level. The client rejects others because of qualities the client is unable to accept in his or her own life.

▶ *Reaction formation:* White (1948) referred to reaction formation as developing characteristics or behaviors that are the opposite of tendencies we do not like in ourselves. In a way, reaction formation is an opposite attitude or behavior to strong unconscious desires. Because we fear the emergence of these desires, we defend our egos by associating ourselves with extreme positions that are directly opposite to what we fear will happen to us. For example, the individual who has a strong unconscious urge or fear of becoming an alcoholic will become a member of an organization that advocates the prohibition of alcohol. Sexual and aggressive urges, if repressed severely, can become transformed into extreme positions of prudishness and passivity. A client's extemporaneous and uncensored art productions many times reveal strong sexual and aggressive urges that are portrayed symbolically. These symbols may be evaluated by the psychosocial occupational therapist and psychiatrist to gain insight into the unconscious feelings that are interfering with the client's adjustment and that subsequently can cause anxiety and stress. The client's extreme, rigid, unyielding positions can be analyzed

through the content expressed in the activity media.

▶ *Regression:* This refers to the individual returning to an earlier stage of development where the needs for security and comfort were met. Regressive behavior many times is equated with dependent and passive characteristics. The artistic creations of the individual client who regresses psychologically, progressively become more primitive and infantile, paralleling a regressive retreat toward childhood and dependency. Regression can also be seen as a positive force in the individual creative artist who uses childlike playful feelings to express humor and primitive thinking.

Kris (1952) introduced the concept of regression in the service of the ego: "the integrative functions of the ego include self-regulated regression and permit a combination of the most daring intellectual activity with the experience of passive receptiveness" (p. 318). What is implied in this concept is that the creative artist is able to express childlike feelings buried in the primary process of the id. The paintings of the Swiss artist Paul Klee have the freedom and humorous adventure of a child, which demonstrates how regression can be a positive and healthy factor in expressing feelings through creative media. The use of finger paints, clay, water colors, paper maché, sand, and water play are excellent media for playful expression. In these instances the adult can play with "free" media and obtain the satisfactions and joys of childhood. The occupational therapist can provide the climate of acceptance for the client to experiment creatively with these media without feeling the shame and guilt of regressing. For the adult with obsessive-compulsive tendencies who strives for perfection, loosening up in a free, unstructured activity can be both gratifying and stress reducing. However, the occupational therapist must prepare the client for the activity by "defusing" the anticipating anxiety of engaging in childlike play.

▶ *Repression:* This concept, which is widely used in our vocabulary, refers to the blocking from consciousness of disturbing thoughts, desires, or experiences that arise in the unconscious. The overly puritanical client represses strong sexual feelings, which can be revealed symbolically in art or ceramic projects. Universal or individual symbols for the phallus or vagina and symbols of penetration are frequently portrayed in clients' art productions that are ordinarily repressed in the unconscious.

▶ *Sublimation:* This defense mechanism is unique in that the individual transforms instinctual energy constructively. Freud (1917/1966) stated that sublimation is a process of displacing sexual energy through socially acceptable channels. "This displaced ability and readiness to accept a substitute must operate powerfully against the pathogenic effort of a frustration. . . . We call this process 'sublimation' in accordance with the general estimate that places social aims higher than the sexual ones, which are at bottom self-interested" (p. 34). In a sense, the process of creating artistic works can be considered sublimation. The strong sexual drives of the creative artist are expressed through art, literature, music, dance, drama, and sculpture. It is extremely important for every individual to have the opportunity to express his or her creative urges. The psychosocial occupational therapist provides this opportunity for exploring with the client through various media that are individually appro-

priate to express strong feelings. Sublimation is one of the most important ego defense mechanisms for the occupational therapist using creative media with clients. If used effectively, it can become a powerful influence in the client's life, helping the client relieve anxiety and bolster his or her self-esteem.

▶ *Turning against the self:* The individual experiences self-hatred and feelings of inferiority in displacing negative feelings to others. This ego defense mechanism is probably the most dangerous to the individual, because it generates feelings of depression and self-depreciation. The psychosocial occupational therapist working with the client who is chronically depressed and expresses feelings of self-hatred uses activities to counteract this negative self-image. The individuality of the activities is important. The individual with depression must be shown that he or she is able to make an impact on the environment. The individual with severe depression gets caught in a vicious cycle of physical immobility, passivity, and hopelessness and feels unable to engage in activities to make decisions or to find satisfaction in his or her life. The psychosocial occupational therapist, at the onset of treating the client, structures activities to break the cycle of depression. A structured multimodal approach using exercise, art activities, music, poetry, dance, movies, and support groups is emphasized to mobilize the individual with depression. As the depression lifts, the psychosocial occupational therapist provides opportunities for the client to make decisions and to change the locus of control from the therapist making all the decisions to the client being empowered to making decisions.

▶ *Undoing:* This ego defense mechanism is characteristic of individuals with an obsessive-compulsive disorder who repeat ritualistic behavior to undo disapproved thoughts or fears. An example of undoing is the housewife who ritualistically washes her hands continually to the point where the skin becomes inflamed. The act can symbolically be a cleansing action to rid oneself of undesirable thoughts, such as Lady Macbeth in *Macbeth*. Atonement, repentance, reparation, and confession are examples of undoing. This ego defense mechanism enables the individual to live with the memories of behaviors that are difficult to tolerate in the conscious mind. Undoing serves to protect the self-esteem of the individual. It provides the individual with an opportunity to repair his ego and to rationalize away past errors and injustices that he or she perceives he or she may have committed. Many times, the client with mental illness may destroy the finished project in occupational therapy so as to undo his or her accomplishments. The client may be fearful of a successful painting, sculpture, or art product, because it may not be consistent with his or her negative self-esteem. The client may have difficulty in accepting compliments from the occupational therapist and may try to maintain a perception of self-devaluation. The completed art object can become an extension of the client that must be carefully appraised by the therapist. The art product can also serve positively to undo the negative self-evaluation of the client and act as a tangible example of the individual's worth.

Psychoanalysis' Impact on Occupational Therapy

Psychoanalytic theory gave the psychosocial occupational therapist a conceptual model for interpreting the creative product of a client with mental illness. Azima and Wittkower (1957), in reviewing the state of the art of psychosocial occupational therapy at that time, proposed that the psychosocial occupational therapist incorporate psychoanalytic concepts in treatment and be aware of the importance of the dynamics of object-relationships. Applying this psychoanalytic concept, the psychosocial occupational therapist was encouraged to try to understand (a) the symbolic meaning of the activity to the client, and (b) how it satisfied psychological needs. Is the activity gratifying on an oral or anal level? Is the activity used to sublimate sexual feelings? Is the activity an unconscious outlet for aggressive or sadomasochistic drives? The occupational therapist uses activities in the psychodynamic framework to discover unconscious drives and feelings. For example, Azima and Wittkower (1957) stated that, "unless an activity or production was used specifically for uncovering of unconscious processes, the function of the activity of the product could not extend beyond the diversional field" (p. 3). In this model, the client's art product is also used to work through unhealthy or destructive impulses. The therapist is encouraged to interpret the client's art product and to use newly conscious insights with the client. However, Azima and Wittkower felt strongly that the psychosocial occupational therapist who uses psychoanalytic principles in treatment should have intensive training in psychopathology and psychotherapy. They also felt that art therapy and play therapy present excellent modalities for the psychosocial occupational therapist for creating spontaneous psychotherapeutic situations that can be used for revealing unconscious drives, defenses, and transference phenomena.

Although they strongly proposed that the psychosocial occupational therapist use a psychoanalytic model for treatment, they also felt that too much emphasis had been placed in the past on the diversional and occupational aspect of activities.

In 1959, Azima and Azima presented an outline of a psychodynamic frame of reference. They divided the functions of occupational therapy into three areas: diagnostic, change detection, and therapeutic. In the *diagnostic stage*, the psychosocial occupational therapist uses unstructured objects (e.g., leather, paint, plasticine, clay) in a free choice situation for the client. The therapist observes the client's mode of approach to the media, the selection of activity object, the attitude toward the therapist and other clients, and the manipulation of objects. The client is encouraged to verbalize about the object in a free manner. The therapist then interprets the client's creative product and verbalizations, analyzing drive states, the ego system, and object-relations.

In the second area, *change detection*, the psychosocial occupational therapist remains sensitive to the mood, behavior, and regression or improvement in the patient as reflected in the client's use of objects. The therapist observes and records positive or negative changes in the client's behavior.

In the third area, *therapeutic function*, the authors presented a model that is appropriate only when the psychosocial occupational therapist is properly trained in psychodynamic principles, viz. psychoanalysis. The psychosocial occupational therapist uses activities to (a) uncover unconscious processes, (b) gratify psychosocial needs, and (c) "strengthen certain ego defenses and provide routes for sublimation of aggressive and libidinal impulses" (Azima & Azima, 1959, p. 219). In this area, the psychosocial occupational therapist applies psychotherapeutic principles to treatment.

The main impact of psychoanalysis for psychosocial occupational therapists was that a systematic theory was presented that could be used by the occupational therapist in interpreting the meaning of the patients' art products. Without special training in this theoretical model, the psychosocial occupational therapist should not try to interpret art products without the aid of another professional trained in the procedures.

Critical Analysis of Psychoanalysis and Its Application to Occupational Therapy

Psychoanalysis has developed in the last 80 years into a very elaborate and costly treatment procedure that is not usually available to the majority of clients who are being treated for mental illness. In addition, there are very few published research studies testing the efficacy of psychoanalysis. Strupp (1973), in discussing psychoanalysis and its discontents, concluded that psychoanalytic psychotherapy has something *unique* to contribute, but there are very few research studies to support its effectiveness. However, psychoanalysis does have an intellectual interest that makes it attractive to analyze a painting by Salvador Dali or interpret the neurotic characters in Arthur Miller's play "Death of a Salesman." Psychoanalytic theory can be useful potentially in understanding the psychodynamics underlying a client's mental illness. It can also generate a hypothesis for establishing a plan of treatment in occupational therapy.

For example, the model presented by Azima and Azima (1959) in the 1950s and later by other occupational therapists, such as Fidler and Fidler (1954) and Mosey (1970), espoused a psychodynamic–psychoanalytic theory that primarily emphasized interpretation of symbols in activities and the use of activities as object-relations. Recently, Piergrossi and Gilbertoni (1995) applied psychoanalytic concepts in describing the clinical treatment of a 10-year-old child with autism and a 16-year-old boy with psychosis. They felt that

> The rich psychoanalytic literature seems to be little known to most occupational therapists who often seem skeptical and critical about a field that has much to offer in understanding the inner significance of doing. The concepts of inner self, therapeutic relationship and emotional movement as presented here are part of a psychoanalytic theory base . . . (p. 38)

Saint–Jean and Desrosiers (1993), occupational therapists from Montreal, have also described the application of psychoanalytic theories in treating an individual with a diagnosis of psychosis. Perhaps the most relevant aspects of psychoanalytic theory to psychosocial occupational therapy is in the area of ego psychology in the identification of defense mechanisms (Freud, 1936/1963), ego adaptation function (Hartmann, 1939, 1964), and stages of ego development (Erikson, 1963). Ego psychology emphasizes an adaptive theory of man that is consistent with one of the main purposes of occupational therapy, that is, facilitating independent living skills.

Eklund (1996, 1999, 2000), a Swedish occupational therapist has incorporated object-relations theory in working with patients with psychosocial disorders. Object-relations arises from psychoanalytic theory and examines the attachment of individuals to family members, friends, and colleagues. Eklund employs the *Percept-genetic Object Relation Test* (PORT; Nilsson, 1993, 1995) as an assessment tool to examine the client's ability to establish relationships and, then, to establish an appropriate treatment plan.

Summary

The main advantage of a psychodynamic theoretical model is in the understanding of a client's symptoms and as a model for gaining insight into interpersonal relationships. It is useful for the psychosocial occupational therapist to use psychodynamic concepts in gaining an in-depth understanding of the client's behavior. However, it provides a limited framework for helping a client to learn the social, vocational, and educational skills that are part of a holistic and comprehensive treatment program. In practice, the psychodynamic model can be used by the occupational therapist in exploring areas of self-concept and self-awareness. A psychodynamic frame of reference can be integrated with other treatment perspectives. For example, the concepts of cognitive–behavior therapy, sensory integration and the occupational frame of reference can be used with a psychodynamic model in providing an eclectic approach.

PSYCHODYNAMIC FRAME OF REFERENCE

Fidlers' Analytic Theory of Occupational Therapy

The Fidlers have had a profound influence on the practice of psychosocial occupational therapy since the 1950s. Gail Fidler obtained her certificate in Occupational Therapy from the University of Pennsylvania in 1942. She had wide experiences in psychosocial occupational therapy in state and county facilities and in U.S. Army hospitals. Ms. Fidler has taught at New York University and Columbia University as well as other universities. She has been a prolific writer and has presented numerous lectures and workshops throughout the United States and internationally. In her distinguished career, which spans over 50 years, she has been a clinician, supervisor, consultant, administrator, professor in occupational therapy, and mentor to many of the leaders in the field. She and her husband, Jay

Fidler, a psychiatrist, authored the first textbook in psychosocial occupational therapy in 1954, *Introduction to Psychiatric Occupational Therapy*. This book and a later edition, *Occupational Therapy: A Communication Process in Psychiatry* (1963), served as the "bible" for students studying psychosocial occupational therapy.

The Fidlers' theories are notedly influenced by the theory of psychoanalysis. Major concepts of psychoanalysis are incorporated into their work (e.g., object-relationships, unconscious, sublimation, body image, regression, need gratification, and ego defenses).

The Fidlers advocated the use of activities to understand the psychodynamics of an individual and psychotherapeutic interventions to resolve basic personality conflicts.

> The use of objects and the processes inherent in the use of such objects do not occur in a vacuum. The patterns of interaction, identification, and shared experiences that surround such involvement, either spontaneously or by design, create a gestalt of experiences. Those experiences in occupational therapy that focus more on participative doing than on things, e.g., play-reading groups, drama, dance, music, newspaper work, provide opportunities for the patient to test his new skills in living, experiment and explore capacities in relationships, learn more effective means of communication, and utilize insights gained. These, then, provide an additional dimension to the psychotherapeutic process. Finally, occupational therapy encompasses thinking, feeling, and participation in a world of objects. Such a setting bears a closer resemblance to actual living situations than any other treatment setting, thus providing a realistic environment in which the patient, when he is ready, can test his developing skills in living. Likewise, the transition from treatment to the normal living situation is minimal. (Fidler & Fidler, 1963, p. 97)

They advocated using activities in a meaningful way where the occupational therapist is sensitive to the psychological needs of the client. In selecting activities, the Fidlers were cognizant of the dilemma facing therapists as to whether the therapist selected, or strongly recommended, activities or allowed the client to use free choice in the selection process. In either case, it is important that an intelligent decision is made by the therapist and the client cooperatively in the activity process. The activity selected, according to the Fidlers, should be tied to the therapeutic needs of the client and not to diversional or recreational goals. In the selection of therapeutic activities, the Fidlers listed several factors that the therapist should consider:

- What motions are involved in the activity (e.g., striking, hammering, cutting, tearing, and rhythmic)?
- What levels of knowledge and skill are involved in the activity?
- What is the pliability and resistiveness of the media used?
- Does the activity involve creativity and originality?
- What is the symbolic nature of the activity?
- In the process of doing the activity, is there an opportunity to release hostility or aggressiveness?
- What level of locus of control does the activity generate (e.g., dependence, independence, or interdependency)?
- Does the activity readily ensure success?
- Does the activity gratify an individual's need to express himself individually?
- What are the traditional gender associations of the activity (e.g., woodworking and homemaking)?
- At what psychosexual level (i.e., oral, anal, and phallic) is the activity?
- How does the activity relate to reality testing?

These and other factors are analyzed by the therapist in the selection of a therapeutic activity. For example, a client selects clay sculpting as a therapeutic activity. The therapist can then analyze the activity into the above components and determine whether it meets the therapeutic needs of the client.

The Fidlers conceptualized the use of activities to help the individual understand his or her unconscious desires and to gain insight and by this process to work through psychological problems. The occupational therapist in this process works in tandem with the psychotherapist in uncovering psychological traumas, repressed emotions, and interpersonal conflicts. The activity was a vehicle for the therapist to explore with the client his or her inner psychological world. The key to whether this process was effective is in the valid interpretation of the symbols and products of the activity. The Fidlers made the implied assumption that psychopathology is fundamentally the result of a lack of self-knowledge and insight on the part of the client and that successful treatment involved working through with the client the motivations and desires that drove the client into neurotic or psychotic patterns of behavior. The activity for the Fidlers was then an intermediate step that eventually was tied to a verbal therapy. For the activity to be successful there was a need for psychotherapeutic follow-up. The Fidlers (1963) described a case of an individual diagnosed with a depression who, through activity, gained insight into his self-concept. Subsequently, through psychotherapy the newfound insights were "more intensively explored and worked through" (p. 85).

In addition to the use of activity as a means of understanding the psychodynamics of the client's mental illness, the Fidlers also used the psychoanalytic concept of transference as another dimension of psychosocial occupational therapy. They listed five general areas that are related to the transference issue:

1. *Image of Self:* How does the client portray himself or herself while relating to the therapist?

2. *Concept of Other:* How does the client perceive others and relate to them?

3. *Ego Organization:* How does the client understand and react to his or her immediate environment?

4. *Unconscious Conflicts:* How does the client express, repress, or suppress feelings in his or her relationship with the therapist and others?

5. *Communication:* How does the client relate to the therapist and others?

In psychoanalytic theory, transference refers to the strong feelings that clients develop toward their therapists that are related to prior relationships with parents, relatives, friends, and authority figures who played prominent roles in their lives. The relationship between the occupational therapist and the client generate a transference phenomena and, in a few instances, countertransference may develop in which the therapist maintains unrealistic feelings toward the client.

The client is evaluated by the therapist in his or her relationship to the therapist, to others, and to the activity. By analyzing these three areas, the therapist is able to gain insight into the underlying psychodynamics that contributed to the mental illness. Through insight, personality change and improvement are gained.

In summary, the Fidlers' major contributions were their ability to translate the psychoanalytic theories formulated by Freud and others to introduce a dimension to psychosocial occupational therapy. The Fidlers presented a model for the occupational therapist to interpret activities on a symbolic level and to analyze the relationship between the therapist and the client.

Mosey's Three Frames of Reference

In 1970, Anne Cronin Mosey authored the book *Three Frames of Reference for Mental Health*. This book has had a strong impact on occupational therapists working in psychosocial settings. Mosey outlined theoretical approaches that occupational therapists could apply in working directly with individuals with psychosocial disabilities.

Mosey has been a frequent writer for the *American Journal of Occupational Therapy*. After receiving her bachelor's degree in Occupational Therapy from the University of Minnesota in 1961, she worked as a psychosocial occupational therapist in Glenwood Hills Hospital in Minneapolis and at New York State Psychiatric Institute through 1966. She has taught at Columbia University and New York University where she was a director of the OT curriculum during the 1970s. She received a master's degree in Psychiatric Occupational Therapy in 1965 and a doctorate in Human Relations in 1968 from New York University.

Mosey (1986) felt strongly that the occupational therapist should be guided by a theoretical frame of reference when working in a psychosocial setting. To Mosey, therapy should not be based on intuitive, atheoretical techniques where the therapist interacts with the client casually and in a laissez-faire manner. The theoretical frame of reference for a therapist is based on consistent, comprehensive concepts, definitions, and principles, guiding the therapeutic interaction with the client. Mosey proposed that when a helping relationship is based on a frame of reference, it can be controlled, studied, and changed. For Mosey, the therapist's frame of reference should guide the therapist in a practical manner

in evaluating and treating the client. The theoretical frame of reference should be based on a psychological theory such as psychoanalysis, behaviorism, or sensory integration. It should include delineation of a function-dysfunction continuum. The frame of reference should guide the therapist in specific areas to evaluate the individual's behavior. And lastly, the frame of reference should guide the therapist in planning and carrying through a treatment program.

In 1970, Mosey identified three frames of reference: analytic, acquisitional, and developmental. The *analytic frame of reference* is based on a psychodynamic conceptual base similar to the theories of the Fidlers (1963). For example, projective techniques are used in the analytic framework to uncover symbolic unconscious processes in the individual that are effecting the client's behavior. Like Fidlers' approach to treatment, the analytic therapist assumes that through insight, the individual will be able to work through conflicts. The *acquisitional frame of reference* is based on the acquisition of skills and competencies that enable the individual to cope and functionally adapt to his or her environment. The *developmental frame of reference* is related to multidimensional stages that an individual passes through in attaining maturity such as in Ayres' (1979) theory of sensory integration. Table 4–5 outlines and describes the dimensions and concepts that differentiate the analytic, acquisitional, and developmental frames of reference.

In response to the questions, which frame of reference should be used for a particular client, and what frame of reference is best, Mosey (1970) indicated "that no frame of reference is more effective or efficient in treating psychosocial dysfunction than any other frame of reference" (p. 219). Mosey also proposed that the best criterion for selecting a frame of reference in treating a client is for the therapist to deter-

Table 4–5. Mosey's Three Frames of Reference

Frame of Reference	Theoretical Base	Function–Dysfunction	Evaluation	Treatment
Analytic	Psychoanalysis (Object-Relation Analysis): *individual's emotional attachment to people and things*	Lack of insight into unconscious processes, producing disabling systems	Projective techniques to uncover unconscious processes	Insight and working through, using • unstructured media • transference relationship established between patient and therapist
Acquisitional	Competency—Incompetency (Action—Consequence): *obtaining skills through reward and punishment*	Lack of skills produces ineffective environmental adaptation	Assess functional abilities to cope with life tasks	Operant conditioning—shaping, modeling, social imitation, desensitization
Developmental	Experimental—Maturation (Recapitulation of ontogenesis): *passing again through the stages of development*	Delay in reaching age-appropriate stage	Observation of individual in perceptual-motor activities, cognition, and interpersonal processes	Stimulation and opportunities for maximum development of patient potential

Source: Adapted from *Three Frames of Reference for Mental Health*, by A. C. Mosey (1970), Thorofare, NJ: Slack.

mine the most compatible approach. It is important for the therapist to have a good understanding and insight into his or her own self-concept and to use a treatment method that is congruent to his or her personality. What is implied is that therapists who are analytical and probing, as compared to therapists who are task oriented and goal directed, should feel more comfortable with the analytic frame of reference than the acquisitional frame of reference. However, for the student who is first learning to apply treatment methods in a psychosocial setting, Mosey suggested that the student become familiar with all three frames of reference under controlled supervision from an experienced therapist. In this way, the student can develop the personal insight and subsequently select a frame of reference with which he or she will be most effective in treating clients.

Mosey started out in a psychodynamic frame of reference and later shifted to a more eclectic approach as described in the following quote:

> In summary, activities therapy is based on the assumption that psychosocial dysfunction is a lack of understanding of the self or the inability to participate in the varied and complex tasks of everyday life or both. As a treatment process, activities therapy is here and now, action-oriented, and involves learning through doing. Emphasis is on mastery of the nonhuman environment, and nonhuman objects are utilized in activities designed to enhance self-awareness and interpersonal relationship. The activities used in activities therapy are similar to typical life experiences of the community. Activities therapy is concerned with growth through action. (Mosey, 1973, p. 6)

BEHAVIORAL THEORETICAL MODELS

Definition/Assumptions/Concepts

Behaviorism (Skinner, 1953; Watson, 1924) is the foundation of behavior management, cognitive-behavioral therapy (Dobson, 1988; Meichenbaum 1977), stress management (Lehrer & Woolfolk, 1993), biofeedback (Schwartz & Associates, 1995), and relaxation therapy (Benson, 1975). All of these are based on the principles of learning theory.

> The roots of behavior therapy include the notion that one learns maladaptive behaviors. Thus, in most cases, one can unlearn them. The model is largely educational rather than medical as such. It applies the principles of operant and respondent conditioning, and cognitive learning to change a wide range of behaviors. . . . Behavioral medicine is another outgrowth of learning theory, psychophysiology, and behavior therapy. (Schwartz & Olson, 1995, p. 6)

In order to apply behavior therapy, cognitive-behavioral therapy, stress management, biofeedback, and relaxation therapy, one must understand the concepts of learning theory.

What is behavior therapy?[1] How did it develop historically? How can the concepts and methods be applied to occupational therapy? In the following pages, the major concepts developed by theorists, scientists, and clinicians who have been associated with the behavior modification movement since the 1920s to the present are presented.

The techniques of behavior therapy are based on the principles of human learning. A major concept is that behavior is learned when it is immediately reinforced. For the behavior therapist all behavior is determined and has causes. Another important principle in behavior thera-

py is that a stimulus elicits a response. Behavior therapy techniques developed from the scientific analysis of behavior in which experiments were simulated in the laboratory in order to establish laws of human behavior. There has been much criticism of behavior modification and behavior therapy. Some of the criticism has been leveled against the mechanistic nature of its concepts. A common attack on behavior therapy is that behavior cannot be determined. Another attack is on the nature of reinforcers used in clinical practice, such as food and verbal approval. Critics see these methods as manipulating the individuals and coercing them to conform to society. In spite of these criticisms, behavior modification is neither good nor bad; it is only a method that has the potential to change human behavior. For the psychosocial occupational therapist, it is a useful tool in helping a client become more independent and learn adaptive skills. Behavior modification techniques can be incorporated into a humanistic and holistic framework in treating a client with psychosocial dysfunction or mental illness.

Historical Development of Behaviorism

Behaviorism as a scientific movement in psychology emerged from the experimental work during the middle of the 19th century of Helmholtz (1867), Fechner (1860/1966), and Müller (1833–1838), German physiologists who were interested in the relationship between sensory functions and neural processes (Spence, 1956). Although behaviorism had its roots in Germany, as did psychoanalysis, it has become primarily associated with psychological research in the United States, "a la Skinnerism." The philosophies of empiricism, logical positivism, and pragmatism were the main avenues of thought that generated scientific psychology. Another major influence on behavioristic psy-

---

[1]Much of the material in this section has been adapted from (Stein, 1982), "A Current Review of the Behavioral Frame of Reference and Its Application to Occupational Therapy."

chology was the classical conditioning experiments performed by Ivan Pavlov (1927).

Classical and operant conditioning are two main streams of behaviorism. *Classical conditioning* involves involuntary behaviors. In Pavlov's (1927) study with dogs, he noticed that dogs salivated when they smelled food. The act of salivating is involuntary and, therefore, classical. The emphasis is on the stimulus. Pavlov's act of pairing another stimulus, bell ringing, with salivation was also classical conditioning. Eventually, the dogs salivated when they heard the bell, regardless of whether food was present. In using classical conditioning with clients who are addicted to alcohol, an aversive stimulus such as the drug Antabuse® (disulfiram) is paired with the desire for alcohol in the presence of an unconditioned stimulus such as anxiety, panic, or phobia. The combination of alcohol and the Antabuse® leads to nausea. Eventually, the mere thought of alcohol results in nausea.

Operant conditioning, on the other hand, involves voluntary behavior and the emphasis is on the reinforcement (Skinner, 1953). When the goal is to obtain a particular behavior from a client, the therapist reinforces the client whenever the behavior is seen. At first, the behavior may be poorly executed; however, the act of reinforcement should help the client's performing the behavior again. By reinforcing behaviors that are closer to the desired goal, the client's behavior is "shaped" by the therapist.

The historical development of behaviorism in the United States began with the functional psychology represented by the thought of John Dewey (1891) and William James (1890). Functional psychology was influenced by Darwin's theory of evolution, which emphasized the adaptive qualities of man. This school of thought stressed the operations of consciousness and the purposeful functions it serves. Operation of consciousness, sense perception, imagination,

and emotion were all regarded as different instances of organic adaption to the environment (Spence, 1956). The psychologists subscribing to functionalism directed their attention at the overt behavior of the organism. There was a trend away from an analysis of introspective data such as in psychoanalysis. Instead of a qualitative, subjective approach, functionalists sought to objectify experimental data. This approach led to the measurement of overt behavior through intelligence tests, performance tasks, and aptitude scales. This is especially evident in the impact Dewey (1900) had on educational thought. *Functionalism* as a psychological theory emphasized the significance of applying psychological theory to the practical areas of learning, child development, and behavioral change. This interest in the application of scientific psychology to social problem solving led to the development of laboratories where experiences were simulated in controlled environments.

Another major influence in behaviorism was the tradition of *British empiricism* (Bergman & Spence, 1941), which advocated that the only way knowledge is gained is through the senses. Strict empiricism as interpreted by the behaviorists is translated into a denial of mental and unconscious experiences that cannot be verified through objective sensory data. The behaviorist's assertion in the empirical tradition is that what we know can be verified by universal affirmation in the laboratory. The philosophy of empiricism later changed to logical positivism, a theory closely associated with Alfred Lord Whitehead (1919) and Bertrand Russell (1965). The logical positivists sought to clarify the language of science and to investigate the conditions under which empirical propositions are meaningful. They held that all meaningful scientific propositions are derived from experience and can be expressed as physicalistic language—operational definitions (Hilgard & Marquis,

1961). The concept of physicalism denied the metaphysical dualism of material and mental states. This important implication stated that psychology must be operational and behavioristic. Logical positivism linked psychology with natural science. The transition of the logical positivism and scientific empiricism shaped the theory of behaviorism in that all constructs used in psychological investigations must be defined operationally. For behaviorists, all laws of empirical knowledge must be built on operational definitions of terms. A distinction was made by the behaviorists between empirical truths (inductive knowledge), which can be verified by scientific experimentation, and logical truths (deductive knowledge), which can be analyzed through rational thought.

Logical empiricism also led to the concept of verifiability in science. The method of verification for logical empiricism involves either direct verification of a proposition through sensory observation or indirect verification of a hypothesis through logical inference. Indirect verification of a hypothesis involved predictability such as the relationship between causes and effects in behavior.

The first psychologist to apply the principles of behaviorism to an understanding of human behavior was Watson (1924), who published a book entitled *Behaviorism*. Later the science of behaviorism became most prominent when Skinner (1938) published the book *The Behavior of Organisms*. As a strict empiricist, Skinner built a theory of human behavior based on controlled observations of animals in the laboratory. Science to Skinner was an attempt to discover order and to show that certain events are causally related. As a determinist, Skinner believed that human behavior can be predicted from a knowledge of the essential variables that influence behavior. With this approach Skinner felt that eventually a science of the nervous sys-

tem based on direct observation would be able to describe neural states and events that immediately precede behavior.

For behaviorists applying Skinner's principles, it was important to identify the independent variables (presumed causes of behavior) that were linked directly to the dependent variables (the specific instances of behavior). For the scientific behaviorist, the relationships established between the independent and dependent variables were the laws of science. The laws of behavior expressed in qualitative terms yielded a comprehensive picture of the organism as a behaving system. Through laboratory studies of animals Skinner (1953) postulated that principles of human behavior can be derived and applied to many aspects of living—education, economics, politics, sociology, and therapy. The process of reductionism in which complex examples of human behavior are analyzed in terms of simpler processes and animal experimentation is essentially a behavioristic theory.

These early experiments with laboratory animals by Skinner and others laid the foundation for the clinical application of behavior modification during the 1950s and 1960s with clients with psychosocial and mental disabilities who were institutionalized. Lindsley (1956), for example, applied operant conditioning techniques to individuals with mental retardation, and Wolpe (1961) reported that systematic desensitization techniques were effective with clients with phobias. During the 1970s, behavior modification techniques were used widely in institutions and in private practice as practical methods of eliminating self-defeating behaviors, such as were seen in delinquency (Jesness, 1975), hyperactivity (Christensen, 1975), alcoholism (Miller, 1972), obesity (Stuart, 1971), and seizures (Daniels, 1975).

Behavior therapy is presently a widely applied methodology that can be used with diverse diagnostic groups in psychosocial occupational therapy. The effectiveness of behavioristic programs is dependent on the therapist's ability to use a consistent approach for a specific behavior that can be operationally defined.

Key Concepts in Behavior Therapy

▶ *Behavior modification* is the application of learning theory based on reward and punishment and involves shaping human performance, emotions, attitudes, and values. For example, a psychosocial occupational therapist working with an individual with chronic schizophrenia will use behavior modification by using a system of reinforcers to shape the individual's learning of ADL skills, such as cooking, shopping, dressing, and grooming.

▶ A *stimulus* is an event that produces a reaction. For example, a musical selection can serve as a stimulus to elicit a relaxed state in a client with severe anxiety.

▶ An *unconditional stimulus* (US) is an event that produces an automatic unconditioned response (UR) in the individual. Reflexes and physiological reactions are unconditioned responses. For example, the digestive system of an individual who is hungry will be stimulated when food is perceived.

▶ A *conditioned stimulus* (CS) is any event that is learned which is associated with an unconditioned stimulus (US) and produces a conditioned response (CR). This concept was first identified by Pavlov (1927) and later refined by Skinner (1938), who called it respondent conditioning. The conditioned stimulus may be aversive, such as when Antabuse® is used with individuals with alcoholism. Antabuse® becomes a noxious drug (US) when it is used with alcohol, inducing the individual to become

nauseous (CR). The individual with the addiction is conditioned to associate alcohol with a noxious drug (US), resulting in a conditioned response of nausea when he or she considers drinking an alcoholic beverage.

▶ *Reinforcement* refers to any set of conditions or events that follows a response and increases or decreases the probability that the response will be made again. For example, when a child with autistic behavior imitates a sound from a therapist, and the therapist reinforces the behavior (e.g., making a sound) by rocking the child in his or her arms. Rocking the child becomes the reinforcement for the desired response of imitation.

Relationship of Behaviorism and Cognitive Behavioral Theory

The term *behavior therapy* was first defined by Wolpe (1961) as the use of established principles of learning to change maladaptive behavior. Cognitive–behavioral therapy is an extension of the key concepts and assumptions of behaviorism and behavioral therapy. While behavior therapies rely on such techniques as reinforcement, punishment, extinction, and stimulus control, usually from an external source, to change behaviors, cognitive-behavioral therapies emphasize "the importance of cognitive processes and private events as mediators of behavior change" (Kazdin & Wilson, 1978, p. 6).

Many of the cognitive-behavioral techniques developed outside the traditional concepts of behavior modification (Kazdin & Wilson, 1978). Although all cognitive–behavior therapies have three basic axioms: (a) "cognitive activity affects behavior, (b) cognitive activity may be monitored and altered, and (c) desired behavior change may be affected through cognitive change" (Dobson, 1988, p. 4), there are differences among them. Ellis (1962, 1979), one of the first cognitive–behavioral theorists, proposed in the theory of Rational-Emotive Therapy that "psychological disorders arise from faulty or irrational thought patterns (Kazdin & Wilson, p. 6). This approach incorporated directive therapy counseling approach and behavioral techniques. Meichenbaum (1977) proposed that cognitive–behavioral therapy be used to help clients develop self-regulation techniques to guide behavior. This approach is frequently used in special education programs with students who have emotional or behavioral disturbance. Beck's (1976) technique, called cognitive therapy, was used primarily with clients who were depressed and emphasized the development of thought patterns that were rational and adaptive. Both behavioral and cognitive tasks (e.g., homework, structured activities, assigning a specific activity schedule) are an essential part of the therapeutic program. Glasser (1965), in his book *Reality Therapy*, used problem-solving methods and stressed the responsibility of the individual. Glasser defines responsibility as "the ability to fulfill one's needs, and to do so in a way that does not deprive others of the ability to fulfill their needs" (Glasser, 1965, p. 13).

Behavioral Medicine

The coming together of a biopsychosocial approach to medicine and the practices of holistic health and behaviorism have led to a new arena of practice and research that is behavioral medicine. Metarazzo (1980) defined *behavioral medicine* as

> an interdisciplinary field dedicated to promoting a philosophy of health that stresses individual responsibility and the application of behavioral and biomedical science, knowledge and techniques to the maintenance of health and the prevention of illness and dysfunction by a variety of self-initiated individuals or shared activities. (p. 813)

Behavioral medicine incorporates the research and clinical studies of physiology, psychiatry, psychology, and physical medicine. Specific treatment techniques derived from behavioral medicine include behavior therapy approaches, such as systematic desensitization (Shalev, Orr, & Pitman, 1992), progressive relaxation (Anshel, 1996), assertiveness training (Aschen, 1997), and finger temperature biofeedback (Moser, Dracup, Woo, & Stevenson, 1997). The treatment techniques in behavioral medicine are noninvasive, rely on the active participation of the client, and are interdisciplinary in nature (Schwartz & Associates, 1995). Physicians, psychologists, social workers, nurses, physical therapists, speech-language pathologists, occupational therapists, and special educators in rehabilitation employ treatment techniques that fall under behavioral medicine.

The specific disorders treated by behavioral medicine techniques include medicine and behavioral problems such as hypertension, chronic headache, seizure disorders, pain, anorexia nervosa, incontinence, chemical dependency, anxiety, sexual disorders, chronic respiratory problems (Doley, Meredith, & Ciminero, 1982; Freeman, Pretzer, Fleming, & Simon, 1990; Gorman, 1996), all of which may have a psychophysiological dimension precipitated by stress reactions. Treatment techniques used in behavioral medicine

> go beyond the traditional germ theory of the etiology and progression diseases. It recognizes the important roles of stress, life-style, habits, and environmental variables in the development, maintenance, and treatment of medical and dental diseases and conditions. (Schwartz & Associates, 1995, p. 6)

Figure 4–2 illustrates the relationship between stress and illness in individuals who are vulnerable. Treatment entails counteracting the stressful reactions through relaxation theory (Benson, 1975), cognitive control techniques (Beck, 1970, 1976; Beck, Rush, Shaw, & Emery, 1979), biofeedback (Schwartz, 1995), and other stress management techniques (Lehrer & Woolfolk, 1993). (See Table 4–6 for a summary of treatment methods and Chapter 10 for a more complete description of stress management techniques.)

Behavioral medicine has much in common with the underlying philosophy of occupational therapy. The philosophies of both behavioral medicine and occupational therapy believe the client is an important factor in the treatment process; the client's compliance with the treatment regimen is essential; relaxation therapy and stress management are key elements; the client as a whole person is emphasized; and that treatment strategies involve a multimodal approach (Lehrer, Carr, Sargunaraj, & Woolfolk, 1993; Schwartz & Associates, 1995; Williams & Gentry, 1977).

Occupational Therapy Treatment Process

How can occupational therapy define its treatment role in health care more adequately and still maintain a humanistic tradition? An occupational therapy treatment model that builds on a generalist role and is consistent with behavioral medicine is holistic and comprehensive in scope. In this model, occupational therapy treatment methods are derived from specific areas of clinical practice.

Before identifying these areas of clinical practice, it is important to examine the question: What is treatment in occupational therapy? A medical definition implies that treatment is any specific procedure used for curing or lessening the effects of a disease or pathological condition. Because occupational therapists work primarily with clients who are disabled, the main goal of treatment is to help the client lessen the effects of his or her disability rather than in to cure the condition. When the medical definition of treatment is extended to occupational therapy, treatment is defined as the application of

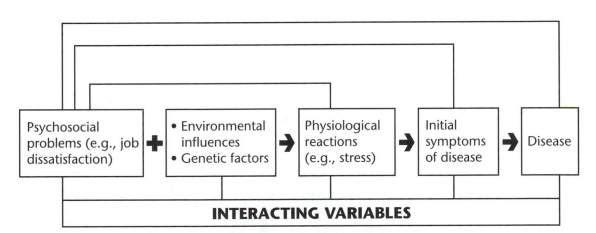

Figure 4–2. This figure depicts the interactions between the variables of stress and disease. A person with psychosocial problems resulting in stress interacts with environmental influences or genetic factors to cause a physiological reaction. This leads to an initial symptom of the disease, and finally to the disease. Each of the variables interacts with each other, leading to additional stress, symptoms, and disease. As the psychosocial problems are reduced, the other manifestations of stress can be relieved.

Table 4–6. Comparison of Behavioral Medicine and Traditional Medicine in Treating Psychophysiological Disorders

Disorder	Estimate of Prevalence	Examples of Behavioral Methods	Traditional Medication	Possible Side Effects of Medication
Essential hypertension	50 million adults in the United States have hypertension (Hall, 1996)	• Biofeedback (McGrady, Olson, & Kroon, 1995) • Relaxation therapy (Benson, 1977) • Lifestyle modifications (Hall, 1996)	Antihypertension drugs	• gastrointestinal irritability • weakness • drowsiness • depression (Berkow, 1992)
Chronic headaches (tension and migraine)	40 million adults in the United States experience chronic headaches (Aronoff, 1985)	• Biofeedback (Schwartz, 1995) • Progressive relaxation therapy (Blanchert et al., 1989) • Cognitive therapy (Holroyd & Andrasik, 1982)	• analgesics • propranolol • amitriptyline • fluoxetine hydrochloride (Mayer, 1996)	• hypotension • depression • fatigue • insomnia • anxiety • gastrointestinal disturbances (Mayer, 1996)
Insomnia	10 to 20% of population experience chronic insomnia (Ehrenberg, 1996)	• Meditation (Woolfolk, Carr–Kaffashan, McNulty, & Lehrer, 1976) • Progressive relaxation and biofeedback (Nicassio, Boylan, & McCabe, 1982) • Paradoxical intention (Turner & Ascher, 1979) • Hypnotic relaxation (Borkovec & Fowles, 1973)	• levodopa • benzodiazepine • opiates or valproate (Ehrenberg, 1996)	• hypotension • hallucinations • addiction • ataxia • cognitive impairments • gastrointestinal disturbances • encephalopathy (Berkow, 1992; Ehrenberg, 1996)
Low back pain ("discomfort in lumbosacral portion of back with or without painful radiation into the hips, buttocks, or legs," Miller & Mathis, 1996, p. 250)	80% of individuals will experience one or more episodes of low back pain sometime in their lifetime (Miller & Mathis, 1996)	• Progressive relaxation and cognitive behavioral therapy (Turner, 1982) • Biofeedback (Sherman & Arena, 1992) • Transcutaneous Electrical Nerve Stimulation (TENS) (Wolfe, 1978) • Acupuncture (Gunn, Milbrandt, Little, & Mason, 1980) • Spinal manipulation therapy (Gibson et al., 1985) • Massage therapy (Pope et al., 1994)	• analgesics • muscle relaxants (e.g., methocarbonol, carisoprodol) • nonsteroid anti-inflammatory drugs (NSAID) • codeine or meperidine (Berkow, 1992)	• respiratory depression • nausea and vomiting • constipation • dysphoria • CNS excitation myoclonus tremulous seizures • addictive (Berkow, 1992)

Table 4–6. Comparison of Behavioral Medicine and Traditional Medicine in Treating Psychophysiological Disorders

Disorder	Estimate of Prevalence	Examples of Behavioral Methods	Traditional Medication	Possible Side Effects of Medication
Alcoholism and substance abuse	• 18 million individuals with addictions in the United States (McMicken, 1996) • 1 million individuals with cocaine addiction • 600,000 individuals with heroin addiction (Schnoll, 1996)	• Autogenic biofeedback (Fahrion, Walters, Coyne, & Allen, 1992) • Communication skills training (Monti, Abrams, & Binkoff, 1990) • Stress inoculation training (Marlatt & Gordon, 1985)	• Antabuse® • benzodiazepines • disulfiram (Berkow, 1992)	• respiratory depression • depression • cognitive disorders (Berkow, 1992)

specific activities or procedures to develop, improve, or restore function in the individual who is disabled.

One of the most important decisions occupational therapists make is in the selection of an activity related to the treatment goal. For example, when the therapeutic goal is to increase social skills in a client with schizophrenia, then the occupational therapist in concert with the client should decide on the best method or activity to accomplish this goal. The occupational therapist and client ideally should use a problem-solving client-centered approach in planning a treatment program. Individual treatment goals are established with the assumption that no single activity is best for all clients. In order to know whether the activity selected is effective in accomplishing the goal, the therapist must use an outcome measure to test the client's functional ability. As an example, a treatment goal to increase social skills would require an outcome measure of social skills. Outcome can be measured or determined by the therapist's clinical evaluation of the client's behavior or performance, the client's self-evaluation of improvement, standardized paper and pencil tests, and observational data from family members or others.

The occupational therapy treatment process consists of the treatment goal, the therapeutic activity or treatment procedure, and the outcome measure of functional ability. The treatment goal represents the core of occupational therapy practice. How are treatment goals usually determined in practice? Treatment goals can be identified by the referring physician, established by the occupational therapist, or expressed by the client. However, many times treatment goals can easily be peripheral to the most important aspects of the client's life. For example, for the client with schizophrenia, treatment goals in occupational therapy can include the following: (a) increase socialization, (b) improve motor performance, (c) foster leisure skills, and/or (d) prepare the client for employment in the community. How does the therapist decide which of these treatment goals is the most important to focus on first? It is conceivable that occupational therapists can spend many hours working with clients on treatment goals that are insignificant. Can occupational therapists agree on clinical areas of practice that can guide them in selecting treatment goals related to the major areas of a client's life? In attempting to answer this question, the occupational therapy literature was searched for a clinical practice model. The most systematic clinical practice model found is in the *Uniform Terminology for Occupational Therapy*, published by the American Occupational Therapy Association (AOTA, 1994). The description of services in this report emphasizes treatment outcomes and occupational therapy's unique contribution in comparison to other health professions. This model serves as a guide to clinical practice and it is used by governmental agencies and private insurance companies for reimbursements. Six areas of occupational therapy treatment were derived from the *Uniform Terminology* to serve as a generalist model in psychosocial practice. (See Figure P–1 for the performance areas and performance components taken from the *Uniform Terminology*.)

A Comprehensive Psychosocial Occupational Therapy Treatment Model

A treatment model is proposed that has the following underlying assumptions:

▶ The model is consistent with the generalist role, where the occupational therapist is prepared to provide comprehensive rehabilitation services to individuals with psychosocial disabilities. The need for primary care workers in the health care system has been recognized by most reformers as most urgent (Mechanic, 1983; Whitbeck, 1981). A generalist, primary care role for the psychosocial occupational therapist presupposes a total assessment of the needs of the individual in the most important areas of his or her life (i.e., work, daily living, interpersonal relationships, leisure). In this model, the occupational therapist defines client's problems in the context of the ability to cope with the disability. It is assumed

that all individuals with disabilities have similar needs to be as independent as possible in the basic areas of life. The functional abilities of those with disabilities, rather than the diagnosis, guide the treatment process. Clients with psychosocial disabilities have to deal with stress, work adjustment, and basic living skills. The generalist role of the occupational therapist defines treatment within specified areas of clinical practice that are representative of a comprehensive approach to rehabilitation.

▶ The major areas of clinical practice identified for the generalist role can be operationally defined. The operational definition of a treatment method infers that the method can be replicated by other therapists (Stein, 1989; Stein & Cutler, 2000). The treatment method is sufficiently detailed so that another therapist can apply it. In this model, the treatment methods used (e.g., biofeedback, relaxation training, and assertiveness training) are operationally defined and can be replicated in practice.

▶ The occupational therapist evaluates the functional abilities of the individual with a psychosocial disability by applying reliable and valid measuring instruments. One of the most challenging parts of occupational therapy treatment is documenting improvement. For example, how can therapists be reasonably certain that what they did has helped the client to increase his or her independence? The tests or measuring instruments that are used in gauging improvement are critical to the treatment process. Reliability, accuracy, and validity are considered in selecting a test instrument to evaluate the client's functional abilities.

▶ The areas of clinical practice represent the major areas of life that are critical to the client with disabilities. Almost every aspect of the individual's life is affected to some extent. The disability threatens the individual's existence and ability to function independently. The disability also presents a continual barrage of stress for the client coping with a dysfunctional role in society. Invariably, pain, whether it is the psychic pain of depression or accompanying pain from stress or the secondary effects of the psychosocial disability, can be a problem for many clients. In most cases, the major areas of life affected by a disability are work, leisure, basic living skills, social interactions, psychological adjustment, motor problems, and stress and pain management. All individuals with psychosocial disabilities must cope with each of these problems in the course of the rehabilitation. How they cope with these problems and how they are treated by therapists are the focus of this proposed model. Rehabilitation of those with disabilities is a shared responsibility in health care. The unique role of the occupational therapist is the ability to skillfully apply activities in the treatment process. Methods, treatment practices, and evaluation procedures are shared by many health care workers.

The eight areas of clinical practice are fundamental to occupational therapy in the proposed model: (a) basic living skills and nutrition, (b) neuromuscular stimulation and exercise, (c) pain management, (d) self-esteem, (e) social skills, (f) stress management, (g) work, and (h) leisure planning. The authors propose these eight areas of clinical practice as a new way to operationally define the practice of psychosocial occupational therapy. We believe that what occupational therapists primarily do can be subsumed under these eight areas of clinical practice. The treatment goals, methods, assessment, and evaluation techniques are introduced

and explained in the remaining chapters of this book. These techniques, related to clients' skill components or life competencies, are examples of the many methodologies that can be applied in occupational therapy practice. This model for practice is intended to be comprehensive in comprising the major psychosocial needs of the client through utilization of the emerging technology in health care.

COGNITIVE BEHAVIORAL THERAPIES (CBT) FRAMES OF REFERENCE

Cognitive Behavioral Therapy

"The introduction of the concept of self-control and self-control strategies for modifying behavior in the early sixties signaled a movement toward more cognitive emphasis in behavior therapy" (Calhoun & Turner, 1981, p. 5). A large portion of CBT involves techniques using self-regulation, such as biofeedback (Brown, 1974; Schwartz & Associates, 1995), progressive relaxation (Jacobson, 1929, 1978), relaxation response and meditation (Benson, 1977), stress inoculation (Meichenbaum, 1985), yoga (Patel, 1973), autogenic training (Linden, 1990), and aerobic exercise (Fillingim & Blumenthal, 1993), psychoeducational[2] (Lillie & Armstrong, 1982). (See Figure 4–3 for the relationship among behaviorism, behavioral therapies, and cognitive–behavioral therapies.)

Definition

Cognitive-behavioral therapy (CBT) *frame of reference* is defined as the application of self-regulation methods and strategies to change think-

---

[2] Within the field of special education as related to emotional and behavioral disturbance, psychoeducational approaches refer to the use of psychodynamic and psychotherapeutic approaches within the school setting.

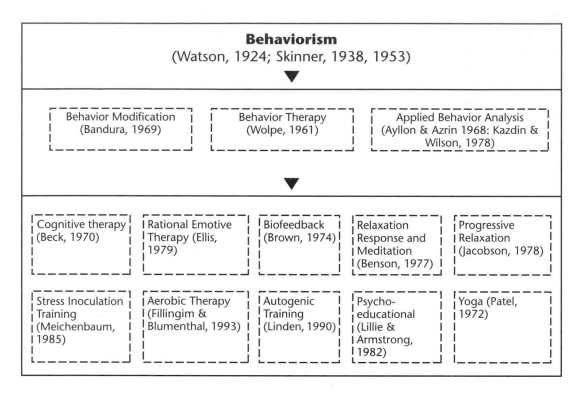

Figure 4–3. Relationship among behavior modification, behavior therapy, and applied behavioral analysis. All of these came from theories of behaviorism developed by Watson (1924) and Skinner (1953), and each is included within the cognitive behavioral therapies. There are many forms of behaviorism within the overall theoretical model.

ing and behavior (Meichenbaum, 1977). Braswell and Bloomquist (1991) conceptualize cognitive-behavioral therapy as "a collaborative, goal-orientated, skills-training, directive approach to psychological treatment" (p. 104). In this frame of reference, the occupational therapist becomes an educator–facilitator (Bruce & Borg, 1993). The assumptions of CBT are listed in Table 4–7, while the principles of CBT are listed in Table 4–8. Both of these are based on the behavioral theoretical model, which suggests that thinking or cognitive activity affects behavior. The key elements in CBT are listed in Table 4–9.

Research and Methodology of CBT

Johnston (1986) was one of the first occupational therapists to report the use of CBT in clinical practice with clients with depression. In her conceptualization of CBT, she stated

> Where as cognitive-behavior skills may not be the traditional skills associated with occupational therapy, they involve basic interpersonal skills, problem solving skills, and self-management skills. As such, they are often prerequisites to the ability to perform effectively in the roles of player, student, or worker. Occupational therapists already have or should have some understanding of how habits and skills are developed or relearned. This information is

Table 4–7. Assumptions of Cognitive-Behavioral Frame of Reference and Implications for Psychosocial Occupational Therapy

- Thinking or cognitive activity affects behavior.
- Behavior can change how we think about ourselves.
- Thinking can be self-regulated.
- Desired behavioral change can occur through structured learning and the acquisition of skills through relaxation therapy and biofeedback.
- Stress management is a key component of cognitive-behavioral therapy (CBT).
- A psychoeducational model using a group format is an essential method for CBT.
- Group activities can be incorporated into CBT.
- Outcome measures are used as pre- and posttests in assessing improvement.
- Triangulation is used in evaluating outcome—self-evaluation, standardized test, and physiological measure.
- Patients are encouraged to practice their newly acquired skills as homework.

Table 4–8. Principles of Cognitive-Behavioral Therapy

- Therapeutic sessions are purposeful and structured for the client, either in a group or individually.
- Client is an active learner and practices methods during sessions.
- New behaviors learned are positively reinforced by the therapist.
- Client is encouraged to actively practice method as homework and to keep a diary or checklist of progress.
- Client is given continuous feedback regarding the ability to cognitively control symptoms and stressors by monitoring physiological responses through biofeedback.
- Therapist and client establish therapeutic alliance and cooperatively select activities that increase positive cognitive control of symptoms and stressors by incorporating copers into a daily schedule of activities.
- Therapist evaluates the client's progress through self-evaluation of compliance.

Table 4–9. Cognitive-Behavioral Approach as a Key Element in the Rehabilitation of the Client with a Psychosocial Dysfunction

- The cognitive-behavioral approach is noninvasive and it does not produce serious side effects, which may occur with psychotropic medication.
- The client is an active participant in the treatment process.
- It is holistic and emphasizes the multifactorial nature of the causes and treatments of a psychiatric disability.
- It places the therapist and client in cooperative relationship in aiding the client to achieve attainable goals that are operationalized and clearly stated.
- It sets up treatment goals that are relevant, understandable, measurable, behavioral, and achievable.
- It is positive in nature and emphasizes what the client can do or has the potential to accomplish rather than focusing on the client's deficits or disabilities.

invaluable in the teaching of cognitive behavioral techniques. Hence, it would seem an appropriate area for occupational therapists to develop interest and expertise. (pp. 55–56)

In spite of this viewpoint, few occupational therapists have reported the use of CBT in their practice. The literature, however, does show that some psychosocial occupational therapists have found CBT effective. Taylor (1988), in a theoretical and review article, compared the use of psychoanalytic and cognitive-behavioral approaches in anger intervention. She proposed an anger intervention model that used a cognitive-behavioral approach with emphasis on stress management and behavior therapy. Sisko Salo-Chydenius (1994), an occupational therapist in Finland, reported the use of a model using CBT in social skills training groups with clients who had long-term severe depression. Likewise, Engel (1994) has found the use of CBT effective in alleviating pain in adults with chronic, recurrent, and nonmalignant pain. Some therapists have reported the incorporation of CBT into psychoeducational groups (Crist, 1986; Lillie & Armstrong, 1982).

Stein has used CBT in his clinical practice as an occupational therapist. Several of his studies are summarized here. These studies took place between 1987 and 1993 in Edmonton General Hospital in Alberta, Canada (Stein, 1987a; Stein & Smith, 1989), Winnipeg, Manitoba (Stein, 1992, 1993, 1994, 1996), and Milwaukee, Wisconsin (Stein, 1990, 1991; Stein & Nikolic, 1989). The major purpose of these studies was to determine if a group of clients with depression, schizophrenia, and alcoholism could reduce their anxiety through a short-term highly structured stress management program. The results demonstrated that clients could reduce their anxiety, either in group or individual therapy. The major implications for these three clinical groups were:

▶ Clients with depression, schizophrenia, and alcoholism can be taught stress management techniques in short-term structured sessions in either group or individual therapy.

▶ Stress management techniques can be used to increase the repertoire of coping skills in managing stress.

▶ The results obtained from the *Stress Management Questionnaire* (Stein, 1987b) can be used to develop individualized programs for clients.

In the development of a stress management program using cognitive-behavioral techniques, Stein (Stein & Smith, 1989) developed a clinical protocol that can be used in either group or individual therapy in a clinical setting. The protocol is based on an eight-session program that involves psychoeducation skill building, relaxation therapy, biofeedback, and role playing. Specific details of the sessions are outlined in Chapter 10. Outcome is measured through the *Stress Management Questionnaire* (Stein, 1987b), the *State-Trait Anxiety Inventory* (Spielberger, 1983), and self-evaluations (see the compliance form in Chapter 10). Compliance is an important aspect of the treatment and is incorporated into the sessions through a diary kept by the client and homework exercises. (See Chapter 10 for more information on this protocol.)

Cognitive Disability Frame of Reference

The Cognitive Disability frame of reference uses a behavioral assessment to determine a client's level of cognitive ability. Allen (1985) defines a cognitive disability as a "restriction in voluntary motor action originating in the physical or chemical structures of the brain, and producing observable limitations in routine task behavior" (p. 31). In the Cognitive Disability frame of reference, treatment can be aimed at (a) expectancy treatment, which relies on the natural process of healing; (b) palliative treatment to reduce symptoms, for example, use of psychotropic drugs; and (c) supportive treatment, which involves sustaining the client's strengths and assets. Allen proposed that individuals with a psychosocial disability have impairments in cognition that can be hierarchically assessed. These impairments are described in Table 4–10.

Table 4–10. Allen's Cognitive Levels of Disabilities

Cognitive Levels	Description of Client Behavior	Treatment Goals
Level 1: Automatic Actions	• does not respond to other people • does not appear to understand language • uses automatic reflexes of swallowing, smelling, toileting, chewing	• reduce pain • reduce muscle contractures • produce responses to sensory stimulation
Level 2: Postural Actions	• aware of other people, but not objects in the environment • imitates movements such as gesturing and simple repetitive movements • attention span for gross motor tasks lasts from 5 to 15 minutes • responds mostly to proprioceptive cues	Gross motor movements such as • walking • bean bag toss • Simple Simon games
Level 3: Manual Actions	• interest in touching, and tactile cues • engages in repetitive activities that are automatized and that are part of a task (e.g., chopping vegetables or stringing beads) • attention span for an activity is about 30 minutes	Completing parts of a task (e.g., preparing part of a meal)
Level 4: Goal-Directed Actions	• use of visual cues and imitation to achieve a goal • can do part of a task, such as part of the laundry • can attend to task for about 1 hour	Can benefit from forward or backward chaining, such as in dressing tasks
Level 5: Exploratory Actions	• learns from trial and error, and initiates new steps or ideas • unable to anticipate changes or to plan differences using symbolic reasoning • difficulty with tasks that may not be automatic (e.g., money management, cooking, traveling)	Designing and completing activities that are within the individual's ability and do not cause multiple errors
Level 6: Planned Activities	• considered absence of disability • uses symbolic cues when planning or anticipating events • can follow complex multiple directions given verbally and in written form • can think abstractly	Engaging in independent activities to plan, design, and complete a project

Sources: Developed from *Occupational Therapy for Psychiatric Diseases: Measurement and Management of Cognitive Disabilities* by C. K. Allen, 1985, Boston: Little & Brown; *Conceptual Foundations of Occupational Therapy* (2nd ed.), by G. Kielhofner, 1997, pp. 127–144, Philadelphia: F. A. Davis; *Psychosocial Occupational Therapy; Frames of Reference for Intervention* (2nd ed.), by M. A. Bruce & B. Borg, 1993, pp. 251–270, Thorofare, NJ: SLACK.

Assumptions

The Cognitive Disabilities frame of reference includes the following assumptions:

▶ Cognition, which includes perception, thinking, and memory, underlies all behavior.

▶ Psychiatric disabilities are due to brain dysfunction or pathology.

▶ Impairment in the brain causes damage to the cognitive processes, resulting in observable behaviors.

▶ There is no difference between a psychiatric disability and neurologic dysfunction.

▶ Assessment of a cognitive disability can be made through observation of an everyday performance of a routine task.

▶ Cognitive abilities in Allen's (1985) frame of reference are organized into six hierarchical levels, which are measured in seven different areas (see Table 4–10).

▶ The most effective treatment for clients who have long-term disabilities that are stable is modification of the environment or the activity. For example, an individual with chronic schizophrenia whose condition has remained stable would benefit from a structured program in day treatment or adult day care, where medications are monitored, leisure activities are structured, self-care activities are taught, and the opportunity for supported employment is provided.

▶ Tasks are selected and modified according to the client's cognitive level using activity analysis and environmental modifications. For example, an individual on Level 4 would be engaged in goal-directed activities in which the activity is organized into several tasks that have two to three steps.

When doing laundry, the tasks might include sorting, putting the soap in the machine, and turning on the machine by moving the dial to "start." These tasks, in turn, would be broken into two to three smaller steps.

▶ Individuals with psychosocial disabilities have difficulties in routine tasks, such as preparing meals, doing laundry, dressing, communicating with others, and using public transportation.

▶ Treatment in occupational therapy is secondary to medication and recovery of function. Skill building is not considered a primary factor in the Cognitive Disabilities frame of reference. "I suggest measurement and management as alternatives to improvement as goals of occupational therapy" (Allen, 1985, p. 32).

Assessment

Allen (1985) developed three tests used for assessment of cognitive function in her Cognitive Disability frame of reference.

▶ The *Routine Task Inventory* (RTI; Allen, 1985) is an observational rating scale in which 14 different tasks (e.g., grooming, dressing, bathing, spending money, preparing food) are evaluated using Allen's six cognitive levels.

▶ *Allen Cognitive Level Test* (ACL; Allen, 1985) is a standardized test that measures functions at levels 4, 5, and 6 in which the client is asked to lace leather.

▶ *Cognitive Performance Task* (Burns, Mortimer, & Merchak, 1994): functional assessment of six areas of ADL skills (dressing, shopping, making toast, telephoning, washing, and traveling) involving verbal directions, performance and cueing or demonstration as necessary, and used to predict independent living skills.

DEVELOPMENTAL THEORETICAL MODEL

Definition, Components, and Assumptions

In general, development is the process of growth. "Growth is a process of organization. It is a unitary and an integrative process. If it were not unitary, the organism would lack wholeness; if it were not integrative, the organism would lack individuality" (Gesell, 1952, p. 64). Typical human growth and maturation occurs in a supportive environment, in a hierarchical, sequential process. The major theories within the developmental theoretical model are outlined in Table 4–11.

Piaget (1929, 1952a, 1952b, 1954) has played an important part in the understanding of how young children develop cognition and in the ways young children learn. Piaget's theories, based on observations of his own children, have influenced the developmental literature in all disciplines. He theorized that development of cognition occurs in four stages, with changes in stages a result of adaptation of the individual to the environmental demands. Each stage is qualitatively different from other stages, meaning that the way in which individuals approach thinking and reasoning is markedly different. During the first stage, *sensorimotor*, infants and toddlers develop an understanding of their environment and surroundings through physical movement and actions. The second stage, *preoperational*, is characterized by the development of the use of symbols (e.g., language) and beginning reasoning. Thinking is combined to the "here and now," and generally requires the use of concrete objects, such as pictures or manipulatives, to comprehend information. During the

third stage, *concrete operations*, children develop the ability to think more abstractly by using mental reasoning rather than physical manipulation. The need for manipulatives or concrete objects is lessened. Children develop the ability to use intellectual operations such as reversibility (half-full and half-empty), conservation, and serial ordering by size, class, or number. In the final stage, *formal operations*, individuals are able to think hypothetically and use symbols and abstract reasoning without any use of concrete objects.

Although Piaget developed a theory of moral development, Kohlberg's (1971) expansion of Piaget's theory is usually given more attention. Kohlberg's theory was developed after many years of interviewing children, adolescents, and adults using a series of vignettes followed by questions regarding moral thinking. Kohlberg conceptualized three levels of moral development, each with two stages. Most children under the age of 9 fall at the first level, stages 1 and 2, which he labeled *preconventional*. At this level, children, who are egocentric and unable to recognize two points of view, follow rules based on (a) the desire to avoid punishment, or (b) the need to satisfy their own needs. In the second level (*conventional* level), consisting of stages 3 and 4, the good of the family or the group is more important than the needs of an individual. "Good behavior," then, pleases and helps others and follows societal authority. The third level, labeled *postconventional, autonomous,* or *principled* and consisting of stages 5 and 6, is characterized by a recognition that rules and standards that are right have been critically examined. Most laws can be changed and modified by the majority; however, universal laws like life and liberty must be upheld regardless of the majority belief. At the highest level are the universal moral principles, such as the Golden Rule, related to human rights and individuality.

Table 4–11. Major Theorists in Development

Stage	Emotional (Freud, 1933)	Social (Erikson, 1950, 1963)	Cognitive (Piaget, 1929)	Motor/Language (Gesell, 1928)	Moral (Kohlberg, 1971)
Infancy and Toddler	Oral • dependent • aggressive	Trust vs. Mistrust	Sensorimotor Age 0–24 months	crawling, sitting • grasping and holding • single words	Pre-moral
	Anal • toilet training	Autonomy vs. Shame, doubt	Preoperational Ages 2–7 years	walking • stacking blocks • two-word sentences	
Early Childhood	Phallic	Initiative vs. Guilt		catching balls and buttoning • copying letters • full sentences	Preconventional • I: Egocentric and heteronomous • II: Concrete individualistic perspective
Middle and Late Childhood	Latency	Industry vs. Inferiority	Concrete Operational Ages 7–11 years	mastery of skills • social clubs • organization of stories	
Adolescence	Genital	Identity vs. Role confusion	Formal operations Age 12 and above	argumentative skills • athletic and sports • peer groups	Conventional • Interpersonal concordance • Social system and consciousness
Early Adult		Intimacy vs. Isolation		vocational and relationship decisions	
Middle Adulthood		Generativity vs. Stagnation			Postconventional or Principled • social contract or utility and individual rights
Late Adulthood		Ego integration vs. Despair			• universal ethical principles

SENSORY INTEGRATIVE THERAPY FRAME OF REFERENCE

The area of perceptual-motor functioning is a basic foundation for Sensory Integration Therapy. Gesell (1928), Piaget (1929), Bender (1938), Schilder (1942), and Werner (1948) were some of the first theorists and researchers to explore and describe the relationship between child development and perceptual functioning. Occupational therapists use perceptual and perceptual-motor tests to assess the effects of dysfunction and impairment. Tests such as the *Test of Visual Perceptual Skills—Revised* (nonmotor; TVPS-R; Gardner, 1996), *Developmental Test of Visual Motor Integration—Fourth Edition* (VMI-4; Beery, 1997), *Bruininks-Oseretsky Motor Perceptual Test* (BOMPT; Bruininks, 1978), and the *Peabody Developmental Motor Scales—Second Edition* (PDMS-2; Folio & Fewell, 2000) are used in this assessment.

The work of Jean Ayres (1972a, 1972b, 1979) on Sensory Integration Therapy is an extension and elaboration of the theories, research, and clinical practice in the perceptual and perceptual-motor areas. Ayres (1954) first expounded her theory on perceptual-motor functioning in the *American Journal of Occupational Therapy* (AJOT) in the article "Ontogenetic Principles in the Development of Arm and Hand Functions." Ayres proposed that neuromuscular principles could be applied in treating clients with brain injuries, such as stroke and cerebral palsy. She theorized that there is a parallelism between the recovery of the client with brain injury and neurological maturation in the typical child. In other words, the presence of abnormal reflexes and motor dysfunctions in clients with neuromuscular disabilities follow a predictable sequence and, consequently, the therapist can use this information to help the client consciously develop the single motor patterns one at a time. This is a landmark article because it laid the framework for the Sensory Integration Therapy frame of reference.

Ayres, the founder of the frame of reference of Sensory Integration Therapy, received her bachelor's degree in Occupational Therapy in 1945. She worked for approximately 8 years primarily with clients with neurological impairments in various hospitals in the Southern California area. She received a master's degree in 1954 and a doctorate in 1961 in Educational Psychology from the University of Southern California. From 1964 to 1966, she worked as a postdoctoral student in brain research at UCLA. She had been a clinician, teacher, and researcher in the fields of occupational therapy, special education, and psychology. The Sensory Integration Therapy frame of reference has been applied to clients with cerebral palsy (Murray & Anzalone, 1997), autism (Ayres & Tickle, 1980; Murray & Anzalone, 1997; Ray, King, & Grandin, 1988; Slavik, Kitsuwa-Lowe, Danner, Green, & Ayres, 1984), learning disabilities (Clark, Mailloux, Parham, & Bissell,1989; Humphries, Wright, Snider, & McDougall, 1992; Murray & Anzalone, 1997), ADHD/ADD (Mulligan, 1996), infants at risk (Gregg, Hafner, & Korner, 1976; Mueller, 1996), schizophrenia (Ayres & Heskett, 1972; Bailey, 1978; Evans & Salim, 1992; Jorstad, Wilbert, & Wirrer, 1977; King, 1974), mental retardation (Murray & Anzalone, 1997), traumatic brain injury (Mercer & Boch, 1983), academic achievement (Polatajko, Law, Miller, Schaffer, & Macnab, 1991; Wilson, Kaplan, Fellowes, Gruchy, & Faris, 1992), handwriting (Price, 1986), and developmentally delayed children (Magrun, Ottenbacher, McCue, & Keefe, 1981).

Definition of Sensory Integration

Ayres (1989) defined sensory integration as

the neurological process that organizes sensation from one's own body and from the environment and makes it possible to use the body effectively within the environment. The spatial and temporal aspects of inputs from different sensory modalities are interpreted, associated, and unified. Sensory integration is information processing. . . . the brain must select, enhance, inhibit, compare, and associate the sensory information in a flexible, constantly changing pattern; in other words, the brain must integrate it. (p. 11)

The American Occupational Therapy Association (1982) defines sensory integration as

the nervous system's process of assimilating and organizing sensory information for functional use. An individual's ability to interact with the environment is influenced by how effectively and efficiently that person is able to process and use information from the tactile, vestibular, proprioceptive, visual, auditory, olfactory, and gustatory systems. (p. 831)

Assumptions (Fisher & Murray, 1991)

▶ There is plasticity within the central nervous system, which is the ability of the brain to change or be modified.

▶ Sensory Integrative (SI) processes occur in developmental sequence.

▶ The brain functions as an integrated whole and is comprised of systems that are hierarchically organized.

▶ "Evincing an adaptive behavior promotes sensory integration, and in turn, the ability to produce an adaptive behavior reflects sensory integration" (Fisher & Murray, 1991, p. 17).

▶ "People have an inner drive to develop sensory integration through participation in sensorimotor activities" (Fisher & Murray, 1991 p. 17).

Theoretical Concepts of Sensory Integration

Jean Ayres, in the Eleanor Clarke Slagle Lecture in 1963, identified five major syndromes of perceptual-motor dysfunction. These major syndromes were later theorized to underlie many of the diagnostic groups that have sensory integrative dysfunction. Factor analytic studies completed between 1965 and 1977 have generally identified the following six patterns of dysfunction (Fisher & Murray, 1991):

▶ *Dyspraxia:* the inability to motor plan, such as performing skilled activities. There is a loss of manual dexterity, especially in handling small objects. Speed of performance is also diminished. This dysfunction is associated with difficulty in tactile discrimination.

▶ *Poor bilateral integration:* described as "a tendency of the hands to avoid crossing the midline of the body when engaged in motor tasks and difficulty in learning to discriminate and identify the right and left sides of the body" (Ayres, 1963, p. 224).

▶ *Tactile defensiveness:* characterized by an individual's lack of tolerance and displeasure in being touched. Individuals with tactile defensiveness show negative emotional response when touched by another person.

▶ *Poor form and space perception:* dysfunction in both visual and tactile modalities, underlying difficulty in such tasks as setting a table, drawing a design, reading, or assembling an object on a production line.

▶ *Auditory–language dysfunction:* Ayres (1979) theorized that children with sensory integration dysfunctions often have difficulties in auditory–language because of the interrelatedness of the sensory systems. Thus, she recommended an evaluation by a sensory integrative therapist whenever a language dysfunction was suspected.

▶ *Poor eye-hand coordination:* a form of dys-praxia resulting in an inability to get the hands to do what the eyes see. Writing difficulties, catching, or drawing are sometimes outgrowths of these difficulties.

Cluster analysis has identified additional areas of deficit (Ayres, 1989). These include (a) *visual figure-ground perception* involving the inability to distinguish an abstract or common figure that is embedded into a design serving as the background for the figure; (b) *visuomotor construction,* affecting the ability to build three-dimensional block designs from a visual model; and (c) *praxis on verbal demand,* resulting in an inability to follow specific motor movements when presented with a verbal command.

Ayres developed a series of neuropsychological standardized tests, *The Southern California Sensory Integration Tests* (SCSIT; 1972b), to measure objectively the presence of these syndromes. After considerable development, these tests were published by Western Psychological Services (Ayres, 1972a, 1972b) and later revised and renamed (*Sensory Integration and Praxis Tests* [SIPT]; Ayres, 1989). The tests were designed to "contribute to the clinical understanding of children from 4 through 8 years of age with mild to moderate learning, behavioral, or developmental irregularities" (Ayres & Marr, 1991, p. 203).

Brief Description of the Sensory Integration and Praxis Tests

The SIPT is made up of 17 tests, each individually administered. The entire battery takes about 1 1/2 hours. An intensive training for administration and interpretation of the test is required, and scoring is by computer, completed through the Western Psychological Services.

The tests are performance based, with only one test requiring reliance on auditory-language comprehension. The tests are divided into four overlapping groups (a) tactile and vestibular-proprioceptive sensory processing; (b) form, space perception, and visuomotor coordination; (c) praxis ability; and (d) bilateral integration and sequencing (Ayres & Marr, 1991).

▶ *Space Visualization* (SV): Form boards are utilized to involve visual perception of form and space, and mental manipulation of objects in space.

▶ *Figure–ground Perception* (FG): Stimulus figures are superimposed and imbedded to require selection of a foreground figure from a rival background.

▶ *Manual Form Perception* (MFP): The test requires matching the visual counterpart of a geometric form held in the hand.

▶ *Kinesthesia* (KIN): With vision occluded, the child attempts to place his or her finger on a point where the examiner had previously placed it.

▶ *Finger Identification* (FI): The child identifies the finger previously touched by the examiner while the child's fingers were hidden from view

▶ *Graphesthesia* (GRA): The child draws a simple design on the back of his or her hand, attempting to copy the design previously drawn at the same place by the examiner.

▶ *Localization of Tactile Stimuli* (LTS): The child is expected to place his or her finger on a spot on his or her arm previously touched by the examiner.

▶ *Praxis on Verbal Command* (PrVC): The individual assumes a number of different positions based on the examiner's verbal commands.

► *Design Copying* (DC): The visual-motor task involves copying a design on a dot grid and in a designated blank space.

► *Constructional Praxis* (CPr): This is a block-building task to assess visual construction skills in accurately copying the three-dimensional pattern.

► *Postural Praxis* (PPr): The individual is required to assume a series of positions or postures demonstrated by the examiner, a process that requires motor planning.

► *Oral Praxis Tests* (OPr): The individual imitates the examiner's movements of the tongue, lips, cheeks, or jaw.

► *Sequencing Praxis Tests* (SPr): The individual's ability to perceive, remember, and do a demonstrated sequence of unilateral and bilateral hand and finger positions is evaluated.

► *Bilateral Motor Coordination* (BMC): Performing this test requires smoothly executed movements of and interaction between both upper extremities.

► *Standing and Walking Balance* (SWB): The kinesthetic test measures the conscious perception of position and movement of the arms and hand with vision occluded.

► *Motor Accuracy* (MAc): The visual–motor task requires that the individual draw a line over a printed line. The motor coordination component is much more demanding than the visual component.

► *Postrotary Nystagmus* (PRN): The duration of the oculomotor reflex following body rotation is recorded. Both atypically high (prolonged) and atypically low (depressed) scores are considered abnormal.

Other scores obtained through analysis of performance on the 17 tests include the following:

► *Space Visualization Contralateral Use* (SVCU): A test of crossing midline is based on the proportion of responses in which the child crosses the midline of the body with the hand to select a block from the contralateral space.

► *Space Visualization Preferred Hand Use* (PHU): This is based on the therapist's observation of which hand is used to pick up the block and place in the form board or the space visualization test.

These tests were originally standardized on children between the ages of 4 to 11 years old. Later investigations have attempted to obtain norms with adults to widen its applicability.

In addition to standardized tests, Ayres also used clinical observations to evaluate sensory integration. Ayres (1972a) posited that postural mechanisms are important areas to assess in children with learning disorders. Other informal clinical observations that are important in diagnosing sensory integration capabilities include the following:

► *Tonic Labyrinth Reflex* (TLR): "a function of the vestibular system manifests itself as increased flexor tone in the extremities when in the prone position and increased extensor tone when in the supine position" (Ayres, 1972a, p. 98). The TLR is normally present in the very young infant. If it is present later on, it indicates sensorimotor dysfunction. The TLR is elicited by placing the individual in the "pivot prone" position when riding a scooter board, for example.

► *Asymmetrical Tonic Neck Reflex* (ATNR): "elicited by stimulation of receptors in joint capsules of the neck . . . [and produces] extensor tone in the muscles of the arm toward which the head is turned [facing] and a relative increase in flex tone [or decrease in extensor tone] in the opposite arm" (Ayres, 1972a, p. 102).

▶ *Muscle tone* refers to the state of the muscles that aids in posture and movement. Abnormal muscle tone can be the result of neurological dysfunction, muscle weakness, or joint degeneration. Hypertonicity and hypotonicity are indicators of abnormality and may indicate neuromuscular dysfunction.

▶ *Extraocular muscle control* refers to the ability of the eyes to follow visual stimulation in a smooth fluid coordinate manner and in coordination with each other. "Overshooting or losing the target, difficulty in changing direction, lagging behind, attempting to move the head instead of the eyes, making faces, blinking frequently or squinting, inattentiveness, difficulty in looking away from the visual stimulus or finding it again, inability of the eyes to work together and especially difficulty in crossing the midline are each suggestive of less than perfect integration" (Ayres, 1972a, p. 110).

▶ *Vestibular system function* refers to the ability to detect motion and gravitational pull. To test function, "the child is either asked to stand on one foot, walk touching the heel of the forward foot to the toe of the foot in place [tandem walk], or to walk on a narrow board" (Ayres, 1972a, p. 111) while his or her eyes are closed.

▶ *Integration of function* of the two sides of the body is evaluated by the degree to which the individual crosses the midline of the body with one hand to assist his or her other hand while engaging in an activity.

▶ *Choreoathetoid movements* are referred to by Ayres (1972a) as involuntary motor incoordination. "It is elicited by asking the child to hold his arms outstretched, fingers

abducted, eyes closed and to count aloud up to ten" (p. 112).

Sensory Integration Treatment Modalities

After developing standardized tests and informal procedures for evaluating sensory integration dysfunction, Ayres introduced treatment methods that are based on the theories of neuromuscular therapy. Ayres acknowledged the work of Kabat and Knott (1948), Fay (1955), Bobath and Bobath (1955), and Rood (1956) as laying the foundation for sensory integration therapy. All of the above theorists advocate the use of therapeutic exercise to the client with a neurological impairment. Ayres' treatment approach is consistent with a therapy that looks for a neurological explanation for dysfunction in individuals with such diagnoses as attentional deficits (ADHD/ADD), learning disability, autism, and schizophrenia. Her treatment methods are based on the premise that sensory integration dysfunction can be treated by providing sensory input to elicit adaptive responses that can enhance the organization of brain mechanisms. In brief, Ayres developed sensory integrative therapy as a remedial approach using motor activities that affect the neurological organization of the brain. In a way, Ayres' approach differs from the work of Bobath and Rood, for example, in that Ayres treatment goals go beyond voluntary control of muscles and primitive reflexes. Ayres' treatment techniques are directed as learning achievement, emotional integration, social development, reading, and language development.

Ayres presents a model for treatment that is based on six hierarchical, sequential steps. Each step is linked to the ontogenetic sequence in normal child development. Table 4–12 outlines the six sequential steps and the specific treatment linked to each of the objectives.

Table 4-12. Specific Treatment Techniques of Sensory Integration Therapy

	Treatment Objectives	Activity Examples	Underlying Theoretical Rationale
Step 1	**Normalizing Tactile and Vestibular Systems**		
	Tactile Stimulation (touch) and Reduction of Tactile Defensiveness (TD)	• rubbing • brushing skin (back, arms, face, legs, and hands) for 1/2 hour before educational experience • enhanced tactile stimulation, such as deep touch pressure, vibrators, and rolling in heavy blankets	"Tactile stimulation can contribute to generalized neurological integration and to enhanced perception in other sensory modalities" (Ayres, 1972a, p. 115).
	Gravitational Insecurity	• swinging or spinning while lying or sitting in net hammock or glider swing • bouncing in a frog swing, mini-trampoline or bounce pad • walking up and down an incline • riding prone on a scooter board on level surface • weight shifting	"Synapses which normally are made as a result of vestibular input and are not being made in child with dysfunction are activated" (Ayres, 1972a, p. 122).
	Proprioceptive Stimulation for Aversive Responses	• enhanced linear vestibular information and resistance to active movements, such as those used with gravitational insecurity or tactile simulation • activities that provide opportunities for linear vestibular-proprioceptive and tactile information: brushing, trampoline activities, hopscotch • orbiting in dual swing • "heavy work activities" such as lifting, carrying, pushing • bilateral motor tasks (catching, throwing, or bouncing balls)	"Observation of the quieting and integrating effect of activity involving prolonged postural muscle contraction against gravity has led to the speculation that the effect may lie through the cerebellum and its inhibiting influence on the reticular activating system as well as through the integration brought directly by enhancing organization through the brain stem locomotion patterns" (Ayres, 1972a, p. 125).
Step 2	**Tonic Postural Extension or Tonic Labyrinthine Reflex (TLR)**		
	Developing and Balancing Tonic Flexion and Extension	• activities that involve movement against resistence or that challenge neck and upper back extensors • riding scooter boards pivot prone position down a ramp • weight shifting when in prone position • net basketball	"Optimal integration of the TLR will be achieved by the child assuming a prone extensory posture" (Ayres, 1972a, p. 146).

Step 3	Developing Equilibrium Reactions	
	Activation of Righting and Equilibrium Reactions	• increased righting response, such as seen in step 2, in prone, sitting, quadruped, kneeling, or standing positions • subtle adaptations to posture, such as being hit by therapy ball while riding on the glider swing or lying on the scooter ball	The activity facilitates equilibrium reactions in all positions.
	Developing Muscle Cocontraction	• alternating pushing and pulling while sitting on scooter board • maintaining flexion against both resistance and gravity, such as holding onto a disc swing or bolster swing	Observation of patients with spinal cord injuries or brain injury showed their inability to cocontract antagonistic muscles. Activities that enable flexion and extension of pairs of muscles are used.
Step 4	Normalizing Ocular Muscle Control	
		• spinning a child to measure ocular control producing postrotary nystagmus • activities to improve visually controlled movements (e.g., tracking, quick localization) • whistles accompanied with movement	Ayres (1972a) posits a constant interaction and interdependence among ocular muscle control, the vestibular system, and the neck muscles.
Step 5	Developing Coordinated Use of Both Sides of the Body (Bilateral Integration)	
		• swinging passively or actively while holding on to ropes (front to back, side to side) • crossing midline to perform activity • "… holding a rope in each hand while sitting on a scooter board and being pulled by ropes … " (Ayres, 1972a, p. 163)	The activities are designed to involve automatic postural mechanisms that require an adaptive interaction of the two sides of the body.
Step 6	Developing Right-left Discrimination and Visual Perception	
		• tossing bean bags through hoops or into boxes while riding a scooter board • juggling using both hands	Ayres (1972a) suggests that right-left discrimination frequently associated with reading disabilities returns only after the occurrence of integration of the body.

Related Models Using the Sensory Integration Therapy Frame of Reference

A model that incorporated a sensory integrative approach to treatment was published by Bachrach, Mosely, Swindell, and Wood (1978) entitled "Developmental Therapy for Young Children with Autistic Characteristics." Their model was intended for children with severe communication and sensory integrative disorders. The underlying premise of their treatment approach was that therapeutic interaction is based on sequential developmental objectives of helping these children begin to experience relationships, social experiences, satisfying behavior processes, and meaningful concepts of the world. The underlying philosophy was one of normalizing the child's experience to help the child become adaptive in everyday activities. The therapeutic program, based on child observation, parent involvement, field experiences, and home programs, contained four stages of progress:

▶ *Stage I*: using activities to stimulate sensory functions

▶ *Stage II*: using activities to facilitate self-confidence

▶ *Stage III*: using activities to understand oneself by group feedback

▶ *Stage IV*: interacting with peer groups in everyday activities

The activities used to accomplish these goals were based on a holistic model using sensorimotor games, interpersonal experiences, play, activities of daily living, music, language, arts and crafts, and other techniques to reach individualized goals.

King (1974) extended a sensory integrative treatment approach to schizophrenia based on the prior observations of Ayres (1972a), Schilder (1933), Leach (1960), and others presenting a biological factor theory. She based her treatment approach on clinical observations of clients with chronic schizophrenia who appeared to have postural disturbances. She ruled out the possibility of long-term institutionalization or medication as causing the unique postural and movement features. These unique factors were characterized by an "S" curve posture, shuffling gait, inability to raise arms above the head, inability to tip the head back, a tendency to hold arms and legs in a flexed position, and a lack of normal hand function. King hypothesized an etiology of schizophrenia based on these observations as the following:

> Some individuals have defective proprioceptive feedback mechanisms, the vestibular component in particular being first under reactive, and second, underactive in its role in the sensorimotor integration process. This defect, whether genetic, developmental, or the result of trauma, constitutes an important etiological or prodromal factor in process and reactive schizophrenia. (p. 530)

King also observed that clients with chronic schizophrenia at the Arizona State Hospital enjoyed simple vestibular stimulation, such as whirling in an office chair or being whirled by the elbow.

Based on these clinical observations and theoretical hypotheses, King implemented an experimental treatment group with 15 clients with chronic schizophrenia. A program of physical activity involved throwing and kicking a ball around a circle, marching to music, stepping over ropes, ducking under the volleyball net, and other similar noncompetitive sports. King noticed spontaneous improvement in the clients in their attitudes, verbalizations, and facial expressions.

Ross and Burdick (1981) developed a group treatment program using the sensory integrative therapy frame of reference with elderly clients with severe psychosocial disturbance. Five stages of treatment were incorporated into each group session:

▶ *Stage I*: The therapist in the opening part of the session used activities to stimulate the sensory systems of the body, such as the reticular activity system (attention and vigilance), the limbic system (emotional), and the cranial nerves (olfactory, auditory, and visual). A vibrator is recommended by Ross and Burdick to stimulate sensory receptors.

▶ *Stage II*: The therapist applied activities that stimulate gross bodily movements. Activities included physical movements on command: touching, picking up marbles with the toes, eye contact exercises, blowing soap bubbles, ball tossing, tug-of-war, mat work, scooter boards, and hand clapping.

▶ *Stage III*: Activities that promoted perceptual integration were encouraged, such as identifying objects and smells, tapping out rhythms, touching body parts reflected in a mirror, completing figure drawings, and pantomiming water play.

▶ *Stage IV*: Therapeutic activities that stimulate cognitive functioning were used. Examples of these activities included poetry reading, number games, telling stories, using arts and crafts, and lip reading.

▶ *Stage V*: Closure activities, such as signing, poetry, storytelling, summarizing events, and circle games were used.

The therapeutic objectives of these five stages were facilitation of focusing on and tracing of objects, crossing the midline, development of body awareness, stimulation of flexibility and equilibrium reflexes, gross motor planning, laterality, alternating movements, stereognosis, form discrimination and constancy, integration of atonic neck reflex, bilateral integration, and promotion of self-esteem and positive self-

image. The activities recommended during these five stages in the group sessions were similar to techniques used in reality orientation.

More recently, Cutler, Stevens-Dominguez, Oetter, and Westby (1992) have extended the theoretical concept of sensorimotor integration to the development of self–regulation (Figure 4–4). Briefly, the development of self-regulation is dependent on the development of automatic functions at the lowest level of the central nervous system, the integration of sensorimotor functions (e.g., suck/swallow/breathe synchrony [Oetter et al., 1993], selective attention, visual searching, oral and motor praxis), and the higher order functions, such as working memory, planning, sustained attention, and use of language for organization. They theorize that children who have not developed adequate sensorimotor integration are unable to self–regulate and use executive control.

Clinical Research Studies of Sensory Integration Therapy Frame of Reference

In 1976 the American Occupational Therapy Association published a monograph entitled *Research in Sensory–Integrative Development* edited by Price, Gilfoyle, and Meyers. The target population selected in these research studies included children with epilepsy, prenatal alcohol and drug exposure, learning disabilities, myelomeningocele, mental retardation, low birth weight, emotional disturbance, cerebral palsy, and multiple disabilities.

In another study, Rider (1973) compared the performance of children with emotional disturbance with typical children on the *Purdue Perceptual–Motor Survey* (Roach & Kephart, 1966) and *The Southern California Sensory Integration Tests* (SCSIT; Ayres, 1972b). On the *Purdue Perceptual–Motor Survey*, significant dif-

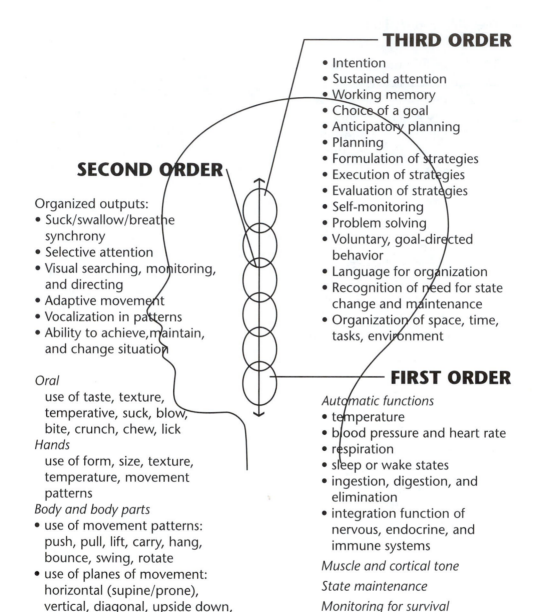

THIRD ORDER
- Intention
- Sustained attention
- Working memory
- Choice of a goal
- Anticipatory planning
- Planning
- Formulation of strategies
- Execution of strategies
- Evaluation of strategies
- Self-monitoring
- Problem solving
- Voluntary, goal-directed behavior
- Language for organization
- Recognition of need for state change and maintenance
- Organization of space, time, tasks, environment

SECOND ORDER

Organized outputs:
- Suck/swallow/breathe synchrony
- Selective attention
- Visual searching, monitoring, and directing
- Adaptive movement
- Vocalization in patterns
- Ability to achieve, maintain, and change situation

Oral
   use of taste, texture, temperative, suck, blow, bite, crunch, chew, lick
Hands
   use of form, size, texture, temperature, movement patterns
Body and body parts
- use of movement patterns: push, pull, lift, carry, hang, bounce, swing, rotate
- use of planes of movement: horizontal (supine/prone), vertical, diagonal, upside down, or backwards

FIRST ORDER

Automatic functions
- temperature
- blood pressure and heart rate
- respiration
- sleep or wake states
- ingestion, digestion, and elimination
- integration function of nervous, endocrine, and immune systems

Muscle and cortical tone

State maintenance

Monitoring for survival

©Cutler, Stevens-Domingues, Oetter, Westby (1992)

Figure 4–4. Development of self-regulation. Three levels of development are necessary for an individual to develop self-regulation: (a) First Order physiological functions needed to survive (e.g., heart rate, sleep/wake cycles, arousal); (b) Second Order development of sensory processes (e.g., sucking, swallowing, use of hands, body parts); and (c) Third Order higher thinking skills (e.g., intention, goal-oriented behavior, planning, problem-solving). These orders loosely correspond to Luria's (1980) levels of cortical development.

ferences between the groups occurred in 11 of the 18 subtests with the typical children scoring significant higher. On the Ayres' battery, the student with emotional disturbance performed significantly poorer than the normal control group of 12 of the 16 tests. Although not statistically significant, the students with emotional disturbance evidenced noticeably more abnormal responses on the other four tests of the SCSIT when compared to the typical children. The investigator concluded that, "The emotionally disturbed children demonstrated more sensory–integrative deficits than non-disturbed children" (p. 320). The investigator then interpreted these results to "suggest that the behaviors which led to the diagnosis of emotional disturbance in these children may have been caused by inadequate reflex maturation or other sensory integrative deficits" (p. 320).

In 1972, Ayres and Heskett published an article entitled "Sensory Integrative Dysfunction in a Young Schizophrenic Girl." This is a case study of a 7-year-old girl with schizophrenia and a learning disorder. The girl had a Verbal I.Q. score on the *Wechsler Intelligence Scale for Children* (WISC) of 57, which placed her in the moderately mentally retarded range. A battery of perceptual tests were administered to the child, and it was concluded that she had a sensory–integrative dysfunction. An intervention program based on the Ayres treatment techniques (see Table 4–12) was applied during a 6-month period. It included rubbing of the skin with a terry cloth, sitting in a suspended net, spinning in a net, rocking in a carpet-covered barrel, riding a scooter board down a ramp, and rolling inside of five inner tubes laced together. At the end of the 6 months of treatment, the investigators tested the subject again and found that her IQ increased from 57 to 72. One year post-treatment, perceptual–motor tests were repeated; improvement was maintained in most areas.

In a later study, Ayres and Tickle (1980) investigated the relationship between hyper-responsivity to touch and vestibular stimuli as predictions of positive responses to sensory integration therapy in children with autism. The investigators were interested in determining the best sensorimotor indicators for improvement in a group of 10 children, ages $3^{1}/_2$ to 13, diagnosed with autism. They found that the children who improved the most showed tactile defensiveness, avoidance of movement, gravitational insecurity, and an orienting response to an air puff. Improvement in the functioning of these children was evaluated qualitatively by observing their behavior in the following areas: (a) language, (b) awareness of the environment, (c) engagement in purposeful activities, (d) self-stimulating behavior, and (e) social and emotional behavior. Each of the 10 children was ranked by the therapists according to the amount of change observed. The criteria for evaluating improvement were not operationally defined.

Herman (1980) presented a case study of a 9-year-old girl with psychotic behavior who was treated using a sensory integrative approach. The child showed symptoms of disordered behavior early in her development. She had difficulty in eating, sleeping, toileting, walking, and using language. She also evidenced severe self-abusive behavior. A treatment program based on King's approach to sensory integration was implemented in occupational therapy. A total program was initiated that emphasized dressing, eating, and other self-care activities. Relaxation sessions to improve breathing, physical exercise, and art therapy were incorporated into a total treatment program providing continual stimulation, interaction, and activity. The child also received speech therapy, special education, and psychotherapy.

After 6 months of intensive treatment, the child showed noticeable improvement in the reduction of self-abusive behavior (head bang-ing), improved motor performance, improved appetite, and improved toileting. The author concluded that the sensory integrative treat-ment program had made a difference.

Bailey (1978) examined three aspects of lan-guage (i.e., number of words, speed of response, and relevance of response) in individuals with chronic schizophrenia and compared changes in these language aspects after providing regular vestibular stimulation. Fourteen adults with nonparanoid schizophrenia were provided sen-sory-stimulating activities 1/2 hour per day, 5 days a week, for 8 weeks. Many of the activities were taken from King's (1974) program. Results showed statistically significant changes in rele-vancy of response, but no changes in the other factors. Bailey suggested,

> The results indicate that the number of words spoken by schizophrenic individuals may not be a useful variable in measuring improvement in language and that the speed of their responses does not improve after eight weeks of sensory-stimulating activities. However, the quality of schizophrenic language, including syntactical style, reference to delusions, bizarre material, abstract versus concrete thinking, and recent and distant recall, does appear to improve with such treatment. (p. 449)

In two studies, Blakeney and her colleagues (Blakeney, Strickland, & Wilkinson, 1983; Reisman & Blakeney, 1991) compared the effica-cy of using sensory integrative activities, follow-ing programs developed by King (1974) and Ayres (1972, 1979). Groups of adults with non-paranoid schizophrenia were compared with control groups in which no sensory integrative activities were used. In both cases, results obtained on the *Nurses Observation Scale of Inpatient Evaluation* (NOSIE–30; Honigfeld, Gillis, & Klett, 1966) showed improvement in the psychiatric and physical status of individuals receiving the sensory integrative activities when compared to the control groups. No improve-ment was noted in other fine or gross motor assessments.

OCCUPATIONAL BEHAVIOR THEO-RETICAL MODEL

Mary Reilly is probably the most cited scholar in the field of occupational therapy. She has been recognized by many leaders in the field and is frequently cited in supporting a theory or justi-fying a research study. She obtained her certifi-cate in Occupational Therapy at the Boston School of Occupational Therapy in 1940. During World War II she was a Chief Occupational Therapist in various army bases and she provided assistance in developing a technical manual and apprentice training course of study (Miller et al., 1988). She later worked with war veterans who were brain damaged at Letterman Army Hospital (Reilly, 1956). Reilly obtained her Ed. D. degree from UCLA in 1959. She published her only book, *Play as Exploratory Learning*, in 1974. While at UCLA she began her association with the University of Southern California, where she was chair of the Occupational Therapy Department until her retirement in 1977. Reilly felt strongly that the profession of occupational therapy should develop comprehensive theories to guide prac-tice (Reilly, 1958).

Occupational Behavior Frames of Reference

The theoretical model of occupational behavior introduced by Reilly (1969, 1974a) is a direct outcome of the philosophical assumptions artic-ulated by the founders of the profession in the early 20th century (Levy, 1993). In a sense the occupational behavior theoretical model reflects the theoretical core of the practice of occupational therapy. It is a holistic and eclectic model that emphasizes the biopsychosocial nature of humans and their need to use occupation in their mastery and adaptation to the environment and the need for a balance in work, play, rest, and sleep. It is also based on the early occupational therapy theorists such as Barton (1918), Meyer (1922), Slagle (1922), and Dunton and Licht (1950). The four Occupational Behavior Frames of Reference, The Model of Human Occupation (Kielhofner, 1997), Occupational Adaptation (Schkade & Schultz, 1993), Occupational Science (Zemke & Clark, 1996), and the Canadian Model of Occupational Performance (CAOT, 1997) are outgrowths of the occupational behavior theoretical model. Figure 4–5 gives quotes from each of these frames of reference within the theoretical model.

Model of Human Occupation (MOHO)

The Model of Human Occupation (MOHO) can be defined as an interactive approach conceptualizing the individual as an open system within a larger environment. General systems theory (Finch, 1967; von Bertalanffy, 1968; see also Bronfenbrenner, 1977) provides the struc-

---

"That man, through the use of their hands as they are energized by mind and will, can influence the state of his own health." (Reilly, 1962, p. 2)

"The achievement theme is our major frame of reference and constitutes a body of knowledge richly supported by the contributions of Robert White [1959], Eric Erikson [1950], and David McClelland [1961]. " (Reilly, 1969, p. 302)

▼   ▼   ▼   ▼

MODEL OF HUMAN OCCUPATION (MOHO) (Kielhofner, 1997)	**OCCUPATIONAL ADAPTION: AN INTEGRATIVE FRAME OF REFERENCE** (Schkade & Schultz, 1993)	**OCCUPATIONAL SCIENCE** (Zemke & Clark, 1996)	**CANADIAN MODEL OF OCCUPATIONAL PERFORMANCE** (CAOT, 1997)
• "The model of human occupation seeks to account for the motivation, performance, and organization of occupational behavior in everyday life." (Kielhofner, 1997, p. 188) • Human occupation system is composed of three systems hierarchically arranged: volitional, habituation, and performance.	• "Individual development proceeds through attempts at relative mastery over occupational challenges." (Schkade & Schultz, 1993, p. 87)	• "Occupations are defined as 'chunks' of activity within the stream of human behavior that are named in the lexicon of the culture, for example 'fishing' or 'cooking' or at a more abstract level, 'playing' or 'working.'" (Yerxa et al., 1989, p. 5) **WORK-PLAY FRAME OF REFERENCE** (Reilly,1974b)	• "Occupational performance refers to the ability to choose, organize, and satisfactorily perform meaningful occupations that are culturally defined and are age appropriate for looking after one's self, enjoying life, and contributing to the social and economic fabric of a community." (CAOT, 1997, p. 30)

Figure 4–5. Occupational Behavior frame of reference. The emphasis in the Occupational Behavior frame of reference is on the relationship between the bio-psychosocial nature of man and healthy aspect of the individual. The frame of reference is derived from the philosophy of Mary Reilly.

tural framework for human occupation. MOHO is a frame of reference that promotes life satisfaction through a healthy balance of work, play, and leisure roles.

A major premise of this model is that individuals change as a function of their interaction with the environment and that there is a reciprocal interaction between the individual and the environment. In this frame of reference, change occurs through a feedback loop: (a) *input* is the energy and knowledge flowing into the individual; (b) *throughput* is the assimilation and organization of information into the individual; (c) *output* includes the actions and behaviors of the individual; and (d) *feedback* is the perceivable effect that the output has on the environment and the individual through reciprocal action. Feedback leads to input, and the cycle begins again.

The major purpose of treatment is to establish an environment that allows the individual to explore and develop competency and mastery of occupational roles. The function of the therapist in this frame of reference is to counsel and to help the client problem-solve ways to alter maladaptive lifestyles and interactions. The ultimate goal is to generalize skills mastered in the clinic to a nontherapeutic setting, such as in a work or home setting.

Assumptions of the Model of Human Occupation

The Model of Human Occupation (MOHO) developed by Kielhofner (1997) contains the following assumptions:

▶ Performance of occupation depends on one's volition (motivation, values, and interests), habituation (occupational roles, daily customs, and routine activities), and mind-brain-body performance subsystem (unified actions in perceptual-motor, communication, and cognitive areas).

▶ As individuals engage in work, play, and daily living tasks, these dynamic interactions change their capacities, beliefs, and occupational roles.

▶ Man is viewed as an open system when the person consistently interacts and self-regulates occupational performance. This view is consistent with the General Systems Theory of Ludwig von Bertalanffy (1968, 1975).

▶ Health is perceived as "the degrees to which the physical, psychosocial and environmental elements of the system work together for function, within the boundaries of health, disease or disability" (Bruce & Borg, 1993, p. 156).

▶ Occupational dysfunction occurs when an individual is unable to meet societal demands for productivity (e.g., in worker or homemaker roles) or cannot engage in leisure or play activities and is no longer able to explain and master the environment (Kielhofner, 1985).

▶ Function–dysfunction continuum contains the following areas, ranging from functional to dysfunctional: (a) achievement (maximum adjustment); (b) competence (mastery of skills); (c) exploration (trying out new skills); (d) inefficacy (decreased function, interest or roles in occupation); (e) incompetence (major loss or limitation of skills and inability to perform tasks of everyday living; and (f) helplessness (highly deficient skills, few or no interests, roles, and disorganized habits) (Kielhofner, 1985).

▶ "The environment has the power to mitigate or exacerbate emotional, functional, and behavioral consequences of impairments" (Kielhofner, 1997, p. 200).

+	+	+
Achievement	Competence	Exploration
−	−	−
Inefficacy	Incompetency	Helplessness

▶ "The model of human occupation emphasizes that, through therapy, persons are helped to engage in occupational behaviors that maintains, restores, reorganizes, or develops their capacities, motives, and lifestyle. Through participation in therapeutic occupations, persons transform themselves into more adaptive and healthy beings" (Kielhofner, 1997, pp. 204–205).

Assessment Techniques Associated with MOHO

Observational measures, self-report questionnaires, and structural interviews have been developed to assess the individual's performance skills, volitional spontaneity or decision making, occupational roles, interests, and activity level. Listed here are some of the tools that Kielhofner and his associates have developed in relationship to MOHO.

▶ *Assessment of Motor and Process Skills* (AMPS; Fisher, 1994): An observational scale measuring performance process and motor skills in occupational roles

▶ *Assessment of Communication and Interactional Skills* (ACIS; Forsyth, Salamy, Simon, & Kielhofner, 1995): An observational scale used to measure communication and interaction skills of clients in social groups

▶ *The Volitional Questionnaire* (De las Heras, 1993): An observational rating scale

designed to identify volitional spontaneity in various environments and used with clients unable to self-report

▶ *The Role Checklist* (Barris, Oakley, & Kielhofner, 1988): A checklist used to examine the value individuals attach to specific occupational roles

▶ *The Interest Checklist* (Matsutsuyu, 1969): A self-report checklist in which clients report interests in which they are presently engaged or would like to be engaged in the future

▶ *Occupational Case Analysis Interview and Rating Scale* (Kaplan & Kielhofner, 1989): Case analysis scale used in short-term psychiatric hospitalization

▶ *The Occupational Performance History Interview* (OPHI; Kielhofner & Henry, 1988; Kielhofner, Henry, & Walens, 1989): A scale used to obtain information about past and present occupational history

▶ *The Worker Role Interview* (Velozo, Kielhofner, & Fisher, 1990): A structured interview designed to examine aspects of life, work, and job settings that affect one's return to work

▶ *Inventory of Occupational Choice Skills* (Shannon, 1974): A checklist of 29 play–chore activities designed for children and adolescents to identify interests and participation in various activities

Research on MOHO

There has been a recent interest in designing qualitative case studies in understanding the client's volitional systems through narrative accounts (Helfrich, Kielhofner, & Mattingly, 1994). Munoz, Lawlor, and Kielhofner (1993) conducted a telephone survey of occupational therapists working in psychiatric facilities. In general the researchers concluded that therapists found major concepts of the MOHO useful for conceptualizing their client's occupational functioning. In addition, it was found that while therapists valued the holistic models, they also incorporated parts of other frames of reference, such as the Cognitive Disabilities (Allen, 1985), the Developmental (Llorens, 1976), the Sensory Integration (Ayres, 1963, 1972a; King, 1974), Psychodynamic (Fidler & Fidler, 1963; Mosey, 1970), and Lifestyle Performance (Fidler, 1982, 1988).

Occupational Adaptation: An Integrative Frame of Reference (OA)

Definition

"The occupational adaptation practice model emphasizes the creation of a therapeutic climate, the use of occupational activity and the importance of relative mastery" (Schultz & Schkade, 1992, p. 917). The three major elements of this frame of reference are the person, the environment, and their interaction.

The Occupational Adaptation frame of reference holds that mental illness affects an individual's ability to reason or problem-solve and that the developmental process of occupational behavior is hindered. Greater dysfunction in the individual leads to an increased decline in occupational performance, eventually resulting in an adaptive response of not engaging in occupations. The role of the therapist in this situation is to provide individual and environmental support for the client so that he or she can begin to master occupations and to engage with the environment.

Assumptions

The OA frame of reference holds the following assumptions (Schkade & Schultz, 1992; Schultz & Schkade, 1992):

▶ Occupation enables human beings to continually adapt to changing needs and conditions in the environment. Adaptation is the process of moving along a continuum from "dysadaptation" to homeostasis and occupational adaptation.

▶ Individuals have an intrinsic motivation to engage in occupation, and this desire leads to adaptation.

▶ Although occupational responses require the involvement of all three performance components, sensorimotor, psychosocial, and cognitive, the relative extent to which each of these component is used varies. The *adaptation gestalt* reflects how the individual uses all three systems to adapt to the environment in a given situation. When the individual inaccurately perceives the demands of the occupational challenge, an improper adaptation gestalt is used. This results in dysfunctional adaptation.

▶ The periods of transition between major stages of development (e.g., infancy, childhood, adolescence, adulthood) require the greatest adaptation. More important aspects of transition are likely to cause greater disruption due to an improper use of an adaptation gestalt. For example, the transition to adolescence is an event that can be highly disruptive in many individuals.

▶ An individual's desire for mastery and the environment's demands for mastery result in the adaptation needed to master the environment.

▶ "Mastery is more than the ability to perform a discrete task; it is a reflection of the client's experience as an occupational being" (Schultz & Schkade, 1992, p. 919).

▶ "Relative mastery is the extent to which the person experiences the occupational response as efficient (use of time and energy), effective (production of the desired results), and satisfying to self and society, that is, it is pleasing not only to the self but also to relevant others as agents of the occupational environment" (Schkade & Schultz, 1992, p. 835).

▶ Adaptation energy is finite and is idiosyncratic to each person. If an individual is highly stressed, then that individual will have less energy available for adaptive responses because of the energy being depleted by the stress (Selye, 1956).

▶ Adaptation energy operates on two levels: simultaneous and parallel processing (Posner, 1973). For example, an individual has a project to complete, but rather than beginning the project, he or she engages in a leisure activity. During the activity, the individual is unconsciously problem-solving the solution to the project.

▶ Individuals have developed a repertoire of adaptive responses to use in all situations. When these responses do not work, the behavior is considered maladaptive. The individual then needs to be taught a new set of behaviors to add to his or her repertoire. Responses can be classified as primitive (i.e., predictive or rigid response), transitional (i.e., exploratory), and mature (i.e., creative problem-solving).

One of the goals of treatment in this frame of reference is to improve occupational functioning as a result of occupational adaptation. The holistic process of treatment includes (a) creating a therapeutic environment, (b) conducting an assessment of the client's condition and occupational environment, (c) developing and implementing an occupational adaptation program, and (d) evaluating outcome (Schkade & Schultz, 1993).

Table 4-13 outlines the model of practice used in the Occupational Adaptation model. In

Table 4–13. Occupational Adaptation Model of Practice

I.	**Assessment and Data Collection**

- What are the occupational environment/roles (OE/R) of the client and which are of the most concern to the client and his or her family?
- What are the performance expectations and the physical, social, and cultural characteristics of the primary OE/R?
- What are the client's sensorimotor, cognitive, or psychosocial strengths?
- What is the level of relative mastery in the primary OE/R, and what facilitates or limits relative mastery in it?

II.	**Programming in Occupational Adaptation**

- What occupational activity and readiness development is necessary to promote adaptation of the client?
- What help will the client need from the therapist to evaluate and change performance?
- What will be the best way to engage the client in the program?

III.	**Evaluation of the Occupational Adaptation Process**

- How is the program affecting the process with regard to energy level, adaptive response mode, or adaptative response behavior?
- What outcomes are seen that reflect changes in the adaptation responses?
- What changes in the program need to be made for optimal change in the adaptation process?

Source: Adapted from *Redefining Psychiatric Rehabilitation: Results of Occupational Therapy Model* by S. Schultz, 1996, April. Paper presented at the 76th Annual Conference and Exposition of the American Occupational Therapy Association, Chicago, IL.

this model, the therapist acts as an objective observer, providing understanding to the uncertainties of the client. The therapist intervenes in the client's skill deficits by providing the client with occupational activities that challenge the client to problem-solve and to make adaptations in the environment. In this manner, the therapist facilitates change by empowering the client to (a) develop a plan to use when given environmental challenges; (b) critiquing and assessing the client's performance; and (c) helping the client to make changes within himself or herself based on the evaluation of his or her performance.

Occupational Science Frame of Reference

The Occupational Science frame of reference is a dynamic model that is still being defined. Blanche & Henny-Kohler (2000), in a discussion of the philosophy of occupational science concluded that "We believe that occupational science and occupational therapy share many philosophical beliefs, one of which is empowering people to become autonomous. Hence, occupational science empowers occupational therapists to become autonomous by inviting them to join in the development of their own science" (p. 109). The philosophy of occupational science is derived from the

> Traditions of occupational therapy as articulated by Adolph Meyer (1922) and Eleanor Clark Slagle (1922), the clinical philosophy of A. Jean Ayres, and the development of the curriculum in occupational therapy at the University of Southern California (USC) by Mary Reilly and her colleagues (1969) [who] provided the foundation for examining the appropriate knowledge base of the field. It was named "occupational science" in 1987 by Paul Bohannan, an anthropologist and Dean of Social Science and Communication, Elizabeth Yerxa and the faculty members and graduate

students at the USC Department of Occupational Therapy. (Yerxa, 1993, p. 5)

Definition

Occupational Science frame of reference is "the study of the human as an occupational being including the need for and capacity to engage in and orchestrate daily occupations in the environment over the lifespan. Because of the complexity of occupation, occupational science synthesizes knowledge from an array of disciplines (biological and social sciences) and organizes it into a systems model" (USC, 1987).

The Concepts of the Occupational Science Frame of Reference

The *American Heritage Dictionary* (1985) definition of occupation is "an activity that serves as one's regular source of livelihood; vocation; an activity engaged in especially as a means of passing time." Other definitions include "occupying or being occupied; what occupies one, means of filling up one's time, temporary or regular employment" (*Concise Oxford Dictionary*, 1911).

Wilcock (1993) has made the following observations about occupation:

> Occupation is purposeful use of "*time, energy, interest and attention*" in work, leisure, family, cultural, self-care and rest activities. It is a "*natural human phenomena*" which is taken for granted because it forms the "*fabric of everyday living*". It includes activities that are "*playful, restful, serious and productive which are carried out by individuals in their own unique ways based on societal influences, their own needs, beliefs and preferences, the kinds of experiences they have had, their environments and the patterns of behavior they acquire over time.*" Occupation which is culturally sanctioned, may be seen as a "*primary organizer of time and resources*" enabling humans to survive, control and adapt to their world, be "*economically self-sufficient*" and to experience social relation-

ships and approval, as well as personal growth. (Wilcock, 1993, p. 1)

Wilcock (1993) views occupational science as a generic term, which would "encompass any humanistic study making a contribution to the knowledge base" (p. 1).

Assumptions of Occupational Science

The assumptions of occupational science are cited from Yerxa (1991, p. 199):

▶ Occupational therapy provides therapeutic intervention to human beings, not to muscles or synapses or superegos.

▶ Human beings are complex, multi-leveled systems who act on and interact with their environments.

▶ Unique human qualities include language, history, culture, and the endowment of life experiences with spiritual meaning.

▶ Occupational therapy is designed to enable people to adapt to the challenges of their environments through the use of their hands, mind, and will (Reilly, 1962).

▶ Occupational therapy, grounded in humanistic values, has an ethical responsibility to persons with chronic conditions.

▶ Human beings have interests, goals, aspirations and plans that, when achieved, provide a valued sense of efficacy.

▶ Occupational therapy is concerned with how occupation enables persons to achieve competence and economic self-sufficiency and to contribute to themselves and others.

▶ Although it may be provided in a medical milieu, occupational therapy is different from and complementary to medicine in its thought process, view of the human being, and scientific foundation.

▶ Occupational therapy's knowledge is based on a synthesis of evolutionary biology, the social sciences, and the humanities; medicine's foundation rests in the physical and natural sciences.

▶ Occupational therapy views the individual as embedded in the stream of time (i.e., evolutionary, developmental, and learning) (Reilly, 1974b).

Research in Occupational Science

The following are examples of the theories and research that are being generated by theorists and researchers in the Occupational Science frame of reference. In general, the major topics are work, leisure, play, temporal adaptation, primate function, habits and skills in daily living, and occupational storytelling (Clark, 1993).

▶ *Household work, leisure, and self-care as well as feminist theory* (Primeau, 1996). "Because occupational science seeks to understand the experience and meaning of one's occupations and how they relate to one's values and sense of purpose in life, occupational scientists must look beyond the conceptual categories of work, leisure, and self care to explore fully the nature of the human as an occupational being" (p. 66).

▶ *Perspectives on play* (Parham, 1996). In this paper, Parham emphasizes that play is more than just social interactions. Rather, play is a "vehicle for integrating multiple developmental skills" (p. 77) and therefore specific aspects cannot be taught in isolation.

▶ *Homelessness and issues of time, space, and geography* (Dear, 1996). The author discusses homelessness in the context of sociospatial networks and describes a program in Los Angeles.

▶ *Balance in occupation* (Christiansen, 1996). In his paper, Christiansen theorizes that "there is great consistency and stability in patterns of time use; daily occupations are influenced by sociocultural patterns, psychological dispositions, and psychological rhythms and by physical and mental capacities. With regard to activity patterns and well-being, however, we have much less empirical evidence on which to rely. We can speculate that biological and social rhythms may be more important to occupational adaptation than previously thought" (p. 447).

▶ *Occupational storytelling* (Clark, Ennevor, & Richardson, 1996). Through autobiographical narratives, "[a]n occupational therapist may assist in enabling a survivor [e.g., stroke] grappling with a disability to reconstruct a bridge to rebuild life again" (p. 374).

▶ *Primate research and relation to occupational science* (Chamove, 1996). Based on the observation that primates engage in specific behaviors, even when those behaviors are not required, Chamove has hypothesized that " 'work' is behavior that individuals would prefer to be doing rather than doing nothing or doing what they are restricted to doing by means of their institutionalized or captive conditions" (p. 177).

Reilly's Work–Play Frame of Reference

"Play being a universal behavior is presumably vital to human existence" (Reilly, 1974b, p. 58). Reilly conceptualized play activity as essential in the development of healthy, mature attitudes toward work and in the formation of interpersonal relationships. Parham (1996) conceptualized play along the work–play dichotomy in which work and play exist on opposing ends of the continuum. In this conceptualization, work is seen as productive, done for extrinsic purposes, and mandatory for sustenance, while play is freely chosen and participated in for its own sake. Adults engage in leisure-time activities, the equivalent of children's play, as respite from work. Reilly (1974b) noted that individuals with emotional disturbance may have not had the rich, enjoyable experiences of play that are so important in normal development. In her conceptual framework, play is an important dimension for the occupational therapist in stimulation of child development, evaluation of personality factors, and psychosocial treatment. In trying to define play, Reilly cited various therapists, including psychoanalytic approaches (Freud, 1920/1953-1974; Kris, 1952), cognitive-Piagetian explanations (Piaget, 1952a, 1952b), cultural anthropological evidence (Roberts, Arth, & Bush, 1959), and historical data (Huizinga, 1955).

Although a definition of play is difficult to find, descriptions of characteristics and functions of play as proposed by many authors give us a feel for what play is (Bundy, 1991). Bruner (1976) stated that first, play "is a means of minimizing the consequences of one's actions and of learning, therefore, in a less risky situation" (p. 38). (See also Reilly, 1974b and Garvey, 1977.) Further, Bruner (1976) stated that "[second], play provides an excellent opportunity to try combinations of behaviour that would, under functional pressure, never be tried" (p. 38). Rubin, Fein, and Vandenberg (1983; as cited by Bundy, 1991) suggested that six characteristics of play are considered by all to be a part of play: "(a) intrinsic motivation; (b) attention to means rather than ends; (c) organism rather than stimulus dominated (what can I do with this object rather than what does this object do?); (d) nonliteral, simulative behavior; (e) freedom from externally imposed rules; and (f) requiring the *active participation* of the player" (p. 49).

Michelman (1974) proposed that play should serve the growth needs of the child with disabilities through careful structuring of the activity and skillful enrichment of the environment. Michelman and others (Florey & Greene, 1997; Parham & Primeau, 1997; Takata, 1974) incorporated Piagetian theory in describing how children learn through experimenting with art media and other activities.

▶ *Sensorimotor, exploratory play*: During the first 18 months to 2 years, children use art, play, and motor explorations in sensory-motor experience. For example, children play with various media such as wood, paper, and water and by so doing they develop their sensory skills and motor performance. Additionally, children imitate others and use simple problem-solving to explore their environment.

▶ *Symbolic and simple constructive*: From 18 months to ages 4 or 5 years, children use intuitive or egocentric thinking and intense feelings in their art programs. In this stage children use symbolic play, including make-believe and pretend, and various media in art activities, in reconstructing reality and expressing feelings. Play shifts from solitary play to parallel play.

▶ *Preoperational or dramatic, complex constructive, and pregame*: Between 4 and 7 years old, children use magical thinking in their creative art and play activities. Play is characterized by a shift from parallel play to associative play, using various media for expression. Play interests include (a) dramatic play, using dress-up and puppetry; (b) collecting objects, especially objects from nature; and (c) arts and crafts,

including simple models and puzzle (Florey & Greene, 1997).

▶ *Concrete operations or games*: Piaget identified the ages between 7 and 11 as the period of concrete operations that translate into art activities as realism and a desire to understand the immediate environment. In this stage the children begin to demonstrate their competency by using media, play, and sports. Games with rules, cooperative play, and building of social groups are important aspects of this stage.

▶ *Formal operations or recreational*: The next Piagetian stage of cognitive development is the period of formal operations, which extends from ages 11 or 12 through adulthood. Symbols are freely used and art is used as a projection of abstract thought. In this stage, individuals incorporate emotional tone in their art productions, which become highly personal. Involvement in service organization, competitive sports, and peer groups are important characteristics of this period.

These five Piagetian stages have a profound influence on the child's development and later self-concept of the adult. The major implications of this theory are that the opportunity to express oneself through play activities and art media is critical in self-actualizing one's potential and in developing one's unique self and personality. Play covers a wide range of activities, including unstructured media such as art, ceramics, and storytelling to structured activities that include a musical instrument, mastering a sport, and solving a puzzle. Play, games, recreation, leisure, and work are all interrelated. Play for a child is like work for an adult and recreation to an adult is like play is to a child (Parham & Primeau, 1997).

Takata (1974) built on Reilly's theory and devised an operational tool to assess the child's play history as a means of evaluation and developing an occupational therapy treatment plan. In Table 4–14 is an example of how *Takata's Play History Questionnaire* can be used in evaluating a child's play behavior.

Another application of Reilly's theory was provided by Knox (1974, 1997a), who constructed a play scale based on observations of typical children. The scale analyzes play using four variables: (a) space management (child's motor activities), (b) material management (use of media), (c) imitation (expressions and creative play), and (d) participation (interpersonal relationships). In a more recent study of play (Knox, 1997b) using observations of children at play and interviews with parents and teachers, Knox found tremendous diversity in children's play in these categories, suggesting that play is an important aspect in children's development. Knox feels that the study of play behavior from a phenomenological perspective is vital in understanding the occupations of children.

Shannon (1967, 1974), a student of Reilly, linked play to the development of occupational choice skills and occupational adjustment. For Shannon, play encourages risk-taking, a trial-and-error learning, and "provides for identification with the worker role through development of self-confidence and competence" (pp. 290–291). He developed an *Inventory of Occupational Choice Skills* intended for use with adolescents with emotional disturbance. The purposes of the inventory, as stated by Shannon are to identify "play deficiencies for their guidance value when considering play enrichment program" (p. 296). Twenty-nine activities were selected on the basis of three factors: (a) self-discovery skills, (b) decision-making skills, and (c) work-role experimentation

skills. Each of the 29 activities was ranked according to its loading on the three factors.

Shannon proposed that an activity program can be planned based on the responses from the *Inventory of Occupational Choice Skills*. The therapist uses the inventory to work cooperatively with the client in choosing a satisfying job. Leisure time activities are used as a bridge in developing vocational interests. In this model the occupational therapist tries to stimulate self-discovery (understanding about one's self), decision-making skills, and work-role experimentations (try-out jobs) by selecting activities that will meet these goals.

Summary of Reilly's Work-Play Frame of Reference

Reilly's theory of work–play as exploratory learning identified the important influences that children's play has on the adolescent and later on the adult's personality. Play activities are important in the development of the child's sensory-motor activities, perception of reality, and self-concept and serve as a vehicle to express emotion. Children deprived of the opportunities for a wide range of play activities are severely limited. By extending this theory to the adult with psychosocial dysfunction, play activities can be used as therapeutic media to help adults explore their occupation capacities and to express their feelings. The relationship between play and work roles and play and job satisfaction is emphasized in this frame of reference. By experimenting with various media, the adult can identify satisfying occupations and occupational roles. What we enjoy as play can be part of our work.

Table 4–14. The Play History: A Case Example

I. General Information

Name: Patricia   Birthdate: 4/10/90   Sex: F

Date: 5/13/96   Informant: Mother

Presenting Problem: "She doesn't follow teacher's directions and is constantly out of her seat" (according to mother)

II. Previous Play Experiences

    A. Type of Play: solitary, parallel, cooperative, other. Describe how child plays.

    Patricia generally plays alone, but may play with her brother on occasion. Her kindergarten teacher reported that she plays cooperatively with one other girl in the class.

    B. Toys and Materials Used: (describe type of materials and purpose of use):

    Patricia likes to play with her dolls, by feeding, dressing, or rocking them. She usually does not play with any other toys.

    C. Gross Physical Play

    Patricia rarely plays outside, but when requested to do so, she will swing or play on playground equipment. She can run and jump, and is able to ride a two-wheeler with training wheels.

    D. Pretend and Make-believe Play

    Patricia plays make-believe with her dolls regularly.

    E. Sports and Games

    Patricia does not enjoy playing any sports or games. Occasionally, she will play hide and go seek with her brother.

    F. Creative Interests

    Other than coloring and make-believe when playing with her dolls, Patricia does not seem to have any creative interests. Her kindergarten teacher reported that she did like to paint at the easel, but did not like to finger-paint.

    G. Hobbies, Collections, Other Leisure Time Activities

    None are reported.

    H. Recreation/Social Activities

    None are reported at this time. She doesn't seem to have any special friends.

III. Actual Play Examination

    A. With *what* does the child play?

    Dolls, play house, play food, play bottles for the dolls, doll clothes

    B. *How* does the child play with toys and other materials?

    Rocks baby doll, takes off clothes, puts on new clothes, asks for water to wash the baby, pretends to cook food and heat the bottle to feed the baby, rocks the baby. All play was pretend, with situations around caring for a baby

    C. What type of play is *avoided*, or liked least?

    Toys, such as trucks, balls, or blocks were avoided. When the examiner attempted to engage Patricia in these activities, she reluctantly agreed to throw the ball a couple of times. She would not play with the trucks or blocks.

    D. With *whom* does the child play?

    Patricia is reported to play with her brother sometimes. When she was observed at recess at school, she did not play with any other children.

Table 4–14. The Play History: A Case Example

III. Actual Play Examination *(continued)*

E. *How* does the child play with other? (Shares, cooperates, parallel play)

Not observed.

F. *What body postures* does the child use during play?

Patricia usually sits when playing with her dolls. When observed on the playground, she lay on the swings, or stood on the merry-go-round hanging on to the inside rungs.

G. *How long* does the child play with objects?

Patricia spent almost 1/2 hour playing with the dolls and the kitchen materials. On the playground, she spent the entire recess time on the playground equipment. Her mother reports that she will play for 2 to 3 hours in her room after school and before dinner.

H. *Where* does the child play?

Patricia's mother reports that she plays in her room, while her teacher reports that she plays on the playground equipment. She did not have any difficulty playing in the playroom at the evaluator's office.

I. *When* does the child play?

Patricia plays during recess periods and after school. She has no time to play. On Saturdays, she plays after breakfast until lunch, then after lunch until dinner. She does spend time helping her mother with housekeeping chores on the weekend.

Source: Adapted from "Play as a Prescription," by N. Takata, 1974, p. 232. In *Play as Exploratory Learning* by M. Reilly (Ed.), pp. 209–246, Beverly Hills, CA: Sage.

Canadian Model of Occupational Performance (CMOP)

Assumptions of the Canadian Model of Occupational Performance

The CMOP is a systems based frame of reference that conceptualizes the interaction and interdependence among the environment, occupational roles, and the person (CAOT, 1991, 1993; Department of National Health and Welfare & Canadian Association of Occupational Therapists, 1986). The environment consists of social, cultural, institutional, and physical aspects. Occupation includes the areas of self-care, leisure, and productivity. The person is perceived as a holistic individual with affective, cognitive, spiritual, and physical dimensions. Major assumptions include (CAOT, 1997):

▶ Occupation refers to groups of activities and tasks of everyday life, named, organ-

ized, and given values and meaning by individual in a culture. Occupation is everything people do to occupy themselves, including looking after themselves (self-care), enjoying life (leisure), and contributing to the social and economic fabric of their communities (productivity).

▶ Occupation has therapeutic effectiveness.

▶ Individuals have intrinsic dignity and worth, are capable of making decisions about life, have the potential to change, and are shaped by their environment.

▶ The environment includes cultural, institutional, physical, and social components.

▶ Health is strongly influenced by having control in everyday occupation and is associated with spiritual meaning, life satisfaction in occupation, and fairness and opportunity in a social context.

▶ Clients are perceived as active partners in the occupational therapy process and are encouraged to take risks in the process of treatment.

Assessment Tool

"The *Canadian Occupation Performance Measure* (COPM; Law et al., 1990, 1991) is built on the model of occupational performance and the framework of client-centered practice" (Chan & Lee, 1997, p. 231).

SUMMARY

For the psychosocial occupational therapist, a theory is essential to guide clinical practice. Theories generate frames of references, which in turn guide clinical practice. Psychosocial occupational therapy is based on theories coming from medicine, psychology, education, and sociology. Four theoretical models have dominated the practice of psychosocial occupational therapy in the last 80 years. They are psychodynamic (Freud, Adler, Erikson, Sullivan), behavioral (Skinner, Pavlov), developmental (Gesell, Luria, Vygotsky), and systems (von Bertalanffy). Frames of reference in psychosocial occupational therapy include Psychodynamic (Fidlers, Azima, Mosey), Cognitive-Behavioral (Stein, Allen), Sensory-Integration (Ayres), and Occupational Behavior (Reilly, Kielhofner, Schkade, & Schultz; Clark, Yerxa). These frames of reference currently guide clinical practice. In reality, when asked, many occupational therapists will state that they use an eclectic approach to treatment, meaning they use a varied approach in selecting treatment techniques and activities. Good practice is based on theory and research evidence. It is critical that what we do as occupational therapists has a rationale based on logical thought. In this chapter, the authors have brought together the theories and frames of references that guide clinical practice in occupational therapy.

REFERENCES

Adler, A. (1956). *The individual psychology of Alfred Adler: A systematic presentation in selections from his writing.* (H. L. Ansbacher & R. R. Ansbacher, Eds. and annotators). New York: Basic Books.

Adler, A. (1974). *Social interest: A challenge to mankind* (J. Linton & R. Vaughan, Trans.). New York: Putnam. (Original work published 1933)

Alexander, F., & Selesnick, S. (1966). *The history of psychiatry: An evaluation of psychiatric thought and practice from prehistoric times to the present.* New York: Harper & Row.

Allen, C. K. (1985). *Occupational therapy for psychiatric diseases: Measurement and management of cognitive disabilities.* Boston: Little, Brown.

American Heritage Dictionary. (1985). Boston: Houghton Mifflin Company.

American Occupational Therapy Association [AOTA]. (1982). Occupational therapy for sensory integrative dysfunction. *American Journal of Occupational Therapy, 36,* 831–832.

American Occupational Therapy Association [AOTA]. (1994). *Uniform terminology for occupational therapy: Application to practice* (3rd ed.). Rockville, MD: Author.

Anshel, M. H. (1996). Effect of chronic aerobic exercise and progressive relaxation on motor performance and affect following acute stress. *Behavioral Medicine, 21,* 186–196.

Aronoff, G. M. (1985). Psychological aspects of nonmalignant chronic pain: A new nosology. In G. M. Aronoff (Ed.), *Evaluation and treatment of chronic pain* (pp. 471–484). Baltimore-Munich: Urban & Schwarzenberg.

Aschen, S. R. (1997). Assertion training therapy in psychiatric milieus. *Archives of Psychiatric Nursing, 11,* 46–51.

Ayllon, T., & Azrin N. (1968). *The token economy: A motivational system for therapy and rehabilitation.* New York: Appleton–Century–Crofts.

Ayres, A. J. (1954). Ontogenetic principles in the development of arm and hand functions. American *Journal of Occupational Therapy, 3*, 3–13.

Ayres, A. J. (1963). The Eleanor Clarke Slagle Lecture: The development of perceptual-motor abilities: A theoretical basis for treatment of dysfunction. *American Journal of Occupational Therapy, 17*, 221–225.

Ayres, A. J. (1972a). *Sensory integration and learning disorders.* Los Angeles: Western Psychological Services.

Ayres, A. J. (1972b). *Southern California Sensory Integration Tests* [SCSIT]. Los Angeles: Western Psychological Services.

Ayres, A. J. (1979). *Sensory integration and the child.* Los Angeles: Western Psychological Services.

Ayres, A. J. (1989). *Sensory integration and praxis tests.* Los Angeles: Western Psychological Services.

Ayres, A. J., & Heskett, W. M. (1972). Sensory integrative dysfunction in a young schizophrenic girl. *Journal of Autism and Childhood Schizophrenia, 2*, 174–181.

Ayres, A. J., & Marr, D. B. (1991). Sensory integration and praxis tests (SIPT). In A. G. Fisher, E. A. Murray, & A. C. Bundy (Eds.), *Sensory integration: Theory and practice* (pp. 203–233). Philadelphia: F. A. Davis.

Ayres, A. J., & Tickle, L. S. (1980). Hyper-responsivity to touch and vestibular stimuli as a predictor of positive response to sensory integration procedures by autistic children. *American Journal of Occupational Therapy, 34*, 374–381.

Azima, H., & Azima, F. (1959). Outline of a dynamic theory of occupational therapy. *American Journal of Occupational Therapy, 13*, 215–221.

Azima, H., & Wittkower, E. (1957). A partial field survey of psychiatric occupational therapy. *American Journal of Occupational Therapy, 11*, 1–7.

Bachrach, A. W., Mosley, A. R., Swindle, F. L., & Wood, M. M. (1978). *Developmental therapy for young children with autistic characteristics.* Baltimore: University Park Press.

Bailey, D. M. (1978). The effects of vestibular stimulation in verbalization in chronic schizophrenics. *American Journal of Occupational Therapy, 32*, 445–450.

Bandura, A. (1969). *Principles of behavior modification.* New York: Holt, Rinehart, & Winston.

Bandura, A. (1977). *Social learning theory.* Englewood Cliffs, NJ: Prentice-Hall.

Barris, R., Oakley, F., & Kielhofner, G. (1988). The role checklist. In B. Hemphill (Ed.), *Mental health assessment in occupational therapy: An integrated approach to the evaluative process* (pp. 73–91). Thorofare, NJ: SLACK.

Barton, G. E. (1918). *Reconstruction.* New York: Macmillan.

Battaglia, M., Gasperini, M., Sciuto, G., Scherillo, P., Diaferia, G., & Bellodi, L. (1991). Psychiatric disorders in the families of schizotypal subjects. *Schizophrenia Bulletin, 17*, 659–668.

Beck, A. T. (1970). Cognitive therapy: Nature and relation to behavior therapy. *Behavior Therapy, 1*, 184–200.

Beck, A. T. (1976). *Cognitive therapy and the emotional disorders.* New York: International Universities.

Beck, A. T., Rush, A., Shaw, B., & Emery, G. (1979). *Cognitive therapy of depression.* New York: Guilford.

Beery, K. E. (1997). *The Developmental Test of Visual-Motor Integration* (4th ed.). Austin, TX: Pro-Ed.

Bender, L. (1938). *A visual motor gestalt test and its clinical use.* New York: The American Orthopsychiatric Association.

Benson, H. (1975). *The relaxation response.* New York: Morrow.

Benson, H. (1977). Systemic hypertension and the relaxation response. *New England Journal of Medicine, 296*, 1152–1156.

Bergman, G., & Spence, K. (1941). Operationalism and theory in psychology. *Psychological Review, 48*, 1–14.

Berkow, R. (Ed.-in-chief). (1992). *The Merck manual of diagnosis and therapy* (16th ed.). Rahway, NJ: Merck Research Laboratories.

Berne, E. (1961). *Transactional analysis in psychotherapy.* New York: Grove Press.

Blakeney, A. B., Strickland, L. R., & Wilkinson, J. H. (1983). Exploring sensory integrative dysfunction in process schizophrenia. *American Journal of Occupational Therapy, 37*, 399–406.

Blanchard, E. B., Appelbaum, R. A., Radnitz, C. L., Jaccard, J., & Dentinger, M. P. (1989). The refractory headache patient: I. Chronic, daily, high intensity headache. *Behavioral Research and Therapy, 27*, 403–410.

Blanche, E. I. & Henny-Kohler, E. (2000). Philosophy, science, and ideology: A proposed relationship for occupational science and occupational therapy. *Occupational Therapy International, 7*, 99-110.

Blum, G. (1953). *Psychoanalytic theories of personality*. New York: McGraw-Hill.

Bobath, K. & Bobath, B. (1955). Tonic reflexes and righting reflexes in diagnosis and assessment of cerebral palsy. *Cerebral Palsy Review, 16*(5), 3-10, 26.

Borkovec, T. D., & Fowles, D. C. (1973). Controlled investigation of the effects of progressive relaxation and hypnotic relaxation in insomnia. *Journal of Abnormal Psychology, 82*, 153–158.

Braswell, L., & Bloomquist, M. L. (1991). *Cognitive-behavioral therapy with ADHD children: Child, family, and school interventions*. New York: Guilford.

Bronfenbrenner, U. (1977). *The ecology of human development*. Cambridge, MA: Harvard University.

Brown, B. B. (1974). *New mind, new body: Bio-feedback: New directions for the mind*. Toronto: Bantam.

Bruce, M. A., & Borg, B. (1993). *Psychosocial occupational therapy: Frames of reference for intervention* (2nd ed.). Thorofare, NJ: SLACK.

Bruininks, R. H. (1978). *Bruininks–Oseretsky Test of Motor Proficiency*. Circle Pines, MN: American Guidance Service.

Bruner, J. S. (1976). Nature and uses of immaturity. In J. S. Bruner, A. Jolly, & K. Sylva (Eds.), *Play—Its role in development and evolution*. New York: Basic Books.

Bundy, A. C. (1991). Play theory and sensory integration. In A. G. Fisher, E. A. Murray, & A. C. Bundy (Eds.), *Sensory integration: Theory and practice* (pp. 46–67). Philadelphia: F. A. Davis.

Burns, T., Mortimer, J. A., & Merchak, P. (1994). Cognitive Performance Test: A new approach to functional assessment of Alzheimer's disease. *Journal of Geriatric Psychiatry and Neurology, 7*, 46–54.

Calhoun, K. S., & Turner, S. M. (1981). Historical perspectives and current issues in behavior therapy. In S. M. Turner, K. S. Calhoun, & H. E. Adams (Eds.), *Handbook of clinical behavior therapy* (pp. 1–11). New York: Wiley.

Canadian Association of Occupational Therapists. (1991). *Occupational therapy guidelines for client-centred practice*. Toronto, ON: Author.

Canadian Association of Occupational Therapists. (1993). *Occupational therapy guidelines for client-centred mental health practice*. Toronto, ON: Author.

Canadian Association of Occupational Therapists. (1997). *Enabling occupation: An occupational therapy perspective*. Ottawa, ON: Author.

Chamove, A. S. (1996). Enrichment in primates: Relevance to occupational science. In R. Zemke & F. Clark, *Occupational science: The evolving discipline* (pp. 177–180). Philadelphia: F. A. Davis.

Chan, C. C. H., & Lee, T. M. C. (1997). Validity of the Canadian Occupational Performance Measure. *Occupational Therapy International, 4*, 231–249.

Christiansen, P. (1975). Effects of combining methylphenidate and a classroom token system in modifying hyperactive behavior. *American Journal of Mental Deficiency, 80*, 266–276.

Christiansen, C. H. (1996). Three perspectives on balance in occupation. In R. Zemke & F. Clark, *Occupational science: The evolving discipline* (pp. 431–451). Philadelphia: F. A. Davis.

Clark, F. A. (1993). Occupation embedded in a real life: Interweaving occupational science and occupational therapy: 1993 Eleanor Clarke Slagle Lecture. *American Journal of Occupational Therapy, 47*, 1067–1078.

Clark, F. A., Ennevor, B. L., & Richardson, P. L. (1996). A grounded theory of techniques for occupational storytelling and occupational story making. In R. Zemke & F. Clark, *Occupational science: The evolving discipline* (pp. 373–392). Philadelpha: F. A. Davis.

Clark, F., Mailloux, Z., Parham, D., & Bissell, J. C. (1989). Sensory integration and children with learning disabilities. In P. N. Pratt & A. S. Allen (Eds.), *Occupational therapy for children* (2nd ed., pp. 457–507). St. Louis: C. V. Mosby.

Concise Oxford dictionary. (1911). New York: Clarendon Press.

Crist, P. H. (1986). Community living skills: A psychoeducational community based program. *Occupational Therapy in Mental Health, 6*(2), 51–64.

Cutler, S. K., Stevens-Dominguez, M., Oetter, P., & Westby, C. (1992). Development of self-regulation. In P. Oetter, E. W. Richter, & S. M. Frick (Eds.), *M. O. R. E.: Integrating the mouth with sensory and postural functions.* Hugo, MN: PDP Press.

Daniels, L. (1975). The treatment of grand mal epilepsy by covert and operant conditioning. *Psychosomatic Medicine, 16*, 64–67.

Darwin, C. (1898). *The origin of species by means of natural selection: Or, the preservation of favored races in the struggle for life* (6th ed.). New York: Appleton.

Dear, M. (1996). Time, space, and the geography of everyday life of people who are homeless. In R. Zemke & F. Clark (Eds.), *Occupational science: The evolving discipline* (pp. 107–114). Philadelpha: F. A. Davis.

De las Heras, C. (1993). *A user's guide to the volitional questionnaire* (2nd ed.). Chicago: The Model of Human Occupation Clearinghouse, Department of Occupational Therapy, University of Illinois.

Department of National Health and Welfare & Canadian Association of Occupational Therapists. (1986). *Intervention guidelines for the client-centred practice of occupational therapy* [Cat. H39-100/1986E]. Ottawa, ON: Author.

Dewey, J. (1891). *Psychology* (3rd rev. ed.). New York: American.

Dewey, J. (1900). *The school and society; being three lectures by John Dewey . . . supplemented by a statement of the University elementary school* (3rd ed.). Chicago: The University of Chicago Press.

Dobson, K. S. (1988). *Handbook of cognitive-behavioral therapies.* New York: Guilford.

Doley, D. M., Meredith, R. L., & Ciminero, A. R. (Eds.). (1982). *Behavioral medicine: Assessment and treatment strategies.* New York: Plenum.

Dubos, R. (1959). *Mirage of health.* Garden City, NY: Doubleday Anchor.

Dunton, W. R., & Licht, S. (1950). *Occupational therapy: Principles and practice.* Springfield, IL: Charles C. Thomas.

Edmundson, M. (1997, July 13). Save Sigmund Freud: What we can still learn from a discredited, scientifically challenged misogynist. *The New York Times Magazine, 147*, 34–35.

Ehrenberg, B. L. (1996). Insomnia and hypersomnia. In J. W. Hurst (Ed.-in-chief), *Medicine for the practicing physician* (4th ed., pp. 1838–1841). Stamford, CT: Appleton & Lange.

Eklund, M. (1996). Patient experiences and outcome of treatment in psychiatric occupational therapy—Three cases. *Occupational Therapy International, 3*, 212–239.

Eklund, M. (1999). Changes in object relations in long-term mentally ill patients treated in a psychiatric day-care unit. *Psychotherapy Research, 9*, 167–183.

Eklund, M. (2000). Applying object relations theory to psychosocial occupational therapy: Empirical and theoretical considers. *Occupational Therapy in Mental Health, 15*, 1–26.

Ellis, A. (1962). *Reason and emotion in psychotherapy.* New York: Lyle Stuart.

Ellis, A. (1970). *The essence of rational psychotherapy: A comprehensive approach to treatment.* New York: Institute for Rational Living.

Ellis, A. (1979). The theory of rational-emotive therapy. In A. Ellis & J. Whiteley (Eds.), *Theoretical and empirical foundations of rational–emotive therapy* (pp. 33–60). Pacific Grove, CA: Brooks/Cole.

Engel, J. M. (1994). Cognitive–behavioral treatment of chronic recurrent pain. *Occupational Therapy International, 1*, 82–89.

Erikson, E. H. (1950). *Childhood and society.* New York: W. W. Norton.

Erikson, E. H. (1963). *Childhood and society* (2nd ed.). New York: W. W. Norton.

Evans, J., & Salim, A. A. (1992). A cross-cultural test of the validity of occupational therapy assessments with patients with schizophrenia. *American Journal of Occupational Therapy, 46*, 685–695.

Fahrion, S. L., Walters, E. D., Coyne, L., & Allen, T. R. (1992). Alternations in EEG amplitude, personality factors and brain electrical mapping after alpha–theta brainwave training: A controlled case study of an alcoholic in recovery. *Alcoholism. Clinical and Experimental Research, 16*, 547–552.

Fay, T. (1955). The origins of human movement. *American Journal of Psychiatry, 3*, 644–652.

Fechner, G. T. (1966). *Elements of psychophysics* (H. E. Adler, Trans., D. H. Howes & E. G. Boring, Eds.). New York: Holt, Rinehart & Winston. (Original work published 1860)

Fidler, G. S. (1982). The lifestyle performance profile: An organizing frame. In B. Hemphill (Ed.), *The evaluative process in psychiatric occupational therapy* (pp. 43–47). Thorofare, NJ: SLACK.

Fidler, G. S. (1988). The lifestyle performance profile. In S. Robertson (Ed.), *SCOPE: Strategies, concepts and opportunities for program development and evaluation* (pp. 35–40). Rockville, MD: American Occupational Therapy Association.

Fidler, G. S., & Fidler, J. W. (1954). *Introduction to psychiatric occupational therapy.* New York: Macmillan.

Fidler, G. S., & Fidler, J. W. (1963). *Occupational therapy; A communication process in psychiatry.* New York: Macmillan.

Fillingim, R. B., & Blumenthal, J. A. (1993). The use of aerobic exercise as a method of stress management. In P. M. Lehrer & R. L. Woolfolk (Eds.), *Principles and practice of stress management* (2nd ed., pp. 443–462). New York: Guilford.

Finch, J. R. (1967). A further extension of general systems theory for psychiatry. In L. von Bertalanffy & A. Rapoport (Eds.), *Yearbook of the Society for General Systems Research, 12,* 103–105.

Fisher, A. G. (1994). *The assessment of motor process skills (Version 8.0).* Unpublished test manual, Colorado State University, Occupational Therapy Department, Fort Collins.

Fisher, A. G., & Murray, E. A. (1991). Introduction to sensory integration theory. In A. G. Fisher, E. A. Murray & A. C. Bundy (Eds.), *Sensory integration: Theory and practice* (pp. 3–26). Philadelphia: F. A. Davis.

Fisher, A. G., Murray, E. A., & Bundy, A. C. (Eds.). (1991). *Sensory integration: Theory and practice.* Philadelphia: F. A. Davis.

Florey, L. L., & Greene, S. (1997). Play in middle childhood: A focus on children with behavior and emotional disorders. In L. D. Parham & L. S. Faxio (Eds.), *Play in occupational therapy for children* (pp. 126–143). St Louis: Mosby.

Folio, M. R., & Fewell, R. R. (2000). *Peabody Developmental Motor Scales- Second edition (PDMS-2).* Austin, TX: Pro-Ed.

Forsyth, K., Salamy, M., Simon, S., & Kielhofner, G. (1995). *A user's guide to the Assessment of Communication and Interaction Skills* (ACIS). (Version 4.0). Unpublished manuscript, Department of Occupational Therapy, University of Illinois at Chicago.

Frankl, V. (1963). *Man's search for meaning.* New York: Washington Square Press.

Freeman, A., Pretzer, J., Fleming, B., & Simon, K. M. (1990). *Clinical applications of cognitive therapy.* New York: Plenum.

Freud, A. (1963). *The ego and the mechanisms of defense* (C. Bains, Trans.). New York: International University Press. (Original work published 1936)

Freud, S. (1953–1974). Three essays on the theory of sexuality. In J. Strachey (Ed. and Trans.), *The standard edition of the complete psychological works of Sigmund Freud* (Vol. 7). London: Hogarth. (Original work published 1905)

Freud, S. (1953–1974). Leonardo da Vinci and a memory of his childhood. In J. Strachey (Ed. and Trans.), *The standard edition of the complete psychological works of Sigmund Freud* (Vol. 11, pp. 63–137). London: Hogarth. (Original work published 1910)

Freud, S. (1966). The development of the libido and the sexual organizations. In J. Strachey (Ed. and Trans.), *The complete introductory lectures on psychoanalysis.* New York: W. W. Norton. (Original work published 1917)

Freud, S. (1953–1974). Beyond the pleasure principle. In J. Strachey (Ed. and Trans.), *The standard edition of the complete psychological works of Sigmund Freud* (Vol. 18, pp. 1–64). London: Hogarth. (Original work published 1920)

Freud, S. (1953–1974). The ego and the id. In J. Strachey (Ed. and Trans.), *The standard edition of the complete psychological works of Sigmund Freud* (Vol. 19, pp. 1–66). London: Hogarth. (Original work published 1923)

Freud, S. (1953–1974). Dostoevsky and parricide. In J. Strachey (Ed. and Trans.), *The standard edition of the complete psychological works of Sigmund*

Freud (Vol. 21, pp. 177–197). London: Hogarth. (Original work published 1928)

Freud, S. (1953–1974). New introductory lectures on psycho-analysis. In J. Strachey (Ed. and Trans.), *The standard edition of the complete psychological works of Sigmund Freud* (Vol. 22, pp. 1–182). London: Hogarth. (Original work published 1933)

Fromm, E. (1941). *Escape from freedom.* New York: Rinehart.

Gardner, M. F. (1996). *Test of Visual Perceptual Skills–Revised* (nonmotor). Burlingame, CA: Psychological and Educational Publications.

Garvey, C. (1977). *Play.* Cambridge: MA: Harvard.

Gesell, A. (1928). *Infancy and human growth.* New York: McGraw-Hill.

Gesell, A. (1952). *Infant development: The embryology of early human behavior.* New York: Harper & Row.

Gibson, T., Grahame, R., Harkness, J., Woo, P., Blagrave, P., & Hills, R. (1985, June 1). Controlled comparison of short-wave diathermy treatment with osteopathic treatment in non-specific low back pain. *Lancet, 1*(8440), 1258-1261.

Glasser, W. (1965). *Reality therapy: A new approach to psychiatry.* New York: Harper & Row.

Gorman, J. M. (1996). *The new psychiatry: The essential guide to state-of-the-art therapy, medication, and emotional health.* New York: St. Martin's.

Gregg, C. L., Hafner, M. E., & Korner, A. (1976). The relative efficacy of vestibular-proprioceptive stimulation and the upright position in enhancing visual pursuit in neonates. *Child Development, 47,* 309–314.

Gunn, C. C., Milbrandt, W. E., Little, A. S., & Mason, K. E. (1980). Dry needling of muscle motor points for chronic low-back pain: A randomized clinical trial with long-term follow-up. *Spine, 5,* 279–291.

Hall, W. D. (1996). Mild, moderate, severe, and resistant hypertension. In J. W. Hurst (Ed.-in-chief), *Medicine for the practicing physician* (4th ed., pp.1080–1085). Stamford, CT: Appleton & Lange.

Hartmann, H. (1939). *Ego psychology and the problem of adaptation.* New York: International Universities.

Hartmann, H. (1964). *Essays on ego psychology.* New York: International Universities Press.

Havighurst, R. J. (1972). *Developmental tasks and education* (3rd ed.). New York: Longman.

Helfrich, C., Kielhofner, G., & Mattingly, C. (1994). Volition as narrative: An understanding of motivation in chronic illness. *American Journal of Occupational Therapy, 42,* 311–317.

Helmholtz, H. (1867). *Handbuch der physiologischen optik* [Handbook of physiology of optics]. Leipzig: L. Voss.

Herman, B. E. (1980). A sensory integrative approach to the psychotic child. *Occupational Therapy in Mental Health, 1*(1), 57–68.

Hilgard, E., & Marquis, D. (1961). *Conditioning and learning.* New York: Appleton–Century–Crofts.

Holroyd, K. A., & Andrasik, F. (1982). Do the effects of cognitive therapy endure? A two year follow-up of tension headache suffers treated with cognitive therapy or biofeedback. *Cognitive Therapy and Research, 6,* 325–334.

Honigfeld, G., Gillis, R. D., & Klett, C. J. (1966). NOSIE—30: A treatment sensitive ward behavior scale. *Psychological Reports, 19,* 180–182.

Horney, K. (1939). *New ways in psychoanalysis.* New York: W. W. Norton.

Huizinga, J. (1955). *Homo ludens: A study of the play element in the culture.* Boston: Beacon.

Humphries, T., Wright, M., Snider, L., & McDougall, B. (1992). A comparison of the effectiveness of sensory integrative therapy and perceptual–motor training in treating children with learning disabilities. *Journal of Developmental and Behavioral Pediatrics, 13,* 31–40.

Jacobson, E. (1929). *Progressive relaxation.* Chicago: University of Chicago.

Jacobson, E. (1978). *You must relax* (4th ed.). New York: McGraw-Hill.

James, W. (1890). *The principle of psychology.* New York: Holt.

Jesness, C. (1975). Comparative effectiveness of behavior modification and transactional analysis programs for delinquents. *Journal of Consulting and Clinical Psychology, 43,* 758–779.

Johnston, M. T. (1986). The use of cognitive–behavioral techniques with depressed patients in day treatment. In American Occupational Therapy Association, *Depression: Assessment and treatment update* (pp. 49–60). Rockville, MD: Author.

Jorstad, V., Wilbert, D. E., & Wirrer, B. (1977). Sensory dysfunction in adult schizophrenia. *Hospital Community Psychiatry, 28*(4), 280–283.

Jung, C. (1961). *Memories, dreams, reflections.* New York: Vintage.

Kabat, H., & Knott, M. (1948). Principles of neuro-muscular reeducation. *Psychological Review, 28,* 107–111.

Kaplan, K., & Kielhofner, G. (1989). *The Occupational Case Analysis Interview and Rating Scale.* Thorofare, NJ: SLACK.

Kazdin, A. E., & Wilson, G. T. (1978). *Evaluation of behavior therapy: Issues, evidence, and research strategies.* Lincoln: University of Nebraska.

Kerlinger, F. N. (1973). *Foundations of behavioral research* (2nd ed.). New York: Holt, Rinehart and Winston.

Kielhofner, G. (1985). Occupational function and dysfunction. In G. Kielhofner (Ed.), *A model of human occupation* (pp. 63–74). Baltimore: Williams & Wilkins.

Kielhofner, G. (1995). *A model of human occupation: Theory and application* (2nd ed.). Baltimore: Williams & Wilkins.

Kielhofner, G. (1997). *Conceptual foundations of occupational therapy* (2nd ed.). Philadelphia: F. A. Davis.

Kielhofner, G., & Henry, A. D. (1988). Development and investigation of the Occupational Performance History Interview. *American Journal of Occupational Therapy, 42,* 489–498.

Kielhofner, G., Henry, A. D., & Walens, D. (1989). *A user's guide to the Occupational Performance History Interview.* Rockville, MD: American Occupational Therapy Association.

King, L. J. (1974). A sensory-integrative approach to schizophrenia. *American Journal of Occupational Therapy, 28,* 529–537.

Knox, S. (1974). A play scale. In M. Reilly (Ed.), *Play as exploratory learning* (pp. 247–266). Beverly Hills, CA: Sage.

Knox, S. (1997a). Development and current use of the Knox Preschool Play Scale. In L. D. Parham & L. S. Fazio (Eds.), *Play in occupational therapy for children* (pp. 35–51). St Louis: Mosby.

Knox, S. (1997b). Play and playfulness in preschool children. In R. Zemke & F. Clark (Eds.), *Occupational science: The evolving discipline* (pp. 81–88). Philadelphia: F. A. Davis.

Kohlberg, L. (1971). *Essays on moral development. Vol 1: The philosophy of moral development.* New York: Harper & Row.

Kris, E. (1952). *Psychoanalytic explorations in art.* New York: International Universities Press.

Law, M., Baptiste, S., Carswell-Opzoomer, A., McColl, M., Polatajko, H., & Pollock, N. (1991). *Canadian Occupational Performance Measure manual.* Toronto, ON: CAOT Publications.

Law, M., Baptiste, S., McColl, M., Opzoomer, A., Polatajko, H., & Pollock, N. (1990). The Canadian Occupational Performance Measure: An outcome measure for occupational therapy. *Canadian Journal of Occupational Therapy, 57,* 82–87.

Leach, W. W. (1960). Nystagmus: An integrative neural deficit in schizophrenia. *Journal of Abnormal Social Psychology, 66,* 305–309.

Lehrer, P. M., Carr, R., Sargunaraj, D., & Woolfolk, R. L. (1993). Differential effects of stress management therapies in behavioral medicine. In P. M. Lehrer & R. L. Woolfolk (Eds.), *Principles and practice of stress management* (2nd ed., pp. 571–605). New York: Guilford.

Lehrer, P. M., & Woolfolk, R. L. (1993). *Principles and practice of stress management* (2nd ed.). New York: Guilford.

Levy, L. L. (1993). Model of human occupation frame of reference. In H. L. Hopkins, & H. D. Smith (Eds), *Willard and Spackman's occupational therapy* (8th ed., pp. 76–79). Philadelphia: Lippincott.

Lillie, M., & Armstrong, H. (1982). Contributions to the development of psychoeducation approaches to mental health service. *American Journal of Occupational Therapy, 36,* 438–443.

Linden, W. (1990). *Autogenic training: A clinical guide.* New York: Guilford.

Lindsley, O. (1956). Operant conditioning methods applied to research in chronic schizophrenia. *Psychiatric Research Reports, 5,* 118–139.

Llorens, L. A. (1972). Problem-solving: The role of occupational therapy in a new environment. *American Journal of Occupational Therapy, 26,* 234–238.

Llorens, L. (1976). *Application of a developmental theory for health and rehabilitation.* Rockville, MD: American Occupational Therapy Association.

Lorenz, K. Z. (1965). *Evolution and modification of behavior.* Chicago: University of Chicago.

Luria, A. R. (1980). *Higher cortical functions in man* (2nd ed., B. Haigh, Trans.). New York: Basic Books.

Magrun, W. M., Ottenbacher, K., McCue, S., & Keefe, R. (1981). Effects of vestibular stimulation on spontaneous use of verbal language of developmentally delayed children. *American Journal of Occupational Therapy, 35,* 101–104.

Marlatt, G. A., & Gordon, J. R. (Eds.). (1985). *Relapse prevention: Maintenance strategies in the treatment of addictive behaviors.* New York: Guilford.

Maslow, A. (1968). *Toward a psychology of being* (2nd ed.). New York: Van Nostrand Reinhold.

Matsutsuyu, J. S. (1969). The Interest Check List. *American Journal of Occupational Therapy, 34,* 368–373.

Mayer, W. B. (1996). Headaches. In J. W. Hurst (Ed.-in-chief), *Medicine for the practicing physician* (4th ed., pp. 1845–1849). Stamford, CT: Appleton & Lange.

McGrady, A., Olson, R. P., & Kroon, J. S. (1995). Biobehavioral treatment of essential hypertension. In M. S. Schwartz & Associates (Eds.), *Biofeedback: A practitioner's guide* (2nd ed., pp. 445–467). New York: Guilford.

McMicken, D. B. (1996). Alcohol: Tolerance, addiction, and withdrawal. In J. W. Hurst (Ed.-in-chief), *Medicine for the practicing physician* (4th ed., pp. 1975–1980). Stamford, CT: Appleton & Lange.

Mechanic, D. (Ed.). (1983). *Handbook of health, health care and the health professions.* New York: The Free Press.

Meichenbaum, D. (1977). *Cognitive behavior modification: An integrative approach.* New York: Plenum.

Meichenbaum, D. (1985). *Stress inoculation training.* Elmsford, NY: Pergamon.

Mercer, L. & Boch, M. (1983). Residual sensorimotor deficits in the adult head-injured patient. A treatment approach. *Physical Therapy, 63*(12), 1988–1991.

Metarazzo, J. D. (1980). Behavioral health and behavioral medicine: Frontiers for a new health psychology. *American Psychologist, 35,* 807–817.

Meyer, A. (1922). The philosophy of occupational therapy. *Archives of Occupational Therapy, 1*(1), 1–10.

Michelman, S. S. (1974). Play and the deficit child. In M. Reilly (Ed.), *Play as exploratory learning* (pp. 157–207). Beverly Hills, CA: Sage.

Miller, B. R. J., Sieg, K. W., Ludwig, F. M., Shortridge, S. D., & Van Deusen, J. (1988). *Six perspectives on theory for the practice of occupational therapy.* Rockville, MD: Aspen.

Miller, P. (1972). The use of behavioral contracting in the treatment of alcoholism: A case report. *Behavior Therapy, 3,* 593–596.

Miller, S. B., & Mathis, D. E. (1996). Low back pain. In J. W. Hurst (Ed.-in-chief), *Medicine for the practicing physician* (4th ed., pp. 250–253). Stamford, CT: Appleton & Lange.

Monti, P., Abrams, D., & Binkoff, J. (1990). Communication skills training: Communication skills training with family and cognitive behavioral mood management training for alcoholics. *Journal of Studies on Alcohol, 51,* 263–270.

Moser, D. K., Dracup, K., Woo, M. A., & Stevenson, L. W. (1997). Voluntary control of vascular tone by using skin–temperature biofeedback–relaxation in patients with advanced heart failure. *Alternative Therapy in Health Medicine, 3,* 51–59.

Mosey, A. C. (1970). *Three frames of reference for mental health.* Thorofare, NJ: SLACK.

Mosey, A. C. (1973). *Activities therapy.* New York: Raven Press.

Mosey, A. C. (1986). *Psychosocial components of occupational therapy.* New York: Raven.

Mueller, C. R. (1996). Multidisciplinary research of multimodal stimulation of premature infants: An integrated review of the literature. *Maternity Child Nursing Journal, 24*(1), 18–31.

Mulligan, S. (1996). An analysis of score patterns of children with attention disorders on the Sensory Integration and Praxis Tests. *American Journal of Occupational Therapy, 50,* 647–654.

Müller, J. (1833–1838). *Handbuch der physiologie des menschen fur vorlesungen* [Handbook of physiology]. Coblenz, Germany: Holscher.

Munoz, J. P., Lawlor, M., & Kielhofner, G. (1993). Use of the model of human occupation: A survey of therapists in psychiatric practice. *The Occupational Therapy Journal of Research, 13,* 117–139.

Murray, E. A., & Anzalone, M .E. (1997). Integrating sensory integration theory and practice with other intervention approaches. In A. G. Fisher, E. A. Murray, & A. C. Bundy (Eds.), *Sensory integration: Theory and practice* (pp. 354–383). Philadelphia: F. A. Davis.

Nicassio, P. M., Boylan, M. B., & McCabe, T. G. (1982). Progressive relaxation, EMG biofeedback and biofeedback placebo in the treatment of sleep-onset insomnia. *British Journal of Medical Psychology, 55,* 159–166.

Nilsson, A. (1993). Preliminärt kodningsschema, interbedömar- och parallelltestreliabilitet hos PORT, Perceptgenetiskt ObjektRelationsTest [Preliminary scoring scheme, interrater and parallel test reliability of the PORT, the Perceptgenetic Object-Relations Test]. *Psykologi I Tillämpning, 11.*

Nilsson, A. (1995). Differentiation between patients with schizopherenia and borderline disorders in the Percept-genetic Object Relations Test, PORT. *British Journal of Medical Psychology, 68,* 287–309.

Oetter, P., Richter, E. W., & Frick, S. M. (1993). *M. O. R. E.: Integrating the mouth with sensory and postural functions.* Hugo, MN: PDP Press.

Parham, L. D. (1996). Perspectives on play. In R. Zemke & F. Clark (Eds.), *Occupational science: The evolving discipline* (pp. 71–80). Philadelphia: F. A. Davis.

Parham, L .D., & Primeau, L. A. (1997). Play and occupational therapy. In L. D. Parham & L. S. Fazio (Eds.), *Play in occupational therapy for children* (pp. 2–21). St Louis: Mosby.

Patel, C. (1973). Yoga and biofeedback in the management of hypertension. *Lancet, ii,* 1053–1055.

Pavlov, I. (1927). *Conditioned reflexes.* New York: Dover.

Perls, F., Hefferline, R., & Goodman, P. (1965). *Gestalt therapy.* New York: Dell.

Piaget, J. (1929). *The child's conception of the world.* London: Routledge and Kegan Paul.

Piaget, J. (1952a). *The origins of intelligence in children* (M. Cook, Trans.). New York: International Universities Press.

Piaget, J. (1952b). *Play, dreams and imitation in childhood.* New York: Norton.

Piaget, J. (1954). *The construction of reality in the child* (M. Cook, Trans.). New York: Basic Books.

Piergrossi, J. C., & Gilbertoni, C. (1995). The importance of inner transformation in the activity process. *Occupational Therapy International, 2,* 36–47.

Polatajko, H. J., Law, M., Miller, J., Schaffer, R., & Macnab, J. (1991). The effect of a sensory integration program on academic achievement, motor performance, and self-esteem in children identified as learning disabled: Results of a clinical trial. *Occupational Therapy Journal of Research, 11,* 155–176.

Pope, M. H., Phillips, R. B., Haugh, L. D., Hsieh, C. Y., MacDonald, L., & Halderman, S. (1994, November 15). A prospective randomized three-week trial of spinal manipulation, transcutaneous muscle stimulation, massage and corset in the treatment of subacute low back pain. *Spine, 19*(22), 2571–2577.

Posner, M. I. (1973). *Cognition: An introduction.* Glenview, IL: Scott Foresman.

Price, A. (1986). Applying sensory integration to handwriting problems. *American Occupational Therapy Association Developmental Disabilities Special Interest Section Newsletter, 9,* 4–5.

Primeau, L. A. (1996). Work versus nonwork: The case of household work. In R. Zemke & F. Clark (Eds.), *Occupational science: The evolving discipline* (pp. 57–70). Philadelphia: F. A. Davis.

Ray, T., King, L. J., & Grandin, T. (1988). The effectiveness of self-initiated vestibular stimulation in producing speech sounds in an autistic child. *Occupational Therapy Journal of Research, 8,* 186–190.

Reich, W. (1949). *Character analysis.* New York: Farrar Strauss & Young.

Reilly, M. (1956). Therapeutically influenced recovery. *American Journal of Occupational Therapy, 10,* 229–232.

Reilly, M. (1958). An occupational therapy curriculum for 1965. *American Journal of Occupational Therapy, 12,* 293–299.

Reilly, M. (1962). Occupational therapy can be one of the great ideas of 20th century medicine. *American Journal of Occupational Therapy, 16,* 1–9.

Reilly, M. (1969). The educational process. *American Journal of Occupational Therapy, 23,* 299–307.

Reilly, M. (1971). Occupational therapy—A historical perspective: The modernization of occupational therapy. *American Journal of Occupational Therapy, 25,* 243–246.

Reilly, M. (1974a). Defining a cobweb. In M. Reilly (Ed.), *Play as exploratory learning* (pp. 57–116). Beverly Hills, CA: Sage.

Reilly, M. (1974b). *Play as exploratory learning.* Beverly Hills, CA: Sage.

Reisman, J. E., & Blakeney, A. B. (1991). Exploring sensory integrative treatment in chronic schizophrenia. *Occupational Therapy in Mental Health, 11*(1), 25–43.

Rider, B. A. (1973). Perceptual-motor dysfunction in emotionally disturbed children. *American Journal of Occupational Therapy, 27,* 316-320.

Roach, E. G., & Kephart, N. C. (1966). *Purdue Perceptual Motor Survey.* San Antonio, TX: The Psychological Corporation.

Roberts, J. M., Arth, M. J., & Bush, R. R. (1959). Games in culture. *American Anthropologist, 61,* 597–605.

Rogers, C. (1942). *Counseling and psychotherapy.* Boston: Houghton Mifflin.

Rood, M. (1956). Neurophysiological mechanisms utilized in the treatment of neuromuscular dysfunction. *American Journal of Occupational Therapy, 10,* 220-225.

Ross, M. & Burdick, D. (1981). *Sensory integration: A training manual for therapists and teachers for regressed psychiatric and geriatric patient groups.* Thorofare, NJ: SLACK.

Rubin, K., Fein, G. G., & Vandenberg, B. (1983). Play. In P. H. Mussen (Ed.), *Handbook of child psychology. Vol 4: Socialization, personality and social development* (4th ed., pp. 693–774). New York: Wiley.

Russell, B. (Ed.). (1965). *On the philosophy of science.* Indianapolis, IN: Bobbs–Merrill.

Saint–Jean, M., & Desrosiers, L. (1993). Psychoanalytic considerations regarding the occupational therapy setting for treatment of the psychotic patient. *Occupational Therapy in Mental Health, 12*(2), 69–78.

Salo-Chydenius, S. (1994). Application of occupational therapy in the treatment of depression. *Occupational Therapy International, 1,* 103–121.

Schilder, P. (1933). The vestibular apparatus in neurosis and psychosis. *Journal of Nervous Mental Disorders, 78,* 1–23, 137–164.

Schkade, J. K., & Schultz, S. (1992). Occupational adaptation: Toward a holistic approach for contemporary practice, Part 1. *American Journal of Occupational Therapy, 46,* 829–837.

Schkade, J. K., & Schultz, S. (1993). Occupational adaptation: An integrative frame of reference. In H. L. Hopkins & H. D. Smith (Eds.), *Willard and Spackman's occupational therapy* (8th ed., pp. 87–91). Philadelphia: Lippincott.

Schnoll, S. H. (1996). Psychoactive substance use disorders. In J. W. Hurst (Ed.-in-chief), *Medicine for the practicing physician* (4th ed., pp. 54–57). Stamford, CT: Appleton & Lange.

Schultz, S. (1996, April). *Redefining psychiatric rehabilitation: Results of occupational therapy model.* Paper presented at the 76th Annual Conference and Exposition of the American Occupational Therapy Association, Chicago.

Schultz, S., & Schkade, J. K. (1992). Occupational adaptation: Toward a holistic approach for contemporary practice, Part 2. *American Journal of Occupational Therapy, 46,* 917–925.

Schwartz, M. S. (1995). Headache: Selected issues and considerations in evaluation and treatment. Part B: Treatment. In M. S. Schwartz & Associates (Eds.), *Biofeedback: A practitioner's guide* (2nd ed., pp. 354–409). New York: Guilford.

Schwartz, M. S., & Associates (Eds.). (1995). *Biofeedback: A practitioner's guide* (2nd ed.). New York: Guilford.

Schwartz, M. S., & Olson, R. P. (1995). A historical perspective on the field of biofeedback and applied psychophysiology. In M. S. Schwartz & Associates (Eds.), *Biofeedback: A practitioner's guide* (2nd ed., pp. 6–18). New York: Guilford.

Selye, H. (1956). *The stress of life.* New York: McGraw-Hill.

Shalev, A. Y., Orr, S. P., & Pitman, R. K. (1992). Psychophysiologic response during script-driven imagery as an outcome measure in posttraumatic stress disorder. *Journal of Clinical Psychiatry, 53,* 324–326.

Shannon, P. D. (1967, January). *Work adjustment and the adolescent soldier.* Unpublished thesis, University of Southern California, Los Angeles.

Shannon, P. D. (1974). Occupational choice: Decision making play. In M. Reilly (Ed.), *Play as exploratory learning* (pp. 285–314). Beverly Hills, CA: Sage.

Sherman, R. A., & Arena, J. G. (1992). Biofeedback in the assessment and treatment of low back pain. In J. V. Basmajian & R. New Yorkberg (Eds.), *Spinal manipulation therapies* (pp. 177–197). Baltimore, MD: Williams & Wilkins.

Skinner, B. F. (1938). T*he behavior of organisms.* New York: Appleton–Century–Crofts.

Skinner, B. F. (1953). *Science and human behavior.* New York: Macmillan.

Slagel, E. C. (1922). Training aides for mental patients. *Archives of Occupational Therapy, 1*(1), 11–18.

Slavik, B. A., Kitsuwa-Lowe, J., Danner, P. T., Green, J., & Ayres, A. J. (1984). Vestibular stimulation and eye contact in autistic children. *Neuropediatrics, 15,* 333–336.

Spence, K. W. (1956). *Behavior theory and conditioning.* New Haven, CT: Yale University.

Spielberger, C. (1983). *Manual for the State-trait Anxiety Inventory.* Palo Alto, CA: Consulting Psychologist.

Stein, F. (1967). Distortion of ego functions in schizophrenia and the implications for occupational therapy. In. R. L. Kleinman (Ed.), *Through youth to age: Occupational therapy faces the challenge* (pp. 177–182). Proceedings of the Fourth International Congress of the World Federation of Occupational Therapists, London. Amsterdam: Excerpta Medica Foundation.

Stein, F. (1982). A current review of the behavioral frame of reference and its application to occupational therapy. *Occupational Therapy In Mental Health, 2,* 35–62.

Stein, F. (1987a). Stress and schizophrenia. *Alberta Psychology, 16,* 10–11.

Stein, F. (1987b). *Stress management questionnaire.* [Available from the author at the University of South Dakota, Occupational Therapy Department, 414 E. Clark St., Vermillion, SD 57069]

Stein, F. (1989). *Anatomy of clinical research: An introduction to the scientific inquiry in medicine, rehabilitation, and related health professions* (Rev. ed.). Thorofare, NJ: SLACK.

Stein, F. (1990, April). *Clinical trials using cognitive–behavioral treatment methodologies with psychiatric patients.* Paper presented at the 10th International Congress of the World Federation of Occupational Therapists, Melbourne, Australia.

Stein, F. (1991, July). *Biofeedback with recovering alcoholics.* Paper presented at the Inter-American Congress of Psychology, San Jose, Costa Rica.

Stein, F. (1992, April). *Evaluating stress management groups in psychosocial practice.* Paper presented at the annual conference of the American Occupational Therapy Association, Houston, TX.

Stein, F. (1993, June). *Clinical research in cognitive–behavioral treatment.* Paper presented at the Annual Conference of the Canadian Occupational Therapy Association, Regina, Saskatchewan.

Stein, F. (1994, April). *Stress management in psychosocial practice.* Paper presented at the 11th International Congress of the World Federation of Occupational Therapists, London, UK.

Stein, F. (1996, April). *Clinical research in cognitive-behavioral treatment.* Paper presented at the annual conference of the American Occupational Therapy Association, Chicago, IL.

Stein, F., & Cutler, S. K. (2000). *Clinical research in occupational therapy (4th ed.).* San Diego, CA: Singular Publishing Group.

Stein, F., & Nikolic, S. (1989). Teaching stress management techniques to a schizophrenic patient. *American Journal of Occupational Therapy, 43,* 162–169.

Stein, F., & Smith, J. (1989). Short-term stress management programme with acutely depressed inpatients. *Canadian Journal of Occupational Therapy, 56,* 185–191.

Strupp, H. H. (1973). Toward a reformulation of the psychotherapeutic influences. *International Journal of Psychiatry, 7,* 18–19.

Stuart, R. (1971). A three-dimensional program for the treatment of obesity. *Behavior Research and Therapy, 9,* 177–186.

Sullivan, H. S. (1953). The interpersonal theory of psychiatry. In H. W. Perry & M. L. Gawel (Eds.), *The collected works of Harry Stack Sullivan, M.D.* (Vol. I). New York: W. W. Norton.

Takata, N. (1974). Play as a prescription. In M. Reilly (Ed.), *Play as exploratory learning* (pp. 209–246). Beverly Hills, CA: Sage Publications.

Taylor, E. (1988). Anger intervention. *American Journal of Occupational Therapy, 42,* 147–155.

Turner, J. A. (1982). Comparison of group progressive relaxation training and cognitive–behavioral group therapy for low back pain. *Journal of Consulting and Clinical Psychology, 50,* 757–765.

Turner, R. M., & Ascher, L. M. (1979). Controlled comparison of progressive relaxation, stimulus control, and paradoxical intention therapies for insomnia. *Journal of Consulting and Clinical Psychology, 47,* 500–508.

University of Southern California [USC]. Department of Occupational Therapy. (1987). *Proposal for a new doctor of philosophy degree in occupational science.* Unpublished manuscript.

Velozo, C., Kielhofner, G., & Fisher, B. (1990). *A user's guide to the Worker Role Interview* (Research version). [Available from the Department of Occupational Therapy, University of Illinois at Chicago, Department of Occupational Therapy (M/D 811), College of Associated Health Professions, 1919 West Taylor Street, Chicago, IL 60612–7250]

von Bertalanffy, L. (1968). *General system theory: Foundations, development, application* (Rev. ed.). New York: George Braziller.

von Bertalanffy, L. (1975). *Perspectives on general system theory.* New York: Braziller.

Vygotsky, L. S. (1962). *Thought and language.* Cambridge: Massachusetts Institute of Technology.

Watson, J. (1924). *Behaviorism.* New York: W. W. Norton.

Werner, H. (1948). *Comparative psychology of mental development* (Rev. ed.). Chicago: Follett.

Whitbeck, C. A. (1981). A theory of health. In A. L. Caplan, H. T. Engelhartd, & J. J. McCartney (Eds.), *Concepts of health and disease: Interdisciplinary perspectives.* Reading, MA: Addison–Wesley.

White, R. (1948). *The abnormal personality.* New York: The Ronald Press.

Whitehead, A. N. (1919). *An enquiry concerning the principles of natural knowledge.* Cambridge: University Press.

Wilcock, A. A. (1993). Editorial. *Journal of Occupational Science, 1,* 1–2.

Williams, R. B., & Gentry, W. D. (1977). *Behavioral approaches to medical treatment.* Cambridge, MA: Balinger.

Wilson, B. N., Kaplan, B. J., Fellowes, S., Gruchy, C., & Faris, P. (1992). The efficacy of sensory integration treatment compared to tutoring. *Physical and Occupational Therapy in Pediatrics, 12,* 1–36.

Winnicott, D. W. (1965). *The maturational processes and the facilitating environment: Studies in the theory of emotional development.* London: Hogarth Press.

Wolfe, S. L. (1978). Perspectives on central nervous system responsiveness to transcutaneous nerve stimulation. *Physical Therapy, 58,* 1443–1448.

Wolpe, J. (1961). The systematic desensitization treatment of neuroses. *Journal of Nervous and Mental Disorders, 132,* 189–203.

Woolfolk, R. L., Carr–Kaffashan, L., McNulty, T. F., & Lehrer, P. M. (1976). Meditation training as a treatment for insomnia. *Behavioral Therapy, 7,* 359–365.

Yerxa, E. J. (1991). Nationally speaking: Seeking a relevant, ethical, and realistic way of knowing for occupational therapy. *American Journal of Occupational Therapy, 45,* 199–204.

Yerxa, E. J. (1993). Occupational science: A new source of power for participants in occupational therapy. *Journal of Occupational Science, 1,* 3–10.

Yerxa, E. J., Clark, F., Frank, G., Jackson, J., Parham, D., Pierce, D., Stein, C., & Zemke, R. (1989). An introduction to occupational science: A foundation for occupational therapy in the 21st century. In J. A. Johnson & E. J. Yerxa (Eds.), *Occupational science: The foundation for new models of practice* (pp. 1–17). New York: Haworth.

Zemke, R., & Clark, F. (Eds.). (1996). *Occupational science: The evolving discipline.* Philadelphia: F. A. Davis.

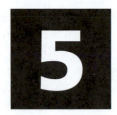

The Occupational Therapy Treatment Process: The Basis for Achieving Positive Mental Health Goals

> *As a communication process, occupational therapy is concerned with action, the meaning of action, its use in communicating feelings and thoughts, and the use of such nonverbal communication of the benefit of the patient.*
>
> —G. S. Fidler & J. W. Fidler, 1963, *Occupational Therapy: A Communication Process in Psychiatry*, p. 19.

Operational Learning Objectives

By the end of this chapter, the learner will:

1. Formulate short- and long-term treatment goals for a client.

2. Identify sequential steps in the treatment process.

3. Identify the purposes of the initial interview.

4. List the general conditions for establishing a supportive environment for the initial interview.

5. Discuss the utilization of the COTA in psychosocial practice.

6. Identify the diagnostic groups outlined in DSM-IV.

7. Identify the components in a comprehensive case study.

8. Identify the psychological landmarks and life crises during infancy and childhood, adolescence, young adulthood, middle and old age.

9. Identify the concepts of positive mental health as the bases for treatment planning.

10. Generate occupational therapy activities that meet treatment objective.

THE PSYCHOTHERAPEUTIC NATURE OF OCCUPATIONAL THERAPY

Psychosocial occupational therapy may be characterized as a discovery treatment process similar to psychotherapy. Like the psychotherapist, the occupational therapist uses diverse methods and activities to help the individual client learn new ways to overcome emotional and behavioral problems, interact with others, increase independent living skills, and self-regulate feelings. The client-therapist relationship is an essential component of both occupational therapy and psychotherapy (Frank, 1958). Psychological theories such as psychodynamic and cognitive behavioral therapy are used in both occupational therapy and psychotherapy as the basis for understanding the client's behavior, formulating treatment goals, and implementing treatment strategies. The major difference between occupational therapy and psychotherapy is in the medium of interaction between therapist and client. The psychotherapist relies on verbal and bodily cues of the client in the interactive exchange, while the occupational therapist uses activities as major treatment modalities. The occupational therapist and psychotherapist perform role functions whose goal is to help the client develop self-esteem, interpersonal competencies, emotional control, and problem-solving skills. Unlike a drug that is directed at a specific neurotransmitter (e.g., dopamine or serotonin) or a surgical procedure that is performed to correct a specific problem, occupational therapy and psychotherapy are interactive processes that rely on the client's active participation. In this process, the client discloses personal information, identifies problems, and tries out new behaviors to cope more effectively with life tasks.

Anthony Storr (1980), a psychiatrist, outlined the steps involved in the practice of psychotherapy. These steps include (a) creating a treatment environment that is friendly to the client; (b) facilitating rapport and client confidence during the initial interview; (c) establishing a pattern in the treatment sessions that places responsibility for improvement on the client; (d) helping the client to gain insight into his/her behavior; (e) remaining objective and nonjudgmental; (f) examining the therapist-client relationship as a focus for improving interpersonal relationships; and (g) establishing criteria for terminating treatment.

How do these factors relate to the treatment process in occupational therapy? How does the psychosocial occupational therapist establish therapeutic goals with the client? What factors are considered in selecting activities or therapeutic modalities? How can the concepts of positive mental health be incorporated into establishing treatment goals in occupational therapy? What is the relationship between the stages of development and the onset of specific mental disorders?

These questions go to the core of the treatment process in occupational therapy. The treatment process can be divided into eight specific sequential steps (Figure 5–1):

1. Initial interview with the client to establish rapport and mutually agreed-on treatment goals as a way of empowering the client in his or her own life

2. Assessment and case study analysis of the client's functional abilities in work, leisure, self-care, and social interactions

3. Establishment of specific short- and long-term goals in treatment (RUMBA—Relevant, Understandable, Measurable, Behavioral, and Achievable)

4. Treatment implementation and working through specific problems in the occupational therapy clinic

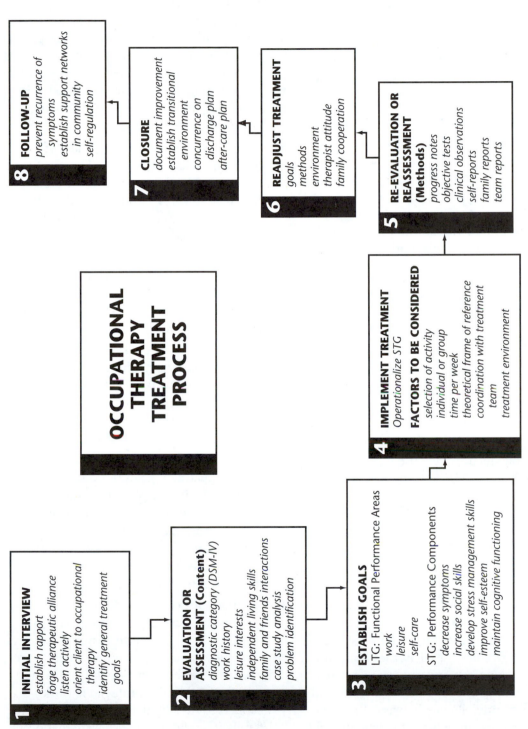

OCCUPATIONAL THERAPY TREATMENT PROCESS

1 INITIAL INTERVIEW
establish rapport
forge therapeutic alliance
listen actively
orient client to occupational therapy
identify general treatment goals

2 EVALUATION OR ASSESSMENT (Content)
diagnostic category (DSM-IV)
work history
leisure interests
independent living skills
family and friends interactions
case study analysis
problem identification

3 ESTABLISH GOALS
LTG: Functional Performance Areas
work
leisure
self-care

STG: Performance Components
decrease symptoms
increase social skills
develop stress management skills
improve self-esteem
maintain cognitive functioning

4 IMPLEMENT TREATMENT
Operationalize STG
FACTORS TO BE CONSIDERED
selection of activity
individual or group
time per week
theoretical frame of reference
coordination with treatment
team
treatment environment

5 RE-EVALUATION OR REASSESSMENT (Methods)
progress notes
objective tests
clinical observations
self-reports
family reports
team reports

6 READJUST TREATMENT
goals
methods
environment
therapist attitude
family cooperation

7 CLOSURE
document improvement
establish transitional environment
concurrence on discharge plan
after-care plan

8 FOLLOW-UP
prevent recurrence of symptoms
establish support networks in community
self-regulation

Figure 5–1. The process of treatment. Notice that treatment begins with an interview and an assessment. Goals are established with the client prior to the treatment, where the short-term goals are operationalized or put into behavioral terms. Following treatment, reassessment occurs through review of progress notes, clinical observations, or reports from other team members, so that readjustment to the treatment or discharge can occur. Follow-up is essential to ensure that the client's symptoms stay in remission.

5. Documentation and reassessment of client's progress

6. Readjustment and recording of treatment goals and priorities, if necessary

7. Plans for closure and discharge into the community

8. Follow-up of the client in the community

The therapist is guided by a holistic approach, which is depicted in Table 5–1. This approach is a step-by-step analysis in planning for initial assessment to discharge.

The content of occupational therapy treatment records for individuals with psychosis were analyzed for treatment goals, interventions, and outcome (Ivarsson, Söderback, & Stein, 2000). The prominent treatment goals that emerged were the ability to manage self-care and the home environment, and the ability to engage in a daily occupation. This conceptual model relied on a client-centered approach where problems were identified by the client before treatment was initiated. In general the treatment process is guided by establishing goals, intervening in treatment, and assessing the outcome. It is important to note that the Americans with Disabilities Act is now becoming increasingly used in following treatment guidelines (U. S. Congress, Office of Technology Assessment, 1994).

INITIAL INTERVIEW

Purposes of the Initial Interview

The overall purposes of the initial interview are to establish rapport with the client, communicate the general purposes of psychosocial occupational therapy, allow the client the opportunity to ask questions, remove any fears or stereotypes the client has of occupational therapy, and forge a therapeutic alliance between the client and the therapist in which the client feels empowered in the process.

The initial interview is a critical stage in the occupational therapy treatment process. It is the starting point for the client and therapist to reinforce the client's will to recovery and improvement. For the occupational therapist, it is an opportunity to orient the client to the purposes of occupational therapy. The initial interview serves the following purposes:

▶ The therapist establishes a climate of unconditional acceptance and rapport with the client. The therapist listens actively to the client, trying to understand the client's feelings and immediate concerns without being overly critical or judgmental.

▶ The therapist gathers historical information from the client that is related to problem findings. The therapist tries to help the client express problems related to functional skills in everyday living in clear and understandable language.

▶ The therapist orients the client to the occupational therapy clinic by taking the client on a tour of the facilities and reducing any preconceived fears about what will occur in occupational therapy.

▶ The therapist describes to the client the general treatment goals of occupational therapy and its relationship to mental health, such as increasing self-esteem through purposeful activities, providing opportunities for self-expression, increasing repertoire of leisure activities, and learning how to self-regulate stress.

▶ The therapist communicates to the client that psychosocial treatment is part of a team process in which the psychiatrist, psychologist, social worker, nurse, vocational counselor, and occupational therapist and other mental health professions work cooperatively with the client and his or her family. The client is made aware that occupational therapy is a treatment procedure

Table 5–1. Holistic Treatment Approach

Step I: Analysis of the Problem

1. What are the major areas that are affected by the disability?
   - self-care
   - work
   - interpersonal skills
   - emotional
   - sleep
   - eating
   - sex
   - other
2. How long has the disability existed? What is the intensity of the disability?
3. Is the disability episodic?
4. How does the individual function during remissions?
5. What are the prime assets and strengths of the individual?
   - intelligence
   - positive attitudes toward receiving therapy
   - motivation to improve
   - interpersonal skills
   - talent or potential in art, music, crafts, computers
   - work experiences
   - educational backgrounds
6. What are the major stressors that trigger symptoms?
7. What are the major symptoms that are precipitated by stress?
8. How does the individual cope with stress?
9. How well does the individual self-regulate symptoms?
10. Does the individual have a holistic approach to health, using exercise, diet, and relaxation?
11. Is the family supportive?

Step II: Planning Treatment

1. Does the individual take an active part in the treatment process?
2. Has a therapeutic alliance between the patient and therapist been established?
3. Are realistic short-term and long-term goals established (RUMBA)?
4. Is the occupational therapy treatment program consistent with the interdisciplinary team?

Step III: Treatment Implementation

1. Is the treatment plan incorporated into a daily schedule?
2. Are activities used as therapeutic media?
3. Has the individual gained insight into the relationship between symptoms and stressors?
4. Has outcome been evaluated through objective measures and self-evaluations (triangulation)?

Step IV: Follow-up in the Community

1. Is there a way to have the client report periodically on his or her ability to function in the community?
2. Is the client able to live independently in the community or is there a need for support in housing, transportation, work, leisure activities, interpersonal skills, and medication?

that has had a long history of involvement in psychiatric practice.

▶ The therapist establishes a future time for evaluating specific functional abilities. The therapist structures continuity in the relationship by giving the client a tentative timetable for the treatment process.

Therapeutic Techniques During Initial Interview

During the initial interview the client may be somewhat confused, anxious, and unable to concentrate, especially if he or she is in the acute phase of an illness. The therapist at this point is supportive and reassuring and not probing or interpretive. For example, the therapist could explore with the client his or her interests in sports, movies, television, music, art, literature, hobbies, and other leisure time pursuits. The occupational therapist emphasizes that the clinic or workshop is an environment to develop self-awareness, social skills, and stress management techniques. The positive, healthy part of the individual is continually reinforced, especially with the client who is acutely depressed or self-deprecating. The occupational therapist may also elicit from the client specific problems that can be worked on in occupational therapy as the basis for a therapeutic contract. To be put into operational terms, problems may have to be restated by the occupational therapist. For example, the client may state, "my friends no longer like me." The therapist may restate the problem to the client as illustrated in the following scenario:

Therapist: "Are you asking for help in developing new ways to relate to other people?"

Client: "Yes, I don't want to lose my friends."

Therapist: "In occupational therapy you will have the opportunity to test out your rela-

tionships while you work on activities. I will try to give you feedback on how you relate to others and perhaps you can learn new skills in your interactions."

Structure of the Initial Interview

These are general considerations for establishing a supportive environment for effective interviewing. Theorists (Bernstein, Bernstein, & Dana 1974; Corey, 1996; Ivey, 1994) discuss the following issues:

▶ *Listening.* The client should feel that he or she is the sole concern of the therapist. The occupational therapist must be an active listener, responsive, and empathetic to the client without passing judgments on the client's behavior. The therapist initially listens more than talks and restates and clarifies points to the client. The therapist uses attending skills, such as culturally and individually appropriate eye contact, body language that encourages talking and sharing, and nonverbal encouragers (e.g., nodding, reinforcing comments, appropriate silences). Additional techniques in interviewing include the use of open questions (i.e., questions that require more than a yes/no answer) to encourage freer discussion of a topic and paraphrasing or summarizing techniques to facilitate clarification of issues.

▶ *Rapport.* A climate of rapport is established by the therapist communicating honestly and with a genuine interest in working with the client on specific problems. Rapport indicates that the client feels an emotional congruence with the therapist, believing that the therapist is attempting to see the world from the client's perspective.

▶ *Freedom from interruption.* The initial interview should take place in a private area or office away from the interruptions of other clients, the telephone, or hospital staff. This condition is extremely important in demonstrating to the client that he or she is respected and important to the occupational therapist. It also demonstrates that the client is treated in an individual manner and that his or her problems warrant individual consideration and attention.

▶ *Psychologic privacy.* The occupational therapist establishes a climate of confidentiality and trust with the client, which implies that information is of a professional nature. Notes that are taken during an interview, manually or through a tape recorder are discussed openly with the client. The purposes of the notes, how they will be used, and who they will be shared with also are made clear to the client during the interview. Occasionally, information divulged in the interview must be disclosed for legal reasons (Corey, 1996). For example, when the client is a danger to himself or herself or others, when abuse is suspected, or when the information is made an issue in a court case, the information must be shared. Likewise, when the client requests that the information be sent to a third party, the therapist must release the records.

▶ *Emotional objectivity.* In psychodynamic terms, the occupational therapist must be aware of any prejudicial attitudes or subjective reactions on the part of the therapist that may develop during the interview. Professional objectivity implies a realistic relationship with the client. A working relationship is established with the client when the therapist shows warmth, empathy, and objectivity. If the therapist develops unrealistic feelings toward the client, such as sexual attraction, hostility, fear, or boredom, then the therapist should examine these feelings with a supervisor so that these feelings do not interfere with the therapeutic relationship or cause acting out by either party (Corey, 1996; Ivey, 1994). Ideally, the therapist teaches the client to be objective about his or her problems.

Guidelines for interviewing are listed in Table 5–2.

Assessment

One of the main purposes of the initial interview is to establish the basis of a working relationship with the client. Assessment of the client's psychological symptoms, personality, and interpersonal problems provide the baseline data for formulating short- and long-term treatment goals. One of the first steps in assessment is the establishment of a diagnosis by the psychiatrist or psychologist. The *Diagnostic and Statistical Manual—IV* (DSM–IV; APA, 1994) is universally accepted by mental health professionals as the standard instrument for generating a diagnosis.

In the initial interview with the client, the psychiatrist usually obtains a mental status examination, which includes observation of the client's appearance and behavior, language and thought disturbances, perceptual distortions, fantasies, intellectual deficits, memory and orientation impairments, and insight into his or her problems (Leon, 1989). Two types of questions are asked during this interview: (a) diagnostic questions, which examine the nature of the complaints or symptoms in order to differentially diagnose the condition or identify other family members who may have had the same condition; and (b) descriptive questions, which involve the behavioral characteristic and mani-

Table 5–2. Basic Concepts in Interviewing

1. Establish a therapeutic alliance with the client by stating that "we are working on your problem together" instead of "I am the authority and you must listen to my words of wisdom."

2. Learn to listen to what the client is saying verbally and nonverbally.

3. Start out with a Rogerian model of nondirective counseling. Be supportive but do not accept the client's self-deprecation or expressions of self-abuse.

4. Assume that the client has the ability to understand what the problem is.

5. Suggest alternatives to self-defeating behaviors to help the client.

6. Establish realistic goals together with the client.

7. Help the client to develop and mature by constantly pointing out the client's assets and improvements.

8. Positive change in a client's behavior is through trial and error. Help the client to explore behavior without being judgmental.

9. Establish the purpose of the interview:

   • information gathering such as learning about the background during the initial interview

   • therapeutic counseling (e.g., discussing client's interpersonal behaviors)

   • periodic evaluation and feedback to client

   • screening for service such as for supportive employment

10. Determine the factors to consider in order to structure the interview as a positive experience for the client.

festations of the condition (Lezak, 1995). The latter category of questions allows for a functional assessment and development of therapeutic goals. From the mental status examination, the mental health professional formulates a tentative psychiatric diagnosis in the form of a short descriptive summary of the client's presenting symptoms and problems.

UTILIZATION OF THE COTA IN PSYCHOSOCIAL PRACTICE

As the history of the Certified Occupational Therapy Assistant (COTA) suggests, chronic long-term care in psychiatry was one of the first areas of employment. Currently, most COTAs work in gerontology, pediatrics, skilled nursing facilities, and psychiatric hospitals. COTA program graduates are filling many expanded career opportunities in traditional and nontraditional roles. These include

▶ activity staff in a residential treatment program for individuals with developmental disabilities

▶ house parent in a residental care facility

▶ teacher's aide in a residential treatment center for adolescents and children with emotional disturbance

▶ administrative assistant in adult day care centers for Alzheimer's disease utilizing RNs, OTRs, and social workers as consultants

▶ co-owner of private practice company with other OTRs

▶ respite care worker for community-based rehabilitation programs

▶ director of activity program and supervisor of volunteers in a skilled nursing facility

▶ community living trainer in a day care program for clients with developmental disabilities

▶ director of activity program in a private psychiatric hospital

▶ activity director in adult community centers

▶ organizational consultant doing staff development training

Specifically, COTAs are involved in a variety of treatment techniques dependent on the ability to be responsive to the client's needs, to have keen observational skills, to be able to set limits on client behavior, and to be a problem solver. They participate in specific treatment techniques such as

▶ participating in a group therapy activity

▶ presenting relaxation or stress management techniques in a group or on an individual basis

▶ directing, teaching, and participating in reality orientation techniques

▶ participating in psychodynamic groups to help clients express feelings

▶ applying group techniques of remotivation or reminiscing to increase relaxation and sociability

▶ leading a variety of sensory motor exercise activity groups

▶ developing and leading a variety of self-image, sexuality, and human potential groups

▶ directing and codirecting multimedia and recreational activities

A COTA should consider the following guidelines when implementing psychosocial treatment using activities:

▶ obtaining initial information about the client through medical records, observa-

tion, and by test data interpreted by the OTR

▶ continually assessing client behavior, problem-solving, interpersonal skills, stress-management, self-regulation of symptoms

▶ conversing with the client regarding skill level, feelings and attitudes toward specific activities, and interests

▶ collaborating with the client and other professionals on the treatment team to establish an activity program

▶ reporting information about the client's behavior, attitudes, and skill level to the supervisor during treatment sessions

▶ planning creative or self-expressive activities to meet the client's needs in collaboration with the client and OTR supervisor

▶ instructing and demonstrating activities (e.g., structured, unstructured, creative, arts and crafts, active, sedentary, individual, social)

▶ aiding client in developing social and interpersonal skills by encouraging interaction among the group

▶ implementing task-oriented groups (e.g., arts and crafts, play and leisure, games, gardening, cooking a meal, preparing a newsletter)

▶ aiding clients in modifying behavior by providing immediate feedback during the therapy session (e.g., encouraging appropriate behavior; ignoring, confronting, or discussing inappropriate behavior; setting limits; discussing feelings; and modeling or direct teaching alternative behaviors)

▶ helping clients to plan recreational activities that are appropriate and meaningful for them (e.g., attending a concert, reading, going on a field trip, having a picnic)

▶ encouraging clients to use community resources and family contacts (e.g., family visits, community service groups, clubs, libraries, volunteering, familiarity with local services)

▶ giving opportunities for practicing skills (e.g., grooming, cooking, applying for jobs, communicating with others, using public transportation, decision-making)

▶ collaborating with the treatment team on recommendations for discharge and follow-up in the community

▶ collaboration with OTRs in assistive technology programs

▶ assisting in wellness and prevention programs

The professional education of COTAs has progressed to a level that enables these practitioners to assume a variety of professional roles in a diversity of practice settings. Opportunities for career advancement and professional development have become increasingly available to COTAs as supervisors and administrators recognize the contributions COTA can make in today's changing health care system. (Cottrell, 2000, p. 411)

The primary objective of the COTA in a psychosocial program is to guide the behavior of a client so that the specific treatment goals are achieved. The COTA is an important part of the treatment program as supervised by the OTR.

DIAGNOSTIC AND STATISTICAL MANUAL (DSM-IV)

Classification systems for psychiatric disorders have undergone many evolutions since first proposed by the Persian physician Rhazes (864–925 A.D.) (Frances, First, & Pincus, 1995). The first edition of the DSM was published by the American Psychiatric Association (APA) in 1952 (DSM–I; APA, 1952). A second edition was published in 1968 (DSM–II; APA, 1968), and a third

edition came out in 1980 (DSM–III; APA, 1980), with a revision of the third edition in 1987 (DSM–III–R; APA 1987). The following goals for applying the DSM–III were listed by the task force members in 1980 and restated in 1983 as the work of the DSM–III–R was begun:

1. clinical usefulness for making treatment and management decisions in varied clinical settings;
2. reliability of the diagnostic categories;
3. acceptability to clinicians and researchers of varying theoretical orientations;
4. usefulness for educating health professionals;
5. maintenance of compatibility with the International Classification of Diseases (ICD–9 CM) published by the World Health Organization;
6. avoidance of new terminology and concepts that break with tradition, except when clearly needed;
7. attempting to reach consensus on the meaning of necessary diagnostic terms that have been used inconsistently, and avoidance of terms that have outlived their usefulness;
8. consistency with data from research studies bearing on the validity of diagnostic categories;
9. suitability for describing subjects in research studies;
10. responsiveness, during the development of the DSM–III–R, to critiques by clinicians and researchers. (APA, 1987, p. xx)

The present classification system, contained in the *Diagnostic and Statistical Manual of Mental Disorders–IV* (DSM–IV; APA, 1994), is widely used by psychiatrists, psychologists, mental health professionals, including occupational therapists. The current revision was worked on by a task force of psychiatrists and psychologists working in 13 subgroups that focused on specific diagnostic categories of mental disorders. These subgroups examined comprehensive literature reviews and client research studies of each disorder. The major purposes of the DSM–IV (APA, 1994) are (a) to provide definitions and descriptions of mental disorders so that clinicians and investigators can do a differential diagnosis, (b) communicate with each other, (c) study the etiology of disorders, and (d) devise treatment programs.

Definition of a Mental Disorder

In the DSM–IV (APA, 1994) a specific mental disorder is conceptualized as a

clinically significant behavioral or psychological syndrome or pattern that occurs in an individual and that is associated with present distress (e.g., a painful symptom) or disability (i.e., impairment in one or more important areas of function) or with a significantly increased risk of suffering death, pain, disability, or an important loss of freedom. In addition, this syndrome or pattern must not be merely an expectable and culturally sanctioned response to a particular event, for example, the death of a loved one. Whatever its original cause, it must currently be considered a manifestation of a behavioral, psychological, or biological dysfunction in the individual. Neither deviant behavior (e.g., political, religious, or sexual) nor conflicts that are primarily between the individual and society are mental disorders, unless the deviance or conflict is a symptom of a dysfunction in the individual as described above. (p. xxi)

The members of the task force for the DSM–IV were cognizant of the difficulty and arbitrariness of defining what a mental disorder is. They acknowledged that there should be no distinction between a mental and physical disorder because both mental and physical disorders are intrinsically linked together and influence each other.

In diagnosing an individual with a mental disorder, the clinician identifies symptoms through interviewing and observing the individual and by collaborative information obtained from relatives and others. The clinician determines how long the individual has had the symptoms and the stressors, if any, that precipitated the episode of mental illness. The clinician also gauges the severity of symptoms, which may range from mild to moderate to severe. For example, the clinician would focus on the areas of behavior in identifying symptoms as shown in Table 5–3. A diagnosis of mental disorder is based on the presence of symptoms in the individual, how long the symptoms have been present, and the identification of any stressors that may have precipitated these symptoms.

Assumptions in DSM–IV

The following nine assumptions are abstracted from DSM–IV:

▶ Mental disorders are categorical based on cardinal symptoms that are observable in the clients. Diagnosis is established from a priori criteria confirmed by clinical experts.

▶ Even though individuals share a diagnostic category, they may display different characteristics. For example, individuals with paranoid schizophrenia present different delusions and various symptoms with the same diagnosis.

▶ There are no completely discrete categories of diagnosis, only probable decisions. For example, in categorizing Borderline Personality Disorder, an individual is diagnosed when five out of nine symptoms are present.

▶ The validity and accuracy of the use of the DSM–IV in arriving at a diagnostic deci-

Table 5–3. Specific Symptoms Related to Major Areas of Behavior

Major Areas of Behavior	Examples of Symptoms
intelligence	• difficulty in problem solving
attention	• inattentive
conduct	• aggressive
emotion	• anxiety
interpersonal relations	• difficulty interacting with others (schizoid behavior)
language	• incoherent verbalizations
memory	• problems with storing and retrieving information
eating	• anorexia
sleeping	• insomnia
toilet habits	• incontinence
menstrual cycle	• dysmenorrhea
thinking	• paranoid delusions
perception	• hallucinations
sexual adjustment	• transvestism

sion is based on the clinical judgment and expertise of the mental health professional. The DSM–IV is a clinical tool that can lead to misdiagnosis by untrained or inexperienced clinicians.

▶ A specific diagnosis does not imply a level of functioning or disability. For example, individuals with the same mental disorders can have a mild, moderate, or severe disability depending on the individual's ability to function in work, self-care, and leisure activities and social interactions.

▶ The diagnosis of a mental disorder does not necessarily give insight into the cause of the disorder. For example, individuals diagnosed with depression have divergent etiologies.

▶ The information in the DSM–IV represents the best thinking at the time of publication. There is no assumption that knowledge of mental disorders is fixed and unchanging. As more research comes forth, the knowledge base will change our understanding of mental disorders. New knowledge may lead to the identification of new disorders or removal of old disorders.

▶ Cultural factors should be considered in determining whether a religious practice or belief is a symptom or an accepted behavior. For example, an individual who believes in UFOs may or may not be mentally ill, depending on whether the belief interferes with an individual's ability to function.

▶ The clinician evaluates the severity of the illness by using the following terms: mild, moderate, and severe (many symptoms result in a marked impairment in social or occupational functions). Partial and full remission are used, and prior history means a past history of a disorder from which an individual fully recovered.

Classifications of Mental Disorders

Mental disorders defined by the DSM–IV are grouped into 16 major classifications, with an additional section labeled "Other Conditions Which May Be a Focus of Attention." An example of other conditions includes stress-related physical illnesses. Descriptions of each disorder are organized into subsections, such as subtypes, diagnostic criteria, probable causes of illness, laboratory findings, and associated medical conditions. In addition, specific information about culture, age and gender differences; prevalence; familial pattern; and differential diagnosis are included for each disorder.

Frances et al. (1995) state the following cautions when using the DSM–IV:

> However, it should always be remembered that assigning a DSM–IV diagnosis represents just one step in the ongoing care of an individual. Although DSM–IV diagnosis conveys pertinent information, other factors (e.g., an individual's personal and family history, previous treatment responses, psychological factors and coping styles, and the influence of the psychosocial environment) are also crucial to treatment planning and must be addressed during the evaluation process. Finally, it is essential to recognize that individuals whose symptoms meet the criteria for a particular diagnosis are not alike in every way; important differences often exist among individuals with the same diagnosis. (p. 24)

Coding of Diagnoses

Coding of diagnoses in the DSM–IV are based on a multiaxial dimension. There are five dimensions, or axes, each of which provides information about a different domain. This allows clinicians to provide information outside of the immediate diagnostic assessment and emphasize the "important role of psychosocial factors in the onset, exacerbation, and manage-

ment of psychiatric disorders" (Frances et al., 1995, p. 70).

The first three axes are diagnostic; the last two are nondiagnostic (Table 5–4). Mental disorders are classified on Axis I and II. Axis I is used to code all the clinical syndromes (see Appendix I: Axis I diagnoses), while personality disorders and mental retardation are coded on Axis II (see Appendix I: Axis II diagnoses). A clinical syndrome is a grouping of symptoms that comprise a diagnostic label, while a personality disorder implies a consistent pattern of behavior that interferes with adjustment in everyday personal interactions. Axis III is used to provide information about clinically relevant general medical or physical conditions secondary to the primary diagnosis, but which have an impact on the individual's adjustment and prognosis. For example, the medical condition may be a physiological cause (e.g., depression occurring as a direct consequence of a stroke) or the precipitating factor (e.g., personality disorder occurring after an amputation). On the other hand, it may be only incidentally involved (e.g., acne in a teenager) or not related at all (e.g., arthritic condition along with a diagnosis of obsessive-compulsive disorder). Axis IV designates psychosocial and environmental problem areas, such as stressors, which affect the individual functioning (see Appendix I: Axis IV). Axis V rates the overall psychological, social, and occupational functioning of the individual, such as superior, good, or poor adjustment to current circumstances (see Appendix I: Axis V). Axes IV and V are important for the clinician in planning treatment programs and predicting outcome of the disorder.

Diagnoses are coded using the categories under Axis I (Clinical Syndromes) and Axis II (Personality Disorders). The numeric codes are based on five digits. The first four digits (Axis I) indicate the diagnostic category, such as cata-

Table 5–4. Multiaxial System Used in the DSM-IV Classification System

Axis	Diagnoses	Description
AXIS I	• Clinical disorders • Other conditions that may be a focus of clinical attention	• All classified mental disorders except those on Axis II • Factors related to the clinical disorder
AXIS II	• Mental retardation • Personality disorders	• Disorders that begin in childhood and persist throughout the lifespan
AXIS III	• General medical conditions	• ICD–9 codes related to the mental disorder
AXIS IV	• Psychosocial and environmental problems	• Life stressors that impact upon the mental disorder
AXIS V	• Global assessment of functioning	• General level of psychosocial and occupational functioning for the past year

Note : From the *Diagnostic and Statistical Manual–IV* (DSM-IV), American Psychiatric Association, 1994.

tonic schizophrenic disorder (295.2x). The fifth digit after the period indicates the state of chronicity. For example, the "4" in 295.24 stands for chronic, with acute exacerbation in a patient who has catatonic schizophrenia. In Axis II (Personality Disorder), for example, code number 301.70 indicates an antisocial personality disorder. It is possible for an individual to have two diagnostic codes on Axis I and Axis II. For example, an individual can be diagnosed 295.32 schizophrenia, paranoid, chronic, on Axis I and 301.20 schizoid personality disorder (premorbid) on Axis II. When there is "insufficient information to know whether or not a presenting problem is attributable to a mental disorder" (DSM–IV; APA, 1994, p. 4), then a V code is given. Additionally, when diagnoses are deferred, either Axis I or II is coded 799.9.

Reliability and Validity of the DSM–III

To objectively evaluate the interrater reliability of the DSM–III, 384 clinicians evaluated a total of 796 adults and children. Two clinicians evaluated the same individual by examining written case records and speaking to family informants. Reliability was tested using a statistical test based on coefficient of agreement. A high reliability was considered to be .70 or above. Reliability was high in the categories of Schizophrenia (.81) and Major Affective Disorders (.80). Reliability was lower with Personality Disorders (.65). The field trials for establishing interrater reliability clearly indicated that there is still much error and arbitrariness in diagnosing a mental disorder.

Is the DSM–IV a valid tool for evaluating a mental disorder? In other words, does the DSM–IV identify a mental disorder correctly and differentiate normal from abnormal behavior? In the DSM–IV there was a constructive attempt to operationally define mental disorders. The authors of the DSM–IV also emphasized that a mental disorder is not a distinct entity that is easily diagnosed. It is implied that the distance from abnormality to normality is on a continuum rather than as discrete independent categories. In analyzing the validity of the DSM–IV, the major variable is still the expertise and experience of the psychiatric clinician. The DSM–IV per se cannot be evaluated without considering the variable of clinician judgment and experience. Schact and Nathan (1977) in appraising a preliminary version of the DSM–III stated that, "The resulting document, then may be likened to a symphony written by a committee—the notes are all there, but the way they are put together reflect the mediocrity inherent in such a process rather than integrated purposes and understanding" (p. 1017).

How can the occupational therapist use the DSM–IV? Basically, the DSM–IV is a tool used by psychiatrists that attempts to standardize the language, definitions, and concepts related to mental disorders. It seems apparent that the psychosocial occupational therapist should understand the system purely from the point of view of relating to the other mental health team members. In addition, Axes IV and V are particularly relevant to the occupational therapist and relate directly to the functional outcome and patient adjustment to environmental stressors. In evaluating the problem areas that lead to difficulty in psychosocial functioning, social relations, self-care, work, and use of leisure time, the occupational therapist can be an essential person and contribute to the overall psychiatric assessment.

CASE STUDY ANALYSIS

The diagnostic study gives a general indication of the client's present problems and symptoms. In understanding the psychodynamics of the client's illnesses, a case study analysis is undertaken by the mental health team. In this case study analysis, the team explores with the client factors in his or her life that predisposed him or her to mental illness and the possible factors or stressors that precipitated illness. (See Figure 10–1 where the diathesis-stress hypothesis is depicted.) A comprehensive history of the client's development and personal history taken from the medical records and interviews with the client and possibly family members serves as the bases for understanding the onset of the ill-

ness. A general outline of a comprehensive case study analysis is described below as a guide for an in-depth study of the client.

Outline of Comprehensive Case Study Analysis

1. *Demographic data:* What is the client's age, gender, marital status, and educational level attained?

2. *Physical characteristics:* What is the client's height and weight, hand dominance, and general appearance?

3. *Health status:* Does the individual have any illnesses, chronic disability or conditions, such as asthma, arthritis, or back pain? Is the individual taking any medications or treatment for any illnesses?

4. *Diet and nutrition:* What are the individual's diet and nutrition patterns, for example, typical meals, foods preferred, and calories consumed? Does the individual engage in binge eating or sporadic eating schedules?

5. *Exercise:* What types of exercises does the individual enjoy, for example, walking, jogging, biking, or swimming? Does the individual exercise daily?

6. *Relaxation:* How does the individual relax? Does the individual use coping activities, such as progressive relaxation, yoga, or meditation daily?

7. *Housing:* What type of housing does the individual live in, such as house, apartment, furnished room, or hotel? Does the individual find this housing adequate?

8. *Family and friends:* How does the individual relate to family members? Does the individual have close friends?

9. *Developmental history:* Were there any significant problems during childhood and

adolescence that affected the illness? Was the individual sexually or physically abused during childhood? What were the prenatal, perinatal, and postnatal development, eating and sleeping patterns, traumatic events during childhood and adolescence, reactions to illnesses, and other significant events affecting behavior?

10. *Academics:* What was the client's level of academic achievement, such as below average, average, or above average? Did the individual have courses or academic subjects he or she enjoyed? Are there any test scores or grades available?

11. *Predisposing factors:* What are the presumed predisposing factors, such as genetics, neurological, or developmental factors that made the individual vulnerable to mental illness? Do other members of the immediate family or close relatives have a history of mental illness?

12. *Precipitating factor:* Were there stressors that triggered an episode of symptoms? Can the individual verbalize factors that led to the exacerbation of the illness?

13. *DSM–IV diagnosis:* What are the primary and secondary diagnoses using DSM–IV axes?

14. *History of psychiatric illness:* At what age was the first episode of mental illness experienced? When did the family, teachers, or educational specialist notice that there might have been some emotional or behavioral difficulties? What is the history of exacerbations and remissions?

15. *Psychiatric treatments:* What treatments were applied in the past, such as psychotherapy, chemotherapy, electroconvulsive treatment (ECT), occupational therapy? What was the effectiveness of each type of treatment?

16. *Evaluation and test findings:* What are the findings from neurological and psychological tests, such as Wechsler intelligence tests (WAIS–III, WISC–III, WPSSI–R), *Minnesota Multiphasic Personality Inventory* (MMPI), magnetic resonance imagery (MRI), electroencephalograph (EEG), electromyograph (EMG)?

17. *Occupational history:* What is the employment history? Which jobs were most fulfilling and which jobs were disliked? What are the work or career aspirations?

18. *Leisure activities:* What are the interests and hobbies of the individual? For example, does the individual engage in participatory or spectator sports, reading, television or movies, arts or crafts, gardening, religious activities, or care of pets?

19. *Self-care:* How independent is the individual in self-care activities, such as transportation, communication, grooming, preparing meals, cleaning one's apartment, and laundering?

The next section includes the major landmarks in human development and their relationship to psychiatric illnesses.

MAJOR STAGES OF LIFE AFFECTING PSYCHOLOGICAL DEVELOPMENT

In the following paragraphs, the developmental tasks in major stages of life (infancy/childhood, adolescence, adulthood) are outlined and discussed. Table 5–5 outlines the major psychiatric disorders noted in each of the stages. As a means of orienting the reader to pertinent issues of each stage, a number of questions about the developmental stages are presented. The reader or therapist may think of additional questions to consider, especially as he or she is working with a specific client.

Table 5–5. Major Psychiatric Disorders

Childhood	*Adolescence*	*Adult*	*Elderly*
• Attention Deficit Hyperactivity Disorder (ADHD)	• Attention Deficit Hyperactivity Disorder (ADHD)	• Affective (mood) disorders	• Affective (mood) disorders
• Autism	• Conduct disorder	• Anxiety or phobias	• Dementia and Alzheimer's disease
• Childhood depression	• Depression	• Personality disorders	
• Conduct disorder	• Eating disorders	• Schizophrenia and psychosis	
• Learning disabilities	• Schizophrenia	• Substance abuse	
• Mental retardation	• Substance abuse		

Source: Names of disorders taken from the *Diagnostic and Statistical Manual-IV,* American Psychiatric Association, 1994.

Prenatal and Perinatal Development

▶ Was the pregnancy accepted by both parents?

▶ What was the physical and psychological health of the mother during pregnancy?

▶ Was the delivery normal?

▶ What was the infant's weight at birth?

▶ Were there any abnormalities in the infant at birth?

Infancy (0–2 years)

▶ What were the patterns in the development of gross and fine motor skills, speech and language, and toileting skills?

▶ How did the child interact and bond with parents or surrogate family?

▶ What were the child's pattern in sleeping?

▶ What was the child's play behavior and favorite toys?

▶ Did the child have any major illnesses or accidents?

▶ Did the child have any problems in eating?

In addition to the above, Erikson (1963) identified infancy as important for developing *trust* in others as when the child establishes a consistent relationship and secure attachment with the mother or surrogate parent. During the second year, Erikson identified *autonomy* as an important developmental task. The child begins to experience his or her own identity and separation from the mother. The emergence of autonomy relates to the child's independence in performing activities of daily living such as toileting, grooming, feeding, and playing through trial and error.

Childhood (3–11 years)

▶ How did the child relate to peers in establishing and maintaining friendships?

▶ How did the child adjust to nursery school, kindergarten, and elementary school?

▶ Were there difficulties in academic or cognitive learning?

▶ How did the child develop physically as far as height, weight, and gross motor skills?

▶ Was speech and language development normal for age?

▶ Did the child have any major illnesses or accidents?

▶ What were the child's favorite play activities, sports, games, and toys?

▶ Were there problems in eating and sleeping?

During this period Erikson (1963) emphasizes the importance of the child's development of *initiative*. The child begins to actively explore the environment and to show a sense of assertiveness in selecting activities and playmates. The child also begins to select what he or she enjoys doing and to decide what to avoid in his or her daily life. Later in this period (8–11 years old), the child begins to develop a sense of *industry* and competence in sports, academic subjects, play activities, games, and other life tasks.

Significant Emotional and Mental Disorders Identified During Infancy and Childhood

Mental retardation due to genetic, organic, and social factors, is diagnosed during the developmental period, which is birth to age 18 (AAMR, 1992). Mental retardation is defined by subaverage adaptive behavior in two or more areas (e.g., communication, leisure, functional academics) and intellectual functioning at least two standard deviations below the mean. Adaptive behavior and intellectual functioning are measured through the use of standardized tests (e.g., AAMR Adaptive Behavior Scales–Second Edition and the Wechsler scales, respectively).

Attention deficit hyperactivity disorder (with and without hyperactivity) (ADHD; DSM–IV,

APA, 1994) is characterized by difficulty in attending to essential sensory information; concentrating on boring, repetitive tasks; disinhibiting impulsive behavior; and using self-regulatory skills (Barkley, 1990). Some individuals also demonstrate a high level of motor activity. The preschool or primary classroom teacher is often the first person to identify children with this disorder, because academic tasks are frequently the first place where concentration is required. The role of the occupational therapist includes helping these children become less impulsive and improving self-regulatory behavior through sensory integrative therapy and behavior management. Social, emotional, and vocational issues are also addressed by the occupational therapist.

Learning disabilities are conditions not usually considered to be psychiatric. Major characteristics of these disorders include an average or above average intelligence level, with a discrepancy between the learner's academic achievement and intelligence. Academic difficulties are seen in reading, math, or written language, as a result of deficits in auditory processing, language or communication, and visual-perception. Children with learning disabilities may also have difficulties with social relationships, psychosocial areas, and fine or gross motor skills. Pediatric occupational therapists often work with speech-language therapists to improve skills in conversation, personal space issues, and nonverbal behaviors important in social interactions.

The therapist's role in an intervention program for the child with LD may change as the child develops, and it depends on the nature and extent of each child's specific disability. With young children, sensory integration, play, and basic socialization and self-help skills may be addressed through early intervention and parent education. As the child progresses into school, sensory integration may continue but additional intervention to promote social play, perceptual motor integration, and writing skills is indicated. By early adolescence the focus of evaluation and treatment may shift to independent living skills, development of compensatory and adaptive techniques, and development of vocational skills, interests, and habits. (Gorden, Schanzenbacher, Case–Smith, & Carrasco, 1996, p. 144)

Autism is a severe disorder of interpersonal relationships, caused by neurological dysfunction, that is usually diagnosed by a pediatric psychiatrist before the child is 3 years old. It is not known how many children in the United States have autism spectrum disorders. Studies done in Europe and Asia since 1985 indicate that there may be as many as 2/1,000 children who have one of the autism spectrum disorders (Center for Disease Control, Division of Birth Defects, Child Development, and Disabilities and Health. Developmental Disabilities Branch, 2001, p. 1). It affects approximately 400,000 persons in the United States (Autism Society of America [ASA], 1996). The specific dysfunctions seen in autism are:

Communication: language develops slowly or not at all; use of words without attaching the usual meaning to them; communicates with gestures instead of words; short attention spans

Social Interaction: spends time alone rather than with others; shows little interest in making friends; less responsive to social cues such as eye contact or smiles

Sensory Impairment: unusual reactions to physical sensations such as being overly sensitive to touch or under-responsive to pain, sight, hearing, touch, pain, smell, taste may be affected to a lesser or greater degree

Play: lack of spontaneous or imaginative play; does not imitate others' actions; doesn't initiate pretend games

Behaviors: may be overactive or very passive; throw frequent tantrums for no apparent reason; may perseverate on a single item, idea or person; apparent lack of common sense; may show aggressive or violent behavior or injure self. (ASA, 1996, p. 3)

The role of the occupational therapist includes teaching social skills, vocational preparation, leisure skills, among others. Huebner (1992), in a review article on autism, summarized the associated disorders and functional and neurological disorders. In her discussion, she suggested a collaborative, multimodal treatment approach when working with individuals with autism. This belief is corroborated by the Autism Society of America (1996):

Because of the spectrum nature of autism and the many behavior combinations which can occur, no one approach is effective in alleviating symptoms of autism in all cases. Various types of therapies are available, including behavior modification, speech/language therapy, sensory integration, vision therapy, music therapy, auditory training, medications and dietary interventions, among others.

Experience has shown that individuals with autism respond well to a highly structured, specialized education and behavior modification program, tailored to the individual needs of the person. A well designed intervention approach will include some level of communication therapy, social skill development, sensory impairment therapy and behavior modification at a minimum, delivered by autism trained professionals in a consistent, comprehensive and coordinated manner. The more severe challenges of some children with autism may be best addressed by a structured education and behavior program which contains a 1:1 teacher to student ratio or small group environment.

Students with autism should have training in vocational skills and community living skills at the earliest possible age. Learning to cross a street safely, to make a simple purchase or to ask assistance when needed are critical skills, and may be difficult, even for those with average intelligence levels. Tasks that enhance the person's independence, give more opportunity for personal choice or allow more freedom in the community are important.

To be effective, any approach should be flexible in nature, rely on positive reinforcement, be re-evaluated on a regular basis and provide a smooth transition from home to school to community environments. A good program will also incorporate training and support systems for the caregivers as well. Rarely can a family, classroom teacher or other caregiver provide effective habilitation for a person with autism unless offered consultation or in-service training by a specialist knowledgeable about the disability.

A generation ago, 90% of the people with autism were eventually placed in institutions. Today, as a result of appropriate and individualized services and programs, even the more severely disabled can be taught skills to allow them to develop to their fullest potential. (ASA, pp. 4–5)

Personality and conduct disorders are characterized by inflexible and maladaptive traits in children that cause significant problems in social, family, and school settings. "The child exhibits repetitive and persistent patterns of behavior that violate social expectations" (Cronin, 1996, p. 399). Common problems that result from personality disorders include overly aggressive and hostile behavior toward peers, withdrawal from activities, overdependence on parents, and antisocial behavior such as truancy, drug abuse, running away from home, sexual acting out, lying, vandalism, shoplifting, and fire-setting (Kauffman, 1997).

Personality and conduct disorders in childhood often lead to difficulties during adolescence and young adulthood. There is a strong relationship between family disorganization in childhood and acting-out behavior during adolescence. The child who is acting-out and who comes from a socially disadvantaged family could further develop feelings of hopelessness and alienation leading to adult crime.

Childhood depression, more common than was previously considered (Birmaher, Ryan, Williamson, Brent, & Kaufman, 1996), is often manifested by behaviors similar to those seen in children with hyperactivity. Thus, the child who is depressed may appear to have difficulty focusing on a task or may be motorically hyperactive. Other behavioral manifestations include irritable or depressed mood for at least part of the day, apathetic attitude toward various activities, weight loss, or difficulty eating or sleeping almost daily.

Anxiety and phobic disorders (DSM–IV) are atypical behaviors in children arising from unwarranted fears. Fears can be associated with animals, being alone, dying, plane travel, and other specific events or objects in the child's environment. The anticipation of encountering an anxiety-provoking situation often precipitates physiological reaction such as sweating, dizziness, headaches, nausea, and other autonomic nervous system responses.

Related Disorders and Symptoms of Childhood Disorders

Mental disorders in children can also be related to a specific problem in daily living or behavior such as eating (anorexia), sleeping (night disturbance), grooming, toilet control (incontinence), underachievement, language and speech disturbances (stuttering), and involuntary movements (tics). The disorders or problems may be related or associated with other major diagnoses. It is important for the occupational therapist to note the presence of any major symptoms or behavior that interfere with the child's adjustment and/or ability to make use of his or her potential (Sholle–Martin & Alessi, 1990).

Adolescence (12–20 years)

▶ Were friendships established with peers?

▶ How did the adolescent girl adjust to menstruation?

▶ How did the adolescent adjust to the emergence of sexual feelings?

▶ How did the adolescent relate to parents or parent surrogate figures?

▶ How did the adolescent achieve in school?

▶ Did the adolescent have special talents in music, art, dance, drama, writing, or other creative areas?

▶ What activities did the adolescent participate in, such as sports, computer clubs, social and political groups, nature and ecology organizations?

▶ What part-time or full-time jobs did the adolescent have during school and summer vacations?

▶ Did the adolescent have a career goal in mind during the academic years?

▶ Who were the adolescent's ego ideals in the popular media or sports, music, film, or theater?

▶ What were the adolescent's major problems in experiencing feelings, social adjustment, and self-identity?

▶ Did the adolescent act out through drug abuse, delinquency, sex, truancy, or running away from family?

According to Erikson (1963), the major task of adolescents is to establish a *sense of identity*. The adolescent begins to have insight into his or her own likes and dislikes and begins to make decisions regarding career choices, friendships, leisure time activities, and other outlets for emotional, social, and sexual expression. It is the transition period from childhood to adulthood.

Significant Mental Disorders During Adolescence

Adolescence is the most turbulent period in human development and it is the most vulnerable period for the onset of mental disorders. The most severe disorder precipitated during adolescence is schizophrenia. For the psychosocial occupational therapist working in a community mental health center or day treatment facility, the majority of the clients will have a diagnosis of affective disorders, substance abuse, conduct disorders, attention deficit hyperactivity disorder (ADHD), and schizophrenia (see Table 5–5). Many of these disorders initially occur during adolescence (DeLisi, 1992; Kaplan, Sadock, & Grebb, 1994; McGlashan, 1988). Occupational therapy intervention may enable the individual to have a more positive outcome (Henry & Coster, 1996).

Schizophrenic Disorders

Definition. Schizophrenia is a severe neurological disorder that interferes with psychosocial, cognitive, and perceptual processing. Many individuals with schizophrenia can benefit from a comprehensive psychosocial rehabilitation program that includes medication, social skills training, supportive employment, supportive housing, group counseling, and a support group. The following behaviors are characteristic of schizophrenia:

▶ passive withdrawal from involvement with the everyday tasks of life

▶ perceptual distortion of reality that is typified by the presence of hallucinations (misperceptions of sensory data) and delusions (false belief systems)

▶ demonstrated cognitive problems and thinking disorders of judgment, decision-making, and reasoning

▶ inappropriate emotional responses

▶ severe anxiety

▶ psychomotor disturbances in the form of bizarre posturing and poorly integrated motor responses

Presumed Causes and Predisposing Factors. There are many theories to explain the onset of schizophrenia; however, there is no total agreement on the specific variables that underlie the disorder (Bellak, 1979; Lehmann, 1985). The major factors that have been implicated in the etiology of schizophrenia include

▶ *Genetics* (Bassett, 1991; Levison & Mowry, 1991): inheritance of personality traits such as schizoid behavior, extreme introversion, hypersensitivity to others, marked proneness to developing anxiety that may make one vulnerable to developing a schizophrenic disorder lifestyle.

▶ *Neurophysiological causes* (Davis, Kahn, Ko, & Davidson, 1991; van Kammen, 1991): Biochemical and neurophysiological abnormalities, such as excess dopamine causing hyperarousal of the autonomic nervous system. These abnormalities generate perceptual distortions of reality, emotional disorders, and psychomotor disturbances that lead to difficulties in adjusting to reality and society.

▶ *Interpersonal factors* (Falloon, Boyd, & McGill, 1984; Rund, Oie, Borchgrevink, & Fjell, 1995; Moenking, Hornung, Stricker, & Buchkremer, 1997) such as inadequate parenting or abuse that interfere with the individual's normal psychological development. The individual with schizophrenia may not develop the self-esteem and coping skills that are necessary in human relationships because he or she was not provided with a consistently supportive family environment, such as in families with high expressed emotion. High expressed emotion refers to parents or family members being overly critical and dissatisfied with the individual who has schizophrenia (Brown, Birley, & Wing, 1972).

Precipitating Factors. Early theorists (Bateson, Jackson, Haley, & Weakland, 1956; Bellak, 1979; Wynne, Rykoff, Day, & Hirsch, 1958) conceptualized that schizophrenic behavior developed during childhood and intensified in adolescence and young adulthood when the life decisions regarding career choices, marriage, and independent living become paramount. A schizophrenic crisis where the symptoms exacerbate is usually related to one of the life stressors, such as the death of a family member, academic or job failure, change in residence, extreme social rejection or isolation, and general disruption and/or disorganization in the family (Hultman, Wieselgren, & Ohman, 1997; Norman & Malla, 1993; Neuchterlein et al., 1992).

Diagnosis. An individual is diagnosed as schizophrenic based on the following data:

▶ Interview with a psychiatrist noting the presence of cardinal symptoms such as delusions, hallucination, inappropriate affect, deterioration of personal care, and a thinking disorder

▶ Psychological test results such as derived from the *Minnesota Multiphasic Personality Inventory* (MMPI) where the individual scores high on the Schizophrenia Clinical Scale

▶ Personal history derived from a social worker's contact with family members who describe the individual's life-patterns indicating lack of social interactions, inadequate coping with life tasks, and a general lifestyle of personal withdrawal and an inability to cope with stress

Subdiagnostic Groups. The American Psychiatric Association subdivides schizophrenia into five types (DSM–IV; APA, 1994).

▶ *Disorganized* type, formerly called hebephrenic, is probably the most regressed category of schizophrenia. It is characterized by inappropriate emotional responses, incoherence, extreme social withdrawal, and individual bizarre behavior.

▶ *Catatonic* type displays a psychomotor disturbance that ranges from immobilized rigidity to posturing to extreme motor excitement.

▶ *Paranoid* type is characterized by thinking disorders and distortions of reality. The individual may be normal in all other aspects of life in spite of having a specific delusional system.

▶ *Undifferentiated* type is similar to the former category of simple schizophrenia. The individual displays delusions, hallucinations, and disorganized behavior but does not have the prominent characteristics of any of the above specific types.

▶ *Residual* type is probably the mildest form of schizophrenia. The major symptoms include inappropriate affect, social withdrawal, eccentric behavior, illogical thinking, and a flight of ideas.

Another form of schizophrenia is *schizoaffective disorder*. This disorder is characterized by psychotic symptoms as in schizophrenia and major mood disorder. Treatment includes medication for the psychosis and the mood disorder and psychosocial rehabilitation.

Comprehensive Treatment Planning. At present the most common method of treatment for individuals with schizophrenia is chemotherapy, which includes tranquilizers, antidepressants, and anti-anxiety drugs (NIMH, 1999). Chemo-therapy is used to relieve the severe symptoms of schizophrenia so that the individual is more accessible to rehabilitation methods that have more lasting results (see Chapter 7 for description of psychotropic drugs) (Grace et al., 1996; Kane, 1995; Menditto et al., 1996). Rehabilitation methods include cognitive-behavioral therapy, group therapy, individual counseling, family therapy, special education, prevocational training, social skills training, and special job placements (Arns & Linney, 1995; Falloon, 1996; Liberman & Kopelowica, 1995; Penn & Mueser, 1996; Peuskens, 1996; Scott & Dixon, 1995). The environments that best facilitate rehabilitation include CMHCs, halfway houses, day treatment centers, and outpatient clinics (Eikelmann & Reker, 1996; Heitger & Saameli, 1995; Mahendran, Ibrahim, & Tan, 1995; Wing & Furlong, 1986).

General Treatment Objectives for Occupational Therapy. Schizophrenia, as a severe disorder in human living, touches on almost every aspect of behavior. Treatment objectives are usually organized under the following major categories; social skills, leisure activity, emotional expression, interpersonal and family relationships, self-care, nutrition, exercise, relaxation training, and vocational adjustment. It is important to note that these are general categories for setting up treatment objectives. In planning treatment the psychosocial occupational therapist works in clinics with the client and mental health team to devise an individualized treatment plan.

Other Disorders of Adolescence

Antisocial Personality Disorders. Antisocial personality disorders (APA, 1994) are an outgrowth of the Conduct Disorder, and are not diagnosed until an individual is age 18. The disorder represents behavior that is in continual conflict with the norms and values of a community. In adolescence, delinquency, alcohol and drug abuse, and violence are behavioral examples of conduct that may lead to a diagnosis of antisocial personality disorders. Without effective therapeutic intervention these individuals could become the institutionalized populations of our society, filling prisons, mental hospitals, alcohol and drug abuse centers, and detention centers.

Eating Disorders. Anorexia nervosa (APA, 1994) is an eating disorder that usually starts during adolescence in which the individual reduces the daily food intake drastically and literally chooses to starve. Bulimia (APA, 1994) is another eating disorder, which is manifested by binge eating and vomiting to prevent weight gain. Individuals with bulimia may fast for one or more days or exercise excessively to compensate for binge eating (APA, 1994). An individual can be both anorexic and bulimic. Females are most commonly affected (95 percent). The disorders are not due to organic causes. As symptoms of a mental disorder they are a result of a psychological adjustment problem. The psychodynamics underlying the disorders as well as the life-threatening symptoms of the self-induced starvation or binge eating become the focal points of therapy.

Young Adult (21–35 Years)

▶ What was the individual's history of occupational choices, jobs, and general vocational adjustment?

▶ Was the individual's separation from the parent family adequate?

▶ How did the individual adjust to sexual needs?

▶ Did the individual establish intimate relationships through friendships or marriage?

▶ What were the individual's leisure-time interests in sports, music, literature, art, and other related areas, either as a spectator or participant?

▶ What were the individual's commitments to community affairs and social interests?

▶ Did the individual experience any major physical illnesses or accidents?

▶ What were the specific stresses during the period, for example, death of a close relative, divorce, loss of job, failure in business, or unstable relationships?

According to Erikson (1963), this period is important in the establishment of *intimacy*. The young adult is at his or her prime of life in physical and intellectual activities. This is the time of life when the individual is putting forth his or her major efforts in life tasks.

Significant Mental Disorders During Young Adulthood

Mood Disorders. DSM–IV (APA, 1994) divides mood disorders into depressive disorders and bipolar disorders. Generally, women tend to be depressed more often than men, and thus have a higher incidence of depression. Bipolar disorders are equally distributed between men and women. It is estimated that one in four women is likely to experience a bout of depression during her lifetime. Of this number about 20 percent will seek professional treatment. Depression in humans is considered to be a normal reaction to loss.

Depression has existed throughout human history. In the 17th century, Robert Burton (1632/1938), an Oxford scholar and recluse, wrote his classical text *The Anatomy of Melancholy*. This work summarized the western world's view of the causes and treatment of depression. To quote Burton:

melancholy is either a disposition or habit. In disposition, it is that transitory melancholy which goes and comes on every small occasion of sorrow, need, sickness, trouble, fear, grief, passion or perturbations of the mind . . . And from these melancholy dispositions, no men (or women) living is free. (p. 125)

These remarkable insights of Burton still ring true 350 years later. Depression is a universal phenomena that is an integral characteristic of human thought and behavior.

Depression is still a significant problem in the 2000s. It is estimated that in any 6-month period over 9 million people in the United States will experience a bout of depression that will require clinical treatment. Clinical depression, as compared to a depressed mood, can last for weeks or months and includes the following symptoms: sleep disturbances, feelings of worthlessness, inability to concentrate, fatigue, eating disorders, indecisiveness, lack of sexual desire, and recurrent thoughts of suicide.

Recent Findings in the Dynamics of Depression. Current research findings (Gotthardt et al., 1995; Jacobs, 1994; Johnson, Monroe, Simons, & Thase, 1994; Lechin et al., 1995; Lechin, Van der Dijs, & Benaim, 1996) have reinforced the concept that depression is a biological reaction that causes symptoms that interfere with the everyday activities of life such as eating, sleeping, interpersonal relationships and the ability to work. A conceptual model for describing the relationship between the vulnerable individual to depression and the onset of symptoms is shown in Figure 5–2.

In this model an individual vulnerable to depression is defined as someone with genetic/environmental factors that predispose him or her to becoming depressed. Blehar, Weissman, Gershon, and Hirschfeld (1988) provide evidence of a genetic factor in unipolar depression.

Damaging environmental factors encountered during the developmental periods in a person's life such as poverty, physical and sexual abuse, parental neglect, and illness can predispose an individual to depression. The presence of a genetic factor to depression and negative environmental factors can lead to a high probability that depression will occur. This vulnerable individual will have a high probability of becoming depressed when stressful events, such as a loss in the family or interpersonal conflicts, occur. This interaction between predisposing factors in the individual and stressful events causes the initial symptoms of depression, such as anxiety, sad mood, guilt, physical complaints, and low self-esteem. If these symptoms are intense they can lead to disturbances in the sleep-activity cycle. The depressed individual's circadian rhythm of work, leisure activities, and sleep is disrupted. Depressed individuals have difficulty sleeping at night, feel fatigued during the day, and are unable to carry out the everyday activities of life. The loss of energy and the disruption in the sleep cycle interfere with the depressed individual's ability to work. Alcohol and/or narcotics are frequently used by depressed individuals as a way of self-medicating their symptoms. If the depressed symptoms are not relieved, the individual begins a process of withdrawal from interactions with others and engenders feelings of hopelessness. This aspect of depression is the most dangerous as the individual experiences suicidal thoughts and an increased apathy with negative expectations. The process intensifies with a more profound depression and intensified symptoms accompanied by sleep disturbances and extreme fatigue. The process and the symptoms seem to feed on itself with the individual experiencing increased unrelenting psychic pain. Suicide becomes a real threat as the individual tries to be relieved of the severe unhappiness and despair.

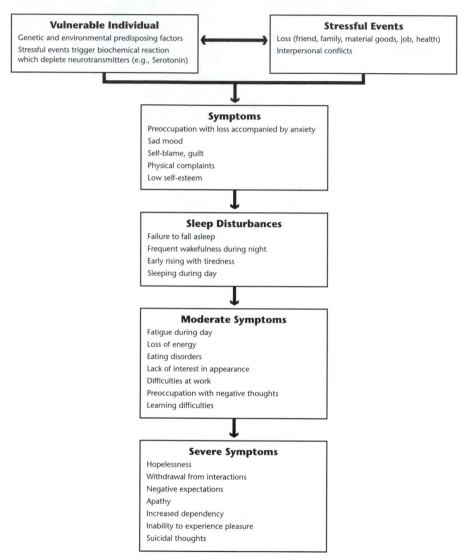

Figure 5–2. Interactive cycle of depression. A vulnerable individual who is presented with stressful events may become depressed. The depression leads to lack of sleep, and this, in turn, leads to more severe depression.

Why are women in our society so prone to depression? Are there genetic, biological, psychological, or sociological factors that predispose women to depression? Theories have been proposed that depression in women is due to the cyclical nature of women's biological functions, hormone differences, and perhaps a stronger innate propensity to bond and therefore to suffer loss more deeply. Some studies indicate that girls are less likely to develop an independent sense of mastery because they are more protected than boys. Other research indicates that because of societal expectations, women have a lower sense of self-efficacy and feel little control over their lives.

Phyllis Chesler (1972) in her classic work *Women and Madness* was one of the first scholars to recognize the vulnerability of women to depression. To quote Chesler:

> National statistics and research studies all document a much higher female to male ratio of depression . . . at all ages. Perhaps more women do get depressed as they grow older—when their already limited opportunities for sexual, emotional and intellectual growth decrease even further. . . . Traditionally, depression has been conceived of as the response to or expression of loss, either of an ambivalently loved other, of the ideal self, or of meaning in one's life. The hostility that should or could be directed outward in response to loss is turned inwards toward the self. Depression rather than aggression is the female response to disappointment or loss. (pp. 41, 44)

In a way Chesler is correct in her analysis because men seem to camouflage their depression through alcohol or violence much more often than women.

In a publication in 1990 edited by McGrath, Keita, Strickland, and Russo and published by the American Psychological Association, the National Task Force on Women and Depression concluded that women are at higher risk for depression that is related to certain cognitive and personality styles such as avoidant, passive, dependent behavior patterns; pessimistic, negative cognitive styles; and focusing too much on dependent feelings instead of action and mastery strategies. This type of behavior implies that many women are easily victimized by individuals in authority roles and are less inclined to challenge others in higher positions. The report also cites the rate of sexual and physical abuse in women as causes of depression. Unhappy marriages are also an underlying cause of depression

in women, especially mothers of young children. Poverty is also seen as a pathway to depression as 75 percent of individuals who are living in poverty in the United States are women and children. The task force also reported that women in high-risk groups include minority women, elderly women, chemically dependent women, women who are lesbians, and professional women. These women are especially prone to depression and need special attention and support. With regard to the treatment of depression, the task members noted that research results support the use of interpersonal therapy and cognitive-behavioral treatment. They also recommended feminist therapy that (a) attends to the issues of power and powerlessness through assertiveness training, (b) encourages egalitarian relationships, and (c) explores sources of depression that are societal, such as sexism. Nothing in their report showed the relationship among exercise, serotonin, and the reduction of depression. Women also seek professional help and counseling more readily than men do. It has also been noted that physicians prescribe antidepressant medications more often to women than men.

The most common forms of treatment for depression are medication and psychotherapy. Both medication and psychotherapy have limitations in that they are expensive, interfere with an individual's everyday life, and may cause dependency. Medications also have significant side effects. On the other hand, there is increasing research evidence that exercise on a regular basis can be a significant factor in reducing the symptoms of depression. The major symptoms of depression (e.g., sad mood, fatigue, sleep and eating disturbances, decreased sexual libido, and cognitive deficits) are all impacted positively by exercise. A number of research studies have related exercise to an increase in serotonin and endorphin (neurotransmitters that have an impact on the symptoms of depression).

Historically, treatment of depression has included both organic remedies such as medication, electroconvulsive therapy, psychosurgery, and psychosocial methods. In the United States, in the 1990s, the medication of choice is Prozac®, a drug that works by preventing the reuptake and depletion of serotonin. Approximately 5 million prescriptions of Prozac® are written each year. Although research studies continue to show that cognitive behavior therapy, relaxation training, and exercise are as effective as drugs in reducing the symptoms of depression, physicians continue to prescribe medications that are expensive, have considerable side effects, and can interfere with the individual's everyday life. For example, in a research study published in 1995 from the School of Medicine, Washington University in St Louis, 82 percent of the participants receiving cognitive therapy improved, while only 29 percent receiving medication improved (Murphy, Carney, Knesevich, Wetzel, & Whitworth, 1995). The evidence seems to be mounting that non-pharmacological treatment of depression is at least as effective as medication.

The research on the effects of exercise is quite powerful and very persuasive (Hays, 1995). However, it is not prescribed as traditional treatment. The American Psychiatric Association (1998) states that depression is one of the most treatable mental illnesses. Between 80 and 90 percent of all depressed people respond to treatment. The treatments listed include medication, psychotherapy, electroconvulsive treatment (ECT), and light therapy. They state, in summary, that medication, psychotherapy, or a combination of the two treatment methods usually relieve symptoms of depression in weeks. Even the most severe forms of depression can respond to treatment rapidly. Nothing about the benefits of exercise is mentioned. The costs of medication are about $40 to $80 a month. Psychotherapy sessions are about $50 to $100 a session. Medication and psychotherapy can last for months or years, costing thousands and thousands of dollars. Exercise, on the other hand, costs practically nothing and has other positive side effects; for example, on the cardiovascular system. In addition, research has shown that exercise also appears to have a positive effect on self-concept, mastery, self-efficacy, independence, body image, and cognitive processing. (See Chapter 12 for research evidence.) Table 5–6, Holistic Treatment of Depression, lists alternative methods to medication and the rationale for treatment.

Anxiety Disorders. According to NIMH (1997), the classification of anxiety disorders is the most common mental illness in the United States with "more than 23 million Americans suffer[ing] from anxiety disorders . . . [manifested by] panic attacks, obsessive thoughts, flashbacks, nightmares, or countless frightening physical symptoms" (p. 1). In general anxiety disorders are distressing to the individual and tend to be part of a reaction to precipitating stressors in the environment. For example, an individual who has been fired from a job may develop anxiety disorder symptoms. Individuals with anxiety disorders may also adapt their behaviors to avoid the anxiety-provoking events. For example, an individual with a fear of flying may avoid traveling by plane; individuals with social phobias who are fearful of performing in public may avoid giving a presentation to a group. Anxiety disorders also include an anticipatory fear that can produce panic when an individual thinks about being in the situation, thus, precipitating a panic attack. For example, an individual with a morbid fear of being buried alive will be extremely anxious when anticipating a tour of a cave. Anxiety disorders can be

Table 5–6. Holistic Treatment of Depression

Effective Treatment	Rationale
Medication	Decrease symptoms
Exercise	Decrease symptoms
Support group	Counteract loneliness
Vocational	Prepare for work and increase job satisfaction
Counseling	Set personal goals
Relaxation therapy	Reduce anxiety
Bibliotherapy	Enable identification with successful recovery
Leisure pursuits	Increase life satisfaction
Education	Explore career and expand knowledge
Volunteer work	Increase meaning in life
Stress management	Self-regulate symptoms of depression
Dietary management	Increase immune response and general health
Creative Arts	Express feelings

mild, moderate, or severe. If the attack is severe, it can cause an individual to be unable to work, engage in leisure activities, or be independent in self-care activities.

Anxiety disorders have a multifactoral etiology. Biological causes include genetic or neurological dysfunction. Psychological factors include environmental stressors, inter- and intrapersonal relationships, and social factors. In short, this category of mental illness is a bio-psycho-social disorder. Treatment for anxiety disorders involve a multimodal approach, including medication, psychotherapy, cognitive-behavioral therapy, group therapy, and psychosocial rehabilitation. The psychosocial occupational therapist can play an important role in treating the individual with an anxiety disorder by using cognitive-behavioral treatments, creative arts, biofeedback, exercise, stress management, relaxation therapy, and vocational rehabilitation.

According to the DSM–IV (APA, 1994), anxiety disorders include the following:

▶ *Panic disorder without agoraphobia (panic attack)*: a sudden onset of intense apprehension, fearfulness, or terror, accompanied by feelings of impending death or becoming mentally ill; symptoms include shortness of breath, rapid heartbeat, chest pain, choking sensation, and other unpleasant physical sensations.

▶ *Panic disorder with agoraphobia*: symptoms of panic attacks accompanied by an extreme fear of being in public places or outside the home. Individuals with extreme agoraphobia become homebound and have a morbid fear of going outside.

▶ *Agoraphobia without history of panic disorder*: presence of symptoms of agoraphobia without sudden panic attacks.

▶ *Specific phobia*: presence of anxiety when experiencing or thinking about an unfounded fear of an object such as a snake or situation, such as being locked in a closet. For example, an individual who is fearful of heights becomes anxious when thinking about a hiking tour of the mountains. Individuals develop numerous fears—fear of flying, snakes, open spaces, or school. The phobia is not diagnosed unless it interferes with an individual's functioning in school, work, social situations, leisure activities, or self-care.

▶ *Social phobia*: the fear of social situations or performing in public. Embarrassment is one of the emotions associated with performance anxiety. This phobia is significant when it interferes with an individual's functioning in school, work, social activities, or relationships.

▶ *Obsessive-compulsive disorder (OCD)*: characterized by an individual's pattern of repetitive thoughts and behaviors that interfere with his or her everyday life. For example, an individual may become obsessed with the thought that he has cancer. The thought persists in spite of reassurance from a physician. Another individual with OCD may wash her hands continuously or for long periods of time.

▶ *Posttraumatic stress disorder (PTSD)*: occurs after a traumatic event such as a devastating flood, fire, war experience, or a rape. The trauma is seen as life-threatening or leaves memories of a devastating event such as witnessing a murder. The individual who has been traumatized may have guilty feelings for surviving as with holocaust victims. Others may try to avoid situations that re-create the traumatic events. Flashbacks, distressing dreams, and difficulty sleeping may accompany PTSD.

▶ *Acute stress disorder*: occurs within 1 month after exposure to an extreme traumatic stressor such as sexual abuse, physical attack, fire, flood, earthquake, war, or any

other event in which an individual is exposed to a life-threatening event. The individual may experience dissociative symptoms that cause a decrease in emotional responsiveness. The traumatic event also may be reexperienced as in PTSD such as in dreams and flashbacks. The individual may try to avoid any association with the traumatic event. The disorder can lead to the more serious diagnosis of PTSD.

▶ *Generalized anxiety disorder*: refers to an individual's persistent worrying for a period of at least 6 months concerning past or anticipated events, relationships, or losses. The individual experiences restlessness, fatigue, difficulty concentrating and attending to information, disturbed sleep, eating, and sexual arousal, irritability, and muscle tension.

▶ *Anxiety disorder due to a general medical condition*: occurs when an individual develops significant symptoms of anxiety when diagnosed with a medical condition such as cancer. The symptoms are a direct result of the individual becoming aware of medical condition. The symptoms include anxiety, panic attacks, or obsessions and compulsions.

▶ *Substance-induced anxiety disorder*: a direct result of the side effects of a medication, drug abuse, or exposure to toxic substances. Symptoms of anxiety, panic, and OCD can be present.

Research Evidence. The research literature is filled with studies in which various treatment modalities were used to treat individuals with anxiety disorders. In general, most of the research included the use of medication and cognitive–behavioral techniques. A sample of recent studies are included below.

▶ *Psychoeducational*: In one study, the participant received education about the interaction between his substance dependence and the posttraumatic stress disorder that occurred as a result of being shot (Polles & Smith, 1995). In another study, the participants received detailed explanation of the "occurrence and maintenance of obsessive thoughts, exposure to obsessive thoughts, response prevention . . . cognitive restructuring, and relapse prevention" (Freeston et al., 1997, p. 405).

▶ *Anger control*: Chemtob, Novaco, Hamada, and Gross (1997) effectively used a 12-session treatment focusing on helping individuals to control anger.

▶ *Social skills, problem-solving, assertiveness, and cognitive restructuring*: A cognitive behavioral group treatment was applied to five adolescents who had social phobias. The treatment included social skills, problem-solving, and assertiveness as part of skills training; cognitive restructuring; behavioral exposure; and homework. Four of the adolescents showed continued improvement after 1 year, the fifth was in partial remission (Albano, Marten, Holt, Heimberg, & Barlow, 1995).

▶ *Cognitive therapy and relaxation therapy*: Cognitive therapy and relaxation therapy were effective in 36 patients with panic disorders who underwent 10 weeks of therapy (Stanley et al., 1996). In another study, Borkovec and Costello (1993) found that applied relaxation and cognitive behavioral therapy were more effective than nondirective therapies when treating patients with a generalized anxiety disorder.

▶ *Biofeedback*: EMG and EEG biofeedback were used successfully with 45 individuals with generalized anxiety disorders, with continued improvement noted at 6 weeks posttreatment (Rice, Blanchard, & Purcell, 1993).

▶ *Meditation*: Kabat–Zinn et al. (1992) used a meditation-based stress reduction program effectively in treating 22 participants with a diagnosis of generalized anxiety disorder, panic disorder, or panic disorder with agoraphobia.

Personality Disorders. Personality disorders are a cluster of disorders that usually begin in adolescent or early adulthood, are stable over time, and lead to distress in the individual or impairment in the individual's ability to work, engage in leisure, or engage in interpersonal relationships. The DSM–IV (APA, 1994) divides these into three clusters based on descriptive similarities:

> Cluster A includes the Paranoid, Schizoid, and Schizotypal Personality Disorders. Individuals with these disorders often appear odd or eccentric. Cluster B includes the Antisocial, Borderline, Histrionic, and Narcissistic Personality Disorders. Individuals with these disorders often appear dramatic, emotional, or erratic. Cluster C includes the Avoidant, Dependent, and Obsessive-Compulsive Personality Disorders. Individuals with these disorders often appear anxious or fearful (pp. 629-630).

Research supporting these clusters has not been conclusive, although it may be useful in educational and research settings (APA, 1994).

A personality disorder is diagnosed when a person's values and behavior deviate markedly from the culture and societal norms. These deviations occur in the way the person thinks, the individual's emotional state, his or her interpersonal relationships, and control of impulses. For example, an individual with an antisocial personality (a) has patterns of behavior that are at variance with the society at large, (b) has not developed the inner controls, and (c) has not incorporated the values of society into his or her thinking or behavior. Approximately 1 to 3 percent of the population are diagnosed with a personality disorder, and approximately 10 percent of clients seen in CMHCs have this diagnosis (Harvard Mental Health Letter, 1996, February).

Cluster A:

▶ *Paranoid personality disorder* is marked by extreme suspiciousness and distrust of others. Attributes hidden motives and agendas of hostility directed by others toward self. Individual is easily offended, tends to misread and distort verbal and nonverbal communications, and is hypervigilant.

▶ *Schizoid personality disorder* is symptomatic of individuals who are withdrawn, introspective, oversensitive, seclusive, and detached from initiating and maintaining close relationships. Individual tends toward working alone and has difficulty expressing feelings.

▶ *Schizotypal personality disorder* is characterized by a desire to be alone. The cognitive style tends to be field independent, where the individual is more interested in activities involving mechanical tasks, such as computer or mathematical games. These individuals tend not to have many close friends and are not usually involved with their families.

Cluster B:

▶ *Antisocial or psychopathic* pertains to antisocial behavior such as violence, criminal activity, physical or sexual abuse, or related behaviors that reflect a lack of moral and ethical standards. Synonymous terms are *sociopathic* and *antisocial reaction.*

▶ *Borderline personality disorder* is marked by an inability to discover meaning in one's life, have a feeling of emptiness, and have difficulty maintaining long-term relationships. Emotional outbursts, sadness, fear, and suicidal ideation are frequently experienced.

▶ *Histrionic personality disorder* is characteristic of individuals who are prone to exaggerate, act out or demonstrate feelings, and show explosive personality reactions. They strive for excitement and surprise in relationships with others. Others characterize these individuals as vain, self-centered, demanding, and shallow.

▶ *Narcissistic personality disorder* is present when an individual shows signs of grandiosity toward self, fantasies of power over others, omniscience, self-importance, vanity, and a strong need for admiration by others and opportunities for exhibiting self. Sometimes the individual shows a lack of empathy and understanding toward others.

Cluster C:

▶ *Avoidant personality disorder* is characterized by social avoidance, lack of friends, inhibition of feelings, feeling of inadequacy, and hypersensitivity to criticism. The individual tends to be a loner and does not seek out social groups or friendships.

▶ *Dependent personality disorder* is characteristic of individuals who cling to other individuals, have difficulties making decisions, lack self-confidence, and are fearful of losing support or approval from others. They tend to be field dependent, in that they have difficulty being objective about their own personality.

▶ *Obsessive-compulsive personality disorder* can be described as an individual having a morbid concern with neatness, orderliness, perfection, and ritualistic or repetitive behavior. Symptoms include extreme preoccupation with details that interfere with task completion, excessive time at work at the expense of leisure, overconscientiousness regarding ethical or legal standards with regard for flexibility in decision making, miserly spending attitude, and the hoarding of objects.

Research Evidence for Treatment Effectiveness. In general, medication, group therapy, individual psychotherapy, and cognitive–behavioral therapy are the main techniques used for individuals with personality disorders. Kazdin (1995) examined 103 children with conduct problems and antisocial personality disorders and found that cognitive-behavior treatment was effective. In another study, Fisher and Bently (1996) found that "cognitive-behavioral group therapy was significantly more effective than [the disease–and–recovery–model] . . . in reducing alcohol use, improving social and family relations, and enhancing psychological functioning" (p. 1244).

Substance Abuse

Many major mental disorders during young adulthood result from alcohol dependence and drug addiction. Drug abuse and alcoholism contribute to school failure and lifelong patterns of low occupational achievement (Substance Abuse and Mental Health Services Administration [SAMHSA], 1997). Incidence and prevalence figures regarding the severity of illicit drug use and alcohol abuse are provided by SAMHSA and reproduced below:

Illicit Drug Use

▶ In 1996, an estimated 13.0 million Americans were current illicit drug users, meaning they had used an illicit drug in the month prior to interview. This represents no change from 1995 when the esti-

mate was 12.8 million. The number of current illicit drug users was at its highest level in 1979 when there were 25 million.

▶ Following a significant increase from 1992 to 1995, between 1995 and 1996 there was a decrease in the rate of past month illicit drug use among youths age 12-17. The rate was 5.3 percent in 1992, 10.9 percent in 1995, and 9.0 percent in 1996. The decrease between 1995 and 1996 occurred in the younger part of this age group, i.e., those age 12 to 15 years.

▶ For those age 18–25 years, the rate of past month illicit drug use increased from 13.3 percent in 1994 to 15.6 percent in 1996. The rate of past month cocaine use also increased in this age group during this period, from 1.2 percent to 2.0 percent.

▶ There were an estimated 2.4 million people who started using marijuana in 1995. This was about the same number as in 1994. The annual number of marijuana initiates rose between 1991 and 1994.

▶ The rate of past month hallucinogen use among youths age 12–17 increased from 1.1 percent in 1994 to 2.0 percent in 1996.

▶ The overall number of current cocaine users did not change significantly between 1995 and 1996 (1.45 million in 1995 and 1.75 million in 1996). This is down from a peak of 5.7 million in 1985. Nevertheless, there were still an estimated 652,000 Americans who used cocaine for the first time in 1995.

▶ There were an estimated 141,000 new heroin users in 1995, and there has been an increasing trend in new heroin use since 1992. A large proportion of these recent new users were smoking, snorting, or sniffing heroin, and most were under age 26. The estimated number of past month heroin users increased from 68,000 in 1993 to 216,000 in 1996.

Alcohol Use

▶ In 1996, 109 million Americans age 12 and older had used alcohol in the past month (51 percent of the population). About 32 million engaged in binge drinking (5 or more drinks on at least one occasion in the past month) and about 11 million were heavy drinkers (drinking five or more drinks per occasion on 5 or more days in the past 30 days).

▶ About 9 million current drinkers were age 12–20 in 1996. Of these, 4.4 million were binge drinkers, including 1.9 million heavy drinkers.

Perceived Risk and Availability of Drugs

▶ The percent of youths age 12–17 that perceived great risk in using marijuana once a month decreased from 1990 (40 percent) to 1994 (33 percent), but remained level from 1994 to 1996.

▶ The percent of youths reporting great risk in using cocaine once a month decreased from 63 percent in 1994 to 54 percent in 1996.

▶ The percent of youths reporting great risk in having five or more drinks once or twice a week decreased from 58 percent in 1992 to 45 percent in 1996. During that same period, the percent reporting great risk in having four or five drinks nearly every day increased from 61 percent to 67 percent.

▶ More than half of youths age 12–17 reported that marijuana was easy to obtain in 1996, and about one quarter reported that heroin was easy to obtain. Fifteen percent of youths reported being approached by someone selling drugs in the month prior to interview. (SAMHSA, 1997, pp. 1–2)

Etiology. Various theories as to the possible causes of alcoholism range from genetic, biological, psychological, and sociological explanation. Risk factors associated with alcoholism include (a) a family history of alcoholism; (b) ratio of 3 to 1, males to females; (c) 20 or 30 years old for males, somewhat later for females; (d) uneven distribution among geographic location, occupation, and cultural or racial differences; and (e) higher frequency if there has been a diagnosis of ADHD or conduct disorder (Goodwin, 1985). Brown, Vik, Patterson, Grant, and Schuckit (1995) found that individuals with alcoholism who experienced high chronic psychosocial stress were more at risk for relapse than those who did not experience the stress. These findings support the stress–vulnerability model of relapse. Some theorists (Blane & Leonard, 1987) support a psychosociological hypothesis that young adults drift into alcoholism because it seems to offer a refuge—an escape from depression, failure, and conflict. The same explanation can be applied to heroin addiction, which is most common among youth who feel hopeless and out of the mainstream of society and are vulnerable in becoming addicted to drugs or alcohol. Leonard and Blane (1987), examined theories of etiology of alcoholism. They concluded that "in a variety of ways, there has been a growing recognition that integrative, multivariate models aimed at highly specific aspects of alcohol use will prove a better understanding of the problems associated with such use" (p. 392).

Treatment Objectives. Medical and psychosocial treatment are the preferred methods in working with individuals with substance and drug dependencies. Medical treatment includes detoxification, use of medication (e.g., Antabuse® or disulfiram, antidepressants, or antipsychotic drugs), hospitalization, and vitamins. Current psychosocial treatment includes psychotherapy, support groups (e.g., Alcoholics Anonymous), residential centers and halfway houses, aversive treatment and cognitive-behavioral treatment emphasizing relaxation training, assertiveness training, and self-control skills (Long, 1995–1997).

The clinical effectiveness for various treatment methods can be found in the research literature and is summarized below.

▶ *Substitution of the addictive substance with another controlled substance* (e.g., using methadone for heroin addiction). Goldstein and Herrera (1995) followed up on 1,019 individuals with heroine addiction who had received methadone treatment. They concluded that methadone was not successful in eliminating the heroine addiction, and that the addiction is a "chronic, lifelong, relapsing disease with a high fatality rate" (p. 139).

▶ *Aversive conditioning* (e.g., use of Antabuse® causing nausea when alcohol is used). In a review of two decades of the use of aversive conditioning to treat drug and alcohol abuse, McLellan and Childress (1985) found mixed results in its effectiveness.

▶ *Detoxification programs in hospitals and outpatient clinics to help individual withdraw from alcohol or drug addiction.* Klijnsma, Cameron, Burns, and McGuigan (1995) found that outpatient detoxification is more cost-effective than inpatient detoxification when treating clients who are alcohol-dependent. Stetter, Zähres, Batra, and Mann (1995) suggested that detoxification alone is not effective, but that treatment must include a medical evaluation, a comprehensive psychiatric diagnosis, and psychotherapeutic treatment aimed at increasing client motivation.

▶ *Social support groups* (e.g., Alcoholics Anonymous, Narcotics Anonymous). George and Tucker (1996) examined the use of AA as a support group. They found that individuals who sought help from a support group were differentiated from those who did not seek help by "alcohol-related psychosocial problems and social network characteristics specific to drinking" (p. 449).

▶ *Therapeutic communities that require individuals with alcohol or drug addiction to change their lifestyle.* Amity is a therapeutic community that provides long-term care for women with addiction and their children. Preliminary research concerning outcome is promising (Stevens & Arbiter, 1995). Motivation and readiness for therapeutic community treatment are important variables in the success of this method (De Leon, Melnick, & Kressel, 1997).

▶ *Cognitive-behavioral treatment.* Graham, Annis, Brett, and Venesoen (1996) in a randomized field trial comparing group and individual cognitive–behavioral treatment methods found both to be effective in preventing relapse over a 12-month period.

▶ *Medication.* Serotonin (5–HT) seems to play an important role in some forms of alcoholism, especially those that are genetically or developmentally mediated. Although results of studies using serotonin selective pharmacotherapy have shown only modest results in reducing alcohol intake, Pettinati (1996) suggested that this treatment is a "viable therapeutic option for alcoholism" (p. 23A).

▶ *Acupuncture.* Gurevich, Duckworth, Imhof, and Katz (1996) used auricular acupuncture over an 11-month period with 47 patients in a psychiatric unit in a general hospital. They concluded that acupuncture is "a safe and inexpensive treatment modality that is easily administered and produces significant results" (p. 165).

▶ *Group therapy.* Martin, Ginnandrea, Rogers, and Johnson (1996) compared the use of psychoeducational approach with a recovery-oriented approach using a patient–counselor collaborative model. Both models were equality effective; however, those in the psychoeducational approach stayed in treatment longer and rated treatment as useful.

▶ *Biofeedback.* Biofeedback has been used successfully in treating individuals with alcohol and drug dependency (Denney, Baugh, & Hardt, 1991; Engstrom & Liebert, 1979; Kurtz, 1974; Page & Schaub, 1978; Rohsenow, Smith, & Johnson, 1985; Steffen, 1975; Townsend, House, & Addario, 1975)

Occupational Therapy Treatment

There have been many misconceptions about the role of occupational therapy in various treatment areas, and alcoholism is no exception. The function of occupational therapy is to view the individual needs of the alcoholic patients to establish a treatment plan based on those individual needs and to provide intervention opportunities. The overall goal is to assist the patient in development of an alcohol-free lifestyle. Short-term goals will support the overall goal and will be directed at specific deficit areas of occupational behavior. Occupational therapy teaches patients a functional, practical approach to living sober. (Rotert, 1989/1993, p. 8)

Van Deusen (1989), in reviewing the research literature, found a relationship between perceptual–motor deficits and individuals with alcoholism. She suggested that there may be a role for occupational therapists in remediating these deficits. Moyers (1997) found that the revised Moyers' Model is consistent with the philosophy of Alcoholics Anonymous (AA) of a spiritual recovery and in addressing the needs of the whole person. Moyers' (1992) model is based on a family-treatment approach based on systems theory and focuses on the reduction of maladaptive role behaviors within the family. AA is an important phase of treatment for the individual with an alcoholic addiction or family members who may be prone to addiction. Table 5–7 describes and identifies the 12 steps of AA. These steps are the core of AA's program.

Middle Adulthood (36–65 Years)

▶ What was the pattern of career and occupational development?

▶ What was the predominant personality characteristic?

▶ How did the individual adjust to physiological changes?

▶ What were the major leisure time activities of the individual?

▶ What were the specific life stressors as indicated in Stein's *Stress Management Questionnaire*?

▶ What were the patterns of changing residences in response to job changes and family needs?

▶ What were the major illnesses and/or major accidents?

This is the period that Erikson (1963) identifies as the psychosocial crises of *generativity* versus *self-absorption*. This is the time of peak achievement and career attainment for most individuals. It is a period when the individual begins to reap the benefits from his previous life experiences. The successful individual is usually a valuable asset in his occupation, profession, or business. It is also a period of preparation for retirement so that the individual may begin to gradually disengage from long-term commitments of occupational climbing.

Table 5–7. The Twelve Steps of Alcoholics Anonymous

The relative success of the A.A. program seems to be due to the fact that an alcoholic who no longer drinks has an exceptional faculty for "reaching" and helping an uncontrolled drinker.

In simplest form, the A.A. program operates when a recovered alcoholic passes along the story of his or her own problem drinking, describes the sobriety he or she has found in A.A., and invites the newcomer to join the informal fellowship.

The heart of the suggested program of personal recovery is contained in Twelve Steps describing the experience of the earliest members of the Society:

1. *We admitted we were powerless over alcohol—that our lives had become unmanageable.*

2. *Came to believe that a Power greater than ourselves could restore us to sanity.*

3. *Made a decision to turn our will and our lives over to the care of God as we understood Him.*

4. *Made a searching and fearless moral inventory of ourselves.*

5. *Admitted to God, to ourselves and to another human being the exact nature of our wrongs.*

6. *Were entirely ready to have God remove all these defects of character.*

7. *Humbly asked Him to remove our shortcomings.*

8. *Made a list of all persons we had harmed, and became willing to make amends to them all.*

9. *Made direct amends to such people wherever possible, except when to do so would injure them or others.*

10. *Continued to take personal inventory and when we were wrong promptly admitted it.*

11. *Sought through prayer and meditation to improve our conscious contact with God as we understood Him, praying only for knowledge of His will for us and the power to carry that out.*

12. *Having had a spiritual awakening as the result of these steps, we tried to carry this message to alcoholics and to practice these principles in all our affairs.*

Newcomers are not asked to accept or follow these Twelve Steps in their entirety if they feel unwilling or unable to do so.

They will usually be asked to keep an open mind, to attend meetings at which recovered alcoholics describe their personal experiences in achieving sobriety, and to read A.A. literature describing and interpreting the A.A. program.

A.A. members will usually emphasize to newcomers that only problem drinkers themselves, individually, can determine whether or not they are in fact alcoholics.

At the same time, it will be pointed out that all available medical testimony indicates that alcoholism is a progressive illness, that it cannot be cured in the ordinary sense of the term, but that it can be arrested through total abstinence from alcohol in any form.

Source : Obtained from Alcoholics Anonymous at *http://www.alcoholics-anonymous.org/english/E_FactFile/ M-24_d6.html.*

Old Age (Over 65)

▶ How did individual adjust to retirement?

▶ What were the patterns of leisure time activities?

▶ What were the major health problems (e.g., cardiovascular, arthritis and joint disabilities, visual and auditory impairments, respiratory, prostate and urinary, gastrointestinal, menopause)?

▶ How is the individual adjusting to death of friends and loved ones?

▶ Is income adequate during retirement?

▶ How does the individual adjust to housing relocations?

▶ Is old age a time for disengagement from occupational tasks or has the individual continued in occupational, avocational tasks, and volunteer work?

▶ How does religion or spirituality play a role in individual's life?

According to Erikson (1963) the major psychosocial crisis confronting the individual during aging is *ego integrity* versus *ego despair*. The individual, during old age, begins to evaluate his or her own life in terms of a wholeness of purpose. Life satisfaction is the final confrontation issue for the aged. The philosophical issue relating to the meaning of a person's life becomes critical at the time of summing up.

Significant Mental Disorders During Old Age

Old age is a period of stress and disorganization for many individuals. It is estimated that approximately 7 percent of the aged population are in nursing homes (Feinleib, Cunningham, & Short, 1994). Mental disorders among the aged are complicated by the loss of physical function. The normal wear and tear on the body takes its toll on the individual. Eyesight becomes weaker, hearing more difficult, range of motion in joints becomes limited, the muscles are not as strong, and the blood vessels begin to lose elasticity (Bowlby, 1993). Along with physical changes, the aged individual may also feel the stress resulting from isolation from relatives and friends, decreased income, inadequate housing, vulnerability to crime, and a lack of usefulness in a society that stresses youth and vitality (Lieberman & Peskin, 1992). Disorders of mental illness among the aged include a range of diagnoses such as schizophrenia; depression; panic, phobic, and obsessive-compulsive disorders, and alcohol and drug abuse (Anthony & Aboraya, 1992). The most severe

mental disorder associated with old age is Alzheimer's disease.

Alzheimer's Disease

Definition: Alzheimer's Disease (AD) is a slowly worsening brain disease. AD is marked by changes in behavior and personality and by a decline in thinking abilities that cannot be reversed. This mental decline is related to a loss of nerve cells, and the links between them. The course of the disease varies from person to person, as does the rate of decline. On average AD lasts from 4 to 8 years after diagnosis; however it can continue for up to 20 years. (National Institute on Aging, 1996, p. 1)

The disease advances in stages from mild memory loss to severe dementia.

In general, dementia refers to a syndrome or group of signs and symptoms that cluster together, such as impairment of short- and long-term memory, plus one of the following cognitive impairments: aphasia (understanding and use of language), apraxia (inability to carry out planned motor tasks), agnosia (inability to recognize objects), and disturbances in executive functioning (problem solving and ability to think abstractly) (APA, 1994). AD is one type of dementia. Other types of dementia can be caused by severe head trauma, arteriosclerosis, Parkinson's disease, Huntington's disease, Pick's disease, later stages of HIV, and Creutzfeldt-Jakob disease (APA, 1994). The impairments in dementia interfere with an individual's ability to work, engage in leisure activities, be independent in self-care, relate to others, and carry on the IADLS such as shopping, driving a car, paying bills, and planning social activities (Trace & Howell, 1991).

Course of the Disease. AD advances in stages, characterized in the beginning by mild forgetfulness, such as not being able to remember names of friends or the words for familiar objects, to the later stages of the disease in which the individual loses all reasoning abilities and becomes completely dependent on a caregiver. The clinical course of the disease is marked in the early stages by obvious repetitions in conversations, disorientation in unfamiliar settings, and failure to remember appointments and responsibilities. "As the disease progresses, remote and highly learned memory traces become lost or inaccessible, and the patient may eventually be unable to recognize even immediate family members" (Raskind & Peskind, 1992, p. 479). Personality changes include apathy, self-centeredness, lack of empathy for others, angry outbursts, and an increased dependency on others. The sleep-wake cycle becomes disturbed and many times the individual wanders in the middle of the night. In very advanced stages of the disease the individual develops muscle rigidity and very slow movements. In the terminal stages of the disease the individual may become mute, unable to walk, incontinent, emaciated, and eventually die from pneumonia (Raskind & Peskind, 1992).

Incidence and Prevalence. Approximately 4 million American adults have a diagnosis of AD, with slightly half of these individuals being cared for at home. Nearly 50 percent of all individuals 85 and older have symptoms of AD (National Institute on Aging, 1996). It is important to note that the number of adults in the population in the United States who will be over the age of 85 will increase dramatically in the next 30 years as the "baby boomers" age. It is predicted that the number of Americans 85 and over will total almost 9 million by the year 2030 (National Institute on Aging, 1996). The prevalence and incidence of AD will rise as the number of aged individuals in the population increases.

Etiology and Risk Factors. "The search for the causes or pathogenesis of AD has focused on three areas: genetics, the beta-amyloid protein and potential environmental toxins" (Raskind & Peskind, 1992, p. 480). Recent findings examining the genetic link to the onset of AD led investigators to conclude that late-onset AD has a substantial genetic cause (Bergem, Engedal, & Kringlen, 1997; Gatz et al., 1997). There is also evidence that supports the link with Down syndrome and AD (Zigman, Schupf, Haveman, & Silverman, 1997). In a review article, the authors concluded that almost all individuals with a diagnosis of Down syndrome over the age of 40 years have neuropathology that is consistent with AD. There is also increasing evidence that lipoproteins, which help carry fats in the blood and are associated with the buildup of amyloid plaques in the brains, are risk factors for AD (Fratiglioni, 1996). Some investigators have found a relationship between the presence of aluminum in the brain and AD. However, there is no conclusive evidence that aluminum or other environmental toxins are implicated in AD (Raskind & Peskind, 1992).

Diagnosis. Assessment and diagnosis for any dementia must include the following (Bowlby, 1993):

▶ a complete medical, developmental, and psychosocial history

▶ a comprehensive medical evaluation, including a neurological evaluation, to identify possible biological or neurological causes

▶ a psychiatric evaluation to determine comorbidity of other disorders, such as mood disorders and psychosis

▶ a social/behavioral evaluation to assess the individual's living situation, independent functioning, psychosocial interactions, and availability of social or familial supports

▶ an evaluation of the individual's independence in self-care and leisure activities

▶ a neuropsychological assessment to examine cognitive functioning, including memory, attention, perceptual, intelligence, executive functioning, judgment, language, and motor skills

Other evaluations and assessment that might be useful include PET scans, MRIs, genetic testing, and tau levels. Recent studies have found that "AD patients had higher tau levels [in the cerebrospinal fluid] at the earliest stages of the disease than health volunteers and people with other neurological diseases" (National Institute of Aging, 1996, p. 17).

Treatment. According to Bowlby (1993)

> While there is no cure for the disease, it is vital to appreciate that there are effective approaches and interventions for the person with ADRD [Alzheimer's Disease and Related Disorders]. The symptoms of ADRD and the factors causing excess disability are amendable to treatment. Specialized treatment and care regimens maximize the self-esteem and functioning and minimize the suffering and dependence of the millions of affected individuals during the long course of their illness. (p. 55)

Recent Research on the Treatment of Alzheimer's Disease

▶ *Pet therapy* has been increasingly used with elderly persons in nursing homes to reduce irritable behavior (Zisselman, Rovner, Shmuely, & Ferrie, 1996). In another study, Darrah (1996) found that "nursing facility administrators identified sensory stimulation, facilitation of resident social interaction, stress reduction, and companionship as the top four therapeutic purposes for using pets and animals in the nursing home" (p. 105).

▶ *Cognitive treatment.* Bach, Bach, Böhmer, Früwalk, and Grilc (1995) found that "application of a reactivating occupational therapy program in addition to functional rehabilitation is significantly more efficient

than the application of functional rehabilitation alone on levels of cognitive performance, psychosocial functioning, and the degree of contentedness with life" (p. 222).

▶ *Reminiscence groups* enable individuals to share memories in order to stimulate reminiscing and reaffirm value for previous life experiences (Bowlby, 1993; Stevens–Ratchford, 1993). Baines, Saxby, and Ehlert (1987) found less cognitive decline among individuals who participated in reminiscence groups than individuals who did not participate, especially when personal objects (e.g., pictures, slides, etc.) were used.

▶ *Sensory stimulation* is "an individual or group activity for the cognitively impaired elderly who have difficulty in relating and responding to their surroundings" (Bowlby, 1993 p. 274). Corcoran and Barrett (1987) found that use of sensory stimulation increased the attention span, postural and motor control, communication, orientation, and social interaction of elderly patients. In another study, improvement was also noted in independence for feeding when provided sensory integration (Hames–Hahn & Llorens, 1989).

Other therapeutic activities described by Bowlby (1993) in *Therapeutic Activities with Persons Disabled by Alzheimer's Disease and Related Disorders* include ADL training, cooking groups, handicraft activities, horticulture, exercise, music, visual and expressive arts.

Caregivers. The family provides a support for the individual with dementia or Alzheimer's disease that is critical to the individual.

> Providing this care is not without cost, however. In particular, those who are caring for the most impaired older persons . . . report very high rates of guilt, demoralization, and depression associated with the great burden of care (Brody, 1989). Caregivers . . . show significant

suppression of a number of immune system paraments, thus making them more susceptible to illness and death from infections, influenza, etc. (Kiecolt–Glaser & Glaser, 1989). (Lebowitz & Niederehe, 1992, pp. 18–19)

Chung (1997), in a qualitative study examining caregivers of individuals with dementia recommended that "occupational therapists should include therapy to family carers as a part of treating individuals with dementia" (p. 66).

FORMULATING SHORT- AND LONG-TERM TREATMENT GOALS

In general the overall treatment goal in psychosocial occupational therapy is to help the client to be as independent and self-actualizing as possible within the areas of work/school, self-care (ADL), leisure, social skills, and self-regulation of dysfunctional symptoms. The degree to which the client is able to work in a satisfying job, establish and maintain meaningful interpersonal relationships by living harmoniously with family and friends, engaging in meaningful leisure activities, and self-regulating daily activities and emotions will depend on the individual's level of functional skills. Short-term goals are linked to improvements in performance components that underlie the major performance areas of work, ADL, and leisure (AOTA, 1994). Short-term treatment goals are formulated to reduce the acute symptoms that interfere with personal adjustment, thereby enabling the client develop skills in interpersonal relationships, self-esteem, and coping mechanisms. (See the Individual Treatment Plan in Chapter 3.)

In many instances the acute symptoms such as severe anxiety or depression and acute delusional and hallucinating disturbances are first controlled by medication. Other short-term goals require psychosocial therapeutic interventions in the client's behaviors and adaptations.

The occupational therapist works with a client in a dynamic framework of refining treatment goals and assessing and reassessing progress. General treatment goals are discussed with the client during the initial interview. Later, specific short-term goals are formulated based on observations by the occupational therapist and objective data gathered from the mental health team members. The occupational therapist tries to coordinate specific treatment objectives with the overall goals that have been established in team meetings.

CONCEPTS OF POSITIVE MENTAL HEALTH AS BASES FOR ESTABLISHING OCCUPATIONAL THERAPY TREATMENT GOALS

A theoretical model for establishing treatment goals is based on the holistic concepts of positive mental health first advanced by Jahoda (1958). Marie Jahoda identified concepts of positive mental health that are relevant for the psychosocial occupational therapist in formulating treatment goals.

Table 5–8 summarizes the mental health concepts defined by Jahoda and includes examples of occupational therapy activities. This conceptual model provides an overall guide for generating occupational therapy activities.

1. A Positive Feeling of Self-Good Initiated by Self-Confidence, Self-Esteem, Self-Acceptance, Self-Reliance, and Self-Respect

These concepts imply that the healthy individual has a good understanding of self and personal resources as well as personal limitations. The individual accepts his or her being and uses his or her potential to fulfill realistic goals. Clark

Table 5–8. Generating Occupational Therapy Activities Based on Jahoda's Positive Concepts of Mental Health

Mental Health Concepts	Treatment Goals	Examples of Occupational Therapy Activities
POSITIVE FEELINGS OF SELF	• Increase feelings of self-acceptance, self-esteem, and development of self-identity	• Opportunity for successful mastery of understanding of self through activities that encourage self-disclosure
SELF-ACTUALIZATION	• Fulfillment of personal and vocational potential	• Vocational rehabilitation and social skills training
INTEGRATION AND UNIFYING OUTLOOK ON LIFE	• Development of goals with client that are consistent with values and abilities	• Values clarification exercises to help client identify personal values, goals, and meaning of life
RESISTANCE TO STRESS	• Stress inoculation training designed to help the client reduce negative results of stress	• Identification of activities that are effective with individual in reducing or minimizing the effects of stress (Stress management)
AUTONOMY	• Ability to self-regulate behavior by independent actions	• Creative media allowing the client opportunity to design and complete original projects
PERCEPTION OF REALITY	• Increase the ability to perceive reality objectively and accurately	• Participation in group activities that provide consensual validation and feedback regarding the perception of reality
EMPATHY	• Ability to understand the feelings of others	• Opportunities for client to assist others, such as in a cooking group or teaching activity
ENVIRONMENTAL MASTERY	• Ability to love • Adequacy in love, work, and play • Adequacy in interpersonal relationships • Efficiency in meeting situational requirements • Capacity for adaptation and adjustment • Efficiency in problem-solving. Shared expression of love • Ability to organize daily life patterns • Ability to establish sharing relationships • Ability to adjust to new situations • Ability to use resources in environment • Ability to resolve everyday problems	• Simulated activities such as role-playing, mock interviews, and psychodrama, in which the client has the opportunity to test abilities in a supportive environment that facilitates growth. Prevocational exploration and work adjustment training can help client to develop new attitudes and behaviors toward work.

Source : Adapted from *Current Concepts of Positive Mental Health,* by M. Jahoda, 1958, New York: Basic Books.

E. Moustakas (1956) in a theoretical study, "True Experiences and the Self," defined the self as "The self is itself alone existing as a totality and constantly emerging. It can be understood only as unique personal experience . . . The self is undifferentiated in time and space. It is being, becoming, moving, undivided from the world of nature or the social world" (pp. 3–4). In a study of self-ideal congruence as an index of adjustment, Turner and Vanderlippe (1965), using the Q-sort technique,[1] defined the healthy individual as someone with a high self-ideal congruence. In other words, the healthy individual has accepted the self as unique and ideal in fulfilling life goals.

Implementing Treatment Goals Through Occupational Therapy

Development of *self-confidence* or *self-esteem* in the individual can be facilitated through activities that foster learning and upon completion represent a finished product or applied skill. For example, photography is an activity in which the individual can develop skills in using a camera, developing negatives, and enlarging photographs and, in the process, develop self-confidence. Related activities include learning a new craft, learning to play a musical instrument, developing skill in a sport, or becoming competent in an adaptive activity, such as driving a car.

▶ *Fostering of self-identity and self-disclosure through activities that enable the individual to learn about himself or herself.* Spontaneous art, poetry, creative writing, dramatics, sculpture, and magazine collage are examples of activities that can be used to help the individual understand his/her own identity. The activities are used as vehicles for exploring the individual's personality and self-identity through creative self-expression.

▶ *Encouraging autonomy and initiative in the individual through activities that may imply risk and assertiveness into areas of uncertainty.* Autonomy also implies a self-directedness in life decisions as well as a control and mastery of one's destiny. Helping the

individual to overcome the fears of everyday life situations can be helpful in personal adjustment (e.g., interviewing for a job, planning an evening entertainment with a friend, becoming a member of a community interest group, seeking an apartment, and selecting an adult education course). These everyday "mundane" activities may panic the individual with mental illness who has not developed the sense of autonomy that is essential for mastering independent living skills. The occupational therapist can encourage autonomy in activities that simulate these life tasks through therapeutic task groups, role playing, and behavioral rehearsal in which each individual tries out personal strategies in a safe situation to reduce the anxiety attached to the behaviors. Another technique that is used is *paradoxical intention* (Frankl, 1963). In this technique, the individual simulates the fearful behavior and, by doing so, obtains control of it. For example, an individual who is fearful of stuttering produces the stuttering.

Outward Bound programs (Ewert, 1982) have been used to encourage autonomy and initiative. These programs entail mountain climbing, hiking, canoe trips, and other activities where the individual must use his or her physical and mental resources to cope with the natural environment. Outward Bound programs also encourage mutual trust as well as testing the individual's resources in activities that involve physical risk, since many of the activities involve cooperation and joint assistance.

---

[1] A psychological test where the subject systematically sorts cards containing personality descriptions into present self and ideal categories.

2. Growth Development and Self-Achievement as Criteria for Mental Health (Self-Actualization)

The ability to actualize one's potentials is one of the basic needs of man. The individual must have a realistic understanding of himself or herself before realizing his or her potential. We fulfill our potentials in our daily occupations and work roles, hobbies and avocations, and interaction with others. We are happiest when we perform at our highest levels of potential, for example, at jobs where we receive recognition from others. The motivation to grow and develop our skills and abilities is a critical process that unfolds as we receive the support and encouragement from significant others, such as parents, teachers, friends, and colleagues. Our potentials are determined by our genetic constitution and our environmental experiences. Related to the concept of self-actualization is hope and striving. In an environment that fosters self-actualization, the individual has opportunities and means to test his or her skills to succeed. On the other hand, self-actualization is deterred in extreme situations such as prisons or institutions, where freedom is severely limited or in hostile environments where the basic needs are marginally met. Maslow (1956), in his classic study of self-actualizing people found "that all subjects felt safe and unanxious, accepted, loved and loving, respect-worthy . . . It may be that self-actualization means basic gratification plus at best, minimum talent, capacity or richness" (p. 162). One of the most important and key concepts of self-actualizing people that Maslow found was "their entirely unique and idiosyncratic-character-structure-expression" (p. 192). In other words, self-actualizing people are self-consistent in their uniqueness. They fulfill their talents in their own individual and personal ways.

3. Integration

Jahoda (1958) states that "integration refers to the relatedness of all processes and attributes in an individual" (p. 36). As a criterion for mental health, integration encompasses the individual's balance of internal forces such as strong feelings, mastery of the environment, and conscience. It is a balance between emotion and rational thinking. Another element of integration involves a unifying outlook on life. The search for the meaning of life is a continual process of reintegrating new experiences with previous learning. The healthy individual sees his or her life in a continual state of growth, refining his or her life experiences to realize an integrated whole. Helping those with mental illness to find direction in their lives is an important treatment goal. The therapist and client work together to resolve the following issues: Who am I? What are my personal goals in life? How can I fulfill my potentials? Values clarification exercises can be potentially helpful to the client in identifying personal values and goals.

4. Resistance to Stress

The research on biofeedback and self-regulation directly relate to the individual's ability to manage stress (Stoyva & Budzynski, 1993). Terms related to this concept include individual resiliency, frustration-tolerance, ability to rebound from failure and rejection, and stress-inoculation (Meichenbaum, 1993). The healthy individual is able to self-regulate stress through exercise, yoga, relaxation, music, meditating, creative activities, or by expressing feelings to friends (Lehrer & Woolfolk, 1993). At one time or another, almost every individual experiences anxiety, depression, personal loss, and failure. The strength of the individual is in learning how to handle the stress so that it is not overwhelming. Jahoda (1958) stated that "Not only does the mentally healthy person tolerate anxiety without disintegration, but . . . the healthy person must be able to produce and experience anticipatory anxiety in order to cope better with subsequent danger" (pp. 42–43). This implies that all stress is not detrimental. In fact the "sheltered" or overprotected individual who encounters little or no stress during childhood and adolescence may not be able to handle stress later in life as well as the individual who has coped with problems early in life. One of the goals of treatment is to help the client to be aware of the factors in the environment that precipitate stress.

5. Autonomy

In Western cultures, we highly value the trait of self-determination and independence. Healthy individuals are in control of their lives and make self-determined decisions. This concept also implies an "inner directedness" for controlling one's destiny. As a treatment goal, the therapist encourages opportunities for the client to express autonomous decisions. Individuals who lack autonomy frequently refer to fate or external forces as controlling their lives. They tend to conform to popular patterns of behavior and are fearful of being different or "standing out" in a crowd. The individual with schizophrenia frequently relinquishes his or her autonomy of action and places himself or herself into the guardianship of someone else or an institution. In this way, the individual with schizophrenia loses the autonomy and independence of behavior. Another threat to autonomy in the individual is in stereotyped and compulsive behavior in which the individual with mental illness is inflexible in her or his behavior and feels driven to perform ritualistic acts. A treatment goal for the individual with compulsive behavior disor-

der is to encourage risk-taking in behavior and to avoid perfectionistic thinking. The therapist must continually emphasize to this client that it is "all right to make a mistake; it means we are making conscious decisions and exercising our autonomy."

The opposite extreme of autonomy in the individual with mental illness is catatonia, where the individual denies his or her self-expression and remains immobile. The occupational therapist can actively work with the client's risk-taking behavior through creative media such as clay and water colors where the client can try new ways to express feelings and construct objects.

6. Perception of Reality

Jahoda (1958) states, "As a rule, the perception of reality is called mentally healthy when the individual sees and corresponds to what is actually there" (p. 49). The perception of reality is a unique and individual response based on accurate sensory awareness. What is perception may be dependent on consensual validation, that is, other individual's accurate agreements. Hallucinations are examples of disturbances of the perceptions of reality where the individual with mental illness sees and hears sensations that are unique. In a way, the individual who is hallucinating is generating internal sensations that are auditory or visual. It is analogous to legitimizing the reality of dreams. Healthy perception is mostly free from sensory distortions; however, the concept of true perception of reality is an issue that philosophers, writers, and psychologists have grappled with for centuries. For example, Cervantes (1609/1964), in a literary context in the book *Don Quixote*, presented the concept of phenomenology as he tried to ascertain the relationship between perceived reality and truth. He raised the question, through his protagonist, Don Quixote: "Are the appearances of objects real or do our senses deceive us?" Don Quixote fights windmills, which he thinks are giants. He makes inns become castles and peasant girls are perceived as beautiful maidens. In contrast to Don Quixote, Cervantes created the character Sancho Panza, who is the typical pragmatist who interprets reality from the vantage point of its effect on life. Distortion-free reality is a relative concept.

A goal of therapy is to help the individual who is mentally ill to become even more aware of the auditory, visual, tactile, kinesthetic, olfactory, gustatory, and vestibular information in the environment. Perception of reality is sharpened as the individual trains his or her sensory organs to become sensitive to external stimuli. We can also increase our sensory knowledge by integrating sensory stimuli through multimodal reinforcement by using multiple senses to verify information. For example, sensory integration therapy relies on the concept of multiple stimulation to reinforce cognitive and affective learning.

7. Empathy or Social Sensitivity

Corey (1996) states:

> empathy is a deep and subjective understanding *of* the client *with* the client. It is a sense of personal identification with the client's experience. Therapists are able to share the client's subjective world by tuning in to their own feelings that are like the client's feelings. Yet therapists must not lose their own separateness. Rogers asserts that when therapists can grasp the client's private world, as the client sees and feels it, without losing the separateness of their own identity, constructive change is likely to occur. (p. 207)

Jahoda (1958) states that empathy requires that an individual treat the feelings of others as "worthy of his [or her] concern and attention" (p. 52) and without distortion. It is an impor-

tant part of interpersonal competency. Empathy is also an issue for health professionals. Empathy involves authenticity, as defined by Yerxa (1967):

> Personal authenticity as an occupational therapist means that the therapist allows himself to feel real emotional as he enters into the *mutual* relation with the client . . . "Being there" also means being able to separate his feelings from the client as a human being from projections of how he would feel if he had experienced the client's disability. For the authentic occupational therapist knows that the client is the only one who can discover his own particular meaning. (p. 8)

For the client-centered therapist, empathy is viewed as *unconditional positive regard* (Rogers, 1977).

8. Environmental Mastery

Jahoda (1958) defines environmental mastery as the ability to love; adequacy in love, work, and play; adequacy in interpersonal relations; efficiency in meeting situational requirements; capacity for adaptation and adjustment; efficiency in problem-solving. This mental health goal is most directly related to occupational therapy. The activities used in occupational therapy are directly related to enabling the client to become independent in living skills, expand leisure interests, develop vocational abilities, facilitate interpersonal relationships, and test out problem-solving skills.

SUMMARY

The occupational therapy treatment process is based on a psychosocial model of evaluation, formulation of treatment goals, treatment implementation, and reassessment. Each individual in this process is unique. A case study analysis helps the therapist to understand the client and to gain insight into the events and relationships in the client's life that led to mental illness. The case study also provides information on the client's strengths and abilities that can be reinforced and supported. The family is an integral part of the treatment process. In this dynamic process, the occupational therapist and client establish short- and long-term treatment goals to meet the individual needs of the client. Treatment progresses as the client begins to develop a heightened sense of self-awareness and insight, identifies feasible life goals, and develops the interpersonal skills and competencies that are necessary for coping with the daily problems of life. Occupational therapy activities are a means to attain treatment goals based on a holistic concept of positive mental health.

REFERENCES

Albano, A. M., Marten, P. A., Holt, C. S., Heimberg, R. G., & Barlow, D. H. (1995). Cognitive-behavioral group treatment for social phobia in adolescents: A preliminary study. *Journal of Nervous and Mental Disorders, 183,* 649–656.

Alcoholics Anonymous. (n.d.). *The twelve steps of alcoholics anonymous.* Retrieved January 30, 2001, from the World Wide Web: *http://www.alcoholics-anonymous.org/english/E_FactFile/M-24_d6.html.*

American Association of Mental Retardation. (1992). *Mental retardation, definition, classification, and systems of supports.* Washington, DC: Author.

American Occupational Therapy Association. (1994). *Uniform terminology for occupational therapy: Application to practice* (3rd ed.). Rockville, MD: Author.

American Psychiatric Association. (1952). *Diagnostic and statistical manual of mental disorders* (DSM–I). Washington, DC: Author.

American Psychiatric Assocation. (1968). *Diagnostic and statistical manual of mental disorders* (2nd ed., DSM–II). Washington, DC: Author.

American Psychiatric Association. (1980). *Diagnostic and statistical manual of mental disorders* (3rd ed. DSM–III). Washington, DC: Author.

American Psychiatric Association. (1987). *Diagnostic and statistical manual of mental disorders* (3rd ed., rev.; DSM–IIIR). Washington, DC: Author.

American Psychiatric Association. (1994). *Diagnostic and statistical manual of mental disorders* (4th ed. DSM–IV). Washington, DC: Author.

American Psychiatric Association. (1998). *Depression.* Retrieved January 31, 2001 from the World Wide Web: *http://www.psych.org/public_info/depression.cfm.*

Anthony, J. C., & Aboraya, A. (1992). The epidemiology of selected mental disorders in later life. In J. E. Birren, R. B. Sloane, & G. D. Cohen (Eds.), *Handbook of mental health and aging* (2nd ed., pp. 27–73). San Diego: Academic Press.

Arns, P. G., & Linney, J. A. (1995). Relating functional skills of severely mentally ill clients to subjective and societal benefits. *Psychiatric Services, 46,* 260–265.

Autism Society of America [ASA]. (1996). *What is autism?* Retrieved January 27, 2001, from the World Wide Web: *http://www.autism-society.org/autism.html#contents.* [1997, September 9].

Bach, D., Bach, M., Böhmer, F., Frühwald, T., & Grilc, B. (1995). Reactiving occupational therapy: A method to improve cognitive performance in geriatric patients. *Age Ageing, 24,* 222–226.

Baines, S., Saxby, P., & Ehlert, K. (1987). Reality orientation and reminiscence therapy. *British Journal of Psychiatry, 151,* 222–231.

Barkley, R. A. (1990). *Attention-deficit hyperactivity disorder: A handbook for diagnosis and treatment.* New York: Guilford.

Bassett, A. S. (1991). Linkage analysis of schizophrenia; Challenges and promise. *Social Biology, 38,* 189–196.

Bateson, G., Jackson, D. P., Haley, J., & Weakland, J. (1956). Towards a theory of schizophrenia. *Behavioral Science 1,* 251–254.

Bellak, L. (Ed.). (1979). *Disorders of the schizophrenic syndrome.* New York: Basic Books.

Bergem, A. L., Engedal, K., & Kringlen, E. (1997). The role of heredity in late-onset Alzheimer disease and vascular dementia: A twin study. Archives of *General Psychiatry, 54,* 264–270.

Bernstein, L., Bernstein, R., & Dana, R. (1974). *Interviewing: A guide for health professionals* (2nd ed.). New York: Appleton-Century-Crofts.

Birmaher, B., Ryan, N. D., Williamson, D. E., Brent, D. A., & Kaufman, J. (1996). Childhood and adolescent depression: A review of the past 10 years, Part II. *Journal of the American Academy of Childhood and Adolescent Psychiatry, 35,* 1575–1583.

Blane, H. T., & Leonard, K. E. (1987). *Psychological theories of drinking and alcoholism.* New York: Guilford.

Blehar, M. C., Weissman, M. M., Gershon, E. S., & Hirschfeld, R. M. A. (1988). Family and genetic studies of affective disorders. A*rchives of General Psychiatry, 45,* 289–292.

Borkovec, T. D., & Costello, E. (1993). Efficacy of applied relaxation and cognitive-behavioral therapy in the treatment of generalized anxiety disorder. *Journal of Consulting and Clinical Psychology, 61,* 611–619.

Bowlby, C. (1993). *Therapeutic activities with persons disabled by Alzheimer's disease and related disorders.* Gaithersburg, MD: Aspen.

Brown, G. W., Birley, J. L. T., & Wing, J. K. (1972). Influence of family life on the course of schizophrenia disorders: A replication. *British Journal of Psychiatry, 121,* 241–258.

Brown, S. A., Vik, P. W., Patterson, T. L., Grant, I., & Schuckit, M. A. (1995). Stress, vulnerability and adult alcohol relapse. *Journal of Studies in Alcohol, 56,* 538–545.

Burton, R. (1938). *The anatomy of melancholy* (R. Dell & P. Jordan–Smith, Eds. and Trans.). New York: Tudor. (Original work published 1632)

Center for Disease Control [CDC]. Division of Birth Defects, Child Development, and Disabilities and Health. Developmental Disabilities Branch. (2001). *Autism among children.* Retrieved January 27, 2001, from the World Wide Web: *http://www.cdc.gov/nceh/cddh/dd/ddautism.htm.*

Cervantes, M. (1964). *Don Quixote* (W. Starkie, Trans.). New York: New American Library. (Original work published 1609)

Chemtob, C. M., Novaco, R. W., Hamada, R. S., & Gross, D. M. (1997). Cognitive-behavioral treatment for severe anger in posttraumatic stress disorder. *Journal of Consulting Clinical Psychology, 65,* 184–189.

Chesler, P. (1972). *Women and madness.* Garden City, NY: Doubleday.

Chung, J. C. C. (1997). Focus on family care givers for individuals with dementia: Implications for occupational therapy practice. *Occupational Therapy International, 4,* 66–80.

Corcoran, M., & Barrett, D. (1987). Using sensory integration principles with regressed elderly patients. *Occupational Therapy in Health Care, 4,* 119–128.

Corey, G. (1996). *Theory and practice of counseling and psychotherapy* (5th ed.). Belmont, CA: Brooks/Cole.

Cottrell, R. P. F. (2000). COTA education and professional development: A historical review. *The American Journal of Occupational Therapy, 54,* 407–412.

Cronin, A. F. (1996). Psychosocial and emotional domains of behavior. In J. Case–Smith, A. S. Allen, & P. N. Pratt (Eds.), *Occupational therapy for children* (3rd ed., pp. 387–429). St. Louis: C. V. Mosby.

Darrah, J. P. (1996). A pilot survey of animal-facilitated therapy in Southern California and South Dakota nursing homes. *Occupational Therapy International, 3,* 105–121.

Davis, K. L., Kahn, R. S., Ko, G., & Davidson, M. (1991). Dopamine in schizophrenia: A review and reconceptualization. *American Journal of Psychiatry, 148,* 1474–1486.

De Leon, G., Melnick, G., & Kressel, D. (1997). Motivation and readiness for therapeutic community treatment among cocaine and other drug abusers. *American Journal of Drug and Alcohol Abuse, 23,* 169–189.

DeLisi, L. (1992). The significance of age of on-set for schizophrenia. *Schizophrenia Bulletin, 18,* 209–215.

Denney, M. R., Baugh, J. L., & Hardt, H. D. (1991). Sobriety outcome after alcoholism treatment with biofeedback participation: A pilot inpatient study. *International Journal of Addiction, 26,* 335–341.

Eikelmann, B., & Reker, T. (1996). [Rehabilitation of psychiatrically ill and handicapped patients— Historical, conceptual and scientific aspects]. *Gesundheitswesen, 58* (Suppl.), 72–78.

Engstrom, D. R., & Liebert, D. E. (1979). Muscle tension and experienced control: Effects of alcohol intake vs. biofeedback on alcoholics and non-alcoholics. *Currents in Alcoholism, 7,* 219–218.

Erikson, E. (1963). *Childhood and society* (2nd ed.). New York: Norton.

Ewert, A. W. (1982). *A study of the effects of participation in an Outward Bound short course upon the reported self-concepts of selected participants.* Unpublished doctoral thesis, University of Oregon, Eugene.

Falloon, I. R. H. (1996). *Psychosocial interventions in schizophrenia: A review.* Armonk, New York: M. E. Sharpe.

Falloon, I. R. H., Boyd, J. L., & McGill, C. W. (1984). *Family care of schizophrenia: A problem-solving approach to the treatment of mental illness.* New York: Guilford.

Feinleib, S. E., Cunningham, P. J., & Short, P. F. (1994). *Use of nursing and personal care homes by the civilian population, 1987.* In Public Health Service, Agency for Health Care Policy and Research, U.S. Department of Health and Human Services, *National medical expenditure survey; Use of nursing and personal care homes by the civilian population, 1987* (Research findings 23). Washington, DC: Government Printing Office.

Fidler, G. S., & Fidler, J. W. (1963). *Occupational therapy; A communication process in psychiatry.* New York: Macmillian.

Fisher, M. S., & Bentley, K. J. (1996). Two group therapy models for clients with a dual diagnosis of substance abuse and personality disorder. *Psychiatric Service, 47,* 1244–1250.

Frances, A., First, M. B., & Pincus, H. A. (1995). *DSM–IV guidebook.* Washington, DC: American Psychiatric Press.

Frank, J. D. (1958). The therapeutic use of self. *American Journal of Occupational Therapy, 12,* 215–225.

Frankl, V. (1963). *Man's search for meaning.* New York: Washington Square Press.

Fratiglioni, L. (1996). Epidemiology of Alzheimer's disease and current possibilities for prevention. *Acta Neurologica Scandinavia, 165*(Suppl.), 33–40.

Freeston, M. H., Ladouceur, R., Gagnon, F., Thibodeau, N., Rhéaume, J., Letarte, H., & Bujold, A. (1997). Cognitive–behavioral treatment of obsessive thoughts: A controlled study. *Journal of Consulting Clinical Psychology, 65,* 403–413.

Gatz, M., Pedersen, N. L., Berg, S., Johansson, B., Johansson, K., Mortimer, J. A., Posner, S. F., Viitanen, M., Winblad, B., & Ahlbom, A. (1997). Heritability for Alzheimer's disease: The study of dementia in Swedish twins. *Journal of Gerontology, 52,* M117–M125.

George, A. A., & Tucker, J. A. (1996). Help-seeking for alcohol-related problems: Social contexts surrounding entry into alcoholism treatment or Alcoholics Anonymous. *Journal of Studies in Alcoholism, 57,* 449–457.

Goldstein, A., & Herrera, J. (1995). Heroin addicts and methadone treatment in Albuquerque: A 22–year follow-up. *Drug Alcohol Dependency, 40,* 139–150.

Goodwin, D. W. (1985). Alcoholism and alcoholic psychoses. In H. I. Kaplan & B. J. Sadock (Eds.), *Comprehensive textbook of psychiatry* (4th ed., pp. 1016–1026). Baltimore: Williams & Williams.

Gorden, C. Y, Schanzenbacher, K. E., Case–Smith, J., & Carrasco, R. C. (1996). Diagnostic problems in pediatrics. In J. Case–Smith, A. S. Allen, & P. N. Pratt (Eds.), *Occupational therapy for children* (3rd ed., pp. 113–162). St. Louis: C. V. Mosby.

Gotthardt, U., Schweiger, U., Fahrenberg, J., Lauer, C. J., Holsboer, F., Heuser, I. (1995). Cortisol, ACTH, and cardiovascular response to a cognitive challenge paradigm in aging and depression. *American Journal of Physiology, 268*(4, Pt. 2), R865–873.

Grace, J., Bellus, S. B., Raulin, M. L., Herz, M. I., Priest, B. L., Brenner, V., Donnelly, K., Smith, P., & Gunn, S. (1996). Long-term impact of clozapine and psychosocial treatment on psychiatric symptoms and cognitive functioning. *Psychiatric Services, 47,* 41–45.

Graham, K., Annis, H. M., Brett, P. J., & Venesoen, P. (1996). A controlled field trial of group versus individual cognitive–behavioural training for relapse prevention. *Addiction, 91,* 1127–1139.

Gurevich, M. I., Duckworth, D., Imhof, J. E., & Katz, J. L. (1996). Is auricular acupuncture beneficial in the inpatient treatment of substance–abusing patients? A pilot study. *Journal of Substance Abuse Treatment, 13,* 165–171.

Hames–Hahn, C., & Llorens, L. (1989). Impact of a multisensory occupational therapy program on components of self-feeding behavior in the elderly. In E. Taira (Ed.), *Promoting quality long term care for older persons* (pp. 63–86). New York: Haworth.

Harvard Mental Health Letter. (1996, February). *Personality disorders: The anxious cluster, part I.* Cambridge, MA: Harvard Medical School.

Hays, K. F. (1995). Psychotherapy and exercise behavior change. *Psychotherapy Bulletin, 30*(3), 29–43.

Heitger, B., & Saameli, W. (1995). [Effectiveness of psychiatric day clinic treatment. An empirical study from the psychiatric service of the Thun regional hospital]. *Schweiz Archives of Neurological Psychiatry, 146*, 33–38.

Henry, A. D., & Coster, W. J. (1996). Predictors of functional outcome among adolescents and young adults with psychotic disorders. *American Journal of Occupational Therapy, 50*, 171–181.

Huebner, R. A. (1992). Autistic disorder: A neuropsychological enigma. *American Journal of Occupational Therapy, 46*, 487–501.

Hultman, C. M., Wieselgren, I. M., & Ohman, A. (1997). Relationships between social support, social coping and life events in the relapse of schizophrenic patients. *Scandinavian Journal of Psychology, 38*, 3–31.

Ivarsson, A-B., Söderback, I., & Stein, F. (2000). Goal, intervention and outcome of occupational therapy in individuals with psychoses. Content analysis through a chart review. *Occupational Therapy International, 7*, 21–41.

Ivey, A. E. (1994). *Intentional interviewing and counseling: Facilitating client development in a multicultural society* (3rd ed.). Belmont, CA: Brooks/Cole.

Jacobs, B. L. (1994). Serotonin, motor activity and depression–related disorders. *American Scientist, 82*, 456–463.

Jahoda, M. (1958). *Current concepts of positive mental health.* New York: Basic Books.

Johnson, S. L., Monroe, S., Simons, A., & Thase, M. E. (1994). Clinical characteristics associated with interpersonal depression: Symptoms, course and treatment response. *Journal of Affective Disorders, 31*, 97–109.

Kabat–Zinn, J., Massion, A. O., Kristeller, J., Peterson, L. G., Fletcher, K. E., Pbert, L., Lenderking, W. R., & Santorelli, S. F. (1992). Effectiveness of a meditation-based stress reduction program in the treatment of anxiety disorder. *American Journal of Psychiatry, 149*, 936–943.

Kane, J. M. (1995). Dosing issues and depot medication in the maintenance treatment of schizophrenia. *International Clinics of Psychopharmacology, 10*(Suppl. 3), 65–71.

Kaplan, H. I., Sadock, B. J., & Grebb, J. A. (1994). *Synopsis of psychiatric behavioral sciences, clinical psychiatry* (7th ed.). Baltimore: Williams & Wilkins.

Kauffman, J. M. (1997). *Characteristics of behavior disorders of children and youth* (6th ed.). Columbus, OH: Merrill.

Kazdin, A. E. (1995). Child, parent and family dysfunction as predictors of outcome in cognitive–behavioral treatment of antisocial children. *Behavioral Research Therapy, 33*, 271–281.

Kiecolt–Glaser, J. K., & Glaser, R. (1989). Psychoneuroimmunology: Past, present, and future. *Health Psychology, 8*, 677–682.

Klijnsma, M. P., Cameron, M. L., Burns, T. P., & McGuigan, S. M. (1995). Out-patient alcohol detoxification—outcome after 2 months. *Alcohol & Alcoholism, 30*, 669–673.

Kurtz, P. (1974). Treating chemical dependency through biofeedback. *Hospital Progress, 55*, 68–70.

Lebowitz, B. D., & Niederehe, G. (1992). Concepts and issues in mental health and aging. In J. E. Birren, R. B. Sloane, & G. D. Cohen (Eds.), *Handbook of mental health and aging* (2nd ed., pp. 3–26). San Diego: Academic.

Lechin, F., Van der Dijs, B., & Benaim, M. (1996). Stress versus depression. *Progress in Neuro-Psychopharmacological and Biological Psychiatry, 20*, 899–950.

Lechin, F., Van de Dijs, B., Orozco, B., Lechin, M. E., Báez, S., Lechin, A. E., Rada, I., Acosta, E., Arocha, L., Jiménez, V., et al. (1995). Plasma neurotransmitters, blood pressure, and heart rate during supine-resting, orthostasis and moderate exercise conditions in major depressed patients. *Biological Psychiatry, 38*, 166–173.

Lehmann, H. E. (1985). Current perspectives on the biology of schizophrenia. In M. N. Menuck & M. V. Seeman (Eds.), *New perspectives in schizophrenia* (pp. 3–31). New York: Macmillan.

Lehrer, P. M., & Woolfolk, R. L. (1993). Specific effects of stress management techniques. In P. M. Lehrer & R. L. Woolfolk (Eds.), *Principles and practice of stress management* (2nd ed., pp. 481–520). New York: Guilford Press.

Leon, R. L. (1989). *Psychiatric interviewing: A primer* (2nd ed.). New York: Elsevier.

Leonard, K. E., & Blane, H. T. (1987). Conclusion. In H. T. Blane & K. E. Leonard (Eds.), *Psychological theories of drinking and alcoholism* (pp. 388–395). New York: Guilford.

Levison, D. F., & Mowry, B. J. (1991). Defining the schizophrenia spectrum: Issues for genetic linkage studies. *Schizophrenia Bulletin, 17*, 491–514.

Lezak, M. (1995). *Neuropsychological assessment* (3rd ed.). New York: Oxford.

Liberman, R. P., & Kopelowica, A. (1995). Basic elements in biobehavioral treatment and rehabilitation of schizophrenia. *International Clinics of Psychopharmacology, 9*(Suppl. 5), 51–58.

Lieberman, M. A., & Peskin, H. (1992). Adult life crises. In J. E. Birren, R. B. Sloane, & G. D. Cohen (Eds.), *Handbook of mental health and aging* (2nd ed., pp. 119–143). San Diego: Academic Press.

Long, P. W. (1995–1997). *Alcohol dependence*. Retrieved October 3, 1997, from the World Wide Web: *http://www.mentalhealth.com/rx/p23-sb01.html*.

Mahendran, R., Ibrahim, K., & Tan, Y. P. (1995). Psychiatric day centres—The Singapore experience. *Singapore Medical Journal, 36*, 644–646.

Martin, K., Giannandrea, P., Rogers, B., & Johnson, J. (1996). Group intervention with pre-recovery patients. *Journal of Substance Abuse Treatment, 13*, 33–41.

Maslow, A. H. (1950). Self-actualizing people: A study of psychological health. *Personality Symposia, 1*, 16.

Maslow, A. H. (1956). Self-actualizing people: A study of psychological health. In C. E. Moustakas (Ed.), *The self: Explorations in personal growth* (pp. 160–194). New York: Harper & Row.

McGlashan, T. H. (1988). Adolescent versus adult onset of mania. *American Journal of Psychiatry, 145*, 221–223.

McGrath, E., Keita, G. P., Strickland, B. R., & Russo, N. F. (1990). *Women and depression: Risk factors and treatment issues*. Washington, DC: American Psychological Association.

McLellan, A. T., & Childress, A. R. (1985). Aversive therapies for substance abuse: Do they work? *Journal of Substance Abuse Treatment, 2*, 187–191.

Meichenbaum, D. (1993). Stress inoculation training: A 20-year update. In P. M. Lehrer & R. L. Woolfolk (Eds.), *Principles and practice of stress management* (2nd ed., pp. 373–406). New York: Guilford Press.

Menditto, A. A., Beck, N. C., Stuve, P., Fisher, J. A., Stacy, M., Logue, M. B., & Baldwin, L. J. (1996). Effectiveness of clozapine and a social learning program for severely disabled psychiatric inpatients. *Psychiatric Services, 47*, 46–51.

Moenking, H. S., Hornung, W. P., Stricker, K., & Buchkremer, G. (1997). Expressed-emotional development and course of schizophrenic illness: Considerations based on results of a CFI replication. *European Archives Psychiatry Clinical Neuroscience, 247*, 31–34.

Moustakas, C. E. (1956). True experiences and the self. In C. E. Moustakas (Ed.), *The self* (pp. 3–14). New York: Harper.

Moyers, P. A. (1992). Occupational therapy intervention with the alcoholic's family. *American Journal of Occupational Therapy, 46*, 105–111.

Moyers, P. A. (1997). Occupational meanings and spirituality: The quest for sobriety. *American Journal of Occupational Therapy, 51*, 207–214.

Murphy, G. E., Carney, R. M., Knesevich, M. A., Wetzel, R. D., & Whitworth, P. (1995). Cognitive behavior therapy, relaxation training, and tricyclic antidepressant medication in the treatment of depression. *Psychological Reports, 77*, 403–420.

National Institute of Mental Health [NIMH]. (1997). *Launch of NIMH anxiety disorders educational program*. Retrieved January 30, 2001, from the World Wide Web: *http://www.cyberpsych.org/nimh.htm*.

National Institute of Mental Health [NIMH]. (1999). *Schizophrenia*. Retrieved January 30, 2001, from the World Wide Web: *http://www.nimh.nih.gov/publicat/schizoph.htm.*

National Institute on Aging. (1996). *Progress report on Alzheimer's disease, 1996.* (NIH Publication No. 96–4137). Washington, DC: National Institutes of Health. Retrieved January 30, 2001, from the World Wide Web: *http://www.alzheimers.org/pr96text.html.*

Neuchterlein, K. H., Dawson, M. E., Gitlin, M., Ventura, J., Goldstein, M. J., Snuyder, K. S., Yee, C. M., & Mintz, J. (1992). Developmental processes in schizophrenic disorders: Longitudinal studies of vulnerability and stress. *Schizophrenic Bulletin, 18,* 387–423.

Norman, R. M. G., & Malla, A. K. (1993). Stressful life events and schizophrenia. I: A review of the research. *British Journal of Psychiatry, 162,* 161–166.

Page, R., & Schaub, L. (1978). EMG biofeedback applicability for differing personality types. *Journal of Clinical Psychology, 34,* 1014–1020.

Penn, D. L., & Mueser, K. T. (1996). Research update on the psychosocial treatment of schizophrenia. *American Journal of Psychiatry, 153,* 607–617.

Pettinati, H. M. (1996). Use of serotonin selective pharmacotherapy in the treatment of alcohol dependence. *Alcoholism and Clinical Experimental Research, 20*(Suppl.), 23A–29A.

Peuskens, J. (1996). Proper psychosocial rehabilitation for stabilised patients with schizophrenia: The role of new therapies. *European Neuropsychopharmacology, 6*(Suppl. 2), S7–S12.

Polles, A. G., & Smith, P. O. (1995). Treatment of coexisting substance dependence and posttraumatic stress disorder. *Psychiatric Services, 46,* 729–730.

Raskind, M. A., & Peskind, E. R. (1992). Alzheimer's disease and other dementing disorders. In J. E. Birren, R. B. Sloane, & G. D. Cohen (Eds.), *Handbook of mental health and aging* (2nd ed., pp. 477–513). San Diego: Academic Press.

Rice, K. M., Blanchard, E. B., & Purcell, M. (1993). Biofeedback treatments of generalized anxiety disorder: Preliminary results. *Biofeedback and Self Regulation, 18,* 93–105

Rogers, C. (1977). *Carl Rogers on personal power.* New York: Delacorte.

Rohsenow, D. J., Smith, R. E., & Johnson, S. (1985). Stress management training as a prevention program for heavy social drinkers: Cognitions, affect, drinking, and individual differences. *Addictive Behavior, 10,* 45–54.

Rotert, D. A. (1993). Occupational therapy in alcoholism. *Occupational Therapy Practice, 4*(2), 1–11. (Original work published 1989)

Rund, B. R., Oie, M., Borchgrevink, T. S., & Fjell, A. (1995). Expressed emotions, communication deviance and schizophrenia. An exploratory study of the relationship between two family variables and the course and outcome of a psychoeducational treatment programme. *Psychopathology, 28,* 220–228.

Schact, T., & Nathan, P. E. (1977). But is it good for the psychologists? Appraisal and status of DSM–III. *American Psychologist, 32,* 1017–1025.

Scott, J. E., & Dixon, L. B. (1995). Psychological interventions for schizophrenia. *Schizophrenia Bulletin, 21,* 621–630.

Sholle–Martin, S., & Allessi, N. E. (1990). Formulating a role for occupational therapy in child psychiatry: A clinical application. *American Journal of Occupational Therapy, 44,* 871–882.

Stanley, M. A., Beck, J. G., Averill, P. M., Baldwin, L. E., Deagle, E. A., & Stadler, J. G. (1996). Patterns of change during cognitive behavioral treatment for panic disorder. *Journal of Nervous Mental Disorder, 184,* 567–572.

Steffen, J. (1975). Electromyographically induced relaxation in the treatment of chronic alcohol abuse. *Journal of Counseling and Clinical Psychology, 43,* 275.

Stetter, F., Zähres, S., Batra, A., & Mann, K. (1995). [Results of integrated inpatient detoxification and motivation treatment of alcohol dependent patients]. *Psychiatrische Praxis, 22,* 189–192.

Stevens, S. J., & Arbiter, N. (1995). A therapeutic community for substance-abusing pregnant women and women with children: Process and outcome. *Journal of Psychoactive Drugs, 27,* 49–56.

Stevens–Ratchford, R. G. (1993). The effect of life review reminiscence activities on depression and self-esteem in older adults. *American Journal of Occupational Therapy, 47,* 413–420.

Storr, A. (1980). *The art of psychotherapy.* New York: Methuen.

Stoyva, J. M., & Budzynski, T. H. (1993). Biofeedback methods in the treatment of anxiety and stress disorders. In P. M. Lehrer & R. L. Woolfolk (Eds.), *Principles and practice of stress management* (2nd ed., pp. 263–300). New York: Guilford Press.

Substance Abuse and Mental Health Services Administration. (1997). *1996 National Household Survey on Drug Abuse.* Retrieved January 30, 2001, from the World Wide Web: *http://www.samhsa .gov/oas/nhsda/pe1996/rtst1006.htm.*

Townsend, R., House, J., & Addario, D. (1975). A comparison of biofeedback-mediated relaxation and group therapy in the treatment of chronic anxiety. *American Journal of Psychiatry, 132,* 598–601.

Trace, S., & Howell, T. (1991). Occupational therapy in geriatric mental health. *American Journal of Occupational Therapy, 45,* 833–838.

Turner, R. H., & Vanderlippe, R. H. (1965). Self-ideal congruence as an index of adjustment. In G. Lindzey & C. S. Hall (Eds.), *Theories of personality: Primary sources and research* (pp. 494–504). New York: John Wiley.

U.S. Congress. Office of Technology Assessment. (1994). *Psychiatric disabilities, employment, and the Americans with Disabilities Act.* OTA–BP–BBS–124. Washington, DC: Government Printing Office. Retrieved January 28, 2001, from the World Wide Web: *http://www.wws. princeton.edu/~ota/disk1/1994/9427.html.*

Van Deusen, J. (1989). Alcohol abuse and perceptual-motor dysfunction: The occupational therapist's role. *American Journal of Occupational Therapy, 43,* 384–390.

van Kammen, D. P. (1991). The biochemical basis of replase and drug response in schizophrenia: Review and hypothesis. *Psychological Medicine, 21,* 881–895.

Wing, J. K., & Furlong, R. (1986). A haven for the severely disabled within the context of a comprehensive psychiatric community service. *British Journal of Psychiatry, 149,* 449–457.

Wynne, L. C., Rykoff, I. M., Day, J., & Hirsch, S. I. (1958). Pseudomutuality in the family relationships of schizophrenics. *Psychiatry, 21,* 205–220.

Yerxa, E. J. (1967). 1966 Eleanor Clarke Slagle Lecture: Authentic occupational therapy. *American Journal of Occupational Therapy, 21,* 1–8.

Zigman, W., Schupf, N., Haveman, M., & Silverman, W. (1997). The epidemiology of Alzheimer disease in intellectual disability: Results and recommendations from an international conference. *Journal of Intellectual Disability Research, 41*(Pt. 1), 76–80.

Zisselman, M. H., Rovner, B. W., Shmuely, Y., & Ferrie, P. (1996). A pet therapy intervention with geriatric psychiatry inpatients. *American Journal of Occupational Therapy, 50,* 47–51.

CHAPTER

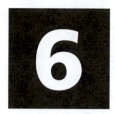

Evaluation and Assessment of the Individual with Psychosocial Dysfunction

> *An integrative approach assures that the client is viewed from a holistic philosophy. This means that using the four areas of human function [adaptive performance, biodevelopmental, facilitating growth and development, and occupational behavior] to assess the client, encourages the therapist to administer a variety of assessments that are based on different theoretical premises.*
>
> —B. J. Hemphill (1988a), An Integrative Approach to the Use of Occupational Therapy Assessments in Mental Health, in B. J. Hemphill (Ed.), *Mental Health Assessment in Occupational Therapy*, p. 4.

Operational Learning Objectives

By the end of this chapter, the learner will:

1. Define evaluation and key concepts in measurement.

2. State major purposes of testing in psychosocial programs.

3. State the differential roles of mental health professionals in testing.

4. Recognize the sources of error in testing or possible factors in the environment, tester, subject, or test instrument that can potentially distort the test results.

5. Understand how to select reliable and valid tests.

6. Identify the skills necessary in administrating, scoring, and interpreting results.

7. Identify the function to be measured within performance areas of work, leisure/play, self-care (ADL), and social skills.

8. Establish a test battery and identify standardized assessment tools.

9. Apply tests to specific psychosocial diagnostic groups.

10. Adapt or modify tests procedures.

11. Interpret evaluation results to client, family, and team members based on results of test and clinical observations, incorporating results into a progress note.

Focusing Questions

▶ What is the evaluation process?

▶ What is assessment?

▶ What is the difference between evaluation and assessment?

▶ Why are evaluation and assessment important in designing psychosocial treatment programs?

▶ What are the major areas that occupational therapists assess in psychosocial practice?

▶ How do occupational therapists select a reliable and valid test?

▶ What factors can result in error in testing?

▶ What are the assessment tools used currently by occupational therapists in psychosocial practice?

▶ What is functional assessment?

▶ Why is functional assessment important?

▶ What is the relationship between functional assessment and the uniform terminology from AOTA?

▶ How are clinical observations used in assessment?

▶ What is the relationship between assessment and cultural environment?

▶ How do we devise a test battery that can be used by a psychosocial occupational therapist?

OVERVIEW AND DEFINITIONS

Client evaluation is an integral part of the treatment process where the psychosocial occupational therapist plans an individual treatment program based on the results of testing. However, the role of the occupational therapist in evaluation is different than that of other mental health professionals. Table 6–1 describes the differential roles of mental health professionals.

In practice, however, client evaluation by psychosocial occupational therapists is not always used systematically to plan and document treatment. There is a wide variation in the types of assessments used by psychosocial occupational therapists. Additionally, the quality of tests used varies in reliability and validity. Occupational therapists should use valid and reliable tests and follow standard administration practices if norms are to be applied in interpreting raw scores. When clinical judgment suggests that the standard administration of a test should not be followed (e.g., when a patient is so depressed that he or she is not responding), then the norms cannot be used. However, this process may tell the clinician more about the client and result in more appropriate treatment goals. Custom-made tests are developed by some occupational therapists needlessly, without doing a careful search of the literature to identify whether there is a published test that can be readily used.

Skills in assessment and measurement should be taught systematically on the undergraduate or graduate level to adequately prepare clinicians. Students should learn about test instruments and have sufficient practice in administering them in both the classroom and field work. They should have the opportunity to be critiqued by their peers or instructors. With this process, students will:

Table 6–1. Examples of Differential Roles in Assessment for Mental Health Professionals

Profession	Traditional Method	Content of Assessment	Purpose of Assessment	Examples of Specific Instruments
OCCUPATIONAL THERAPIST	• behavioral observation	• functional skills in self-care, leisure/play, work, and social interactions	• enabling independent living	• *Role Checklist* (Barris, Oakley, & Kielhofner, 1988) • *Kohlman Evaluation of Living Skills* (KELS; Thomson, 1992)
PSYCHIATRIC NURSE	• clinical observation	• interpersonal interactions	• documenting patient interactions	• *Parachek Geriatric Rating Scale* (Parachek & King, 1986)
PSYCHIATRIST	• psychiatric interview	• abnormal behavior	• establishing diagnostic category	• *Diagnostic and Statistical Manual* (DSM-IV; American Psychiatric Association, 1994)
PSYCHOLOGIST	• standardized objective and projective tests	• personality • intelligence • aptitude	• interpreting personality characteristics and behavior	• *Minnesota Multiphasic Personality Inventory* (MMPI; Hathaway & McKinley, 1943) • *Wechsler Scales* (The Psychological Corporation)
REHABILITATION COUNSELOR	• simulated work tasks	• vocational	• identifying feasible occupations	• *Valpar tests* (Valpar Corporation) • work samples
SPECIAL EDUCATOR	• norm-referenced tests (NRTs) • criterion-referenced tests (CRTs)	• academic achievement	• identifying academic strengths and weaknesses	• *Woodcock-Johnson-III®* *Tests of Achievement–III* (WJ-III; Woodcock, McGrew, & Mathers, 2000)) • *Wechsler Individual Achievement Tests* (WIAT-2; Psychological Corporation, 2000) • *Comprehensive Inventory of Basic Skills -- Revised* (CIBS; Brigance, 2000)
SOCIAL WORKER	• family interview	• family dynamics	• interpreting social interactions	• *Index of Family Relations* (Hudson, 1982)

Source: Adapted from "Research Analysis of Occupational Therapy Assessments Used in Mental Health," by F. Stein, 1988. In *Mental Health Assessment in Occupational Therapy: An Integrative Approach to the Evaluative Process,* by B. J. Hemphill, Thorofare, NJ: SLACK.

▶ have knowledge of available tests

▶ know where to look for bibliographies of tests (e.g., books, test catalogs, Internet through ERIC)

▶ select an appropriate test instrument or test battery for a performance area and specific performance component within a target population

▶ evaluate the validity and reliability of tests (Search *Tests in Print–V* [Murphy, Impara, & Plake, 1999] for current review of test)

▶ incorporate test results into a psychosocial program including development of appropriate treatment goals

▶ determine skills necessary to give tests following standard administration

▶ score and interpret tests accurately

▶ report test results to clients, families, and interdisciplinary staff

Definition of Evaluation

Clinical evaluation is the process of systematically observing the characteristics of individuals in a standardized manner. An evaluation usually includes a battery of tests, which may be completed in one or more sessions, and the therapist's objective observations. The results of the evaluation, recorded in the client's record, should summarize the strengths and weaknesses. These results are used in designing a treatment program, formulating treatment goals, or recommending discharge or termination of services. The evaluation process is summative. Assessment, on the other hand, is ongoing and provides the therapist with a continuous record of client progress. Assessment is considered formative and enables the therapist to readjust treatment goals and practices (Table 6–2). Examples of questions in evaluation are:

▶ What are the self-care skills of a client with a psychosocial dysfunction?

Table 6-2. Definitions and Characteristics of Evaluation, Assessment, Test Instruments, and Clinical Observations

	Definition	Purpose	Frequency
Evaluation	Overall judgment of individual's behavior, characteristics, aptitudes, and present functioning that is gained through specific tests, clinical observations, and procedures	To determine skills, aptitude, and behavior of client before initiating therapy, establishing long-term goals, and determining continued need for treatment	Completed at initial interview and at discharge
Assessment	Critical appraisal of client's functional abilities in everyday tasks. Includes clinical observations, tests, facility-generated procedures, and client interviews	To generate short-term goals, determine need for modification of treatment, and document progress	Continual process of assessing client at each therapy session
Test	Tool used to obtain information for a specific area of a client's functioning	Serves as an integral part of evaluation and/or assessment	Used as needed in the evaluation and assessment process
Clinical Observation	Method of observing client's verbal and nonverbal behavior	To understand a client's approach and motivation in learning a task. These are incorporated into the assessment process and SOAP notes	Used during treatment sessions

▶ How well does a client with schizophrenia perform in a simulated work situation?

▶ Is this client prepared to live independently in the community?

▶ Has the client improved over the course of treatment?

Examples of questions in assessment are:

▶ How effective is biofeedback in increasing relaxation in a client with depression?

▶ How effective are specific activities used in sensory integration therapy in increasing attention span?

▶ How effective is an exercise program in helping the client to gain self-esteem?

Basic Concepts in Psychosocial Testing

To understand testing and evaluation, some key concepts must be defined. What is a test? How do we measure reliability and validity? What are potential sources of error in testing? What are measures of central tendency and variability? These key concepts are listed in Table 6–3.

The evaluation/assessment process is ongoing and is used to objectively appraise the client's assets and weaknesses or his or her improvement in a specific performance area or component. In order to objectively appraise performance or improvement, criteria must be set. How do you determine the criteria? One way is to examine the norms established for a specific test. For example, when considering typical levels of anxiety, the therapist must have norms or the universally accepted criteria for interpreting a client's raw score. Another way is to examine outcome criteria. Outcome criteria are used to evaluate client progress. For example, the occupational therapist identifies measurable criteria, such as interpersonal skills, self-esteem, or self-

care. Then, the client's pretest scores are compared to the posttest scores to measure the progress made by the client.

Purpose of Testing

The purposes of psychosocial testing are to (a) plan treatment goals, (b) determine prognosis, (c) establish baseline data, (d) document patient progress before and after intervention, (e) document progress for reimbursement purposes, (f) motivate the client, and (g) carry out clinical research.

▶ *Planning treatment programs.* Evaluation of client's strengths and weaknesses allows the therapist to plan a treatment program that will be beneficial and therapeutic. For example, the *Kohlman Evaluation of Living Skills* (KELS; Thomson, 1992) or the *Canadian Occupational Performance Measure* (COPM; Chan & Lee, 1997; Law et al., 1994) enable therapists to identify capabilities of clients in order to plan appropriate treatments. The planning of treatment programs involve formulating both short- and long-term treatment objectives. Short-term objectives serve to reduce acute symptoms; long-term objectives serve in the planning of major lifetime adjustments. For example, the short-term objectives for an individual with high anxiety would include reducing the level of stress and anxiety. Long-term objectives would include planning ways the individual can be successful in a working environment even when there are anxious moments.

▶ *Determine prognosis.* The evaluation serves to help the therapist determine prognosis of the episode of illness and the client's potential for improvement. The therapist seeks to answer the question "Is the disability chronic or progressive"?

Table 6–3. Key Definitions in Tests and Measurements

- A *test* is essentially an objective and standardized measure of a sample of behavior (Anastasi & Urbina, 1997).

- A *measurement scale* is a system of assigning scores to a trait or characteristic.

- *Reliability* is the extent to which the test gives consistent results when administered by different therapists on different occasions. The major types used to measure reliability is test-retest; however, other forms, such as split half and equivalency forms are also used.

- *Validity* is the extent to which a test measures what it is designed to measure. Types of validity include face, content, concurrent, predictive, and construct.

- *Content* or *face validity* is the extent to which the test matches the content of the task of material. For example, examining a test on self-concept to see if the language used is consistent with the purpose of the test is content validity.

- *Predictive validity* is the extent to which a test can predict success or accuracy over a period of time. For example, predicting a client's ability to live in the community after discharge from the hospital is predictive validity.

- *Construct validity* is the extent to which the test measures a theoretical construct. For example, generating test items based on a theoretical construct (e.g., *Southern California Test of Sensory Integration*).

- *Concurrent validity* is the degree of correlation with another standardized instrument. For example, a new test of stress is correlated with a test of stress that has an established high reliability and validity.

- The *sources of error in measurement* are derived, for example, from the unreliability of the instrument, bias of the test administrator, unreliability of the client, and undesirable test environment.

- *Percentile* is a point in a distribution that defines where a given percentage of the cases fall. For example, the 89th percentile is the point where 89% of the cases are at or below that score.

- *Percentage* is the number of cases per hundred.

- *Raw score* is the score obtained directly on the test before transforming into a more meaningful comparison (e.g., z-score, percentile, standard score).

- *Standard score* describes the individual's performance on the test as the distance from the mean using standard deviation units. For example, with a standard score (z-score) of -1, in a distribution of a mean of 100 and a standard deviation of 15, the score is expressed as 85.

- *Normal curve* is a bell-shaped distribution where the mean, mean, and mode all fall at the 50th percentile and 0 z-score, and where 68.26% of the cases fall between -1 and +1 standard deviation units (z-scores). Many human characteristics, such as height and weight, are normally distributed.

- *Measures of central tendency* include the mean (average score), mode (the most frequent score), and the median (the 50th percentile or middle score).

- *Measures of variability* include the standard deviation (the degree of dispersion in the scores), and the range (the difference between the highest and lowest scores).

▶ *Document progress.* One way to do this is to use pre- and posttesting after treatment intervention. For example, a therapist may use an anxiety scale, such as the *State-Trait Anxiety Inventory* (Spielberger, 1983), on admission and discharge to measure the reduction of symptomatology in the client. Progress needs to be monitored frequently so that changes in treatment can be made if no improvement is seen.

▶ *Make a diagnosis.* Testing is used to differentially describe symptoms in a client to arrive at an accurate diagnosis. The DSM–IV criteria are used in establishing a diagnosis.

▶ *Psychodynamic formulations.* Members of the mental health team use evaluation and assessment to understand some of the motivations and dynamics underlying the client's behavior. For example, the *Magazine Picture Collage* (Lerner & Ross, 1977) may be used by the occupational therapist to identify personality characteristics. The MMPI (Hathaway & McKinley, 1943), one of the personality instruments commonly used by the psychologist, can also be helpful to the occupational therapist in planning short- and long-term treatment goals.

▶ *Evaluate effectiveness of clinical treatment.* Using pre- and posttesting, and assessing improvement over the course of treatment, enables the therapist to assess the efficacy of treatment. If little or no progress is seen, the therapist should re-evaluate the client and seek another treatment method.

▶ *Motivate the client.* The therapist shares the test results with the client and provides immediate feedback about his or her progress. In so doing, the therapist seeks the client's active participation in the treatment process.

Assumptions Underlying Evaluation and Testing

What are some of the assumptions in clinical evaluation and assessment that guide a clinician? The major assumptions are outlined below.

▶ Evaluation is essential in the treatment process in assessing and reassessing the client. It is used to determine abilities in performance areas and performance components.

▶ Evaluation is used as an outcome measure.

▶ Adequate evaluation is based on using reliable and valid tests. The degree of accuracy in measurement depends on the degree of reliability (consistency) and validity (accuracy).

▶ Evaluation always has some error. The error is derived from improper or changes in the administration of the test; lack of motivation, anxiety, or negative mood of the client; adverse environmental conditions; and the psychometric properties of the test.

▶ Evaluation can provide data for (a) the medical record and documenting client progress (SOAP note), (b) eligibility for reimbursement, and (c) clinical research.

The evaluation of outcome in psychosocial practice depends on the quality of the test instrument. What are the characteristics of a good test instrument in psychosocial practice?

Characteristics of a Good Test in Psychosocial Practice (Stein, 1988)

▶ Are norms established for the test variable? For example, what is considered for an individual to be classified as depressed on a given test? What are the norms for anxiety?

▶ What are the operational purposes of the test? For example, can the test be used to measure outcome, plan treatment goals, or document progress?

▶ What variables are measured by the test? For example, does the test purport to measure independent living skills, leisure interests, social skills, or health status?

▶ How does the test or instrument gather information?
  ▶ *client self-evaluation*
  ▶ *formal observation*

▶ *projective tests*

▶ *biofeedback or physiological measures*

▶ *standardized performance tests*

▶ *therapist rating scales*

▶ Does the test have a standardized procedure for administering it? Are there clearly written directions for the client taking the test?

▶ Is there a clearly written manual for the therapist and are there tables for interpreting raw scores?

▶ Does the therapist need special training in administering, scoring, and interpreting the test?

▶ Are there research studies to support the use of the test in clinical practice?

Scales of Measurement

When we evaluate a client's progress, we are essentially measuring a variable. Measurement can be broken down into two areas: categorical or continuous. Categorical measurement consists of (a) classifying variables, such as the diagnosis given a patient; or (b) ranking levels of performance, such as evaluating the degree of independence in self-help skills. Continuous measurement consists of assigning numbers to (a) characteristics, such as intelligence or (b) abilities, such as social skills. These numbers are broken down into equal integrals (i.e., interval scale) and may have an absolute zero point (i.e., ratio scale).

Qualification Levels

Qualification levels are set by the APA Standards for Educational and Psychological Testing.

▶ Level A requires no special qualification.

▶ Level B requires at least a bachelor's degree in psychology, counseling, or a closely related field and relevant training.

▶ Level C requires (a) a graduate degree in clinical or counseling psychology, school psychology, counseling or a closely related field and training, (b) membership in a professional association that requires training and experience in the ethical and competent use of testing (e.g., American Psychological Association [APA], National Association of School Psychologists [NASP]), or (c) license or certification from an agency that requires training in testing. Almost all test publishing companies adhere to this policy (Davis, 1974).

METHODS USED IN OCCUPATIONAL THERAPY EVALUATIONS

What methods are most commonly used in psychosocial occupational therapy to evaluate client performance and progress? Historically, psychosocial occupational therapists have used a number of evaluation methods in the clinic. The most basic methods are:

▶ *Clinical observation:* This procedure focuses on nonverbal and verbal cues that the therapist observes while a client is working on an activity. Examples of nonverbal cues include facial expressions, body language, gestures, and expressions of pain, sadness, pleasure, anxiety, and anger. Verbal cues include comments made by the client as an aside or to family members who may be present, to other clients, and directly to the therapist. An example of an observational test is the *Functional Assessment Scale* (FAS; Breines, 1988).

▶ *Initial interview:* This method provides an opportunity to establish a therapeutic alliance between the therapist and client during the process of initially evaluating the client's personal strengths and weaknesses, interests, and level of motivation. An example is the *Worker Role Interview* (WRI; Velozo, Kielhofner, & Fisher, 1990).

▶ *Self-report inventories*: Checklists and surveys filled out by the client either alone or in company of the therapist comprise this method. The information obtained is "self-reported" by the client. Examples are the *Stress Management Questionnaire* (SMQ; Stein, 1987), the *Hamilton Depression Inventory* (HDI; Reynolds & Kobak, 1995), *State-Trait Anxiety Inventory* (STAI; Spielberger, 1983).

▶ *Functional tasks*: Simulated tasks are used to evaluate the client's ability to carry out activities of daily living and self-care activities with or without assistance. Such activities might involve personal hygiene, feeding or cooking, and driving an automobile. Examples of tests include *Kohlman Evaluation of Living Skills* (KELS; Thomson, 1992) and *The Milwaukee Evaluation of Daily Living Skills* (MEDLS; Leonardelli, 1988).

▶ *Standardized tests*: These are published and unpublished tests that have a standardized procedure, normative data, reliability, and validity data. Examples of such tests include the *Bay Area Functional Performance Evaluation* (BaFPE; Williams & Bloomer, 1987) or the *Allen Cognitive Levels* (ACL; Allen, 1985).

▶ *Behavioral assessment*: These assessments rate the client as he or she performs the task in an unstructured manner or non-standardized setting. Examples include the *Independent Living Skills Evaluation* (ILSE; Johnson, Vinnicombe, & Merrill, 1980) and the *Jacobs Prevocational Skills Assessment* (JPSA; Jacobs, 1985).

▶ *Machine monitoring*: This procedure involves the recording of physiological and motor responses, such as in biofeedback training and muscle re-education. Examples of machine monitoring include the EMG, heart rate monitor, blood pressure cuff, and finger temperature trainer.

▶ *Work sampling*: Work samples are well-defined activities that are similar to those performed on an actual job. They can be used to assess an individual's vocational aptitude, worker characteristics, and vocational interests (Nadolsky, 1974). Examples of work samples include tests published by Valpar (Valpar Corporation).

▶ *Projective testing*. This method involves using unstructured but standardized procedures to gain insight into the client's personality structure and dynamics of behavior. Examples of these tasks include the *Magazine Picture Collage* (MPC; Lerner, 1982).

▶ *Computerized assessment*. A number of instruments have been adapted for the computer for ease of scoring and analysis. Examples of these include the *Stress Management Questionnaire* (SMQ; Stein, Bently, & Natz, 1999), the computer-assisted questionnaire on *Adolescent Risk-Taking Behaviors* (Black, Gordon, & Santelli, 1999); and the *OT FACT* (Smith, 1999). The latter tool is a system for analyzing ADL and IADL skills and which provides a comprehensive summary of a client's abilities using the *Uniform Terminology* (AOTA, 1994).

MODULE FOR LEARNING

TEST ADMINISTRATION

Environmental Considerations

Consideration should be given to arranging a test environment for administrating any test. The environment should be quiet and without distractions. There should be enough room for the tester and testee to simulate a realistic testing situation. Lighting, temperature, and noise are factors that affect the validity of the results. The room should have a table on which to work and chairs that are ergonomically correct. Prior to administering the test, the tester should read through the test manual and examine the test materials. Any additional materials that might be needed should be collected and available.

Administrative Considerations

When a student is learning to administer a new test, he or she should become familiar with (a) the purposes of the test and (b) the directions for giving the test. Good test administration requires practice in giving the test. Following are some guidelines for developing these skills:

▶ *Become familiar with test directions and purposes of the test.* Read the manual thoroughly before practicing administration of the test. Of utmost importance are understanding the purposes of the test and learning the specific directions, such as positioning of the test materials, following the wording verbatim, and accurate timing.

▶ *Arrange test materials neatly on the table with a stopwatch or clock if needed.* Make sure that all test materials are available before testing begins and that there is enough room on the table for the client to take the test.

▶ *Position yourself and the client comfortably.*

Usually the examiner will sit across from the client. Accommodate the client if he or she is in a wheelchair. Consider the ergonomic aspect of the chair and table in relationship to the client.

▶ *Establish rapport with the client.* Before giving the test, establish a nonthreatening and friendly environment for the client so that anxiety and lack of motivation are reduced. Some testers establish rapport by asking clients about neutral topics. For example, the examiner might ask, "What do you enjoy doing?" "What do you like to do most?" or "What are your favorite pasttime activities?"

▶ *Be sure to answer any questions the client may have before administering the test.* Some clients may be concerned about the purpose of the testing, how long the testing will take, or how the results of the test will be used. The evaluator may have to initiate the questions, for example, by asking the client, "Do you have any questions about the test and its purposes?" or "Do you know why you're here?" This should help to prevent the client from interrupting the test administration with questions and may alleviate some of the client's anxiety.

▶ *Speak clearly and directly in explaining directions for the test.* Use the exact words in the testing manual. Read the directions as if you are talking to the client. There is no need to memorize the directions. Consider the client's ability to process information when reading the directions.

▶ *Demonstrate to the client what has to be done and follow the directions verbatim.* In a performance test, be prepared to demonstrate to the client what has to be done. The examiner should practice taking the performance test and saying the directions before administering the test.

▶ *If the subject has a question, be noncommittal and reassuring.* If a client asks how he or she is doing, be encouraging and say things like, "You're doing a good job," "You're working well." Never tell the client whether the item was correct or incorrect. Scoring should be done after the test is completed. The examiner should take notes during the evaluation pertaining to the client's anxiety, fatigue, motivation, and attitude toward the test. Any unusual behavior should be noted; for example, obsessively looking at one's watch, tracing letters before reading or copying, or reading aloud. Be sure to inform the client before testing that notes will be taken.

▶ *Have an objective attitude during testing.* Maintain a professional, objective, and noncommittal demeanor during the evaluation. Good eye contact, friendly reassurance, and appropriate dress are all important and can potentially affect the results of the evaluation.

Scoring and Interpretation of the Test

Another essential skill in giving the test is scoring and interpretation. The evaluator must read the manual carefully to determine how to score the test. In some tests, the raw score is converted to a standard score using conversion tables based on age, gender, or occupation. The examiner must be careful to use the correct conversion table. An interpretation of the test requires the examiner to identify ranges of scores. These ranges should be found in the manual.

In addition to finding ranges of scores, interpretation involves hypothesizing why a client may have performed in a particular manner. For

example, was the client motivated to do his or her utmost during the test? Did the client understand what was to be done? Did the client receive a low score because of difficulties in reading? Was the client able to stay on task during the performance evaluation or was he or she distracted during the task? Does the client do better when allowed to verbalize while performing the task or can the client perform adequately without verbalizing? These behaviors can give insight into the client's learning style.

Essential Questions in Analyzing Test Instruments

As a learner practices administering various test instruments, he or she may want to keep a record of the description, purposes, and skills necessary for giving the test. Table 6-4 includes a form that may be helpful for analyzing a test instrument.

Self-Evaluation

In learning how to administer tests, students should be able to describe their current strengths and weaknesses in administrating, scoring, and interpreting. This information can be used to help the student improve in test-giving skills. A form to help students structure their learning experience is found in Table 6–5.

COMMUNICATING RESULTS

Discussing Results with the Client

Clients may be very anxious when they come to learn the results of tests. Anxiety can be reduced by asking the client what questions he or she has about the testing or about the results. If these questions are addressed first, the client usually is more attentive when discussing more difficult issues.

When giving results to a client, the therapist

Table 6–4. Analysis of Test Instrument

1. Name of the Test

2. Name and Address of Publisher

3. Cost if Known

4. Target Population

5. Purposes of the Test

6. What are specific variables measured within the test (e.g., occupational interest, degree of anxiety, personality type, cognitive level)?

7. How is the test administered (e.g., performance, paper/pencil, self-report, observation)?

8. What is the average time taken to complete the test?

9. What skills are necessary in administering the test?

10. What factors could interfere with obtaining valid results (e.g., behaviors, motivation, time of day, fatigue, environment)?

11. How are test results reported (e.g., description of raw score ranges, qualitative description, percentiles, standard scores)?

Table 6–5. Self-Evaluation of Skills in Administering, Scoring, and Interpreting Test Results

Skill	Points Possible	Points Earned	Reflective Comments on Areas of Strength and Areas to Improve
Establishing rapport	12	_____	
Answering client's questions before testing	8	_____	
Preparation and arranging test materials	8	_____	
Following directions from test manual	15	_____	
Demonstrating performance tests	11	_____	
Use of stopwatch or clock	8	_____	
Professional and objective demeanor	8	_____	
Scoring (including converting raw scores to standard scores)	15	_____	
Interpreting results to testee	15	_____	

wants to identify the areas of strength as well as areas to be improved. We recommend that the areas of strength be addressed first. The areas of improvement can serve as short-term treatment goals. Thus, following a discussion of results, the therapist may wish to formulate or establish short-term treatment goals with the client.

Discussing Results with the Treatment Team

When results are reported to the treatment team, there are a number of considerations. First, the results of the test in relationship to the norms must be given. This includes standard scores, percentiles, or qualitative terms (e.g., severely depressed). Second, the client's behavior during the test session should be reported. This behavior could affect the validity of the test results and may provide insight into the dynamics of the client's diagnosis. Strengths and weaknesses of the client based on test results are a third consideration. Short- and long-term treatment goals are derived from the strengths and weaknesses, as are implications for therapeutic methods. Finally, the test results need to be incorporated into the total team's goals for the client.

SUGGESTED TEST BATTERY FOR PSYCHOSOCIAL ASSESSMENT

In a psychosocial setting, occupational therapists will be selecting specific tests in an evaluation. In a comprehensive evaluation, the occupational therapist will want to test more than one function. A test battery includes selection of tests measuring several functions, performance areas, and performance components. In Table 6–6 we have suggested commonly used tests in the performance areas of work, self-care, and leisure, and in the performance components of cognitive functioning, social skills, and psychosocial functioning.

Other Sources for Locating Appropriate Tests

▶ Anastasi, A., & Urbina, S. (1997). *Psychological testing* (7th ed.). Englewood Cliffs, NJ: Prentice Hall.

▶ Asher, I. E. (1996). *Occupational therapy assessment tools: An annotated index* (2nd ed.). Rockville, MD: American Occupational Therapy Association.

▶ Cole, B., Finch, E., Gowland, C., & Mayo, N. (1994). *Physical rehabilitation outcome measures.* Toronto, Ontario: Canadian Physiotherapy Association in cooperation with Health and Welfare Canada and the Canada Communication Group–Publishing, Supply and Services, Canada.

▶ Fischer, J., & Corcoran, K. (1995). *Measures for clinical practice: A sourcebook* (2nd ed.). New York: Free Press.

▶ Hemphill, B. J. (Ed.). (1982). *The evaluative process in psychiatric occupational therapy.* Thorofare, NJ: SLACK.

▶ Hemphill-Pearson, B. J. (1999). *Assessments in occupational therapy mental health: An integrative approach.* Thorofare, NJ: SLACK.

▶ Lewis, C. B., & McNerney, T. (1994). *The functional tool box: Clinical measures of functional outcomes.* Washington, DC: Learn.

▶ Murphy, L. L, Impara, J. C., & Plake, B. S. (Eds.) (1999). *Tests in print V: An index to tests, test reviews and the literature on specific tests.* Lincoln, NE; Buros Institute.

▶ Power, P. W. (2000). *A guide to vocational assessment* (3rd ed.). Austin, TX: PRO-ED.

▶ Reed, K. L. (2001). Appendix C: Assessments developed entirely or in part by occupational therapy personnel. In K. L. Reed (Ed.), *Quick reference to occupational therapy* (2nd ed; pp. 863–933). Gaithersburg, MD: Aspen.

▶ Stein, F. & Cutler, S. K. (1996). *Clinical research in allied health and special education.* San Diego: Singular Publishing Group.

▶ Stein, F., & Cutler, S. K. (2000). *Clinical research in occupational therapy* (4th ed.). San Diego: Singular Publishing Group.

▶ Van Deusen, J., & Brunt, D. (1997). *Assessment in occupational therapy and physical therapy.* Philadelphia: Saunders.

TABLE 6–6. Suggested Test Battery: Performance Areas

Performance Area	Variables Measured	Examples of Tests
Work	• Work habits	• *Canadian Occupational Performance Measure* ([COPM] Law et al., 1994)
	• Occupation	• *Jacobs Prevocational Skills Assessment* ([JPSA], Jacobs, 1991)
		• *Occupational Questionnaire* (Smith, Kielhofner, & Watts, 1986)
		• *Role Checklist* (Oakley, Kielhofner, Barris, & Reicheler, 1986)
	• Vocational interests	• *Strong-Campbell Interest Inventory* ([SCII], Strong, Campbell, & Hansen, 1985)
	• Aptitude	• *Valpar* (Brown, McDaniel, Couch, & McClanahan, 1994)
Leisure/Play	• Interests	• *Canadian Occupational Performance Measure* ([COPM], Law et al., 1994)
	• History	• *NPI Checklist* (Matsutsuyu, 1969)
		• *Occupational Questionnaire* (Smith, Kielhofner, & Watts, 1986)
		• *Role Checklist* (Oakley, Kielhofner, Barris, & Reicheler, 1986)
Self-care	• Independent living	• *Bay Area Performance Functional Evaluation* ([BaPFE], Williams & Bloomer, 1987)
	• Health maintenance and safety	• *Canadian Occupational Performance Measure* ([COPM], Law et al., 1994)
	• Personal hygiene	• *Functional Assessment Scale* ([FAS], Breines, 1988)
	• Communication skills	• *Health Status Questionnaire* ([HSQ]–12, version 2.0; Health Outcomes Institute, 1995)
	• Pain	• *ILB Checklist*
		• *Independent Living Skills Evaluation* ([ILSE], Johnson, Vinnicombe, & Merrill, 1980)
		• *Kohlman Evaluation of Living Skills* ([KELS], Thomson, 1992)
		• *Milwaukee Evaluation of Daily Living Skills* ([MEDLS] Leonardelli, 1988b)
		• *Parachek Geriatic Rating Scale* (Parachek & King, 1986)
		• *Short-Form McGill Pain Questionnaire* ([SF-MPQ], Melzack, 1987)
		• *Street Survival Skills Questionnaire* ([SSSQ], Linkenhoker & McCarron, 1973)

TABLE 6–6. Suggested Test Battery: Performance Areas

Performance Area	Variables Measured	Examples of Tests
Cognitive Integrations and Cognitive Components	• Level of cognitive skill	• *Allen Cognitive Levels* ([ACL], Allen, Earhart, & Blue, 1992)
		• *Bay Area Performance Functional Evaluation* ([BaPFE], Williams & Bloomer, 1987)
		• *Cognitive Adaptive Skills Evaluation* ([CASE], Masagatani, Nielson, & Ranslow, 1981; 1994)
		• *Loewenstein Occupational Therapy* Cognitive Assessment ([LOTCA], Itzkovich, Elazar, Averbuch, & Katz, 1990)
		• *Mini–Mental State* ([MMS], Folstein, Folstein, & McHugh, 1975)
		• *Short Portable Mental Status Questionnaire* ([SPMSQ], Pfeiffer, 1975)
Psychosocial Skills and Psychological Components	• Social skills	• *Geriatric Rating Scale* (Plutchik, et al., 1970)
	• Self-expression	• *Katz Adjustment Scale* (Katz & Lyerly, 1963)
	• Social adjustment	
	• Social interactions	
	• Self-concept	• *Geriatric Depression Scale* (Yesavage et al., 1983)
	• Depression	• *Hamilton Depression Inventory* ([HDI], Reynolds & Kobak, 1995)
	• Stress management/coping skills	• *Holmes-Rahe Life Change Index* (Holmes & Rahe, 1967)
	• Anxiety	• *Life Satisfaction Index K* (Koyano & Shibata, 1994)
		• *Magazine Picture Collage* (Lerner, 1982)
		• *Profile of Mood States* ([POMS], McNair, Lorr, & Droppleman, 1971)
		• *State-Trait Anxiety Inventory* ([STAI], Spielberger, 1983)
		• *Stress Management Questionnaire* (Stein, 1987)
		• *Stress Audit Questionnaire* (Miller, Smith, & Mehler, 1988)
		• *Zung Self-Rating Depression Scale* ([ZSRDS], Zung, 1965)
	• Time management	• *Barth Time Construction* (Barth, 1985)

TEST SUMMARIES OF
COMMONLY USED TESTS
IN PSYCHOSOCIAL PRACTICE

Category	Cognitive
Test Name	*Allen Cognitive Levels* (ACL; Allen, 1985, Earhart & Allen, 1988)
Publisher	S & S Arts and Crafts, P.O. Box 513, Colchester, CT 06415-0513
Testing Level	C: Knowledge of Allen's cognitive levels
Purpose	Screening tool to classify people into one of six cognitive levels based on Allen's theory
Target Population	Clients with psychiatric or cognitive impairment
Description	Craft activity requiring a client to copy leather lacing stitches demonstrated by the examiner
Variables Measured	Six cognitive levels: automatic actions, postural actions, manual actions, goal-directed actions, exploratory actions, and planned actions
Format	Task analysis using demonstrations and instruction
Materials	Kit includes leather pattern, laces, needles, thread. Needle-nosed pliers are required
Scoring	Cognitive level measured based on the ability to complete stitches after demonstration

Reliability	Interrater	$r = .99$
Validity	Content	Based on Allen's theory
	Concurrent	Described by author as discriminating among individuals who are schizophrenic or depressed, and nonpatient populations
	Construct	
	Predictive	

References	Allen, C. K. (1982). Independence through activity: The practice of occupational therapy (psychiatry). *American Journal of Occupational Therapy, 36,* 731–739. Allen, C. K. (1985). *Occupational therapy for psychiatric diseases: Measurement and management of cognitive disabilities.* Boston: Little, Brown. Allen, C. K., Earhart, C. A., & Blue, T. (1992). *Occupational therapy treatment goals for the physically and cognitively disabled.* Rockville, MD: American Occupational Therapy Association. Unsworth, C. (1999). Allen's Cognitive Level Test. In C. Unsworth (Ed.), *Cognitive and perceptual dysfunction: A clinical reasoning approach to evaluation and intervention* (pp. 86–87, 91–92). Philadelpha: F. A. Davis.

Category	Psychosocial: Time Management	
Test Name	***Barth Time Construction*** (Barth, 1985)	
Publisher	Unpublished scale. Available from Model of Human Occupation Clearinghouse, Department of Occupational Therapy (M/C 811), College of Associated Health Professions, 191 W. Taylor Street, Chicago, IL 60612–7250	
Testing Level	A: interpretation by any occupational therapist	
Purpose	Assess time-management skills	
Target Population	Adults or adolescents with psychosocial dysfunction, although it may be used with any individual, adolescent through geriatric	
Description	"Color-coded time chart in which the patient depicts the use of time for a week within 12 categories of activities" (Barth, 1988, p. 117)	
Variables Measured	Qualitative summary of interests based on the Model of Human Occupation Frame of Reference	
Format	Paper and pencil test	
Materials	Test booklet	
Scoring	Qualitative scoring, which can be used in planning treatment	
Reliability	Test-retest	$r = .92$ (range of .82 to .92) over a 3-week period
Validity	Content	Based on *a priori* and clinical basis by experienced occupational therapists
References	Barth, T. (1985). *Barth Time Construction.* New York: Health Related Consulting Services. Barth, T. (1988). Barth Time Construction. In B. J. Hemphill (Ed.), *Mental health assessment in occupational therapy: An integrative approach to the evaluative process* (pp. 117–129). Thorofare, NJ: SLACK.	

Category	Psychosocial Skill; Cognitive; Self-Care
Test Name	***Bay Area Functional Performance Evaluation*** (BaFPE; 2nd ed.; Williams & Bloomer, 1987)
Publisher	Maddock, Inc., 6 Industrial Road, Pequannock, NJ 07440
Testing Level	B: Any occupational therapist
Purpose	Assessment of cognitive, affective, and performance skills in daily living tasks and social interaction skills
Target Population	Adults with psychosocial dysfunction. Can be used with individuals with neurological dysfunction and mental retardation
Description	Two subtests: Task Oriented Assessment (TOA), consisting of five performance tasks assessing functional skills, and Social Interaction Scale (SIS), in which the client is observed in five defined social situations. The two subtests can be administered separately
Variables Measured	Ten functional components (e.g., paraphrasing, productive decision making, and motivation); Seven social interactions (e.g., ability to work with peers, verbal communication, response to authority figures)
Format	TOA: timed performance tasks SIS: behavioral observation and self-report, which is optional
Materials	Kit with materials, scoring sheet, and manual with directions
Scoring	Rating of performance or social interaction according to well-defined behavioral guidelines used (from 1 (markedly dysfunctional) to 4 (almost always functional or appropriate)). Clinical observations are also used.
Reliability	Interrater	r = exceeds .90 in TOA , .75 to .79 in SIS
Validity	Content	Based on the compatibility with several frames of reference, especially the Model of Human Occupation
References	Houston, D., Williams, S. L., Bloomer, J., & Mann, W. D. (1989). The Bay Area Functional Performance Evaluation: Development and standardization. *American Journal of Occupational Therapy, 43*, 170–182. Klyczek, J. P. (1999). The Bay Area Functional Performance Evaluation. In B. J. Hemphill-Pearson, *Assessments in occupational therapy mental health: An integrative approach* (pp. 87–107). Thorofare, NJ: SLACK

Category	Self-Care; Work; Leisure
Test Name	*Canadian Occupational Performance Measure* (COPM; Law, Baptiste, Carswell–Opzoomer, McColl, Polatajko, & Pollock, 1991)
Publisher	Canadian Association of Occupational Therapists, 110 Eglinton Ave. West, 3rd Floor, Toronto, Ontario, Canada M4R1A3
Testing Level	A: Any occupational therapist
Purpose	Outcome measured designed to detect changes in client's perception of occupational performance. Identifies problem areas, client perception of and satisfaction with performance, and measures changes over time.
Target Population	Clients with disabilities. Can be used with children as young as 7.
Description	Unstructured interview-based rating scale. Based on the Model of Occupational Performance. Typically requires 30 to 40 minutes to give.
Variables Measured	Three subareas are measured (self-care, productivity, and leisure), with total scores obtained for performance and satisfaction. Based on the Canadian Model of Occupational Performance.
Format	Unstructured interview, which can be used with the client or caretaker.
Materials	Rating scale, manual, score sheet. Pencil must be supplied.
Scoring	Rating scale scored from 1 (lowest) to 10 (highest)
Reliability	Test-retest	$r = .63$ for performance, .84 for satisfaction ($N = 27$)
Validity	Criterion	$r = -.14$ to .38 with FIM; $-.13$ to .40 with SPSQ

References	Baptiste, S., & Rochon, S. (1999). Client-centered assessment: The Canadian Occupational Performance Measure. In B. J. Hemphill- Pearson, *Assessments in occupational therapy mental health: An integrative approach* (pp. 42–57). Thorofare, NJ: SLACK.
	Chan, C. & Lee, T. M. C. (1997). Validation of Canadian Occupational Performance Measure. *Occupational Therapy International, 4,* 231–249.
	Law, M., Baptiste, S., Carswell, A., McColl, M. A., Polatajko, H., & Pollock, N. (1994). *Canadian Occupational Performance Measure* (2nd ed.). Toronto, Ontario: Canadian Association of Occupational Therapists.
	Law, M., Polatajko, H., Pollock, N., McColl, M. A., Carswell, A., & Baptiste (1994). Pilot testing of the Canadian Occupational Performance Measure: Clinical and measurement issues. *Canadian Journal of Occupational Therapy, 61*(4), 191–197.

Category	Cognitive	
Test Name	***Cognitive Adaptive Skills Evaluation*** (CASE; Masagatani, 1994, Rev. ed.)	
Publisher	Available from the author: Gladys Masagatani, Eastern Kentucky University, Department of Occupational Therapy, Dizney 103, Richmond, KY 40475–3135	
Testing Level	B: occupational therapist familiar with theories of Piaget and Mosey	
Purpose	Survey functional skills to examine individual's cognitive skills while performing a task and responding to interview questions	
Target Population	Clients with psychosocial dysfunction; can be used with adults and adolescents with developmental delays or cognitive dysfunction	
Description	Skills inventory using observation during task performance and interview: Client is asked to make a calendar.	
Variables Measured	Performance summary using defined behavioral criteria based on analysis of task completion and responses to interview questions	
Format	Observation of task completion and interview questions	
Materials	Writing implements (pen and pencil), paper, ruler, sample calendar, written directions, protocol, evaluation summary sheet	
Scoring	Qualitative score based on therapist observations	
Reliability	Interrater	Reported as high if raters understand theories of Piaget and Mosey
Validity	Content	Based on theories of Piaget and Mosey and by trial administration to identify behaviors
References	Masagatani, G. N. (1994). *Cognitive Adaptive Skills Evaluation manual* (Rev. ed.). Unpublished manuscript. [Available from Gladys Masagatani, Eastern Kentucky University, Department of Occupational Therapy, Dizney 103, Richmond, KY 40475–3135]. Masagatani, G. N. (1999). In B. J. Hemphill-Pearson, *Assessments in occupational therapy mental health: An integrative approach* (pp. 280–284). Thorofare, NJ: SLACK.	

Category	Self-Care
Test Name	*The Comprehensive Occupational Therapy Evaluation* (COTE; Brayman, Kirby, Meisenheimer, & Short, 1976) *KidCOTE* (children's version of the COTE; 1995)
Publisher	Unpublished test. See reference below.
Testing Level	B: Any occupational therapist
Purpose	Provide a standardized way to report patient behaviors and to aid in developing and evaluating a treatment plan
Target Population	Adults with psychosocial disorders. KidCOTE is appropriate for children ages 5 to 12 receiving occupational therapy services.
Description	Behavioral observation scale
Variables Measured	Adult version: 26 behaviors in 3 areas: general behaviors, interpersonal behaviors, and task behaviors. Child version: 27 behaviors in 4 areas: general behaviors, sensory motor performance, cognitive behaviors, and psychosocial behaviors.
Format	Observational form. The KidCOTE is a summary form for standardized tests used in assessment of perceptional skills.
Materials	Various occupational therapy arts and crafts activities
Scoring	Adult version: Rating scale ranging from 0 to 4. Higher scores indicate inability to perform the task independently.
Reliability	Interrater	Adult version: r = .76 to 1.00, with average of .95 *KidCOTE*: r = .96 to 1.00, with average of .98
Validity	Predictive	Review of medical records for discharged patients reflected observed functioning levels
References	Brayman, S. J., Kirby, T. F., Meisenheimer, A. M. & Short, M. J. (1976). The comprehensive occupational therapy evaluation scale. *American Journal of Occupational Therapy, 30,* 94–100. Kunz, K. R., & Brayman, S. J. (1999). The Comprehensive Occupational Therapy Evaluation. In B. J. Hemphill-Pearson, *Assessments in occupational therapy mental health: An integrative approach* (pp. 260–274). Thorofare, NJ: SLACK.

Category	Self-Care
Test Name	*Functional Assessment Scale* (FAS; Breines, 1988)
Publisher	Geri-Rehab, Inc., 15 Hibbler Road, Lebanon, NJ 08833
Testing Level	A: No training required
Purpose	Scale designed to rate self-care function in patients who are institutionalized
Target Population	Individuals who are hospitalized or institutionalized (e.g., nursing homes)
Description	Outcome scale designed to measure progress or decline in individuals or groups on a bi-weekly basis. Could be used as an observational tool for raters not familiar with the client.
Variables Measured	Provides a single level of function, ranging from 1 "total care" to 10 "prepared to live independently"
Format	Checklist-type rating scale
Materials	Protocol and writing utensil
Scoring	Items are scored from 1 to 10 based on a criteria stated in the protocol
Reliability	Test-retest	$r = .95$ per level and .93 per item
Validity	Content	Review from panel of experts and from field testing suggested high level of validity
References	Breines, E. (1988). The Functional Assessment Scale as an instrument for measuring changes in levels of function for nursing home residents following occupational therapy. *Canadian Journal of Occupational Therapy, 55,* 135–140.

Category	Psychosocial Functioning
Test Name	*Geriatric Depression Scale* (Yesavage, Brink, Rose, Lum, Huang, Adey, & Leirer, 1983)
Publisher	Unpublished; see reference below
Testing Level	A: No training required
Purpose	Assess level of depression
Target Population	Elderly population
Description	Easily administered survey used as screening instrument to evaluate depression. Can be self-administered, or administered by clinician
Variables Measured	Level of depression (normal, mild, severe)
Format	Self-administered paper-pencil test. Can also be administered by a clinician or physician.
Materials	Test, pencil, and scoring criteria
Scoring	Higher points reveal higher level of depression.

Reliability (only on LSR)	Split-half	$r = .79$
	Interrater	$r = .87$

Validity	Concurrent	•$r = .64$: based on in-depth interview and ratings by judges using the LSR •$r = .55$ and .58 using the LSR and LSI–A or LSI–B, respectively

References	Yesavage, J. A., Brink, T. A., Rose, T. L., Lum, O., Huang, V., Adey, M., & Leirer, V. O. (1983). Development and validation of a geriatric depression screening scale: A preliminary report. *Journal of Psychiatric Research, 17,* 37–49.

Category	Psychosocial Function
Test Name	***Geriatric Rating Scale*** (GRS; Plutchik, Conte, Lieberman, Baker, Grossman, & Lehrman, 1970)
Publisher	Unpublished; see reference below
Testing Level	A: No training required
Purpose	Assessment of readiness to leave a hospital setting
Target Population	Elderly patients in a clinical setting, including those with psychotic disorders or organic mental disease
Description	28-item rating scale in the following areas: physical disability, apathy, communication failure, and socially irritating behavior
Variables Measured	Level of intellectual functioning. Levels of education (grade school, high school, post secondary school) is taken into account
Format	Observational based behavioral rating scale
Materials	Rating scale, pencil
Scoring	3-point Likert scale, evaluating behavior in self-care, use of time, need for assistance, or interpersonal behavior. Total summed score, with higher scores indicating greater impairment
Reliability	Interrater	$r = .87$
	Internal consistency	Determined by factor analysis, ranging from .75 to .90
	Test-retest	$r = .65$ over a 1 year period
Validity	Reportedly discriminated between clinical and nonclinical groups
References	Plutchik, R, Conte, H., Lieberman, M., Baker, M., Grossman, J., & Lehrman, N. (1970). Reliability and validity of a scale for assessing the functioning of geriatric patients. *Journal of the Geriatric Society, 18,* 491–500.

Category	Psychosocial Functioning
Test Name	*Hamilton Depression Inventory* (HDI; Reynolds & Kobak, 1995)
Publisher	Psychological Assessment Resources, Inc. (PAR), P.O. Box 988, Odessa, FL 33556
Testing Level	B: Interpretation needs background in personality theory
Purpose	Self–report measure designed to screen for symptoms of depression
Target Population	Adults
Description	Self–report questionnaire. Four versions: The Full-Scale HID contains 23 items; HDI–17 contains 17 items, HDI—Melancolia, contains 9 items, and the HDI–SF, contains 9 items. The latter form is recommended only when time constraints preclude the use of the full questionnaire. Fifth grade reading level. Computer scoring available
Variables Measured	Symptoms of depression as defined by the DSM–IV. An overall score defines the level of depression.
Format	Self-report questionnaire containing multiple choice questions (5 responses, ranging from no symptom to severe symptoms)
Materials	Protocol, scoring sheet
Scoring	Total score obtained by adding the item score and comparing to a cutoff score. In addition, critical scores on particular items suggest further evaluation regardless of the cutoff score
Reliability	Test-retest	Reported as "very high" in professional manual
Validity	Correlation	Highly correlated with *Hamilton Depression Rating Scale* (HDRS), clinical interviews of depression, and related constructs
References	Reynolds, W. M., & Kobak, K. A. (1995). *Hamilton Depression Inventory (HDI) professional manual.* Odessa, FL: PAR.

Category	Self–Care
Test Name	***Health Status Questionnaire*** (HSQ, version 2.0; Health Outcomes Institute, 1995)
Publisher	NCS 5605 Green Circle Dr. Minnetonka, MN 55343-4400
Testing Level	A.
Purpose	Designed to measure aspects of physical and emotional health.
Target Population	Adults, Adolescents age 14 and older
Description	Self–report questionnaire, containing 39 items and taking 5 to 10 minutes to complete
Variables Measured	Overall health, functional status, and well being
Format	Self-report multiple-choice questionnaire in which the individual rates (a) health perception, (b) physical, social, and role functioning, (c) mental health, and (d) depression.
Materials	World Wide Web version
Scoring	Hand or computer scoring
Reliability	Not available
Validity	Not available
References	Health Outcomes Institute. (1995). *HSQ,* Verson 2.0. Retrieved May 17, 2001, from the World Wide Web: http://www.assessments.ncs.com/assessments/download/medicalcat/HSQ.pdf

Category	Self-Care
Test Name	***Independent Living Skills Evaluation*** (ILSE; Johnson, Vinnicombe, & Merrill, 1980)
Publisher	Community Living Experiences, Inc., The Independent Living Project, 291 North Tenth Street, San Jose, CA, 95112
Testing Level	B: Any occupational therapist
Purpose	Assess levels of living skills in areas necessary for independent community living
Target Population	Adults (age 18 and above) with chronic psychosocial dysfunction who are living in independent living arrangements or living independently
Description	Self-report and behavioral rating scale assessing 10 major areas of independent living skills
Variables Measured	10 major categories: money management, shopping and consumer education, meal preparation and storage, house cleaning and maintenance, medication management and health care, community resources and transportation, communication and interpersonal relations, problem-solving and decision-making, vocational and personal growth
Format	Behavioral rating scale and self-report, followed by discussion between therapist and client regarding skill level
Materials	Protocol and manual
Scoring	Each item is scored from 1 (lowest) to 4 (optimal) based on well-defined behavioral guidelines. Low scores are used to determine behavioral objectives used.
Reliability	Has not been done
Validity	Has not been done
References	Johnson, T. P., Vinnicombe, B. J., & Merrill, G. W. (1980). The Independent Living Skills Evaluation. *Occupational Therapy in Mental Health, 1*(2), 5–18. Stein, F. (1988). Research analysis of occupational therapy assessments used in mental health. In B.J. Hemphill (Ed.), *Mental health assessment in occupational therapy: an integrative approach to the evaluative process* (pp. 223–247). Thorofare, NJ: SLACK.

Category	Work
Test Name	*Jacobs Prevocational Skills Assessment* (JPSA; Jacobs, 1985)
Publisher	Available from K. Jacobs (1985), *Occupational therapy: Work–related programs and assessments*, Boston, Little, Brown, & Co.
Testing Level	B: Training required to give test
Purpose	Clinical test used to assess performance in specific work-related skills, behaviors, and habits
Target Population	Adolescents through adults; specifically designed for students with learning disabilities; can be adapted to use with individuals with psychosocial dysfunction
Description	Performance instrument containing 15 simulated work tasks. Although time is recorded, there are no time limits imposed.
Variables Measured	Three major areas (physical capacities, work behavior, and work aptitudes) related to specific work skills
Format	Performance test of client's prevocational abilities
Materials	Kit containing test items, checklist, manual
Scoring	Each work task is scored separately. Items are scored based on the ability to perform the task and the time involved. Results are used to plan a therapy program
Reliability	Not reported
Validity	Not reported
References	Jacobs, K. (1985). *Occupational therapy: Work–related programs and assessments.* Boston: Little, Brown. Jacobs, K. (1991). The Jacobs Prevocational Skills Assessment. In K. Jacobs, *Occupational therapy: Work-related programs and assessments* (2nd ed., pp. 61–136). Boston: Little, Brown

Category	Psychosocial Function
Test Name	*Katz Adjustment Scale* (Katz & Lyerly, 1963)
Publisher	Unpublished scale; see reference below
Testing Level	A: interpretation by any occupational therapist
Purpose	Assesses the ability of clients after intervention to return to the community by providing a description of social behavior
Target Population	Adults with psychosis prior to and after hospitalization
Description	Rating scale completed by the client and by a close relative regarding social adjustment
Variables Measured	Five subscales: measuring recent symptoms and social behavior; perceptions of and expectations of level of performance on socially expected acts; and level of and satisfaction with free-time activities
Format	Paper and pencil test
Materials	Two test booklets and scoring system
Scoring	Individual scoring of items on a 3- to 4-point scale, with comparisons between two raters. Yields a profile of adjustment from two perspectives
Reliability	Internal consistency	$r = .61$ to $.87$ among item clusters
Validity	Concurrent	Evident in agreement between client and relative
	Discriminative	Preliminary studies indicate adequate discrimination between well-adjusted and poorly adjusted individuals.
References	Katz, M. M., & Lyerly, S. B. (1963). Methods for measuring adjustment and social behavior in the community: I. Rationale, description, discriminative validity and scale development. *Psychological Reports, 13,* 503–535.

Category	Self-Care (Independent Living Skills)
Test Name	*Kohlman Evaluation of Living Skills* (KELS; 3rd ed.; Thomson, 1992)
Publisher	American Occupational Therapy Association 4720 Montgomery Lane Bethesda, MD 20824–1220
Testing Level	B: Any occupational therapist
Purpose	Quick assessment to provide information about a person's ability in everyday functioning in daily living skills, independent living, and work/leisure
Target Population	Clients with acute psychiatric disorders, elderly patients in acute care hospitals; adolescent through elderly. Must be used cautiously with individuals hospitalized for more than 1 month
Description	Criterion-referenced assessment tool that provides space for recommendations for intervention and treatment
Variables Measured	17 living skills in areas of self-care, safety/health, money management, transportation/telephone, work/leisure
Format	Interview, observation, and completion of simple tasks
Materials	Kit includes three-ring binder, common everyday materials used as stimulus, protocol, and manual
Scoring	Categories include "independent" and "needs assistance"; criteria for scoring are included for each item. Yields single cutoff score identifying patients who can live independently in the community
Reliability	Interrater	r = .84 to 1.00
Validity	Concurrent	r = .78 to .89 with Global Assessment Scale; -.84 with BaFPE
	Predictive	Successfully predicted which geriatric patients could live independently
References	Thomson, L. K. (1992). *The Kohlman Evaluation of Living Skills* (KELS; 3rd ed.). Rockville, MD: American Occupational Therapy Association. Thomson, L. K. (1999). *The Kohman Evaluation of Living Skills.* In B. J. Hemphill-Pearson, *Assessments in occupational therapy mental health: An integrative approach* (pp. 231–242), Thorofare, NJ: SLACK.

Category	Psychosocial Functioning	
Test Name	*Life Satisfaction Index K* (LSI-K; Koyano & Shibata; 1994)	
Publisher	Unpublished; see reference below	
Testing Level	A: No training required	
Purpose	Quick measure of one's self-perception of well-being	
Target Population	Elderly population	
Description	Nine-item, self-administered test using a Likert scale, with maximum score of 9. Take 3-5 minutes to administer, 5 minutes to score	
Variables Measured	Cognitive/short-term, cognitive/long-term, and emotional/short-term well-being	
Format	Self-administered paper-pencil test	
Materials	Test, pencil, and scoring criteria	
Scoring	Items are scored either 0 or 1 and totaled. Higher scores indicate higher satisfaction.	
Reliability	Correlation coefficient between total score on LSI-K and second order factor score = .99	
Validity	Construct	Analysis of Covariance Analysis (ANCOVA) and factor analysis revealed three components contained in subjective well-being
References	Koyano, W., & Shibata, H. (1994). Development of a measure of subjective well-being in Japan: Construct validity and reliable of the Life Satisfaction K. In L. J. Fritten (Ed.), *Facts and research in gerontology: Dementia and cognitive impairments* (Suppl. 2; pp. 181–187). New York: Springer.	

Category	Life Roles: Work, Leisure, Self-Care
Test Name	*Loewenstein Occupational Therapy Cognitive Assessment* (LOTCA; Katz, Itzkovich, Averbuch, & Elazer, 1989)
Publisher	Western Psychological Corporation
Testing Level	B: Anyone with knowledge of neuropsychological models
Purpose	• Assessment of individuals in orientation, perception, visuomotor organization, cognitive operations • Identify a baseline prior to treatment • Determine therapeutic goals • Screen for need for further assessments
Target Population	Age 6 through adult. Used for adults with traumatic brain injury, psychosocial disorders, and cognitive deficits
Description	Performance test divided into subscales that measure area of cognitive processing based on a neuropsychological model
Variables Measured	Four areas: orientation, visual and spatial perception, visuomotor organization, and thinking. Each area is divided into subtests
Format	Performance test divided into subscales that measure area of cognitive processing based on a neuropsychological model
Materials	Portable kit that includes a manual and associated testing materials
Scoring	Items are rated from 0 (low) to 4 or 5 (high) based on ability to complete the task
Reliability	Interrater Internal consistency	Reported as adequate
Validity	Criterion construct	Reported as adequate for individuals with mild/moderate disabilities
References	Katz, N., Itzkovich, M., Averbuch, S., & Elazer, G. (1989). Loewenstein Occupational Therapy Cognitive Assessment (LOTCA) battery for brain-injured patients: Reliability and validity. *American Journal of Occupational Therapy, 43,* 184–192. Itzkovich, M., Elazar, B., Averbuch, S., & Katz, N. (1990). *Loewenstein Occupational Therapy Cognitive Assessment.* Los Angeles: Western Psychological Services.

Category	Psychosocial Functioning
Test Name	*Magazine Picture Collage* (MPC; Lerner, 1982)
Publisher	Unpublished; see reference below
Testing Level	B: Interpretation needs background in personality theory
Purpose	Diagnostic instrument to examine aspects of personality and self, including ego functions and organization. Considered to be tangible expression of the client's feelings
Target Population	Clients with psychiatric or cognitive impairment
Description	Unstructured craft activity where the client selects pictures from a magazine and pastes them on colored construction paper
Variables Measured	Formal variables (colors, performance of task [cutting, pasting, neatness], how the pictures are placed on the paper); content variables (themes, number and description of people selected, use of animals or objects); patient-therapist variable (how the patient interprets the following of directions and the time taken to complete task)
Format	Craft activity used as a projective technique for interpretation of client's personality
Materials	Glossy magazines with a variety of colored photograph (people, animals, and landscape scenes), colored paper (12 x 18 inches), paste or glue, scissors
Scoring	Qualitative scoring system where therapist interprets client's product in terms of personality characteristics. The manner in which the client completes the collage is a part of the interpretation.
Reliability	Interrater	$r = .92$ on formal, .94 on the content
Validity	Content	Based on psychodynamic theoretical model (Azima & Azima, 1959).
References	Lerner, C. J. (1982). Magazine Picture Collage. In B. Hemphill (Ed.), *The evaluative process in psychiatric occupational therapy* (pp. 139–154, 361–362). Thorofare, NJ: SLACK. Lerner, C. J., & Ross, G. (1977). The Magazine Picture Collage: Development of an objective scoring system. *American Journal of Occupational Therapy, 31*, 156–161.

Category	Self–Care
Test Name	***Short-Form McGill Pain Questionnaire*** (SF-MPQ; Melzack, 1987)
Publisher	Unpublished test; see references below
Testing Level	A: No training required.
Purpose	Designed to measure client's perception of pain
Target Population	Adults
Description	Self-report questionnaire, completed in 2 to 5 minutes
Variables Measured	Sensory, affective, and total pain. The Present Paint Intensity (PPI) is based on the sum of the intensity rank values, whereas the Visual Analog Scale (VAS) depicts level of pain on a continuum.
Format	Self-report questionnaire
Materials	Questionnaire, pencil
Scoring	Intensity rank scores are summed. Qualitative scoring obtains a Present Pain Intensity (PPI) and Visual Analog Scale (VAS).
Reliability	Reliability of reporting pain varies from day to day.
Validity	Concurrent	Comparisons with McGill Pain Questionnaire were high.
References	Melzack, R. (1987). The short–form McGill Pain Questionnaire. *Pain, 30*, 191–197.

Category	Cognitive
Test Name	***Short Portable Mental Status Questionnaire*** (SPMSQ; Pfeiffer, 1975)
Publisher	Unpublished; see reference below
Testing Level	A: No training required
Purpose	Quick assessment of the degree of intellectual impairment
Target Population	Elderly patients in the home or in clinical setting
Description	Response-driven examination with questions asked by the evaluator and answered by the client. Can be given in 10 minutes
Variables Measured	Level of intellectual functioning. Levels of education (grade school, high school, post secondary school) is taken into account
Format	Question and answer
Materials	Questionnaire, pencil, scoring sheet
Scoring	Number of errors, based on specific criteria
Reliability	Test-retest	$r = .82$ and .83 after 4-week interval on two groups of patients
Validity	Face	Comparison of 141 clients with 997 elderly living in the community showed adequate face value.
References	Pfeiffer, E. (1975). A short portable mental status questionnaire for the assessment of organic brain deficit in elderly patients. *Journal of the American Geriatrics Society, 23*, 433–441.

Category	Self-Care (Independent Living Skills)	
Test Name	*Milwaukee Evaluation of Daily Living Skills* (MEDLS; Leonardelli, 1988b)	
Publisher	SLACK Publishing Co.	
Testing Level	B: Any occupational therapist	
Purpose	Assessment of behavior and skills needed for adequate functioning in the client's living situation	
Target Population	Adults with chronic mental illness who are inpatients or outpatients in a CMHC	
Description	Behavioral observation of specific tasks	
Variables Measured	20 subtests, measuring basic living skills, safety, communication, and transportation	
Format	Completing of simple tasks in above areas	
Materials	Materials include equipment provided within the kit and personal items of the client (e.g., dressing, shaving materials), protocol, manual	
Scoring	Each item is scored separately, with scores ranging from 0 (unable to perform) to 4 (performs all skills).	
Reliability	Interrater	$r = .4$ to 1.0 for 17 of 20 subtests; most at .8 or above
Validity	Content	Based on literature review and evaluation by experts
References	Haertlein, C. L. (1999). The Milwaukee Evaluation of Daily Living Skills. In B. J. Hemphill-Pearson (Ed.), *Assessments in occupational therapy mental health: An integrative approach* (pp. 245–257), Thorofare, NJ: SLACK. Leonardelli, C. A. (1988). *The Milwaukee Evaluation of Daily Living Skills* (MEDLS). Thorofare, NJ: SLACK.	

Category	Cognitive	
Test Name	***Mini-Mental State*** (MMS; Folstein, Folstein, & McHugh, 1975)	
Publisher	Unpublished; see reference below	
Testing Level	A level: No training required	
Purpose	Quantitative measure of cognitive performance that can be given quickly	
Target Population	Geriatric patients with neurological deficits, especially those with short attention spans	
Description	Standardized questionnaire given orally. Can be given in 5 to 10 minutes. Two parts: oral (22 pts. max.); performance (9 pts. max)	
Variables Measured	Five areas of cognition: orientation, memory, attention and calculation, recall, and following oral and written instructions	
Format	Oral questionnaire administered by examiner	
Materials	Questionnaire, wristwatch, pencil, and blank paper (4 sheets)	
Scoring	Sum of the maximum value of each question, total of 30 possible	
Reliability	Test-retest	$r = .887$ over 24-hour period, .92 with two examiners. $r = .98$ for clinically stable patients in 2-week interval
Validity	Concurrent	$r = .776$ with VIQ on WAIS, .66 on PIQ on WAIS
	Construct	Discriminated between diagnostic categories, cognitive disorders from typical individuals, and improvements in clients who were improving
	Predictive	Scores below 20 found only in patients with dementia or delirium, not in elderly or those with personality disorder or neurosis
References	Folstein, M. F., Folstein, S. E., & McHugh, P. R. (1975). Mini-mental state: A practical method for grading the cognitive state of patients for the clinician. *Journal of Psychiatric Research, 12,* 189–198.	

Category	Leisure
Test Name	***NPI Interest Checklist*** (Matsutsuyu, 1969; Rogers, Weinstein, & Firone, 1978)
Publisher	Unpublished scale. Available from Model of Human Occupational Clearninghouse, Department of Occupational Therapy (M/C 811), College of Associated Health Professions, 191 W. Taylor Street, Chicago, IL 60612–7250
Testing Level	A: Interpretation by any occupational therapist
Purpose	Identify interest levels in leisure activities
Target Population	Adults with psychosocial dysfunction, although it may be used with any individual, adolescent through geriatric
Description	Checklist containing activities in five categories: basic domestic arts, manual skills, cultural/education, physical sports, and social recreation. Items are identified by no, casual, or strong interest.
Variables Measured	Qualitative summary of interests based on the Model of Human Occupation frame of reference
Format	Paper and pencil test
Materials	Test booklet
Scoring	Qualitative scoring, which can be used in planning treatment
Reliability	Test-retest	$r = .92$ (range of .82 to .92) over a 3-week period
Validity	Content	Based on *a priori* and clinical basis by experienced occupational therapists
References	Matsutsuyu, J. (1969). The Interest Checklist. *American Journal of Occupational Therapy, 23,* 368–373. Rogers, J., Weinstein, J., & Firone, J. (1978). The Interest Checklist: An empirical assessment. *American Journal of Occupational Therapy, 32,* 628–630. Rogers, J. C. (1988). The NPI Interest Checklist. In B. J. Hemphill (Ed.), *Mental health assessment in occupational therapy: An integrative approach to the evaluative process* (pp. 93–114). Thorofare, NJ: SLACK.

Category	Life Roles: Work, Leisure, Self-Care
Test Name	*Occupational Performance History Interview* [1] (OHPI-II; Kielhofner et al., 1998)
Publisher	Model of Human Occupation Clearing House, University of Illinois at Chicago, Department of Occupational Therapy (M/C 811), College of Associated Health Professions, 1919 West Taylor Street, Chicago, IL 60612–7250
Testing Level	B: Any experienced interviewer
Purpose	Obtain information about an individual's work, self-care, and leisure performance history
Target Population	Adults with psychosocial disorders
Description	Semistructured interview
Variables Measured	Five thematic areas: activity/occupational choice; critical life events, daily routine, occupational roles, occupational behavior settings
Format	Semistructured interview, which leads to completion of a rating scale and historical time line
Materials	User's manual helps interviewer generate question; rating scale
Scoring	Rating scale ranges from 1 to 4, with 1 being extremely occupationally dysfunctional.
Reliability	Interrater	Reported by authors as high
Validity	Construct	Reported as high, with $r = .90 -.96$.
References	Kielhofner G., & Henry, A. D. (1988). Development and investigation of the occupational performance history interview. *American Journal of Occupational Therapy, 42,* 489–498. Henry, A. D., & Mallinson, T. (1999). The Occupational Performance History Interview. In B. J. Hemphill-Pearson, *Assessments in occupational therapy mental health: An integrative approach* (pp. 59–70). Thorofare, NJ: SLACK.

[1]This test has been translated into eight languages and is distributed by the American Occupational Therapy Association.

Category	Life Roles: Work, Leisure
Test Name	*Occupational Questionnaire* (OQ; Smith, Kielhofner, & Watts, 1986)
Publisher	Model of Human Occupation Clearing House, University of Illinois at Chicago, Department of Occupational Therapy (M/C 811), College of Associated Health Professions, 1919 West Taylor Street, Chicago, IL 60612–7250
Testing Level	A: Any occupational therapist
Purpose	Self-inventory of daily activities and volitional issues for those activities
Target Population	Adults and adolescents
Description	Questionnaire completed by the respondent regarding the typical activities at 1/2 hour intervals
Variables Measured	Activity patterns, classification of activities (e.g., work, leisure, ADL), and ranking of activities according to value, interest, and personal causation
Format	Worksheet divided into 1/2 hour intervals beginning at 5:00 A.M.
Materials	Worksheet
Scoring	Results are summarized into percentages (e.g., time spent on an activity, interest or value of activity).
Reliability	Test-retest	r = .68 for typical day's activities, .87 for agreement on type of activity, .77 for personal causation, .81 for values, and .77 for interests
Validity	Concurrent	Comparison with the *Household Work Study Diary* showed correlations between .82 and .97.
References	Smith, N. R., Kielhofner, G., & Watts, S. J. H. (1986). The relationships between volition, activity pattern, and life satisfaction in the elderly. *American Journal of Occupational Therapy, 40,* 278–283.

Category	Psychosocial Function	
Test Name	***Parachek Geriatric Rating Scale*** (3rd ed.; Parachek & King, 1986)	
Publisher	Center for Neurodevelopmental Studies 5340 West Glenn Drive Glendale, AZ 85301	
Testing Level	B: Some training needed	
Purpose	Screening tool to assist mental health workers in treatment planning for elderly patients, derived from the *Plutchik Geriatric Rating Scale*	
Target Population	Elderly patients	
Description	10 item observation-based behavior rating scale completed by support staff or mental health practitioner	
Variables Measured	Level of physical capabilities, self-care skills, and social interaction skills	
Format	Set of items that are rated by staff on a Likert Scale	
Materials	Scale and treatment manual	
Scoring	Total score in each area provides general level of functioning	
Reliability	None reported	
Validity	Criterion	$r = .88$ with the *Plutchik Geriatric Rating Scale*, .77 with initial diagnostic classification
	Concurrent	
References	Miller, E. R., & Parachek, J. F. (1974). Validation and standardization of a goal-oriented, quick-screening geriatric scale. *Journal of the American Geriatrics Society, 22,* 278–283. Parachek, J. F., & King, L. J. (1986). *Parachek Geriatric Rating Scale* (3rd ed.). (Available from Center for Neurodevelopmental Studies, 5340 West Glenn Drive, Glendale, AZ 85301.)	

Category	Self-Care
Test Name	***Performance Assessment of Self-Care Skills (PASS), Version 3.1*** (Rogers & Holm, 1988)
Publisher	Unpublished; see reference below.
Testing Level	A: No training required
Purpose	Interactive or dynamic assessment of mobility, ADL, and IADL
Target Population	Adult clients in the home or occupational therapy clinic. Has been used with clients with a variety of diagnoses (eg., schizophrenia, Alzheimer Disease, depression)
Description	26 criterion referenced subtasks performed by the client following a series of standardized instructions
Variables Measured	Level of independence, quality and performance of outcome, and safety in performing the tasks, based on a 4-point scale
Format	Performance tasks with standardized instructions
Materials	Common household items, either in a clinical or home kit transported in a rolling suitcase. In the home, the client's household items are used.
Scoring	A rubrics ranging from 0 to 3 (3 being high) enables the examiner to rate the variables. Independent scores on a 9-point scale, with 9 indicating inability to perform tasks without assistance. Scoring allows the therapist to identify the point of breakdown.
Reliability	• Test-retest: over a 1- to 3-day period, *r* ranged from .82 to .97 • Interrater reliability: ranged from 88% to 97%
Validity	• Content: established by comparing PASS with several established tests of IADL, mobility, and ADL • Construct: established in clinical studies using a number of diagnostic groups
References	Rogers, J. C., & Holm, M. B. (1988). *Performance assessment of self-care skills* (ver. 3.1). Available from J. C. Rogers and M. B. Holm, School of Health and Rehabilitation Sciences, University of Pittsburgh, Pittsburgh, PA. Holm, M. B. & Rogers, J. C. (1999). Performance assessment of self-care skills. In B. J. Hemphill-Pearson, *Assessments in occupational therapy mental health* (pp. 117–124), Thorofare, NJ: SLACK.

Category	Psychosocial Functioning
Test Name	***Profile of Mood States*** (POMS; McNair, Lorr, & Droppleman, 1971)
Publisher	Educational and Industrial Testing Service San Diego, CA 92107
Testing Level	B: Understanding of psychosocial issues
Purpose	Examine the dimensions of mood in a client
Target Population	Adults
Description	65-item adjective checklist reflecting measurement in terms of primary mood states. Especially sensitive to individuals with alcohol addiction
Variables Measured	Six mood dimensions: tension-anxiety, depression-dejection, confusion, anger-hostility, vigor, and fatigue
Format	Self-report questionnaire in which respondent rates the adjective on a scale from 1 (not at all) to 5 (extremely) based on the previous 7 days
Materials	Questionnaire, pencil
Scoring	Scores are obtained by summing factors and adding a constant. Summed scores are compared to either male or female norms.
Reliability	Internal consistency	r = range from .74 to 92
	Test-retest	r = ranges from .61 to .69 after a 1-month interval
Validity	Predictive	Sensitive in clinical change studies
References	McNair, D. M., Lorr, M., & Droppleman, L. F. (1971). *Profile of Mood States*. San Diego: Educational and Industrial Testing Service.

Category	Life Roles (Work/Leisure/Family)	
Test Name	***Role Activity Performance Scale*** (RAPS; Good-Ellis, Fine, Haas, Spencer, & DiVittis, 1987)	
Publisher	Unpublished; see reference below.	
Testing Level	B: Experienced in interviewing	
Purpose	Identify performance over the previous 18 months in 12 primary role functions	
Target Population	Adult clients with psychosocial dysfunction	
Description	Assesses 12 role domains including work, education, home management, relationships (family, parental, social, and marital), leisure, self-management, health, hygiene and appearance, and rehab treatment	
Variables Measured	Changes in level of functioning in each of the role domains	
Format	Semi-structured interview and rating scales	
Materials	Paper-pencil evaluation or verbal interview	
Scoring	6-point rating with operational definitions	
Reliability	Interrater reliability:	Ranged from .82 to .99 across four raters
Validity	Content:	Independent expert review of content to determine • reflection of roles • relevancy to occupational therapy
References	Good-Ellis, M., Fine, S. B., Spencer, J. H., & DiVittis, A. (1987). Developing a Role Activity Performance Scale. *American Journal of Occupational Therapy, 41,* 232–241. Good-Ellis, M. A. (1999). The Role Activity Performance Scale. In B. J. Hemphill-Pearson, *Assessments in occupational therapy mental health* (pp. 205–226), Thorofare, NJ: SLACK.	

Category	Life Roles (Work/Leisure/Family)	
Test Name	*Role Checklist* (Barris, Oakley, & Kielhofner, 1988)	
Publisher	Unpublished scale. Obtain from Frances Oakley, MS, OTR/L, FAOTA, Occupational Therapy Service, National Institutes of Health, Building 10, Room 6S-235, 10 Center Drive MSC 1604, Bethesda, MD 20892-1604	
Testing Level	A: Interpretation by any occupational therapist	
Purpose	Identify major roles in one's life	
Target Population	Adolescent or Adult	
Description	Checklist containing 10 roles (student, worker, volunteer, care giver, home maintainer, friend, family member, religious participant, hobbyist/amateur, participant in organizations, or other). Roles in past, present, or future are identified and then ranked in importance.	
Variables Measured	Qualitative summary of roles based on the Model of Human Occupation frame of reference	
Format	Paper and pencil test	
Materials	Test booklet	
Scoring	Qualitative scoring which can be used in planning treatment	
Reliability	Test-retest	$r = .82$ (median) over a 2-week period
Validity	Content	Based on literature review and consulation with experts
References	Oakley, F., Kielhofner, G., Barris, R., & Reichler, R. K. (1986). The Role Checklist: Development and empirical assessment of reliability. *Occupational Therapy Journal of Research, 6,* 157–169. Barris, R., Oakley, F., & Kielhofner, G. (1988). The Role Checklist. In B. J. Hemphill (Ed.), *Mental Health assessment in occupational therapy: An integrative approach to the evaluative process* (pp. 75–91). Thorofare, NJ: SLACK. Dickerson, A. E. (1999). The Role Checklist. In B. J. Hemphill-Pearson (Ed.), *Assessments in occupational therapy mental health: An integrative approach* (pp. 175–191). Thorofare, NJ: SLACK.	

Category	Psychosocial Function (Anxiety)	
Test Name	***State-Trait Anxiety Inventory*** (STAI; Spielberger, 1983)	
Publisher	Mind Garden, 1690 Woodside Rd., Suite 202, Redwood City, CA 94061 (www.mindgarden.com)	
Testing Level	B: Must understand construct of anxiety	
Purpose	To assess how anxious an individual feels at a given moment (state) or in general (trait)	
Target Population	Adults with or without psychosocial dysfunction. (Other forms are available for adolescents or children.)	
Description	20 item self-rating scale, ranging from 1 to 4. Can be given in group or individually. Takes between 10 to 20 minutes. Two forms	
Variables Measured	State of anxiety (i.e., feeling at a given moment) and trait of anxiety (i.e., how a person generally feels)	
Format	Self-rating pencil-paper scale	
Materials	Scale, manual, scoring grid	
Scoring	Total score for both state and trait	
Reliability	Test-retest	$r = .27$ to $.62$ for State, upper $.70$ for Trait over 20 to 104 days
	Internal consistency	$r = .80$ and $.90$ for both State and Trait Anxiety
Validity	Construct	Based on experimental research of the construct
	Concurrent	High correlations with other self-report anxiety inventories and personality tests
References	Spielberger, C. D. (1983). *Manual for the State-Trait Anxiety Inventory.* Palo Alto, CA: Consulting Psychologists Press. Spielberger, C. D. (1985). Assessment of state and trait anxiety: Conceptual and methodological issues. *The Southern Psychologist, 2,* 6–16.	

Category	Self-Care (Independent Living)
Test Name	*Street Survival Skills Questionnaire* (SSSQ; Linkenhoker & McCarron, 1979; 1993)
Publisher	McCarron-Dial Systems, P.O. Box 45628, Dallas TX 75245
Testing Level	B: Needs training on how to administer and score tests
Purpose	Assessment of specific aspects of adaptive behavior needed for independent living
Target Population	Adolescents and adults with developmental disabilities, including psychosocial dysfunction
Description	Individually administered test consisting of community and living skills divided into 9 sections related to a specific area of adaptive behavior (e.g., basic concepts, functional signs, public services, health and safety, measurement)
Variables Measured	Variable, depending on the particular work sample. Examples include range of motion, speed of assembly, motor coordination.
Format	Norm-based pictorial multiple-choice test, individually administered
Materials	Binder containing 9 subtests of picture plates, scoring forms, curriculum guides, planning chart. Can be computer scored
Scoring	Raw scores are converted to scaled scores for comparison with the normed group. Norms are available for different populations.
Reliability	Test-retest	$r = .99$ for total test, .81 to .95 on subtests
	Internal consistency	$r = .95$ for total test, .69 to .96 on various subtests
Validity	Content	Sample of items developed after literature review, interviews with staff, analysis of behaviors, and statistical analysis.
References	Linkenhoker, D., & McCarron, L. T. (1979). *Adaptive behaviors: Street Survival Skills Questionnaire* (SSSQ). Available from McCarron-Dial Systems, P. O. Box 45628, Dallas, TX 75245. Dial, J., Freemon, L., McCarron, L., & Swearingen, S. (1979). Predictive validation of the McCarron–Dial Evaluation System. *Vocational Evaluation and Work Adjustment Bulletin, 12,* 11–18. Linkenhoker, D., & McCarron, L. T. (1993). *Adaptive behaviors: Street Survival Skills Questionnaire* (SSSQ; Rev. ed.). Available from McCarron-Dial Systems, P.O. Box 45628, Dallas, TX 75245.

Category	Psychosocial Functioning	
Test Name	***Stress Audit Questionnaire*** (Miller & Smith, 1983, 1988)	
Publisher	Biobehavioral Institute 13309 Beacon Street, Suite 202 Brookline, MA 02146	
Testing Level	B: needs understanding of biobehavioral model of stress	
Purpose	Operationalization of biobehavioral model of stress into a self-report questionnaire	
Target Population	Adults	
Description	238-item instrument that "samples the magnitude and types of stress experienced or anticipated . . . and assesses relative vulnerability to stress" (Miller, Smith, & Mehler, 1988)	
Variables Measured	14 scales, with 3 facets of stress: (a) Situational stress items, organized into six scales (family, individual roles, social being, environment, financial, and work/school), (b) symptom items, organized into seven physiological system scales (muscular system, parasympathetic nervous system, sympathetic nervous system, emotional, cognitive, endocrine, and immune system), and (c) vulnerability factors	
Format	Self-report questionnaire in which respondents are requested to rate items from 1 (almost always) to 5 (almost never) regarding the amount of stress encountered during the last 6 months and the anticipation of stress over the next 6 months	
Materials	Protocol, pencil, manual	
Scoring	Results are summed, and converted into a *T*-score (mean of 50, standard deviation of 10).	
Reliability	Test-retest	$r = .81$ for symptoms, .92 for sources after 1 week; .70 for symptoms and .72 for sources after 6 weeks
	Internal consistency	$r = .70$ and .90; Cronbach's Alpha shows scores between .87 and .93
Validity	Concurrent	Comparison with the *State-Trait Anxiety Inventory* showed .42 in state and .59 in trait.
References	Miller, L. H., & Smith, A. D. (1983). Stress Audit Questionnaire. *Your Life and Health, 98,* 20–30. Miller, L. H., Smith, A D., & Mehler, B. L. (1988). *The Stress Audit manual.* Brookline, MA: Biobehavioral Institute.	

Category	Psychosocial Function
Test Name	***Stress Management Questionnaire*** (SMQ; Stein, 1987)
Publisher	Unpublished questionnaire. Available from F. Stein, Department of Occupational Therapy, University of South Dakota, 414 E. Clark Street, Vermillion, SD 57069
Testing Level	B: Any occupational therapist
Purpose	Assess an individual's symptoms precipitated by stress, stressors that cause a stress response, and coping activities used to manage stress
Target Population	Typical adults and adults (18 and above) with disabilities, including those with schizophrenia, depression, or alcohol abuse
Description	Self-report paper and pencil test
Variables Measured	Three categories of responses: • Symptoms of stress (physiological, cognitive, emotional, and behavioral) • Stressors (e.g., interpersonal, intrapersonal, time demands, mechanical breakdowns, performance, financial) • Copers to manage stress (e.g., creative, construction, exercise, self-care, social, sports)
Format	Paper and pencil test
Materials	Protocol and standard directions
Scoring	Qualitative ranking of top 10 responses in each category from 1 to 10. Results are used to design a treatment program.
Reliability	Split-half	$r = .63$ to $.87$
	Test-retest	$r = .85$ to $.89$ on concurrence of ranks
Validity	Concurrent	$r = .28$ to $.67$ six stress management scales
References	Stein, F. (1987). *The Stress Management Questionnaire* (SMQ). Unpublished test instrument. Stein, F., & Nikolic, S. (1989). Teaching stress management techniques to a schizophrenic patient. *American Journal of Occupational Therapy, 43,* 162–169. Bentley, D. E., & Stein, F. (1994, July). *The stress management questionnaire: Development and work in progress.* Paper presented at the annual conference of the National Consultation on Career Development (NATCOM), Ontario.

Category	Work: Interest Inventory
Test Name	***Strong–Campbell Interest Inventory*** (SCII; Strong, Campbell, & Hansen, 1985)
Publisher	Consulting Psychologist Press 3803 East Bayshore Rd P.O. Box 10096 Palo Alto, CA 94303
Testing Level	A: Need some knowledge of vocational counseling to interpret
Purpose	Assess occupational interests for individuals who are oriented toward college graduation and professional occupations
Target Population	Adolescents through adults
Description	Self-inventory of occupational interests, using Holland's (1959) theory of career development
Variables Measured	Holland's Model of Realistic, Investigative, Artistic, Social, Enterprising, and Conventional themes
Format	Self-record inventory containing 325 three-response items; computerized scoring required (disk available through CPP)
Materials	Record book
Scoring	Provides scores in 193 areas: 6 general occupational themes, 23 basic interest scale, 162 occupational scales, 2 specific scales. Also includes 26 administrative indices
Reliability	Test-retest	$r = .70$ to $.92$ over a 2-week to 3-year period
Validity	Extensive studies to support, concurrent, predictive, and construct validity over a 40-year period
References	Strong, E. K., Campbell, D. P., & Hansen, J. (1985). *The Strong-Campbell Interest Inventory.* Minneapolis, MI: National Computer Systems.

Category	Work
Test Name	*Valpar* (Valpar Corp)
Publisher	Valpar Corp 3801 E. 34th, Suite 105 Tucson, AZ 85713
Testing Level	B: Needs training on how to administer and score tests
Purpose	Assessment of aptitude in several different skill areas
Target Population	General population, individuals needing rehabilitation, ages adolescent through adult
Description	19-separate independent work samples, ranging from fine motor dexterity to planning and organization tasks
Variables Measured	Variable, depending on the particular work sample. Examples include range of motion, speed of assembly, motor coordination
Format	Work samples, manipulative tasks
Materials	Individual kits contain all materials needed for each task
Scoring	Weighted combination of time and errors, with separate reporting forms for each sample. Separate norms for different populations

Reliability	Test-retest	Consistently reported as high; different for each task
Validity	Concurrent	Related to Wechsler scales, dexterity tests, interest inventories and achievement tests

References	Brown, C., McDaniel, Couch, R. & McClanahan, M. (1994). *Vocational evaluation systems and software: A consumer's guide.* Menomonie: Stout Vocational Institute, University of Wisconsin.

Category	Work
Test Name	***Worker Role Interview*** (WRI; Velozo, Kielhofner, & Fisher, 1990)
Publisher	Model of Human Occupation Clearing House University of Illinois at Chicago Department of Occupational Therapy (M/C 811) College of Associated Health Professions 1919 West Taylor Street, Chicago, IL 60612–7250
Testing Level	A: Any occupational therapist
Purpose	"Designed to identify the system and environmental variables that may influence the ability of the injured worker to return to work" (Kielhofner, Mallinson, & de las Heras, 1995, p. 223).
Target Population	Adults with work injuries
Description	Semi-structured interview of work attitudes and behavioral observations during work capacity assessment
Variables Measured	6 major variables within the Model of Human Occupation frame of reference: personal causation, values, interests, roles, habits, and work environment
Format	Semi-structured interview and behavioral observations
Materials	Worksheet
Scoring	4-point rating scale on 17 items based on a specific rating scale. Total score identifies the success in returning to work.
Reliability	Test- retest	$r = .95$ for a total score, .86 to .94 for the content areas over a 6- to 12-day interval
	Interrater reliability	$r = .81$ for three raters (range of .46 to .92 for six content areas)
Validity	Content	Validated by extensive literature review of factors influencing return to work.
References	Velozo, C., Kielhofner, G., & Fisher, A. (1990). *A user's guide to the Worker Role Interview (Research version)*. Chicago: Department of Occupational Therapy, University of Illinois at Chicago.

Category	Psychosocial Functioning	
Test Name	*Zung Self-Rating Depression Scale* (ZSRDS; Zung, 1965)	
Publisher	Unpublished; see reference below.	
Testing Level	A: No training required	
Purpose	Assess level of depression	
Target Population	Adult clients with depressive disorders	
Description	Self-administered, brief quantitative scale consisting of 20 questions, 10 positive and 10 symptomatically negative. Client rates each item from "little of time" to "most of time."	
Variables Measured	Level of depression, ranging from infrequently to frequently	
Format	Paper-pencil test. Client reads the description and circles responses ranging from "little of time" to "most of time."	
Materials	Questionnaire, pencil	
Scoring	Points are calculated according to a rating of 1 to 4, with negative and positive items scored in opposite way. Points are summed, and divided by 80 (total possible points). Result is percentage of depression. Scores above .63 indicate depression; scores between .38 and .71 may suggest another psychiatric problem.	
Reliability	Test-retest	• Administration pre- and posttest treatment revealed changes in means from .74 to .39. • Administration to a control group revealed a mean score of .33, with a range of .25 to .43
Validity	Content	High correlation with clinical evaluation, self-rating depressive disorder, self-rating score on Zung, and EEG responses during sleep
References	Zung W. K. (1965). A self-rating depression scale. *Archives of General Psychiatry, 12,* 63–70.	

REFERENCES

Allen, C. K. (1982). Independence through activity: The practice of occupational therapy (psychiatry). *American Journal of Occupational Therapy, 36,* 731–739.

Allen, C. K. (1985). *Occupational therapy for psychiatric diseases: Measurement and management of cognitive disabilities.* Boston: Little, Brown.

Allen, C. K., Earhart, C. A., & Blue, T. (1992). *Occupational therapy treatment goals for the physically and cognitively disabled.* Rockville, MD: American Occupational Therapy Association.

Anastasi, A., & Urbina, S. (1997). *Psychological testing* (7th ed.). Englewood Cliffs, NJ: Prentice Hall.

Asher, I. E. (1996). *Occupational therapy assessment tools: An annotated index* (2nd ed.). Rockville, MD: American Occupational Therapy Association.

American Occupational Therapy Association. (1994). *Uniform terminology for occupational therapy: Application to practice* (3rd ed.). Rockville, MD: Author.

Baptiste, S., & Rochon, S. (1999). Client-centered assessment: The Canadian Occupational Performance Measure. In B. J. Hemphill-Pearson, *Assessments in occupational therapy mental health: An integrative approach* (pp. 42–57). Thorofare, NJ: SLACK.

Barris, R., Oakley, F., & Kielhofner, G. (1988). The Role Checklist. In B. J. Hemphill (Ed.), *Mental health assessment in occupational therapy: An integrative approach to the evaluative process* (pp. 75–91). Thorofare, NJ: SLACK.

Barth, T. (1985). *Barth Time Construction.* New York: Health Related Consulting Services.

Barth, T. (1988). Barth Time Construction. In B. J. Hemphill (Ed.), *Mental health assessment in occupational therapy: An integrative approach to the evaluative process* (pp. 117–129). Thorofare, NJ: SLACK.

Bentley, D. E., & Stein, F. (1994, July). *The stress management questionnaire: Development and work in progress.* Paper presented at the annual conference of the National Consultation on Career Development (NATCOM), Ontario.

Black, M. M., Gordon, J., & Santelli, J. (1999). Adolescent Risk-Taking Behaviors: Computer-assisted questionnaire. In B. J. Hemphill-Pearson, *Assessments in occupational therapy mental health: An integrative approach* (pp. 310–319). Thorofare, NJ: SLACK.

Brayman, S. J., Kirby, T. F., Meisenheimer, A. M. & Short, M. J. (1976). The comprehensive occupational therapy evaluation scale. *American Journal of Occupational Therapy, 30,* 94–100.

Breines, E. (1988). The Functional Assessment Scale as an instrument for measuring changes in levels of function for nursing home residents following occupational therapy. *Canadian Journal of Occupational Therapy, 55,* 135–140.

Brigance, A. (2000). *Comprehensive Inventory of Basic Skills–Revised* (CIBS-R). North Billerica, MA: Curriculum Associates.

Brown, C., McDaniel, Couch, R., & McClanahan, M. (1994). *Vocational evaluation systems and software: A consumer's guide.* Menomonie: Stout Vocational Institute, University of Wisconsin.

Chan, C., & Lee, T. M. C. (1997). Validation of Canadian Occupational Performance Measure. *Occupational Therapy International, 4,* 231–249.

Cole, B., Finch, E., Gowland, C., & Mayo, N. (1994). *Physical rehabilitation outcome measures.* Toronto, Ontario: Canadian Physiotherapy Association in cooperation with Health and Welfare Canada and the Canada Communication Group—Publishing, Supply and Services, Canada.

Davis, F. B. (Chair). (1974). *Standards for education and psychological tests.* Prepared by a joint committee of the American Psychological Association, American Educational Research Association, and National Council on Measurement in Education. Washington, DC: American Psychological Association.

Dial, J., Freemon, L., McCarron, L., & Swearingen, S. (1979). Predictive validation of the McCarron-Dial Evaluation System. *Vocational Evaluation and Work Adjustment Bulletin, 12,* 11–18.

Dickerson, A. E. (1999). The role checklist. In B. J. Hemphill-Pearson (Ed.), *Assessments in occupational therapy mental health: An integrative approach* (pp. 175–191, Thorofare, NJ: SLACK.

Earhart, C. A., & Allen, C. A. (1988). *Cognitive disabilities: Expanded activity analysis.* Los Angeles County/University of Southern California Medical Center.

Fischer, J., & Corcoran, K. (1995). *Measures for clinical practice: A sourcebook* (2nd ed.). New York: Free Press.

Folstein, M. F., Folstein, S. E., & McHugh, P. R. (1975). Mini-mental state: A practical method for grading the cognitive state of patients for the clinician. *Journal of Psychiatric Research, 12,* 189–198.

Good-Ellis, M., Fine, S. B., Spencer, J. H., & DiVittis, A. (1987). Developing a Role Activity Performance Scale. *American Journal of Occupational Therapy, 41,* 232–241.

Good-Ellis, M. A. (1999). The Role Activity Performance Scale. In B. J. Hemphill-Pearson (Ed.), *Assessments in occupational therapy mental health* (pp. 205–226), Thorofare, N.J.: SLACK.

Haertlein, C. L. (1999). The Milwaukee Evaluation of Daily Living Skills. In B. J. Hemphill-Pearson (Ed.), *Assessments in occupational therapy mental health: An integrative approach* (pp. 245–257), Thorofare, NJ: SLACK.

Hathaway, S. R., & McKinley, J. C. (1943). *The Minnesota Multiphasic Personality Inventory* (Rev. ed.). Minneapolis: University of Minnesota Press.

Health Outcomes Institute. (1995). *HSQ-2, Version 2.0.* Retrieved May 17, 2001, from the World Wide Web:http://assessments.ncs.com/assessments/download/medicalcat/HSQ.pdf.

Hemphill, B. J. (Ed.). (1982). *The evaluative process in psychiatric occupational therapy.* Thorofare, NJ: SLACK.

Hemphill, B. J. (1988a). An integrative approach to the use of occupational therapy assessments in mental health. In B. J. Hemphill (Ed.), *Mental health assessment in occupational therapy* (pp. 1–20). Thorofare, NJ: SLACK.

Hemphill, B. J. (Ed.). (1988b). *Mental health assessment in occupational therapy.* Thorofare, NJ: SLACK.

Henry, A. D., & Mallinson, T. (1999). The Occupational Performance History Interview. In B. J. Hemphill-Pearson (Ed.), *Assessments in occupational therapy mental health: An integrative approach* (pp. 59–70). Thorofare, NJ: SLACK.

Holm, M. B., & Rogers, J. C. (1999). Performance assessment of self-care skills. In B. J. Hemphill-Pearson (Ed.), *Assessments in occupational therapy mental health: An integrative approach* (pp. 117–124), Thorofare, NJ: SLACK.

Holmes, T. H., & Rahe, R. H. (1967). The Social Readjustment Rating Scale. *Journal of Psychosomatic Research, 11,* 213–218.

Houston, D., Williams, S. L., Bloomer, J., & Mann, W. D. (1989). The Bay Area Functional Performance Evaluation: Development and standardization. *American Journal of Occupational Therapy, 43,* 170–182.

Hudson, W. W. (1982). *The clinical measurement package: A field manual.* Chicago: Dorsey.

Itzkovich, M., Elazar, B., Averbuch, S., & Katz, N. (1990). *Loewenstein Occupational Therapy Cognitive Assessment.* Los Angeles: Western Psychological Services.

Jacobs, K. (1985). *Occupational therapy: Work-related programs and assessments.* Boston: Little, Brown.

Jacobs, K. (1991). The Jacobs Prevocational Skills Assessment. In K. Jacobs, *Occupational therapy: Work-related programs and assessments* (2nd ed., pp. 61–136). Boston: Little, Brown.

Johnson, T. P., Vinnicombe, B. J., & Merrill, G. W. (1980). The Independent Living Skills Evaluation. *Occupational Therapy in Mental Health, 2*(1), 5–18.

Katz, M. M., & Lyerly, S. B. (1963). Methods for measuring adjustment and social behavior in the community: I. Rationale, description, discriminative validity and scale development. *Psychological Reports, 13,* 503–535.

Katz, N., Itzkovich, M., Averbuch, S., & Elazer, G. (1989). Lowenstein Occupational Therapy Cognitive Assessment (LOTCA) battery for brain-injured patients: Reliability and validity. *American Journal of Occupational Therapy, 43,* 184–192.

Kielhofner, G., & Henry, A. D. (1988). Development and investigation of the occupational performance history interview. *American Journal of Occupational Therapy, 42,* 489–498.

Kielhofner, G., Mallinson, T., Crawford, E., Nowak, M., Rigby, M., Henry, A., & Walens, D. (1998). *A* user's manual for the Occupational Performance History Interview, Version 2. Chicago: Model of Human Occupation Clearinghouse, University of Illinois.

Klyczek, J. P. (1999). The Bay Area Functional Performance Evaluation. In B. J. Hemphill-Pearson (Ed.), *Assessments in occupational therapy mental health: An integrative approach* (pp. 87–107). Thorofare, NJ: SLACK.

Koyano, W., & Shibata, H. (1994). Development of a measure of subjective well-being in Japan: Construct validity and reliable of the Life Satisfaction K. In L. J. Fitten (Ed.). *Facts and research in gerontology: Dementia and cognitive impairments* (Suppl 2; pp. 181–187). New York: Springer.

Kunz, K. R., & Brayman, S. J. (1999). The Comprehensive Occupational Therapy Evaluation. In B. J. Hemphill-Pearson (Ed.), *Assessments in occupational therapy mental health: An integrative approach* (pp. 260–274). Thorofare, NJ: SLACK.

Law, M., Baptiste, S., Carswell–Opzoomer, A., McColl, M., Polatajko, H., & Pollock, N. (1991). *Canadian Occupational Performance Measure manual.* Toronto: Canadian Association of Occupational Therapists.

Law, M., Baptiste, S., Carswell, A., McColl, M. A., Polatajko, H., & Pollock, N. (1994). *Canadian Occupational Performance Measure* (2nd ed.). Toronto, Ontario: Canadian Association of Occupational Therapists.

Law, M., Polatajko, H., Pollock, N., McColl, M. A., Carswell, A., & Baptiste, S. (1994). Pilot testing of the Canadian Occupational Performance Measure: Clinical and measurement issues. *Canadian Journal of Occupational Therapy, 61*(4), 191–197.

Leonardelli, C. A. (1988). *The Milwaukee Evaluation of Daily Living Skills* (MEDLS). Thorofare, NJ: SLACK.

Lerner, C. J. (1982). Magazine Picture Collage. In B. Hemphill (Ed.), *The evaluative process in psychiatric occupational therapy* (pp. 139–154, 361–362). Thorofare, NJ: SLACK.

Lerner, C. J., & Ross, G. (1977). The Magazine Picture Collage: Development of an objective scoring sys-

tem. *American Journal of Occupational Therapy, 31*, 156–161.

Lewis, C. B., & McNerney, T. (1994). *The functional tool box: Clinical measures of functional outcomes.* Washington, DC: Learn.

Linkenhoker, D., & McCarron, L. T. (1979). *Adaptive behaviors: Street Survival Skills Questionnaire* (SSSQ). (Available from McCarron-Dial Systems, P.O. Box 456289, Dallas, TX 75245.)

Linkenhoker, D., & McCarron, L. T. (1993). *Adaptive behaviors: Street Survival Skills Questionnaire* (SSSQ) (Rev. ed.). (Available from McCarron-Dial Systems, P.O. Box 456289, Dallas, TX 75245.)

Masagatani, G. (1994). *Cognitive Adaptive Skills Evaluation manual* (Rev. ed.). Unpublished manuscript. (Available from Gladys Masagatani, Eastern Kentucky University, Department of Occupational Therapy, Dizney 103, Richmond, KY 40475–3135.)

Masagatani, G. N. (1999). The Cognitive Adaptive Skills Evaluation. In B. J. Hemphill-Pearson (Ed.), *Assessments in occupational therapy mental health: An integrative approach* (pp. 280–284). Thorofare, NJ: SLACK.

Masagatani, G. N., Nielson, C. S., & Ranslow, E. R. (1981). *Cognitive Adaptive Skills Evaluation manual.* New York: Haworth.

Matsutsuyu, J. (1969). The Interest Checklist. *American Journal of Occupational Therapy, 23*, 368–373.

McNair, D. M., Lorr, M., & Droppleman, L. F. (1971). *Profile of mood states.* San Diego: Educational and Industrial Testing Service.

Melzack, R. (1987). The short–form McGill Pain Questionnaire. *Pain, 30*, 191–197.

Miller, E. R., & Parachek, J. F. (1974). Validation and standardization of a goal-oriented, quick-screening geriatric scale. *Journal of the American Geriatrics Society, 22*, 278–283.

Miller, L. H., & Smith, A. D. (1983). Stress Audit Questionnaire. *Your Life and Health, 98*, 20–30.

Miller, L. H., Smith, A. D., & Mehler, B. L. (1988). *The Stress Audit manual.* Brookline, MA: Biobehavioral Institute.

Murphy, L. L., Impara, J. C., & Plake, B. S. (Eds.). (1999). *Tests in print V: An index to tests, test reviews, and the literature on specific tests.* Lincoln, NE: Buros Institute.

Nadolsky, J. M. (1974). The work sample in vocational evaluation: A consistent rationale. *Vocational Evaluation and Work Adjustment Bulletin, 7,* 2–5.

Oakley, F., Kielhofner, G., Barris, R., & Reichler, R. K. (1986). The Role Checklist: Development and empirical assessment of reliability. *Occupational Therapy Journal of Research, 6,* 157–170.

Parachek, J. F., & King, L. J. (1986). *Parachek Geriatric Rating Scale* (3rd ed.). [Available from Center for Neurodevelopmental Studies, 5340 West Glenn Drive, Glendale, AZ 85301.]

Pfeiffer, E. (1975). A short portable mental status questionnaire for the assessment of organic brain deficit in elderly patients. *Journal of the American Geriatrics Society, 23,* 433–441.

Plutchik, R., Conte, H., Lieberman, M., Baker, M., Grossman, J., & Lehrman, N. (1970). Reliability and validity of a scale for assessing the functioning of geriatric patients. *Journal of the Geriatric Society, 18,* 491–500.

Power, P. W. (2000). *A guide to vocational assessment* (3rd ed.). Austin, TX: Pro-Ed.

Reynolds, W. M., & Kobak, K. A. (1995). *Hamilton Depression Inventory (HDI), professional manual.* Odessa, FL: PAR.

Rogers, J. C. (1988). The NPI Interest Checklist. In B. J. Hemphill (Ed.), *Mental health assessment in occupational therapy: An integrative approach to the evaluative process* (pp. 93–114). Thorofare, NJ: SLACK.

Rogers, J. C., & Holm, M. B. (1988). *Performance assessment of self-care skills* (ver. 3.1). [Available from J. C. Rogers and M. B. Holm, School of Health and Rehabilitation Sciences, University of Pittsburgh, Pittsburgh, PA.]

Rogers, J., Weinstein, J., & Firone, J. (1978). The Interest Checklist: An empirical assessment. *American Journal of Occupational Therapy, 32,* 628–630.

Smith, N. R., Kielhofner, G., & Watts, S. J. H. (1986). The relationships between volition, activity pattern, and life satisfaction in the elderly. *American Journal of Occupational Therapy, 40,* 278–283.

Smith, R. O. (1999). OT FACT applications in mental health. In B. J. Hemphill-Pearson (Ed.), *Assessments in occupational therapy mental health: An integrative approach* (pp. 289–307). Thorofare, NJ: SLACK.

Spielberger, C. D. (1983). *Manual for the State-Trait Anxiety Inventory.* Palo Alto, CA: Consulting Psychologists Press.

Spielberger, C. D. (1985). Assessment of state and trait anxiety: Conceptual and methodological issues. *The Southern Psychologist, 2,* 6–16.

Stein, F. (1987). *The Stress Management Questionnaire (SMQ).* Unpublished test instrument. [Available from F. Stein, University of South Dakota, School of Medicine, Occupational Therapy Dept., 404 E. Clark Street, Vermillion, SD. 57069]

Stein, F. (1988). Research analysis of occupational therapy assessments used in mental health. In B .J. Hemphill (Ed.), *Mental health assessment in occupational therapy: An integrative approach to the evaluative process* (pp. 223–247). Thorofare, NJ: SLACK.

Stein, F., Bentley, D. E., & Natz, M. (1999). Computerized assessment: The Stress Management Questionnaire. In B. J. Hemphill-Pearson (Ed.), *Assessments in occupational therapy mental health: An integrative approach* (pp. 321–337). Thorofare, NJ: SLACK.

Stein, F., & Cutler, S. K. (1996). *Clinical research in allied health and special education.* San Diego: Singular Publishing Group.

Stein, F., & Cutler, S. K. (2000). *Clinical research in occupational therapy.* San Diego: Singular Publishing Group.

Stein, F., & Nikolic, S. (1989). Teaching stress management techniques to a schizophrenic patient. *American Journal of Occupational Therapy, 43,* 162–169.

Strong, E. K., Campbell, D. P., & Hansen, J. (1985). *The Strong-Campbell Interest Inventory.* Minneapolis, MI: National Computer Systems.

The Psychological Corporation. (2000). *Wechsler Individual Achievement Test–2.* San Antonio, TX: Author.

Thomson, L. K. (1992). *The Kohlman Evaluation of Living Skills* (3rd ed.). Rockland, MD: American Occupational Therapy Association.

Thomson, L. K. (1999). The Kohman Evaluation of Living Skills. In B. J. Hemphill-Pearson (Ed.), *Assessments in occupational therapy mental health: An integrative approach* (pp. 231–242), Thorofare, NJ: SLACK.

Unsworth, C. (1999). Allen's Cognitive Level Test. In C. Unsworth (Ed.), *Cognitive and perceptual dysfunction: A clinical reasoning approach to evaluation and intervention* (pp. 86–87, 91–92). Philadelphia: F. A. Davis.

Van Deusen, J., & Brunt, D. (1997). *Assessment in occupational therapy and physical therapy.* Philadelphia: Saunders.

Velozo, C., Kielhofner, G., & Fisher, G. (1990). *A user's guide to the worker role interview* (research version). Unpublished manuscript, University of Illinois at Chicago.

Williams, S., & Bloomer, J. (1987). *Bay Area Functional Performance Evaluation* (2nd ed.). Novato, CA: Consulting Psychologists Press.

Woodcock, R. W., McGrew, K. S., & Mathers, N. (2000). *Woodcock Johnson, Tests of Achievement–III® (WJ-III).* Chicago: Riverside Publishing.

Yesavage, J. A., Brink, T. A., Rose, T. L., Lum, O., Huang, V., Adey, M., & Leirer, V. O. (1983). Development and validation of a geriatric depression screening scale: A preliminary report. *Journal of Psychiatric Research, 17,* 37–49.

Zung, W. K. (1965). A self-rating depression scale. *Archives of General Psychiatry, 12,* 63–70.

CHAPTER

7

Medications Related to Psychosocial Issues

> *In recent years a considerable number of drugs have been intro-
> duced which, though they do not have a causal influence, are so
> effective symptomatically that their use has become very wide-
> spread.*
>
> — P. H. Hoch (1959), Drug therapy. In S. Arieti (Ed.),
> *American Handbook of Psychiatry,* Vol. 2, p. 1541.

Operational Learning Objectives

By the end of this chapter, the learner will:

1. Discriminate between the terms "trade drug" and "generic drug."

2. Identify common trade and generic names for specific medications used in drug treatment.

3. Define important terms related to drug and medication issues.

4. Differentiate among Schedule I, II, III, IV, and V drugs.

5. Understand major classifications of drugs used in psychiatric and other neurological disorders.

6. Understand the mechanisms of drugs.

7. Distinguish between drugs given for different diagnoses.

8. Identify adverse effects for specific drugs.

9. Understand how to observe adverse effects.

10. Understand interactions between foods, herbs, and drugs.

Since the 1950s, when the chance discovery that the use of drugs could alleviate some of the somatic symptoms of persons with mental illness, the use of drugs and medications in therapeutic treatment has expanded extensively (Opler, 1992). In the majority of psychiatric facilities in which occupational therapists are employed, including community-based facilities, approximately 90 percent or more of the patients will be receiving some type of psychotropic drug. Although fewer in number than adults, an increasing number of children receive drugs to control for the symptoms of ADHD, conduct disorders, and emotional disorders. According to *USA Today* (1997), "'about 2.8% of people under 19—1.5 million—are on the stimulant drug,' says Daniel Safer of Johns Hopkins University Medical School" (p. 1). Consequently, psychosocial occupational therapists need to have a basic understanding of medication issues. In this chapter, we will attempt to answer the following questions:

▶ What do occupational therapists need to know about major drugs?

▶ What are the different classifications of drugs?

▶ Which drugs are effective in reducing symptoms with specific mental illnesses?

▶ How does a physician or psychiatrist decide to use medication in treatment and how does he or she choose the medication?

▶ How do drugs work?

▶ What is a drug receptor?

▶ What is drug absorption?

▶ What is the effect of a drug on a fetus?

▶ What are the physiological barriers to drug absorption?

▶ What is drug biotransformation?

▶ What factors affect drug biotransformation?

▶ What are the clinical signs of drug toxicity?

▶ How are drug levels measured in an individual?

▶ What does bioavailability mean and how do drugs with similar compounds differ?

▶ What are drug antagonists and drug agonists?

▶ How does a physician decide the frequency and dosage of the drug?

▶ What is a "drug holiday"?

▶ What happens if a client misses a dosage?

▶ How do drugs interact with foods, herbs, and other drugs?

▶ How does physical activity and sleep affect the actions of drugs?

▶ What is meant by a half-life of a drug?

▶ What are some of the general effects of abrupt withdrawal of medication?

▶ Can some drugs be abruptly withdrawn safely?

▶ What are the major side effects or adverse effects of specific drugs?

▶ What are some of the abbreviations used regarding medication (e.g., p.r.n., p.o., s.c., b.i.d., t.i.d)

DEFINITIONS AND TERMS

What is a drug? *Taber's Cyclopedic Medical Dictionary* (1993) defines a drug as "any substance that when taken into the living organism, may modify one or more of its functions" (p. 576). Drugs are considered non-food substances and they are monitored by the Food and Drug Administration (FDA). Subtances that can claim nutrient value can avoid FDA regulation. Drugs are used in psychosocial illnesses to modify the functioning of an individual with mental illness by ameliorating the symptoms of the illness. Any discussion of the way in which drugs work necessitates an understanding of basic terms and concepts. The reader may find it helpful to refer to the definitions in Table 7–1 in further understanding the mechanisms of drugs are described in the text.

Table 7–1. Essential Terms and Concepts in Medication Issues

Allergic reactions to a drug are systemic responses in which the immune system reacts as if a foreign substance has been introduced into the organism. Respiratory and cardiovascular symptoms can arise from allergic reactions.

An **agonist** is a substance that mimics the effects of a neurotransmitter, hormone, or other chemical, usually because it acts on a receptor.

An **antagonist** is a substance or drug that blocks the effect of a neurotransmitter, hormone, or other chemical at a receptor while causing no effect itself. A functional antagonist acts opposite the agonist to "cancel" the agonist's actions.

Anticholinergic effects (blocking parasympathetic impulses) are side effects or adverse affects of some drugs. Adverse effects include dry mouth, blurred vision, constipation, urinary retention, increased heart rate, increased blood pressure, and reduced sweating.

Bioavailability is the rate and extent of absorption of the active molecules into the body so that the drug can act in a therapeutic way. Even though a generic drug has the same amount of the therapeutic compound as the trade drug, the bioavailability may be different, thus affecting the way in which the generic drug works.

Bolus is usually a large concentrated amount of a drug given through oral or intravenous injection.

Chemical name refers to the chemical compound of a specific drug. This name is used in scientific literature or research studies.

A **drug** is a substance, which when taken into the body, modifies one or more bodily functions.

Drug dependency or addiction is a compulsion or biological craving for a drug. The drug can produce a desired psychological effect that creates the dependency or its withdrawal can create discomfort or pain.

A **drug holiday** is an interval when the physician or psychiatrist prescribes that a specific drug be stopped for a period of time so that the patient can be evaluated for toxic reactions, to allow the patient to recover from adverse effects, or to minimize the development of side effects as well.

Drug interactions are the effects that occur when two or more drugs are taken concurrently. Interactions can have antagonistic, additive, cumulative, or super additive results.

The **effective dose** (ED) indicates the percentage of people that show the desired effect of a drug at a given dosage.

The **generic name** refers to the legal or official name of a drug. The generic name is sometimes categorized as the nonproprietary name of a drug, meaning that it is not trademarked by a commercial drug company. The name is assigned by the United States Adopted Name Council (USAN) when it becomes available to the public.

The **pharmocological half-life** refers to the time it takes for 1/2 of the drug effect to be lost. This may be different from the biological half-life, which refers to the amount of time required for half of the drug to be excreted from the body or hepatic biotransformation to occur.

The **lethal dose** (LD) indicates the percentage of the population who would die from taking a given drug at a given dosage.

Monamine oxidase inhibitors (MAOIs) are a class of antidepressant drugs. Nardil®, Marplan®, and Parnate® are the most commonly used MAOIs. Some severe side effects such as hypertension can occur with MAOIs when dietary restrictions are not followed.

Neuroleptic drugs are a class of psychotrophic drugs specifically intended to treat individuals with psychosis such as schizophrenia.

Norepinephrine Dopamine Reuptake Inhibitors (NDRI) are a class of antidepressents that inhibit the reuptake of dopamine and neorepinephrine into presynaptic neurons. For example, Wellbutrin® is an NDRI.

Parenteral route of administration refers to the introduction of a drug into the body in a manner other than through the gastrointestinal system. For example, intravenous, intramuscular injection, or subcutaneous administration as through a patch, are all parenteral routes of administration.

Table 7–1. Essential Terms and Concepts in Medication Issues

Pharmacodynamics refers to the actions of drugs on the body.

Pharmacokinetics refers to the metabolism of drugs in the body. Specifically, this is the way in which drugs are absorbed, distributed, bound, inactivated, and excreted.

Pharmacotherapeutics is the study of how drugs are used in "treatment, prevention, or diagnosis of disease" (Malone, 1989, p. 2).

Placebos are totally inert substances that cause no physiological change, but are administered as though they were medicines (McKim, 1986). A placebo effect occurs when people believe they are being administered a drug that will have an effect, even though there is no drug-related explanation for the improvement. Placebos can have a positive effect and cause improvement. In a double-blind study, the participants receive either a placebo or medication. The researchers or physicians are unaware of which patients are in which group or whether the medication is a drug or a placebo.

Psychotrophic drugs are intended to affect an individual's mood, behavior, and other aspects of mental activity, such as depression or anxiety.

Routes of administration are the methods used to get the drug into the body. The two major routes of administration are enteral and parenteral.

Serotonin-2 Antagonist/Reuptake Inhibitors (SARI) are a class of second-generation antidepressants that result in down-regulation of ß-adrenergic receptors.

Selective Serotonin Reuptake Inhibitors (SSRIs) are a class of antidepressant drugs that work by keeping serotonin in the synapse so that it is not depleted. Prozac®, Zoloft®, and Paxil® are drugs that are SSRIs.

Side effects of a drug are the adverse effects of a drug such as nausea, fatigue, blurred vision, and dizziness.

The **therapeutic index** (TI) of a drug is used to measure the safety of a drug and is determined by the ratio between ED_{50} and LD_{50}. The higher the index, the safer the drug. It is a relative value that may be of limited value clinically.

Tolerance refers to the decreasing effect of a drug after repeated administrations. In these cases, individuals need a larger dosage to obtain the same drug effect.

The **trade name** is the proprietary or brand name of a drug that a company registers with the U.S. Patent Office.

Naming the Drug

Drugs are usually given three names. The *chemical name* of the drug is the stated chemical compound that gives a complete description of the molecular structure of the drug. This name is rarely used except in the experimental laboratory where it is being tested. The *generic* or *nonproprietary name*, considered the legal or official name, specifies a particular chemical compound. This name, assigned when the chemical compound has been found to have therapeutic usefulness (Poe, 1989), is usually used in scientific literature or research studies. The *trade* or *brand name* (also called the proprietary name) is the name given to the drug by the company that manufactures it and which holds the patent. For example, Prozac® is the trade name for fluoxetine

hydrochloride, the generic or nonproprietary name. Usually, names that are meaningful and simple to remember are used as the trade name, undoubtably to make it easier for consumers to remember the name. After the patent for a specific drug has expired, other companies are free to manufacture the drug and give it another proprietary name. Thus, there may be several trade or brand names for a single generic drug. For example, ibuprofen is known as Motrin® when produced by Upjohn, and Nuprin® when produced by Bristol–Myers. Frequently, doctors prescribe medication by the trade name (McKim, 1986; Poe, 1989; Ray & Ksir, 1987).

Recently, there has been a trend to use a generic drug rather than the drug specified by the trade name, on the theory that the drugs with similar compounds are equivalent in how they affect an individual. However, this may not be universally true (Ray & Ksir, 1987), because the drugs may be prepared in somewhat different ways in spite of their equivalent chemical structure. Chemically equivalent drugs contain identical amounts and dosages of the active ingredient. Biological equivalents are drugs that when given in the same amount provide equal availability (i.e., bioavailability) of the active ingredient. Clinical equivalents are equivalent drugs which, when given in the same amount, provide the same therapeutic effect. Generic drugs and trade name drugs can differ in any of these ways (Ray & Ksir, 1987). Thus, 25 mg of desipramine (generic name) may not be clinically equivalent to 25 mg of Norpramin® (trade name), and thus may result in obvious or subtle difference in clinical effects.

Categorization of Drugs

Drugs are organized into various classes based on the particular function of the drug. Because this book is about psychosocial issues, our discussion will be limited to psychotherapeutic drugs used in the care and management of psychosocial disorders. The major classifications of drugs used in psychosocial disorders, as well as some examples of drugs in each classification, are found in Table 7–2. For more information, the reader is referred to a comprehensive text on pharmacology, or psychopharmacology such as the following:

▶ Bezchlibnyk-Butler, K. Z. , & Jeffries, J. J. (2000). *Clinical handbook of psychotropic drugs* (10th ed.). Seattle: Hogrefe & Huber.

▶ Ciccone, C. D. (1996). *Pharmacology in rehabilitation* (2nd ed.). Philadelphia: F. A. Davis.

▶ Craig, C. R., & Stitzel, R. E. (1997). *Modern pharmacology with clinical applications* (5th ed.). Boston: Little, Brown.

▶ Gitlin, M. J. (1996). *The psychotherapist's guide to psychopharmacology*. New York: The Free Press.

▶ Hardman, J. G., Limbird, L. E., Molinoff, P. B., Ruddon, R. W., & Gilman, A. G. (Eds.).

Table 7–2. Schedule of Controlled Substances

Schedule I	Drugs considered as the highest risk for abuse with use restricted to approved research studies, and generally not considered medically useful in the United States.
	Examples: LSD, heroin, marijuana, cocaine
Schedule II	High risk for abuse and addiction, but considered to have some medical usefulness.
	Examples: morphine, secobarbital, methamphetamine, methaqualoe
Schedule III	Mild to moderate risk for physical dependence and/or strong risk for psychological dependence.
	Examples: nonamphetamine stimulants, some narcotic preparations (e.g., paregoric), opioids combined in limited dosage with other non-narcotic drugs (e.g., codeine) or barbiturates not in Schedule II
Schedule IV	Limited potential for physical dependence and/or psychological dependence.
	Examples: benzodiazephines, antidepressants, and some stimulants
Schedule V	Lowest potential for abuse or physical and psychological dependence.
	Examples: cough medicines with opioids such as codeine, antidiarrhea preparations

Source: Adapted from *Pharmacology in Rehabilitation* (2nd ed.) by C. D. Ciccone, 1996, Philadelphia: F. A. Davis; and *Drugs, society, and Human Behavior* (4th ed.) by O. Ray & C. Ksir, 1987, St. Louis: Times Mirror/Mosby.

(1996). *Goodman and Gilman's: The pharmacological basis of therapeutics* (9th ed. Rev.). New York : McGraw-Hill, Health Professions Division.

▶ Katzung, B. G. (2000). *Basic and clinical pharmacology* (8th ed.). New York: McGraw- Hill.

▶ Malone, T. (Ed.). (1989). *Physical and occupational therapy: Drug implications for practice.* Philadelphia: Lippincott.

▶ Preston, J., O'Neal, H. H., & Talaga, M. C. (2000). *Handbook of clinical psychopharmacology for therapists.* Oakland, CA: New Harbinger.

In addition to the general classifications of drugs based on function, drugs that are under the Comprehensive Drug Abuse Prevention and Control Act (also known as the Controlled Substances Act) have the potential for physical or psychological dependence. These drugs are classified into five "schedules" based on their capacity for abuse (Umhauer, Their–Spain, & Spain, 1986). (See Table 7–2.) Penalties for possession or distributing these drugs illegally are administered in a court of law. Additionally, the drugs listed in Schedule I and II are restricted in production. Interestingly, Ritalin®, or methlyphenidate, is considered a Schedule II drug, and is therefore restricted in production, resulting in several recent news stories about the nonavailability of the drug for children with ADHD.

PHARMACOKINETICS

Pharmacokinetics refers to the biotransformation of drugs, specifically in the way the drug is administered, absorbed, distributed, bound, activated, inactivated, and excreted (McKim, 1986; Poe, 1989; Taber, 1989). Pharmacodynamics, which refers to drug action, is concerned with how quickly and how much of the drug arrives at the intended tissue, organ, or body structure and how the patient responds to the particular drug (Poe, 1989). A basic understanding of both pharmacokinetics and pharmacodynamics is necessary for occupational therapists working in psychosocial settings as the drugs can affect the way the patient responds to treatment. A careful observation of patients and clients before and during drug therapy is essential, so that potential negative side effects of the drug can be identified and rectified.

Administration and Absorption

The more efficiently a drug is administered, the more quickly it will begin to work within the individual. Efficient administration means that a large concentration of the drug must get to the site of action, (i.e., the intended tissue, organ, or body structure) as quickly as possible and must remain at the site of action for a sufficient length of time to become therapeutic. The method of administration is dependent on the nature and characteristics of the specific drug and the rate of absorption required.

Drugs are administered in two major ways: (a) *enterally*, or through the intestines, or (b) *parenterally*, or routes other than the intestines (e.g., injections, topical, and transdermal) (Ciccone, 1996; McKim, 1986; Poe, 1989). Within these two major routes, there are many modifications or variations.

The simplest and safest method of administration is orally, designated as *peroral* or *p.o.* (McKim, 1986). Although this method has several advantages, it may not be the most efficient manner of administration. Drugs given orally go directly to the stomach where they must withstand the action of stomach acids, digestive enzymes, and interference by food in the stomach (Ciccone, 1996; McKim, 1986; Ray & Ksir, 1987). If a drug is taken in a capsule or tablet form, it must first dissolve and mix with the content of the stomach and intestines. For most drugs, absorption is more efficient in the intestines rather than in the stomach; thus the rate of absorption is affected by the speed at which the drug can get to the intestines (McKim, 1986). "Enteric-coated" tablets are made so that they will not dissolve until they get into the small intestine (Poe, 1989). Until the drug is absorbed into the bloodstream, the drug is considered to be outside the body and therefore not medicinally useful (Ciccone, 1996; McKim, 1986). Drugs taken orally must be lipid soluble in order to pass through cells that line the walls of the stomach or gastrointestinal tract and into capillaries to enter the bloodstream. The amount and rate of absorption are affected by several factors, such as the amount of food in the stomach, visceral blood flow, intestinal infection, the solubility, or the acidity of gastric juices. Thus, although the oral method is commonly used, there is less predictability of effect than in other methods of administration (Benet, 1992; Gram, 1994a, 1994b; Katzung, 1992b; McKim, 1986; Yamamoto et al., 1985).

Once in the bloodstream, the drug is distributed to the liver, where it will be transformed into metabolites. This process is called *first-pass effect* (Benet, 1992). The drug remaining after the first-pass metabolism is free to go to the site of action. The dosage in oral administration, therefore, must be large enough to ensure that a therapeutic amount reaches the targeted tissue (Ciccone, 1996).

In spite of the disadvantages of oral administration, there are advantages to this method (Ciccone, 1996). First, as mentioned above, the method is safe and is the easiest to administer, especially when the individual must administer the drug to himself or herself. Second, the

amount of drug entering the bloodstream is fairly well controlled, thus preventing the large changes in the blood metabolism that may be seen with other types of administrations (Ciccone, 1996).

Other enteral routes include *sublingual* administration, which occurs by placing the drug under the tongue, or *buccal* administration, placing the drug between the gum and the cheek. In these cases, the drug is absorbed through the buccal membranes in the mouth, entering the bloodstream from the oral cavity (Gram, 1994a; McKim, 1986). From there, the drug goes to the heart, and eventually the targeted tissue, thereby bypassing the liver and the first-pass effect. A fourth method using enteral routes occurs through rectal administration, using a suppository. When a patient is unconscious, or when vomiting occurs as a result of the drug, this method is preferable (Poe, 1989). On the other hand, this method may result in irritation of the rectal membranes, and/or less absorption of the drug (Benet & Sheiner, 1985).

Parenteral routes of administration are preferable to enteral administration when it is important to get the drug to the site of action quickly. Likewise, when the patient is unable to take the drug by mouth, or the drug is not lipid soluble, a parenteral route of administration is used (Poe, 1989). In this type of administration, the drug is injected directly into the bloodstream, resulting in rapid absorption and transport to the site of action. Parenteral routes involving injection, and therefore a syringe and needle, require the drug to be in a solution or micro-suspension. When the normal state of a drug is a dry powder or crystalline form (the word "drug" is derived from French *drogue*, meaning a dry powder), it must be dissolved in some liquid before injection. The liquid is called a *vehicle*. Often a weak salt solution, called a saline solution, is used, because it is composed of the same concentration of body fluids (0.9 percent sodium chloride) and it does not irritate the body tissues. When the drug does not dissolve in water, alcohol is used. Alcohol, however, is not totally inert and may cause behavioral changes (McKim, 1986). A disadvantage of injections is the need for a sterile technique to prevent infection or illness. Additionally, training is required in administering of injections.

The most common parenteral route is intravenous (*I.V.*) injection into a peripheral vein. A more dangerous *I.V.* method is intra-arterial injection, where the drug is injected directly into an artery (Ciccone, 1996). Use of an *I.V.* has several advantages: (a) a *bolus* can be delivered, resulting in a high concentration of drug getting to the brain quickly; (b) the drug is absorbed into the tissues more quickly; (c) the drug action has a faster onset; (d) the amount and rate of administration can be easily regulated; and (e) irritating material can be injected. Roughly 7 seconds are needed to get the drug to the brain (Ferraro, personal notes, June 1–9, 1989). On the other hand, there are disadvantages (Ciccone, 1996; Gram, 1994a; McKim, 1986; Poe, 1989; Ray & Ksir, 1987): (a) a sterile technique is necessary to prevent infection; (b) the amount of drug must be strictly regulated to prevent too much from being administered; (c) side effects that occur from the bolus may be difficult to control or counteract; and (d) when intravenous injections are frequent, the vein wall loses strength and elasticity in areas and may collapse.

Subcutaneous injections (*s.c.*) place the drug between the skin or cutaneous tissue of the arm or thigh and the muscle. This method is used when a local or systemic response is desired, such as when checking for the presence of tuberculosis, administering a local anesthesia, or administering insulin. Two major disadvantages of this method are the limited amount of a drug that can be administered, and the possible irritation of the tissues (Ciccone, 1996).

Intramuscular injections (*I.M.*) are used more frequently than subcutaneous injections, partly because of its greater efficiency. As with other parenteral routes, the gastrointestinal tract is avoided, resulting in more rapid absorption of the drug into the bloodstream. Intramuscular injections are used most frequently when (a) a slower rate of absorption than would occur with an *I.V.* is desired, (b) when a larger amount of a drug is needed than can be given with an *s.c.*, or (c) when the drug is water-insoluble (Ferraro, personal communication, June 1–9, 1989; Poe, 1989). Additionally, this method provides a higher level of reliability and precision in the amount of drug absorbed and allows for larger amounts of the drug than would be seen with an *s.c.* administration (Gram, 1994a). Generally, the deltoid muscle of upper arm or gluteus maximus muscle of the buttocks is used because of their size (McKim, 1986). Most immunizations are given in the deltoid muscle (McKim, 1986), while *p.r.n.'s*[1] are given to agitated patients in the gluteus maximus muscle. The deltoid muscle allows for more rapid absorption because of larger blood vessels (McKim, 1986; Ray & Ksir, 1987).

Two less frequent administration sites using the parenteral route are intraperitoneal (*I.P.*) injection, where the drug is inserted into the peritoneal cavity, and intrathecal injection, where the drug is injected directly into the spinal subarachnoid space. The *I.P.* injection may be subject to a first-pass effect. The latter is used when it is necessary for the drug to bypass the blood-brain barrier (BBB) and go directly to the nervous system. Examples of drugs used in this manner are antibiotics, anticancer drugs, or narcotic analgesics (Ciccone, 1996).

---

[1]Meaning *pro re nata*, as circumstances may require, as needed, or as necessary.

The administration of inhalants use a parenteral route of administration, because the procedure avoids the gastrointestinal tract. Although the amount of drug reaching the bloodstream is affected by the amount of the drug getting to the lungs, and is therefore unpredictable (Ciccone, 1996), this method of administration is highly efficient (McKim, 1986). The large surface within the lungs and the enormous number of capillaries available enable the drug to reach the bloodstream, and thus the brain, quickly. The gaseous drug is diffused into the blood through the capillaries. Because excess amounts are exhaled, control of the drug is relatively simple. On the other hand, as the concentration of the drug is reduced, absorption becomes slower. Drugs that might irritate the respiratory tract cannot be administered in this manner (McKim, 1986). The use of inhalation requires patient training.

Finally, both the topical and transdermal administrations use parenteral routes. Topical administrations are applied directly to the skin. Transdermal patches are applied directly to the skin, but are intended to be absorbed by the body. Transdermally administered drugs must be able to penetrate the skin and must not be metabolized by enzymes in the skin (Finnen, Herdman, & Shuster, 1985; Kao, Patterson, & Hall, 1985). Transdermal patches require frequent reposition to avoid skin irritation and unpredictable drug absorption.

Drug Distribution

Once the drug has been administered, it must be absorbed and distributed. Four characteristics are required for drugs to be absorbed (Ray & Ksir, 1987): (a) the drug must be in solution; (b) the drug must be lipid soluble (McKim, 1986; Ray & Ksir, 1987); (c) the drug must be in a suitably high concentration; and (d) the drug molecule must be small enough to pass through pores in a membrane (McKim, 1986). Microsuspensions or lipid soluble drugs may be absorbed by mechanisms other than passive processes. The rate of absorption, and resulting distribution, depends on a number of factors (Ciccone, 1996; Gram, 1994a; McKim, 1986; Poe, 1989; Ray & Ksir, 1987). These factors include (a) the solubility of the lipid-soluble drugs, (b) the permeability of the capillaries or specific tissues, (c) the amount of lipid content, (d) the ionization of the drug, (e) the binding properties of the drug to protein, and (f) specific transport systems. Drug molecules with higher lipid solubility are more easily distributed than water-soluble drug molecules. The latter will frequently stay outside the cell, to be metabolized and excreted through body waste (Gram, 1994a; McKim, 1986; Ray & Ksir, 1987). Lipid solubility is affected by the degree of ionization; increased ionization results in decreased solubility. As with water-soluble drugs, molecules that have increased ionization remain outside the cell and are often eliminated before they can reach the site of action (Ray & Ksir, 1987). Only those drug molecules not bound to protein are free to be distributed. Drug molecules bound to a protein are stored in cell membranes until they are needed.

All administration methods, except intravenous injection, which places the drug directly into the bloodstream, require that the drug be transported to the bloodstream. In many cases, the transport system is "passive," meaning that no energy is required in the transport. Diffusion across membranes, filtration through intercellular channels, and bulk flow through intercellular pores are examples of passive transport. In each of these cases, a concentration gradient is the driving force behind the transport system. The drug crosses the membrane in order to equalize the drug concentration on either side of the membranes (Gram, 1994a; McKim, 1986; Poe, 1989).

A second transport system is called *active transport* because of the expenditure of energy (Poe, 1989). In this system, membrane proteins are used to carry the drug across the membrane (Almers & Stirling, 1984; Hobbs & Albers, 1980). Transport is only in one direction, toward the bloodstream. Thus, an active transport system can work against the concentration gradient by increasing the concentration of a drug rather than allowing for diffusion. Drugs that are nonlipid soluble, or ionized, are transported in this way. A third transport system, called *facilitated diffusion*, is similar to the active transport system in that drugs are transported by attaching themselves to a protein; however, because no energy is expended, there is no ability to transport the drug against the concentration gradient (Ciccone, 1996; Gram, 1994a).

Physiological Barriers to Drug Absorption

The *blood-brain barrier* (BBB) "consists of a single row of brain capillary endothelial cells that are joined by continuous tight intercellular junctions . . . [suggesting] that to gain access to the brain from the capillary circulation, drugs must pass through cells rather than between them" (Gram, 1994a, p. 31). The use of active transport systems allows specific drugs to enter the central nervous system in a restricted manner and with a slowed absorption rate (Ciccone, 1996). In general, there is no attempt to equalize the concentration of the drug on either side of the barrier (Gram, 1994a). When there is cerebral trauma, however, the blood-brain barrier is weakened, and substances normally excluded are admitted (Gram, 1994a; McKim, 1986). A similar situation is seen in the *placenta barrier*, except that this barrier is poorly constructed and the drug eventually enters into the fetus.

How much of the drug is absorbed into the blood is related to the route of administration and the ability of the drug to cross the barriers. This action is referred to as *bioavailability*. As noted previously, drugs with similar compounds may have different levels of bioavailability.

Drug Metabolism and Elimination

Drugs can be removed from the body by two different ways: biotransformation or excretion (Malone, 1989). "Metabolism [biotransformation] is a major mechanism by which drug action is terminated" (Gram, 1994b, p. 33). In the biotransformational process, the drugs are inactivated and transformed into metabolites, a more water-soluble compound (Ciccone, 1996; Malone, 1989; Ray & Ksir, 1987). "Chemical changes that occur during drug metabolism are usually due to oxidation, reduction, hydrolysis, or conjugation of the original compound" (Ciccone, 1990, p. 28). Although the liver is primarily responsible for metabolism, metabolism can also occur in the lungs, kidneys, the lining of the gastrointestinal tract, and the skin (Ciccone, 1996). When there is liver damage, metabolism is slowed or hindered. In these cases, there must be adjustments to the dosages of the drug to prevent toxicity or accumulation of the drug in the body (Ciccone, 1996).

The rate of biotransformation can be affected by the age of the individual, the amount of time a person takes a specific drug, diet, environment, smoking, and alcohol use (Ciccone, 1996). The prolonged use of a drug results in an increased efficiency of the liver to metabolize the drug because of an increase in the amount of enzyme. This process, known as *enzyme induction*, results in the drug being metabolized more quickly than would normally occur (Ferraro, personal communication, June 1–9, 1989; Ciccone, 1996). In other cases, metabolism will be slowed. "When two drugs that use the same enzyme are introduced into the body, the metabolism of each will be depressed because both will be competing for the enzyme" (McKim,1986, p. 34). Age affects the rate of metabolism. At birth, the enzyme systems are not fully functional, and in the elderly, the enzymes may lose some of their efficiency. Drug and diet interactions, such as with herbals and dietary supplements, can be dangerous. Use of MAO-inhibitors when taken with certain foods can be deadly (Ciccone, 1996). For example, foods high in tyramine content (e.g., beer, wine, salami, cheeses, chicken liver, lima beans, yeast) interact with MAOIs causing severe hypertension, headache, and sedation. In some cases, death may result from these interactions (Preston et al., 2000).

Once the drug is metabolized, it is excreted. The kidney is the primary organ for excretion; however, excretion also occurs through the lungs, sweat glands, saliva, and feces (McKim, 1986). Drugs that have been administered through the lungs are usually excreted through the lungs. The kidneys filter impurities from the blood, such as metabolites and unwanted substances. These impurities are then excreted through urine. The kidneys work most efficiently when there is a high concentration of the drug in the blood (McKim, 1986). Most drugs are removed by first order kinetics; that is, a fraction of the drug is removed per unit of time. "Because of this trailing off, the rate of excretion for most drugs can be determined in terms of a half-life" (McKim, 1986, p. 33). The *half-life*, then, is the amount of time required for half of the drug to be excreted from the body.

An exception to the half-life excretion is alcohol. Alcohol and a few other drugs are removed by zero order kinetics, which means a constant amount of the drug is removed per hour. In this case, the rate of excretion is dependent on the level of the metabolized alcohol, called alcohol dehydrogenase. When the alcohol dehydrogenase is above a minimum level, then the enzymes work at a constant rate and the "excretion curve . . . is a straight line" (McKim, 1986, p. 33).

The rate of drug elimination is also affected by the ability of a given organ or tissue to eliminate a drug (Ciccone, 1996). This process is called *clearance*.

> Clearance is actually the amount of plasma from which the drug can be totally removed per unit time. For example, a drug such as tetracycline with a clearance equal to 130 ml/min means that this drug would be completely removed from approximately 130 ml of plasma each minute. (Ciccone, 1990, p. 32)

Drug Effects

Drugs are administered to individuals in order to obtain some behavioral effect. The specific behavioral effect of a drug is determined by the location where the action takes place (e.g., the site of action) and the way in which the drug works. Two types of effects are usually examined: the desired effects, and the side effects.

Desired effects are the therapeutic reasons for giving the drug. Side effects occur as a result of the drug acting in ways other than the desired effect or as an exaggeration of the therapeutic effect. For example, an antidepressant is given to increase mood and relieve the effect of depression. Some side effects of many antidepressants include dry mouth, blurred vision, weight gain or loss, or drowsiness. Side effects can be negative or positive. For example, the antidepressant may cause the client to be drowsy. If he or she has had difficulty sleeping, the fact that the antidepressant will cause drowsiness will be a positive side effect.

The effectiveness of a drug is determined by weighing the benefits of the drug against the negative effects or costs (cost–benefit ratio). A physician may chose to prescribe a drug that has many side effects because the benefits outweigh the costs. Thus, an antipsychotic may be prescribed because of its benefit in reducing hallucination and psychotic symptoms, even though the side effects include sensitivity to sunlight (requiring sunscreen), lowered threshold for seizures, dry mouth, and extrapyramidal symptoms (e.g., tardive dyskinesia, dystonia, parkinsonian-like movements).

Mechanisms of Action and Processes

"Drugs can affect physiochemical processes, neuron functioning, and ultimately thoughts feelings and other behaviors" (Ray & Ksir, 1987, p. 93) through several mechanisms of action at the cellular level (Gitlin, 1996). Neurons differ in shape, location, function, and type of neurotransmitter, and this affects the way a particular drug works (Ciccone, 1996; Ray & Ksir, 1987). [Readers who do not have a basic understanding of neuronal functioning at the cellular level are advised to obtain a basic text in biological psychology, such as *Biological Psychology* by James W. Kalat, 1998.] First, the drug can bind to the receptor site of the postsynaptic neuron and (a) mimic the neurotransmitter by increasing or decreasing the electrical response of the postsynaptic neuron or (b) block the neurotransmitter from the receptor without having any influence on the electrical response of the neuron. In the first case, the drug is said to be an agonist; in the latter case, an antagonist. Typical antipsychotic drugs are antagonists because, although they do not influence the postsynaptic receptor, they block dopamine from attaching to it. Second, the drug can cause more neurotransmitter to be released by stimulating the presynaptic neurons. Stimulants, such as caffeine or Ritalin® stimulate the release of dopamine and norepinephrine. Third, the drug can prevent the reuptake or reabsorption of the neurotransmitter into the presynaptic neuron, thereby enabling the neurotransmitter to have a longer acting time. Selective serotonin reuptake inhibitors (SSRIs), such as Prozac® and Zoloft® are examples. Fourth, the drug can cause the number of postsynaptic receptors to increase or decrease or can affect the sensitivity of the receptors by changing its shape. Neurotransmitters bind to receptors with the same shape. A change in shape can result in decreased or increased sensitivity. Monamine oxidase inhibitors (MAOIs) work by inhibiting the primary degradation pathway for monoamines. Finally,

> the amount of neurotransmitter available could theoretically be altered by providing more or less of the precursor ingredients. L-tryptophan is a naturally occurring amino acid that is metabolized into serotonin. Thus ingesting large amounts of l-tryptophan might result in an increase in serotonin. (Gitlin, 1996, p. 30)

Drug-Response Relationships

How do physicians determine the drug dosage or the frequency of administration? What happens when dosages are increased? What happens when a client forgets to take a medication dose? These questions can be answered by examining the drug-response relationships.

The most basic concept in understanding drug-response relationships is the *dose-response curve* (DRC).

> In simple terms the dose-response curve . . . refers to the fact that as the amount of the drug administered is varied, there may be a change in a monitored behavior. A basic point is that since the effects of a drug can be studied on many behaviors or responses, there are many different dose-response curves for the same drug. (Ray & Ksir, 1987, p. 83)

In general, low dosages of a drug produce no observable response. The *threshold* or *minimal dosage level*, reached as the drug dosage is increased, is the point at which observable responses can be seen. If the dosage is below the threshold level, the concentration of the drug is not high enough to be of any therapeutic value. Thus, the dosage must be high enough to be therapeutically valuable and have therapeutic effect. Above the threshold level and with increased dosages, the magnitude of the response continues until the *maximal efficacy* is reached. Above this level there is no change in observable responses, even with an increase in dosage (Ciccone, 1996; Ferraro, personal communication, June 1–9, 1989; Ray & Ksir, 1987).

> Dose-response curves are used to provide information about the dosage range over which the drug is effective, as well as the peak response that can be expected from the drug. In addition, the characteristic shape of the dose-response curve and the presence of the plateau associated with maximal efficacy can be used to indicate specific information about the binding of the drug to cellular receptors. (Ciccone, 1990, p. 8)

In some cases, as drug dosages are increased, the effect of the drug changes, and new response patterns are involved. For example, when people drink alcohol, the initial response is slower reaction times. As more alcohol is consumed, the individual's ability to walk straight or smoothly is affected, and the individual is said to become ataxic. With additional alcohol consumption, some individuals would become comatose (Ray & Ksir, 1987). The three response systems, reaction time, balance, and arousal, are affected differentially with increasing levels of alcohol. In another example, the effect of increased dosages of depressants range from relaxation from anxiety to sedation, to coma, and finally to death (Ferraro, personal communication, June 1–9, 1989).

The drug effect, determined by the onset time, is affected by the drug level and system responsiveness. Onset time refers to the latency between administration of the drug and the onset of the desired effect. The type of administration, the solubility of the drug to lipids, the absorption rate, the drug circulation, and the binding of the drug all affect onset time. The peak response time refers to the amount of time needed to obtain maximal effectiveness of the drug. The duration time refers to the length of the drug effect and is related to the half-life of the drug. Information about these characteristics can be obtained from the *Physicians' Desk Reference* (PDR, 1999) or from the manufacturer.

Dose-response curves (DRCs) or log dose scales (which linearize the response pattern) are usually plotted on a log scale, because a "small change in low doses can have a big effect, but an equally small change in a large dose has no effect" (Ray & Ksir, 1987, p. 6). Usually, the DRC is a continuous variable; however, occasionally the effect is binary or discrete. For example, when giving an anesthetic, the dose-response curve is discrete: the patient is either anesthetized or not (Ray & Ksir, 1987).

According to Ray and Ksir (1987), the following four questions should be asked about drug dosage:

> First, what is the effective dose of a drug for a desired goal? . . . what dose of the drug will be lethal to the individual? . . . What is the safety margin—how different are the effective dose and the lethal dose? Finally, at the effective dose level, what other effects, particularly adverse reactions, might develop? (p. 85)

Effective dosages, abbreviated ED, indicate the percentage of people who show the desired effect at a given dosage. For example, ED_{25} means that 25 percent of individuals taking the drug at that dosage will show the desired effect (Ray & Ksir, 1987). The *median effective dose,* designated at ED_{50} indicates the dosage at which 50 percent of the population respond in a particular way (Ciccone, 1996; McKim, 1986). *Lethal dosages*, abbreviated LD, are designated in the same way. LD_3 refers to the dose at which 3 percent of the people taking the drug would die. Lethal dosages are determined through animal studies. Toxic dosages are more commonly used than lethal dosages.

The *safety margin* refers to the difference between an acceptable level of effectiveness (e.g., ED_{50}, ED_{90}) and LD_1 (Ray & Ksir, 1987). Obviously, the acceptable level varies depending on the drug and the desired effect. Another way of measuring the safety margin is by examining the *therapeutic index* (TI). This is determined by the ratio between ED_{50} and LD_{50}. Higher indices are safer than lower indices (Ciccone, 1996).

Dosages usually are given in milligrams or milliliters, because the metric system is used. In research papers, doses are reported in terms of milligrams per kilogram of body weight (McKim, 1986). According to Poe (1989) liquid preparations of drugs are called (a) *solutions* when one or more drugs are dissolved in water, (b) *elixirs* or *tinctures* when dissolved in alcohol, or (c) *suspensions* when finely divided particles that will not dissolve are placed into liquid. In the latter case, the preparation must be shaken before administering the drug. Solid preparations include *capsules* enclosed in a gelatin shell or tablets.

> Tablets are solid dosage forms that contain other ingredients (in addition to the medication) to hold them together until they are taken. Tablets are sometimes coated with sugar or other coatings to prevent the patient from tasting the drug and other times are simply compressed tablets (such as most aspirin). One particular type of tablet is made such that it will not dissolve until the drug is in the small intes-

tine. These are referred to as *enteric-coated* tablets. *Sustained-release* preparations are usually capsules or tablets and are made such that not all of the drug is released for absorption at one time. These preparations may enhance compliance because the drug does not have to be administered as often. (Poe, 1989, p. 3)

Potency

"Potency refers only to the amount of drug that must be given to obtain a particular response" (Ray & Ksir, 1987, p. 86). More potent drugs require less dosage to obtain the desired effect. Potency does not refer to the effectiveness of a drug or to the maximum efficacy of the drug (Ferraro, personal communication, June 1–9, 1989).

Drug Interactions

Drug interactions occur in several ways. First, the administration of a second drug can reduce the effect of the first drug. In these cases, the second drug is said to be an *antagonist*, and the drug effect is called *antagonism*. Second, administration of a second drug can increase the effect of the first drug. This effect is called an *additive effect*. For example, taking a barbiturate while drinking alcohol produces additive and, frequently, lethal effects. Third, additional doses of the same drug taken before the first dose has deactivated results in a *cumulative effect* (Ray & Ksir, 1987). In some cases, clients are instructed not to administer a missed dosage because of the cumulative effect of the double dosage. Finally, if the administration of two drugs results in a greater effect than would be expected from adding the individual effects of the drugs, the result is said to be *potentiation* or *super additive effect* (McKim, 1986).

PHARMOCODYNAMICS

While pharmacokinetics refers to the metabolism of drugs, pharmacodynamics refers to the action of the drug on individuals. Specifically, pharmacodynamics refers to the concept of tolerance, physical dependency or addiction, and psychological dependency.

Tolerance

> In the year 63 B.C. Mithradates VI, King of Pontus, tried to commit suicide by poisoning himself. Mithradates was a great leader and a great warrior: he had defeated the Roman legions and spread his influence over Asia Minor, but in 63 B.C. he had been defeated by the Roman emperor Pompey and his son had just led a successful revolt against him. To end it all, the king took a large dose of poison, but it had no effect on him. He was finally forced to have one of his Gallic mercenaries do the job. What was the source of the king's resistance to poison? Well, it appears as though Mithradates was also a good pharmacologist. Throughout his life he lived in great fear of being poisoned, so to protect himself he repeatedly took increasing doses of poison until he could tolerate large amounts without ill effects. This effect has been called *mithradatism* (Lankester, 1889) after the king or *tolerance* as we know it today. (McKim, 1986, p. 53)

Tolerance refers to "the decreased effectiveness of a drug that results from the continued presence of the drug in the body, or the necessity of increasing the dose of a drug in order to maintain its effectiveness after repeated administrations" (McKim, 1986, p. 53). The mechanism of tolerance is dependent on the (a) nature of the drug, (b) the frequency of administration, and (c) the interval between doses (Ferraro, personal communication, June 1–9, 1989; McKim, 1986). Some drugs show tolerance to some effects, but not to other effects. Once a drug is discontinued, tolerance disappears. *Cross tolerance* occurs when the tolerance of one drug results in the reduced effect of another drug. Cross tolerance is usually seen in drugs that are from the same class (McKim, 1986). *Reverse tolerance* occurs when the individual becomes sensitized to the drug after repeated administrations. The individual begins to report effects that may not have been there previously. Possibly this occurs because of a placebo effect, the anticipation of an expected response causes the response to occur (Ferraro, personal communication, June 1–9, 1989).

Tolerance depends on three types of mechanisms (Ferraro, personal communication, June 1–9, 1989):

▶ *Dispositional or metabolic tolerance* refers to the increased efficiency of the liver to metabolize a drug after the drug has been taken for a period of time. This occurs because of *enzyme induction* in which the liver begins to produce additional enzymes and is able to metabolize the drug faster. In order to obtain the same effect, the dosage of drug needs to be increased.

▶ *Cellular or pharmacodynamic tolerance* occurs because of changes at the cellular level that affect the drug effect over time and with repeated doses. Changes made by the drug include (a) decreasing the permeability of the cell, (b) modifying the shape of the receptor so there is less binding, (c) decreasing the number of receptors, or (d) reducing the sensitivity of the receptor. Tolerance at this level can be overcome by (a) increasing the amount of drug or (b) increasing the frequency of the drug administration.

▶ *Behavioral, conditioned, or learned tolerance* refers to the psychological effect the drug has on the individual and is a function of both classical and operant conditioning.

With operant conditioning, the individual learns new ways to compensate for the effect of the drug. Tolerance can be environmentally specific, reflecting that learning of a new behavior took place in one environment, but not in another. Behavioral or learned tolerance can also occur at different rates, with simple behaviors learned quickly and more complex behaviors learned more slowly.

Physical Dependency or Addiction

Physical dependence refers to a physiological state where the "discontinuance of a drug causes *withdrawal symptoms*" (McKim, 1986, p. 55). Withdrawal symptoms are usually the opposite of the drug effects, and occur because the discontinuance of the drug leaves the body in a state of disequilibrium. Before the body is able to adjust to the lack of the drug, it must undergo withdrawal from its previous adjustment to the drug. An example of withdrawal symptoms is the occurrence of diarrhea with a drug that has previously caused constipation (Ferraro, personal communication, June 1–9, 1989; McKim, 1986).

The intensity of withdrawal symptoms varies between drugs and ranges from barely noticeable to death. Dose size and frequency of administration also affect the intensity level. Symptoms can be stopped by giving another drug in the same class or category. Thus, the withdrawal symptoms seen in heroin can be stopped by giving methadone. This effect is called *cross dependence*. Although withdrawal symptoms generally occur several hours after the drug dosage is stopped, administration of an antagonist drug can produce the symptoms almost immediately (McKim, 1986).

Psychological Dependency

Contrary to popular belief, psychological dependency is not addiction. However, it is an important part of some drug's addiction process. Addiction is a physical dependency on a drug. Although physical dependency leads to withdrawal symptoms when a drug is discontinued, psychological dependency does not. Psychological dependency occurs when an individual thinks he or she needs a drug, but shows no withdrawal symptoms when the drug is removed. Psychological dependency can occur with drugs that have no tolerance effect; it can also occur with drugs that do have tolerance effects. Individuals can be both physically and psychologically dependent on a drug. Except for the absence of withdrawal symptoms, the behavior may be similar in both cases (Ferraro, personal communication, June 1–9, 1989).

CLASSES OF DRUGS

In the remaining portion of the chapter, drugs and drug categories used in the treatment of psychosocial disorders are described. Following a brief overview of the various classes is a description of a sample of the more common drugs used (Table 7–3). Most of the information about the drugs has been obtained from the *Physician's Desk Reference 2000* (PDR, 1999). Other references that may be helpful include:

▶ *Clinical Handbook of Psychotropic Drugs* (10th ed.), K. Z. Bezchlibnyk-Butler & J. J. Jeffries, 2000

▶ *Handbook of Clinical Psychopharmacology for Therapists*, J. D. Preston, M. C. Talaga, & J. H. O'Neal, 2000

▶ *The PDR Pocket Guide to Prescription Drugs* (4th ed.), D. W. Sifton (Ed.-in-chief), 2000

▶ *Pharmacology in Rehabilitation* (2nd ed.), C. D. Ciccone, 1996

▶ *Physical and Occupational Therapy: Drug Implications for Practice*, T. Malone, 1996

▶ *Psychiatric Medications: A Guide for Mental Health Professionals*, K. J. Bender, 1990

▶ *The Psychotherapist's Guide to Psychopharmacology*, M. J. Gitlin, 1996

▶ *Saunders Drug Handbook for Health Professionals, 2000*, R. J. Kizior & B.B. Hodgson, 2000

▶ *Psychopharmaology*, monthly periodical

Antianxiety or Anxiolytic Drugs (Sedative-Hypnotics)

Drugs that are classified as sedative-hypnotics are used to relax the patient and promote sleep. As the name implies, sedative drugs exert a calming effect and serve to pacify the patient. At a high dose, the same drug tends to produce drowsiness and to initiate a relatively normal state of sleep (hypnosis). At still higher doses, some sedative-hypnotics (especially the barbiturates) will eventually bring on a state of general anesthesia. Because of their general CNS-depressant effects, some sedative-hypnotic drugs are also used for other functions such as treating epilepsy or producing muscle relaxation. (Ciccone, 1990, p. 61)

Antianxiety (anxiolytics) drugs, formerly called tranquilizers and used to reduce anxiety, and hypnotics, used to produce sleep, actually come from the same class of drugs, the sedative-hypnotics. Prior to the development of benzodiazepines, barbiturates were commonly used to reduce anxiety and relax muscles. Because of their addictive nature, this category of drugs has been generally replaced by the benzodiazepines (Ciccone, 1996). An atypical antianxiety drug, buspirone (BuSpar®) is unrelated to other sedative-hypnotics, but is useful in counteracting anxiety.

Although many clients choose to use stress-management techniques, cognitive-behavioral techniques, and alternative treatment therapies to control anxiety, the use of benzodiazepines may occasionally be of benefit (Preston et al., 2000). (See Chapters 10 through 12 for information on specific techniques for reducing anxiety.) Benzodiazepines' mechanism of action appears to increase the inhibitory effects of GABA, a neurotransmitter, at the postsynaptic allosteric site. The effect of this produced decreased arousal and increased relaxation (Ciccone, 1996). Although less than the barbiturates, the benzodiazepines have tolerance capability and physical dependence may occur. Withdrawal symptoms range from sleep disturbances when the drug has been taken for a short time to "psychosis and seizures if the drug is abruptly stopped" (Ciccone, 1990, p. 65) with long-term administration. Fatalities have been reported due to the seizures. For these reasons, it is important for the dosage to be decreased slowly when discontinuing the medication. Side effects of benzodiazepines include impaired memory, drowsiness, and disinhibition (Bender, 1990) and increased liver damage because of the long half-lives and consequential buildup of the drug in the system (Preston et al., 2000).

Antidepressants and Mood Stabilizers

Antidepressants are used in the treatment of major depressive disorders or unipolar depression. The earliest antidepressants were tricyclics (TCAs), such as Norpramin® (desipramine), Tofranil® (imipramine), and Elavil® (amitriptyline). Although these drugs are helpful in elevating mood and decreasing anxiety and insomnia, the maximal efficacy is often not seen for 2 to 3 weeks (Allen, 1989). Additionally, these drugs

Table 7–3. General Categories of Psychotherapeutic Drugs

Generic Name (specifies the chemical without using the chemical name)	Trade Name (brand or proprietary name)	DSM–IV Diagnoses (what diagnoses should receive the drug)	Symptoms Relieved (intended therapeutic use of drug)	Possible or Common Side Effects (detrimental or adverse effects caused by the use of drugs)
Antianxiety or anxiolytic drugs (Benzodiazepines)				
lorazepam	Ativan®	Anxiety disorders	• anxiety	• may be habit forming
chlordiazeproxide	Librium®	Alcoholism withdrawal	• agitation	• agitation
temazepam	Restoril®		• panic disorder	• anticholinergic symptoms
oxazepam	Serax®		• insomnia	• rapid heartbeat
clorazepate	Tranxene®		• muscle relaxation	• sexual dysfunction
alprazolam	Xanax®		• epilepsy • sedation, amnesia, and anesthesia	• drowsiness • motor incoordination or ataxia • confusion and memory loss • physical dependency and withdrawal syndrome • dry mouth • blurred vision
diazepam	Valium®	All of above and epileptic seizures	All of the above and epileptic seizure activity	All of the above
clonazepam	Klonopin®, Rivotril®			
buspirone	BuSpar®	Anxiety disorders		• dry mouth • fatigue or dizziness • headache • nausea
Antidepressants				
MAO Inhibitors (MAOIs)				
isocarboxazid	Marplan	Atypical depression (e.g., showing hypochondriasis, somatic anxiety, irritability)	• reduce depression • increase mood • reduce phobias	• hypotension • dry mouth • liver damage • lethal cardiovascular effects if dietary restrictions are ignored • tremors • blurred vision • cardiac dysrhythmias • dizziness • fatigue or drowsiness • weight gain • sexual disturbances • headaches
phenelzine sulfate	Nardil®			
tranylcypromine sulfate	Parnate®	Those unresponsive to other antidepressants Social phobias		

Table 7–3. General Categories of Psychotherapeutic Drugs

Generic Name (specifies the chemical without using the chemical name)	Trade Name (brand or proprietary name)	DSM–IV Diagnoses (what diagnoses should receive the drug)	Symptoms Relieved (intended therapeutic use of drug)	Possible or Common Side Effects (detrimental or adverse effects caused by the use of drugs)
Selective Serotonin Reuptake Inhibitors (SSRI)				
citalopram	Celexa®	Major depressive disorder (MDD)	• reduce depression	• nervousness or agitation
fluvoxamine	Luvox®	Obsessive compulsive disorder (OCD)	• reduce obsessive and compulsive behaviors	• anxiety with and without insomnia
paroxetine	Paxil®	Panic disorder	• some reduction of anxiety	• nausea or dyspepsia
fluoxetine	Prozac®	Posttraumatic stress disorder (PTSD)		• diarrhea
sertraline	Zoloft®			• anorexia or weight loss
				• tremor
				• rashes
				• dizziness, impaired balance
				• headaches
Tricyclics (TCAs)				
imipramine	Tofranil® or Janimine®	Mood disorders (MDD, cyclic depression, etc.)	• elevate mood	• fast or irregular heart beat
doxepin	Adapin® or Sinequan®	Panic disorders	• increase physical activity	• dry mouth
amitriptyline	Elavil® or Endep®	Generalized anxiety disorder	• improve appetite	• blurred vision
trimipramine	Surmontil®	Posttraumatic stress disorder (PTSD)	• improve sleep	• sleepiness or insomnias
desipramine	Norpramine® or Pertofrane®	Obsessive-compulsive disorder (OCD)		• constipation
				• urinary retention
				• weight gain
protriptyline	Vivactil®	Eating disorders		• dizziness
nortriptyline	Triptile Pamelor®, Ventyl®, or Aventyl®	Enuresis (imipramine)		• tremors
		ADHD		• hypotension
				• headaches
amoxapine	Asendin®			• seizures
maprotline	Ludiomil®			• sexual disturbances
Neuroepinephrine Reuptake Inhibitors (NDRIs)				
bupropion	Wellbutrin®	MDD	• elevate mood	• headaches
		Depressed phase of bipolar affective disorder	• increase physical activity	• insomnia
				• agitation or anxiety
		Seasonal affective disorder (SAD)	• improve eating and sleep disturbances	• dry mouth
				• urinary frequency
				• short-term memory loss

Table 7–3. General Categories of Psychotherapeutic Drugs

Generic Name (specifies the chemical without using the chemical name)	Trade Name (brand or proprietary name)	DSM–IV Diagnoses (what diagnoses should receive the drug)	Symptoms Relieved (intended therapeutic use of drug)	Possible or Common Side Effects (detrimental or adverse effects caused by the use of drugs)
Serotonin–2 Antagonist/Reuptake Inhibitors (SARI)				
nefazodone	Serzone®	MDD	• elevate mood	• drowsiness
trazodone	Desyrel®	Depressed phase of bipolar affective disorder	• decrease sleep disturbances	• confusion, disturbed concentration • fine tremor • dysphasia or stuttering
Anti-Parkinsonian Agents				
propranolol	Inderal®	Acute dyskinesias or dystonias	• reduce muscular side effects caused by neuroleptics (antipsychotics) • improve muscle control • reduce stiffness • reduce extrapyramidal symptoms • reduce parkinsonian symptoms	• dry mouth
diphenhydramine	Benadryl®	Pseudoparkinsonian effects		• blurred vision
benztropine mesylate	Cogentin®			• constipation
amatadine	Symmetrel®	Akathisia		• dry eyes
biperiden	Akineton®	Akinesia		• flushed skin • vomiting or nausea • confusion • disorientation • memory impairment
Antimanic				
lithium carbonate	Lithane®	Acute mania	• modulate mood swings	• tremor
	Eskalith®	Bipolar mood disorders	• reduce mania	• thirst or dry mouth • excessive urination
	Lithotabs®			• weight gain • fatigue • nausea or vomiting • diarrhea • disturbances in cardiac rhythm • renal damage • thyroid • skin disorders • sexual disturbance in men

Table 7–3. General Categories of Psychotherapeutic Drugs

Generic Name (specifies the chemical without using the chemical name)	*Trade Name* (brand or proprietary name)	*DSM–IV Diagnoses* (what diagnoses should receive the drug)	*Symptoms Relieved* (intended therapeutic use of drug)	*Possible or Common Side Effects* (detrimental or adverse effects caused by the use of drugs)
Antipsychotic or Neuroleptic				
thiothixene	Navane®	Schizophrenia	Decrease symptoms of psychosis, including	• extrapyramidal symptoms, such as dystonia, parkinson-like
chlorpromazine	Thorazine®	Schizoaffective disorder		
		Mania	• agitation	
thioridazine	Mellaril®	Psychotic depression	• paranoia	• Neuroleptic Malignant Syndrome sedation
mesoridazine	Serentil®	Haldol® is used to treat	• delusions	
trifluoperazine	Stelazine®	Tourette's syndrome	• hallucinations	• anticholinergic symptoms (dry mouth, constipation, difficulty urinating)
molindone	Moban®		• bizarre behavior	
loxapine	Loxitane®		• thought disorder	
haloperidol	Haldol®		Does not control negative symptoms such as apathy	• postural hypotension
risperdal	Risperdal®			• weight gain
clozapine	Clozaril®			• tardive dyskinesia (TD)
olanzapine	Zyprexil®			• photosensitivity (sensitivity to sun)
quetiapine	Seroquel®			• impotence and disturbance in sexual function
Psychostimulants				
methylphenidate	Ritalin®	Attention deficit disorder with and without hyperactivity	• increase sustained attention	• weight loss
amicinonide	Cylert®			• decreased appetite
dextroamphetamine sulfate	Dexadrine®		• increase concentration	• insomnia
	Adderal®		• reduce motor activity	• fatigue or drowsiness

Table 7–3. General Categories of Psychotherapeutic Drugs

Generic Name (specifies the chemical without using the chemical name)	Trade Name (brand or proprietary name)	DSM–IV Diagnoses (what diagnoses should receive the drug)	Symptoms Relieved (intended therapeutic use of drug)	Possible or Common Side Effects (detrimental or adverse effects caused by the use of drugs)
Sedatives-Hypnotics				
Barbiturates				
pentobarbital	Nembutal®	Anxiety disorder	• anesthesia	• may be habit forming
secobarbital	Seconal®		• epilepsy and seizures	• drowsiness and lethagy
amobarbital	Amytol®			• constipation
				• blurred vision
				• edema
				• vertigo or dizziness
				• paradoxical dysphoria
				• hyperactivity
				• cognitive disorganization and confusion
				• fatigue
				• nausea and vomiting
				• headache
				• syncope (fainting)
				• ataxia
Anticonvulsant				
phenytoin	Dilantin®	Epileptic and seizure disorders	reduce or control seizures	• liver problems
carbamazepine	Tegretol®			• sleepiness
phenobarbital	Luminal®			• nausea
valproic acid	Depakene®			• vomiting
primidone	Mysoline®			• skin problems
clonazepam	Klonopin®			• dizziness
gabapentin	Nuerontin®			• diplopia
felbamate dicarbamate	Felbatol®			• blurred vision
lamotrigine	Lamictal®			
vigabatrin	Sabril®			

Source: Adapted from "Psychiatry" by C. K. Allen, 1989, in T. Malone, *Physical and occupational therapy: Drug implications for practice* (pp. 207–228), Philadelphia: Lippincott; *Attention Deficit Hyperactivity Disorder: A Handbook for Diagnosis and Treatment* by R. A. Barkley, 1990, New York: Guilford; *Pharmacology in Rehabilitation* by C. D. Ciccone, 1990, Philadelphia: F. A. Davis; *The Psychotherapist's Guide to Psychopharmacology* (2nd ed.) by M. J. Gitlin, 1996, New York: The Free Press; *Saunders Drug Handbook for Health Professionals 2000,* by R. J. Kizior & B. B. Hodgson (Eds.), Philadelphia: Saunders; *Physicians' Desk Reference*® (PDR; 51st ed.), 1997, Montvale, NJ: Medical Economics Company. *Handbook of Clinical Psychopharmacology for Therapists,* by J. Preston, H. H. O'Neal, & M. C. Talaga, 1994, Oakland, CA: New Harbinger; "The Use of Drugs and Other Somatic Treatments," by L. A. Opler, 1992, in F. I. Kass, J. M. Oldham, H. Pardes, & L. B. Morris, *The Columbia University College of Physicians and Surgeons Complete Home Guide to Mental Health* (pp. 63–91), New York: Henry Holt.; and *The PDR Pocket Guide to Prescription Drugs,* by D. W. Sifton (Ed.-in-chief), 2000, New York: Pocket Books.

have side effects such as sedation and dry mouth, blurred vision, and constipation. The latter effects are referred to as "anticholinergic" effects because they are caused from the blockage of the acetylcholine (ACh) transmitter (Bender, 1990). TCAs work by blocking the reuptake of the amine neurotransmitters (e.g., dopamine, norepinephrine) into the presynaptic neuron. This primary mechanism probably stimulates a secondary compensatory change in neurotransmitters, which results in relieving the depression.

Another type of early antidepressant was the MAOIs, so-called because they inhibited the monoamine oxidase enzyme. This enzyme metabolizes the amine neurotransmitters, and inhibition of the enzyme resulted in a longer time of action for the transmitters (Ciccone, 1996). The major difficulty with using MAOIs is the interaction with drugs that stimulate the sympathetic nervous system (directly or indirectly) or foods that are high in tyramine content (e.g., cheese, nuts).

The introduction of a second-generation of antidepressants has alleviated some of the undesirable effects seen in the first-generation. Selective serotonin reuptake inhibitors (SSRIs), such as Prozac®, and an atypical group (e.g., Wellbutrin®) have fewer anticholinergic or sedative effects, and onset of effect is quicker (Ciccone, 1996; Gitlin, 1996).

Bipolar disorders are effectively treated by a mood stabilizer such as lithium, valproate, or carbamazepine. Lithium carbonate (Lithane®) is most commonly prescribed because of its effect on the mania phase of the disorder (Gitlin, 1996). The mechanism of action is not certain (PDR, 1999) and frequent blood levels must be taken to reduce the chance of toxic reactions (Gitlin, 1996).

Antipsychotic or Neuroleptic

This class of drugs is used when there are symptoms of psychosis, such as agitation, paranoia, delusions, hallucinations, bizarre behavior, or thought disorder. The mechanism of action is to block the dopamine receptors on the postsynaptic neuron (Ciccone, 1996). The time required to reduce symptoms varies, with confusion and agitation subsiding after a few hours or days. More severe symptoms (e.g., hallucinations or delusions) require a longer treatment period before the effective dosage is reached (Preston et al., 2000). Side effects that occur with all antipsychotic drugs include (a) extrapyramidal symptoms, such as slowed motor movements, tremors, decreased facial expressions, muscle spasms, and restlessness; (b) anticholinergic symptoms, such as dry mouth, constipation, urinary retention, blurred vision; and (c) hypotension or lowered blood pressure. Most also increase sensitivity to sunlight, requiring clients to wear sunscreen to prevent sunburn.

Tardive dyskinesia (TD) is of gravest concern when using antipsychotic drugs. It can result from prolonged dosages over time, but is preventable by using the lowest effective doses for the shortest time possible. Common signs of TD include involuntary movements such as "tongue thrusting, chewing movements, lip smacking, and eye blinking" (Gitlin, 1996, p. 407). TD is irreversible, even with discontinuation of the drug. Clozapine, is effective without resulting in TD; however, it requires drug dosing based on blood counts.

Neuroleptic Malignant Syndrome (NMS) is a dangerous rare side effect that may occur soon after initial administration. Signs of NMS include muscle rigidity, confusion tremors, fever, and possible liver damage. Treatment includes discontinuing all antipsychotic medicine and providing emergency care (Ciccone, 1996; Gitlin, 1996; Opler, 1992; Preston et al., 2000).

Psychostimulants

Psychostimulants, such as Ritalin®, are widely used with children and adolescents to help them sustain attention and improve concentration. Their mechanism of action involves increasing the amount of dopamine by stimulating the dopamine receptors. Typical side effects include weight loss, inability to sleep, poor growing patterns, and lack of appetite. Frequently, children on psychostimulants are given drug holidays. For example, many children take the medication only when in school where they are required to concentrate and attend to difficult material. Often, a dosage is given at lunch time so that the student's attention continues into the afternoon. When possible, a sustained or timed-release, rather than a noon dosage is given. Although the medication does help students attend, other therapies, such as skills training, relaxation, and cognitive-behav-ioral, are necessary components of treatment and should be incorporated into the behavior management program (Barkley, 1990).

SUMMARY

Occupational therapists who work with clients in psychosocial settings will encounter many individuals who are taking medications. An understanding of pharmacokinetics and pharmacodynamics is important when working with these clients, because the effects of the drugs will impact on the therapy sessions. Occupational therapists will need to watch for signs of abnormal or toxic reactions to various drugs. When questions arise about drug effects, it is important to notify the physician as soon as possible.

Category of Drugs	Antidepressant: Tricyclic (TCA)
Trade or Proprietary Name	Adapin® Sinequan® Zonalon®
Generic or Nonproprietary Name	doxepin hydrochloride
Primary Use (DSM–IV Diagnosis)	Treatment of depression and/or anxiety • associated with alcoholism • associated with organic disease • with psychotic episodes associated with anxiety, such as manic-depressive
Effects	May require several weeks before it is fully effective
Symptoms Relieved	• reduces anxiety, tension, fears, apprehension, or worry • elevates mood • reduces somatic symptoms • increases physical activity
Possible or Common Side Effects	• dry mouth • drowsiness • headache • increased appetite and weight gain • tiredness or weakness • nausea • unpleasant taste • blurred vision • constipation, urinary retention, or diarrhea • bradycardia • sexual dysfunction
Cautions	• adds to effects of alcohol and other CNS depressants (e.g., cold medicines, cough syrup) • use when an MAO Inhibitor is being or has been used within the previous 2 weeks is contraindicated • contraindicated during acute recovery period for myocardial infarction • contraindicated with patients with glaucoma or tendency to urinary retention

Category of Drugs	Psychostimulant
Trade or Proprietary	Adderal®
Generic or Nonproprietary Name	none; contains dextroamphetamine sulfate, dextroamphetamine saccharate, amphetamine sulfate, and amphetamine asparate
Primary Use (DSM–IV Diagnosis)	Treatment of attention deficit hyperactivity disorder or narcolepsy
Effects	Longer lasting than other psychostimulants such as Ritalin®
Symptoms Relieved	• reduces psychotic thoughts • decreases agitation or hyperactivity • increases mood • reduces nausea or vomiting
Possible or Common Side Effects	• insomnia • decreased appetite • stomach pain, headache • irritability • weight loss • dizziness • dry mouth • diarrhea • constipation • metallic taste in mouth
Cautions	• do not use during or within 14 days following the administration of an MAOI • may exacerbate symptoms in psychotic children, tics, and Tourette}s syndrome • may lower the seizure threshold • contraindicated in persons with advanced ateriosclerosis, symptomatic cardiovascular disease, moderate to severe hypertension, hyperthyroidism, glaucoma, agitation, or history of drug abuse

Category of Drugs	Antidepressant: Dibenzoxazepine
Trade or Proprietary Name	Asendin®
Generic or Nonproprietary Name	amoxapine
Primary Use (DSM-IV Diagnosis)	Treatment of endogenous depression and anxiety with • neurotic or reactive depressive disorders • psychotic symptoms (other than schizophrenia) • anxiety or agitation
Effects	• initial clinical effect may occur within 4 to 7 days to 2 weeks
Symptoms Relieved	• increased mood • lessened anxiety or agitation • increased sleeping • increased appetite
Possible or Common Side Effects	• drowsiness • dizziness • dry mouth • headache • increased appetite or weight gain • tiredness or weakness • nausea • unpleasant taste • blurred vision • constipation or difficulty urinating • eye pain • arrhythmias • nervousness
Cautions	• adds to effects of alcohol and other CNS depressants (e.g., cold medicines, cough syrup) • contraindicated when an MAO Inhibitor is being or has been used within the previous 2 weeks • contraindicated with acute phase of myocardial infarction, history of urinary retention, diabetes mellitus, seizures • contraindicated with history of schizophrenia

Category of Drugs	Antidepressant: SSRI
Trade or Proprietary Name	Celexa™
Generic or Nonproprietary Name	citalopram
Primary Use (DSM-IV Diagnosis)	Treatment of Major Depressive Disorder (MDD)
Effects	• initial clinical effect may occur within 4 to 7 days to 2 weeks
Symptoms Relieved	• increased mood • lessened anxiety or agitation • increased sleeping • increased appetite
Possible or Common Side Effects	• dry mouth • nausea • insomnia • sexual dysfunction • drowsiness
Cautions	• adds to effects of alcohol and other CNS depressants (e.g., cold medicines, cough syrup) • contraindicated when an MAO Inhibitor is being or has been used within the previous 2 weeks • on long-term therapy, perform liver/renal function tests

Category of Drugs	Antipsychotic
Trade or Proprietary Name	Clozaril®
Generic or Nonproprietary Name	clozapine
Primary Use (DSM–IV Diagnosis)	• management of schizophrenia that has failed to respond to typical antipsychotic drug treatment
Effects	• may require 2 weeks to obtain optimal effect
Symptoms Relieved	• reduction of psychosis
Possible or Common Side Effects	• drowsiness or sedation • increased saliva • tachycardia • dizziness • constipation • extrapyramidal symptoms, including Neuroleptic Malignant Syndrome (NMS) • transient temperature elevation • headache • tremor • nausea • hypotension • restlessness or agitation • sweating • dry mouth
Cautions	• contraindicated with clients who have uncontrolled epilepsy • risk of agranulocytosis (acute condition of decreased white blood cells [WBC]) requires baseline count of WBC, as well as weekly testing and 4 weeks of posttesting following administration • drug administration determined by effect and WBC • should not be given with other drugs known to suppress bone marrow function • alcohol should not be used with this drug

Category of Drugs	Antiparkinsonian Agent
Trade or Proprietary Name	Cogentin®
Generic or Nonproprietary Name	benztropine mesylate
Primary Use (DSM–IV Diagnosis)	• therapeutic use for all forms of parkinsonism • concomitant use with antipsychotics to reduce extrapyramidal symptoms
Effects	• may not observe effect for 2 to 3 days
Symptoms Relieved	• improve muscle control • reduce stiffness • control severe reactions to other medications
Possible or Common Side Effects	• constipation • vomiting or nausea • dry mouth • drowsiness • increased sweating/urination • toxic psychosis (confusion, disorientation, memory impairment), especially in the elderly • blurred vision • urinary retention
Cautions	• monitoring of drug should be continual because of cumulative action • should not be used with antacids such as Tums® or Maalox® • large doses may result in muscle weakness • caution indicated when client is driving or operating machinery, because the use may slow responses or impair judgment • should be used cautiously in hot weather, due to increased sweating and loss of body fluids • use of sunscreen due to photosensitivity • contraindicated with angle closure glaucoma, intestinal disorders, myasthenia gravis, and children under 3

Category of Drugs	Antipsychotic, Antiemetic
Trade or Proprietary Name	Compazine®
Generic or Nonproprietary Name	prochlorperazine
Primary Use (DSM-IV Diagnosis)	Treatment of • psychotic disorders • severe nausea and vomiting • short-term treatment of generalized non-psychotic anxiety
Effects	• response usually noted in a day or two
Symptoms Relieved	• emotional withdrawal • conceptual disorganization • anxiety and tension • hallucinations • hyperactivity and uncooperativeness
Possible or Common Side Effects	• hypotension • dizziness or fainting • amenorrhea • skin reactions and sensitivity to heat • drowsiness • blurred vision • extrapyramidal symptoms, including motor restlessness, dystonia, pseudoparkinsonism, and tardive dyskinesia • Neuroleptic Malignant Syndrome (NMS) • tardive dyskensia (TD) • anticholinergic symptoms such as constipation, dry mouth, fluid retention, difficulty urinating, nasal congestion
Cautions	• antiemetic action may mask signs of overdosage of other drugs and obscure diagnosis of Reye's syndrome or intestinal obstruction • CNS depressant effect that may affect the ability to operate large machinery, drive a car, or react quickly • use cautiously with alcohol withdrawal or history of seizures

Category of Drugs	Antidepressant: SARI
Trade or Proprietary Name	Desyrel®
Generic or Nonproprietary Name	trazodone hydrocloride
Primary Use (DSM–IV Diagnosis)	Major Depressive Disorder (MDD)
Effects	• effects usually seen within 7 to 28 days
Symptoms Relieved	• elevates mood • reduces anxiety • relieves sleep disturbance
Possible or Common Side Effects	• drowsiness • dry mouth • dizziness/lightheadedness • blurred vision • nausea or vomiting
Cautions	• adds to effects of alcohol and other CNS depressants (e.g., cold medicines, cough syrup) • may cause sleepiness or drowsiness • close monitoring when used with patients with cardiac disease • should be taken with food

Category of Drugs	Antidepressant: Tricyclic (TCA)
Trade or Proprietary Name	Elavil® Endep®
Generic or Nonproprietary Name	amitriptyline
Primary Use (DSM–IV Diagnosis)	Treatment of mental depression with endogenous etiology
Effects	• may require several weeks before it is fully effective
Symptoms Relieved	• elevates mood • increases physical activity • improves appetite • improves sleep
Possible or Common Side Effects	• dizziness • drowsiness, unusual tiredness or weakness • dry mouth • blurred vision • orthostatic hypotension • headache • increased appetite or weight gain • unpleasant taste • constipation and urinary retention • tachycardia • arrhythmias • eye pain • increased sweating • nervousness • insomnia
Cautions	• adds to effects of alcohol and other CNS depressants (e.g., cold medicines, cough syrup) • contraindicated when an MAO Inhibitor is being or has been used within the previous 2 weeks • contraindicated for use with individuals with heart conditions, hyperthyroid, or seizures • should be discontinued when surgery is impending

Category of Drugs	Antipsychotic, with tricyclic antidepressant
Trade or Proprietary	Etrafon® Triavil®
Generic or Nonproprietary Name	perphenazine and amitriptyline
Primary Use (DSM–IV Diagnosis)	Treatment of psychotic disorders with associated depression
Effects	• may require several weeks before it is fully effective
Symptoms Relieved	• depressed activity • reduction of psychotic symptoms • depressed appetite • mood elevator
Possible or Common Side Effects	• hypotension • dizziness or fainting • dry mouth • blurred vision • constipation, urinary retention, or diarrhea • sensitivity to sun (photosensitivity) • craving for sweets • decreased sexual ability and menstrual changes • tardive dyskinesia • extrapyramidal reactions • Neuroleptic Malignancy Syndrome (hyperpyrexia; muscle rigidity; autonomic instability, including irregular pulse or blood pressure, tachycardia, diaphoresis, cardiac dysrhythmias
Cautions	• adds to effects of alcohol and other CNS depressants (e.g., cold medicines, cough syrup) • contraindicated when an MAO Inhibitor is being or has been used within the previous 2 weeks • do not use with history of seizures or glaucoma • contraindicated with bone marrow depression or severe CNS depression

Category of Drugs	Antipsychotic
Trade or Proprietary Name	Haldol®
Generic or Nonproprietary Name	haloperidol
Primary Use (DSM–IV Diagnosis)	Treatment of • manifestations of psychotic disorders • tics and vocal utterances of Tourette's disease • severe behavior problems involving aggressiveness • short-term treatment of hyperactivity with agressiveness or mood lability
Effects	May not reach maximum effectiveness for several weeks, but is fastest acting of the antipsychotics
Symptoms Relieved	Reduction in hallucination or other psychotic symptoms
Possible or Common Side Effects	• blurred vision • constipation • dry mouth • swelling or soreness of female breasts • increased weight • extrapyramidal symptoms including parkinson-like symptoms, akathisia, dystonia • tardive dyskinesia (TD), or Neuroleptic Malignancy Syndrome • insomnia, lethargy, drowsiness, or depression • exacerbation of psychotic symptoms, • grand mal seizures
Cautions	• close monitoring necessary when combined with Lithium • may impair mental and physical ability to perform tasks such as driving or operating machinery • increases action of alcohol and other drugs that depress the CNS system

Category of Drugs	Antimanic
Trade or Proprietary Name	Lithium Carbonate® Eskalith-CR® or Eskalith® Lithonate® or Lithotabs®
Generic or Nonproprietary Name	lithium carbonate
Primary Use (DSM–IV Diagnosis)	Treatment and maintenance treatment of manic episodes of Bipolar Disorder
Effects	May take 3 weeks to be effective
Symptoms Relieved	• manic phase of Bipolar Depression • stabilizes mood swings in Bipolar Depression
Possible or Common Side Effects	• fine hand tremor • increased urination • diarrhea or loss of bladder control • excessive thirst or dry mouth • mild nausea • dizziness • confusion • slurred speech • irregular heartbeat or pulse
Cautions	• may reduce alertness, and thus impair mental or physical abilities • may interact adversely with antipsychotics (e.g., Haldol®) or diuretics • early signs of toxicity may include diarrhea, vomiting, drowsiness, muscular weakness, lack of coordination or ataxia, giddiness, blurred vision, or tinnitus • long-term administration can affect thyroid and kidney functions • blood levels should be monitored monthly • contraindicated for clients with renal or cardiovascular disease, or for women who are pregnant • should not be taken with antiemetics

Category of Drugs	Antipsychotic
Trade or Proprietary	Loxitane®
Generic or Nonproprietary Name	loxapine hydrocloride or loxapine succinate
Primary Use (DSM–IV Diagnosis)	• management of manifestations of psychotic disorders • reduction of anxiety with depressive disorders
Effects	May require 7 to 10 days to be effective
Symptoms Relieved	• decreased excitement or hypermobility • reduction of tension • decreased agitation
Possible or Common Side Effects	• blurred vision • confusion • drowsiness • dizziness or fainting • slurred speech • insomnia • allergic reaction, such as rash or itching • neuromuscular reactions (parkinsonian-like symptoms, motor restlessness, or dystonias) • tardive dyskinesia (TD) • nasal congestion • constipation or urinary retention • nausea or vomiting • nasal stuffiness • weight gain or weight loss
Cautions	• adds to effects of alcohol and other CNS depressants (e.g., cold medicines, cough syrup) • contraindicated in individuals with seizure disorders because it lowers threshold of seizures

Category of Drugs	Antidepressant: Tetracyclic
Trade or Proprietary Name	Ludiomil®
Generic or Nonproprietary Name	maprotiline hydrocloride
Primary Use (DSM–IV Diagnosis)	Treatment of major depressive disorder, including depressive phase of bipolar disorder
Effects	• may not reach maximum effectiveness for 2 to 3 weeks
Symptoms Relieved	• increases mood • reduces anxiety • reduces panic attacks
Possible or Common Side Effects	• drowsiness or fatigue • dry mouth • blurred vision • constipation or urinary retention • postural hypotension • excessive sweating • increased appetite • disturbed concentration • increased restlessness • increased sensitivity to light • nausea or vomiting
Cautions	• adds to effects of alcohol and other CNS depressants (e.g., cold medicines, cough syrup) • withdrawal symptoms on discontinuation, including seizures, impaired concentration, and lightheadedness • use of sunscreen recommended • contraindicated in individuals with history of seizures

Category of Drugs	Antipsychotic
Trade or Proprietary	Mellaril®
Generic or Nonproprietary Name	thioridazine or thioridazine hydrochloride
Primary Use (DSM–IV Diagnosis)	Treatment of • manifestations of psychotic disorders • moderate to marked depression and anxiety • severe behavior disorders involving aggressiveness
Effects	• may take up to 6 weeks before it is fully effective
Symptoms Relieved	• decreased excitement or hypermobility • reducing tension • decreasing agitation
Possible or Common Side Effects	• drowsiness • reduced cognitive performance • dry mouth • lethargy • blurred vision • constipation or urinary retention • nausea or vomiting • nasal stuffiness • decreased sexual ability and menstrual changes • impotence or altered menstrual states • tardive dyskinesia (TD)
Cautions	• adds to effects of alcohol and other CNS depressants (e.g., cold medicines, cough syrup)

Category of Drugs	Antipsychotic
Trade or Proprietary Name	Moban®
Generic or Nonproprietary Name	molindone hydrochloride
Primary Use (DSM–IV Diagnosis)	Management of psychotic disorders, especially schizophrenia
Effects	May take up to 6 weeks to see effect
Symptoms Relieved	• spontaneous motor movement and aggressiveness • bizarre stereotypical behaviors • increases mood
Possible or Common Side Effects	• transient drowsiness or dizziness • dry mouth • constipation, urinary retention, or diarrhea • blurred vision • nasal congestion • extrapyramidal symptoms, including motor restlessness, dystonias, pseudo-parkinsonism, and tardive dyskinesia (TD) • Neuroleptic Malignant Syndrome (NMS) • photosensitivity (use sunscreen)
Cautions	• adds to effect of alcohol or other CNS depressants • contraindicated with severe CNS depressant, severe cardiovascular disorders, or history of seizures • increases risk of seizures

Category of Drugs	Antipsychotic
Trade or Proprietary Name	Navane®
Generic or Nonproprietary Name	thiothixene
Primary Use (DSM-IV Diagnosis)	Management of psychotic disorders
Effects	May require up to 6 weeks before optimal response
Symptoms Relieved	• psychosis • nausea or vomiting
Possible or Common Side Effects	• extrapyramidal reactions, including tardive dykinesia (TD) or Neuroleptic Malignancy Syndrome (NMS; akathisia; hyperpyrexia; muscle rigidity; autonomic instability, including irregular pulse or blood pressure, tachycardia, diaphoresis, cardiac dysrhythmias) • constipation • decreased sweating • drowsiness • increased appetite or weight gain • dry mouth • blurred vision • skin rash
Cautions	• antiemetic action may mask signs of overdosage of other drugs and obscure diagnosis of Reye's syndrome or intestinal obstruction • adds to effects of alcohol and other CNS depressants (e.g., cold medicines, cough syrup) • contraindicated with history of seizures • sunscreen required due to photosensitivity

Category of Drugs	Antidepressant: Tricyclic (TCA)
Trade or Proprietary Name	Norpramin® Pertofrane®
Generic or Nonproprietary Name	desipramine hydrochloride
Primary Use (DSM–IV Diagnosis)	Treatment of • mental depression • mood elevator
Effects	• may require 2 to 4 weeks before it is fully effective
Symptoms Relieved	• elevates mood • increases physical activity • improves appetite • improves sleep
Possible or Common Side Effects	• dry mouth • tiredness or weakness • dizziness/drowsiness • orthostatic hypotension • tachycardia • increased appetite or weight gain • nausea • unpleasant taste • headache • eye pain • increased sweating • constipation • blurred vision
Cautions	• adds to effects of alcohol and other CNS depressants (e.g., cold medicines, cough syrup) • may cause dizziness or fainting • use is contraindicted when an MAO Inhibitor is being or has been used within the previous 2 weeks • contraindicated with cardiovascular disease or myocardial infarction

Category of Drugs	Antidepressant: Tricyclic (TCA)
Trade or Proprietary Name	Pamelor® Aventyl®
Generic or Nonproprietary Name	nortriptyline
Primary Use (DSM–IV Diagnosis)	Treatment of mental depression
Effects	• may require 2 or more weeks before it is fully effective
Symptoms Relieved	• elevates mood • increases physical activity • improves appetite • improves sleep
Possible or Common Side Effects	• dry mouth • blurred vision • constipation and urinary retention • tiredness or weakness • dizziness/drowsiness • tachycardia • arrhythmias • weight gain • headache • eye pain • increased sweating
Cautions	• adds to effects of alcohol and other CNS depressants (e.g., cold medicines, cough syrup) • may cause dizziness or fainting • use is contraindicted when an MAO Inhibitor is being or has been used within the previous 2 weeks

Category of Drugs	Antidepressant: Monoamine Oxidase Inhibitors (MAOI)
Trade or Proprietary Name	Parnate®
Generic or Nonproprietary Name	tranylcypromine sulfate
Primary Use (DSM–IV Diagnosis)	Treatment of Major Depressive Episode without Melancholia for hospitalized clients
Effects	May show relief over depression in 1 week, but require 3 weeks to show maximum improvement
Symptoms Relieved	• reduces depression
Possible or Common Side Effects	• dry mouth • weakness • irritability • agitation or restlessness • sleep loss • postural hypotension • GI upset • hypertensive crises, including occipital headache, neck stiffness, nausea, vomiting, sweating, dilated pupils, photophobia • constipation and urinary retention • increased perspiration and/or chills • dependency with prolonged use
Cautions	• should not be used with other MAO Inhibitors or dibenzazepine-related entities • restrict foods and preparations containing tyramine dopamine, L-tryptophan, or alcohol • use is contraindicated when sympathomimetic drugs are being used • contraindicated with individuals with cardiovascular disorders, hypertension, history of headaches • avoid using with meperidine (Demerol®)

Category of Drugs	Antidepressant: Selective Serotonin Reuptake Inhibitor (SSRI)
Trade or Proprietary Name	Paxil®
Generic or Nonproprietary Name	paroxetine hydrochloride
Primary Use (DSM-IV Diagnosis)	Management of Major Depressive Disorder (MDD)
Effects	• may see therapeutic effect within 1 to 4 weeks
Symptoms Relieved	• increased mood • improved sleep • decreased anxiety
Possible or Common Side Effects	• nausea • somnolence • headache • dry mouth • weakness • constipation • dizziness • insomnia • diarrhea • excessive sweating • tremor • decreased appetite • agitation or nervousness • ejaculatory disturbance or other male genital disturbances
Cautions	• contraindicated with an MAOI, or within 14 days of discontinuing an MAOI • do not use with history of mania, seizures, metabolic or hemodynamic diseases, or history of drug abuse • may result in severe renal or hepatic impairments

Category of Drugs	Antipsychotic
Trade or Proprietary Name	Prolixin®
Generic or Nonproprietary Name	fluphenazine decanoate
Primary Use (DSM–IV Diagnosis)	• management of schizophrenia • management of psychotic disorders
Effects	Generally relieve symptoms within 96 hours, but maximum effect may take up to 6 weeks
Symptoms Relieved	• reduces psychosis, hallucinations • increases self-care, concentration, and interest in surroundings
Possible or Common Side Effects	• hypotension • restlessness, excitement, or bizarre dreams • salivation, sweating, or excessive urination • dry mouth • constipation or urinary retention • drowsiness, dizziness, or fainting • nasal congestion • blurred vision • may result in extrapyramidal reactions, including tardive dykinesia (TD) or Neuroleptic Malignancy Syndrome (hyperpyrexia; muscle rigidity; autonomic instability, including irregular pulse or blood pressure, tachycardia, diaphoresis, cardiac dysrhythmias)
Cautions	• adds to effects of alcohol and other CNS depressants (e.g., cold medicines, cough syrup) • contraindicated with severe CNS depressant or bone marrow depression • use cautiously with history of seizures

Category of Drugs	Antidepressant: Selective Seretonin Reuptake Inhibitor (SSRI)
Trade or Proprietary Name	Prozac®
Generic or Nonproprietary Name	fluoxetine hydrochloride
Primary Use (DSM–IV Diagnosis)	Management of • Major Depressive Disorder (MDD) • Obsessive-Compulsive Disorder (OCD) • panic disorder • bulimia
Effects	• some effect may be seen in 6 to 8 hours, although effects from changes in doses may not be seen for 4 to 6 weeks • relatively slow elimination results in drug action weeks after dosage has been discontinued
Symptoms Relieved	• increased mood • resumption of sleep • reduction of anxiety
Possible or Common Side Effects	• headache • loss of strength • anxiety or nervousness • drowsiness • nausea • diarrhea • decreased appetite • insomnia
Cautions	• caution when using with motor vehicles or heavy machinery, because use may impair judgment, thinking, or motor skills • contraindicated with an MAOI, or within 14 days of discontinuing an MAOI • allow 5 weeks after discontinuing before beginning drugs that might interact with Prozac®, including MAOIs

Category of Drugs	Antipsychotic
Trade or Proprietary Name	Serentil®
Generic or Nonproprietary Name	mesoridazine besylate
Primary Use (DSM–IV Diagnosis)	Treatment of • schizophrenia • organic brain disorders • alcoholism • psychoneuroses
Effects	May not reach maximum effectiveness for up to 6 weeks
Symptoms Relieved	• emotional withdrawal • conceptual disorganization • anxiety and tension • hallucinations • hyperactivity and uncooperativeness
Possible or Common Side Effects	• orthostatic hypotension • dizziness or fainting • dry mouth • blurred vision • lethargy • constipation, urinary retention, or diarrhea • nasal congestion • hypotension and tachycardia • with chronic use can result in tardive dyskinesia (TD), or Neuroleptic Malignant Syndrome (NMS)
Cautions	• may increase CNS depressant effect, respiratory depression, or hypotensive effects • contraindicated with bone marrow depression or subcortical brain damage • use sunscreen due to possible photosensitivity

Category of Drugs	Antipsychotic
Trade or Proprietary Name	Stelazine®
Generic or Nonproprietary Name	trifluoperazine hydrochloride
Primary Use (DSM–IV Diagnosis)	• short-term treatment of psychotic disorders • generalized anxiety disorders
Effects	May require 2 to 3 weeks before optimal response
Symptoms Relieved	• reduces psychotic thoughts • decreases agitation or hyperactivity • increases mood • reduces nausea or vomiting
Possible or Common Side Effects	• extrapyramidal reactions, including tardive dyskinesia (TD) or Neuroleptic Malignancy Syndrome (NMS; hyperpyrexia; muscle rigidity; autonomic instability, including irregular pulse or blood pressure, tachycardia, diaphoresis, cardiac dysrhythmia) • hypotension • drowsiness, dizziness, or fainting • dry mouth • blurred vision • lethargy • constipation, urinary retention, or diarrhea • nasal congestion • photosensitivity (sunscreen required)
Cautions	• adds to effects of alcohol and other CNS depressants (e.g., cold medicines, cough syrup) • contraindicated in individuals with liver damage • lowers seizure thresholds; should not be used with Amipaque® • periodic checking of hepatic and renal functions and blood counts recommended

Category of Drugs	Antipsychotic
Trade or Proprietary Name	Thorazine®
Generic or Nonproprietary Name	chlorpromazine
Primary Use (DSM–IV Diagnosis)	• management of psychotic disorders or manic phase of bipolar disorder • treatment of severe behavioral and aggressive disorders
Effects	• may not reach maximum effectiveness for up to 6 weeks
Symptoms Relieved	• psychotic symptoms • aggressive behaviors
Possible or Common Side Effects	• drowsiness or dizziness • photosensitivity (sunscreen is essential) • defective color vision or night vision • blurred vision • dry mouth • neuromuscular reactions: dystonia, motor restlessness, pseudo-parkinsonism, or tardive dyskinesia (TD) • tachycardia • suppressed white blood cell count (WBC) • nasal congestion • constipation and urinary retention • impotence • Neuroleptic Malignancy Syndrome (hyperpyrexia; muscle rigidity; autonomic instability, including irregular pulse or blood pressure, tachycardia, diaphoresis, cardiac dysrhythmia)
Cautions	• contraindicated with individuals with chronic respiratory disorders or acute respiratory infections because of CNS depressant effect • may lower convulsive threshold, resulting in seizures • may interfere with metabolism of Dilantin®, precipitating Dilantin® toxicity

Category of Drugs	Antidepressant: Tricyclic (TCA)
Trade or Proprietary Name	Tofranil® Tofranil–PM® Janimine®
Generic or Nonproprietary Name	imipramine hydrochloride
Primary Use (DSM–IV Diagnosis)	• treatment of depression, especially endogenous depression • childhood nocturnal eneuresis
Effects	May notice relief of depression within 2 to 3 days, but may not have maximal effect for 2 to 3 weeks
Symptoms Relieved	• elevates mood • increases physical activity • improves appetite • improves sleep
Possible or Common Side Effects	• dry mouth • blurred vision • constipation and urinary retention • tiredness or weakness • dizziness/drowsiness • tachycardia and arrhythmias • increased appetite or weight gain • disturbed concentration • headache • eye pain • increased sweating
Cautions	• adds to effects of alcohol and other CNS depressants (e.g., cold medicines, cough syrup) • may cause dizziness or fainting • use is contraindicted when an MAO Inhibitor is being or has been used within the previous 2 weeks • contraindicated when there is significantly impaired liver or renal function, or with sulfite sensitivity

Category of Drugs	Antidepressant: Tricyclic (TCA)
Trade or Proprietary Name	Vivactil®
Generic or Nonproprietary Name	protriptyline hydrochloride
Primary Use (DSM–IV Diagnosis)	Treatment of depression
Effects	May show reduction of depression within 2 to 5 days, with maximum effectiveness within 2 to 3 weeks (faster than other TCAs)
Symptoms Relieved	• elevates mood • increases physical activity • improves appetite • improves sleep
Possible or Common Side Effects	• dry mouth • drowsiness or fatigue • postural hypotension • blurred vision • constipation and urinary retention • tachycardia and arrhythmias • increased appetite or weight gain • headache
Cautions	• use is contraindicated when an MAO Inhibitor is being or has been used within the previous 2 weeks • contraindicated when there is significantly impaired liver or renal function, or with sulfite sensitivity • contraindicated with individuals with cardiovascular disorders, seizures, tendency for urinary retention, or glaucoma • frequent tests for liver/renal dysfunction essential

Category of Drugs	Antidepressant: NDRI
Trade or Proprietary Name	Wellbutrin® Zyban® Wellbutrin–SR®
Generic or Nonproprietary Name	bupropion
Primary Use (DSM–IV Diagnosis)	Management of • Major Depressive Disorder (MDD) • depressed phase of bipolar disorder
Effects	Generally seen within 3 to 5 days
Symptoms Relieved	• increases mood • reduces anxiety • reduces panic attacks
Possible or Common Side Effects	• constipation • weight loss or weight gain • nausea or vomiting • anorexia • dry mouth • headache • increased sweating • tremor • sedation or insomnia • altered hearing • dizziness • agitation
Cautions	• adds to effects of alcohol and other CNS depressants (e.g., cold medicines, cough syrup) • withdrawal symptoms on discontinuation, including seizures, impaired concentration, and lightheadedness • contraindicated in individuals with seizures • with long-term therapy, perform liver/renal function tests periodically

Category of Drugs	Anxiolytic or antianxiety
Trade or Proprietary Name	Xanax®
Generic or Nonproprietary Name	alprazolam
Primary Use (DSM–IV Diagnosis)	Treatment of • generalized anxiety with or without depression • panic disorder, with and without agoraphobia
Effects	Generally seen within 3 to 5 days
Symptoms Relieved	• increases mood • reduces anxiety • reduces panic attacks
Possible or Common Side Effects	• drowsiness or lightheadedness • irritability • clumsiness • unsteadiness • increased or decreased appetite • weight gain or weight loss • constipation • fatigue • toleration or dependency
Cautions	• adds to effects of alcohol and other CNS depressants (e.g., cold medicines, cough syrup) • withdrawal symptoms on discontinuation, including seizures, impaired concentration, and lightheadedness • perform periodic liver/renal function tests with long-term therapy

Category of Drugs	Antidepressant: Selective Serotonin Reuptake Inhibitor (SSRI)
Trade or Proprietary Name	Zoloft®
Generic or Nonproprietary Name	sertraline hydrochloride
Primary Use (DSM-IV Diagnosis)	Management of • major depressive disorder (MDD) • panic disorder • obsessive-compulsive disorder (OCD)
Effects	• may take several days to see effect
Symptoms Relieved	• improves mood • improves energy level • reduces anxiety and panic attacks
Possible or Common Side Effects	• changes in appetite • decreased sexual drive • dizziness or drowsiness • constipation or diarrhea • dry mouth • headache, increased sweating • inability to sleep • nausea or stomach pain with vomiting • tremors • anxiety or nervousness • flushed skin or palpitations
Cautions	• avoid use of alcohol • contraindicated with MAOI or within 14 days of discontinuing MAOI • may cause liver or renal dysfunction

REFERENCES

Allen, C. K. (1989). Psychiatry. In T. Malone, *Physical and occupational therapy: Drug implications for practice* (pp. 207–228). Philadelphia: Lippincott.

Almers, W., & Stirling, C. (1984). Distribution of transport proteins over animal cell membranes. *Journal of Membrane Biology, 77*, 169–186.

Barkley, R. A. (1990). *Attention deficit hyperactivity disorder: A handbook for diagnosis and treatment.* New York: Guilford.

Bender, K. J. (1990). *Psychiatric medications: A guide for mental health professionals.* Newbury Park, CA: Sage.

Benet, L. Z. (1992). Pharmacokinetics I: Absorption, distribution and elimination. In B. L. Katzung (Ed.), *Basic and clinical pharmacology* (5th ed., pp. 35–48). Los Altos, CA: Lang.

Benet, L. Z., & Sheiner, L. B. (1985). Pharmacokinetics: The dynamics of drug absorption, distribution and elimination. In A. G. Gilman & L. S. Goodman (Eds.-in-chief), *Goodman and Gilman's: The pharmacological basis of therapeutics* (7th ed.). New York: Macmillan.

Bezchlibnyk-Butler, K. Z. & Jeffries, J. J. (2000). *Clinical handbook of psychotropic drugs* (10th ed.). Seattle: Hogrete & Huber.

Ciccone, C. D. (1990). *Pharmacology in rehabilitation.* Philadelphia: F. A. Davis.

Ciccone, C. D. (1996). *Pharmacology in rehabilitation* (2nd ed.). Philadelphia: F. A. Davis.

Craig, C. R., & Stitzel, R. E. (1997). *Modern pharmacology with clinical applications* (5th ed.). Boston: Little, Brown.

Finnen, M. J., Herdman, H. L., & Shuster, S. (1985). Distribution and subcellular localization of drug metabolizing enzymes in the skin. *British Journal of Dermatology, 113*, 713–721.

Gitlin, M. J. (1996). *The psychotherapist's guide to psychopharmacology* (2nd ed.). New York: The Free Press.

Gram, T. E. (1994a). Drug absorption and distribution. In C. R. Craig & R. E. Stitzel (Ed.), *Modern pharmacology* (4th ed., pp. 19–32). Boston: Little, Brown.

Gram, T. E. (1994b). Metabolism of drugs. In C. R. Craig & R. E. Stitzel (Eds.), *Modern pharmacology* (4th ed., pp. 33–46). Boston: Little, Brown.

Hardman, J. G., Limbird, L. E., Molinoff, P. B., Ruddon, R. W., & Gilman, A. G. (Eds.). (1996). *Goodman and Gilman's: The pharmacological basis of therapeutics* (9th ed., Rev.). New York : McGraw-Hill, Health Professions Division.

Hobbs, A. S., & Albers, R. W. (1980). The structure of proteins involved in active membrane transport. *Annual Review of Biophysics and Bioengineering, 9*, 259–291.

Hoch, P. H. (1959). Drug therapy. In S. Arieti (Ed.), *American handbook of psychiatry* (pp. 1541–1551). New York: Basic Books.

Kalat, James W. (1998). *Biological psychology* (6th ed.). Pacific Grove, CA: Brooks/Cole Publishing.

Kao, J., Patterson, F. K., & Hall, J. (1985). Skin penetration and metabolism of topically applied chemicals in six mammalian species, including man: An in-vitro study with benzo(a)pyrene and testosterone. *Toxicology and Applied Pharmacology, 81*, 502–516.

Katzung, B. G. (1992). *Basic and clinical pharmacology* (5th ed.). Los Altos, CA; Lang.

Katzung, B. G. (1992b). Basic principles. In B. L. Katzung (Ed.), *Basic and clinical pharmacology* (5th ed., pp. 1–9). Los Altos, CA: Lang.

Katzung, B. G. (2000). *Basic and clinical pharmacology* (8th ed.). New York: McGraw- Hill.

Kizior, R. J., & Hodgson, B. B. (2000). *Saunders drug handbook for health professionals, 2000.* Philadelphia: W. B. Saunders.

Lankester, E. R. (1889). Mithradatism. *Nature, 40*, 149.

Malone, T. (Ed.). (1989). *Physical and occupational therapy: Drug implications for practice.* Philadelphia: Lippincott.

McKim, W. A. (1986). *Drugs and behavior: An introduction to behavioral pharmacology.* Englewood Cliffs, NJ: Prentice-Hall.

Opler, L. A. (1992). The use of drugs and other somatic treatments. In F. I. Kass, J. M. Oldham, H. Pardes, & L. B. Morris (Eds.), *The Columbia University College of Physicians and Surgeon's complete home guide to mental health* (pp. 63–91). New York: Henry Holt.

Physicians' desk reference 2000™ (PDR; 54th ed.). (1999). Montvale, NJ: Medical Economics Company.

Poe, T. E. (1989). Pharmacology. In T. Malone (Ed.), *Physical and occupational therapy: Drug implications for practice* (pp. 1–35). Philadelphia: Lippincott.

Preston, J., O'Neal, H. H., & Talaga, M. C. (2000). *Handbook of clinical psychopharmacology for therapists.* Oakland, CA: New Harbinger.

Ray, O., & Ksir, C. (1987). *Drugs, society, and human behavior* (4th ed.). St. Lewis: Times Mirror/Mosby.

Sifton, D. W. (Ed.-in-chief). (2000). *The PDR pocket guide to prescription drugs* (4th ed.). New York: Pocket Books..

Taber, C. W. (1989). *Taber's cyclopedic medical dictionary* (16th ed.). Philadelphia: F. A. Davis.

Umhauer, M. A., Their–Spain, S., & Spain, J. W. (1986). History, legislation and standards. In M. K. Mathewson (Ed.), *Pharmacotherapeutics: A nursing process approach.* Philadelphia: F. A. Davis.

USA Today. (1997, April 1). *Ritalin use up among youth* [Online]. Retrieved February 3, 2001, on the World Wide Web: *http://www.usatoday.com/life/health/child/drugs/lhcdr003.htm.*

Yamamoto, A., Utsumi, E., Hamaura, T., Nakamura, J., Hashida, M., & Sezaki, H. (1985). Immunological control of drug absorption from the gastrointestinal tract: Effect of local anaphylaxis on the intestinal absorption of low molecular weight drugs in the rat. *Journal of Pharmacobiodynamics, 8,* 830–840.

CHAPTER

8

Applying the Group Process to Psychosocial Occupational Therapy

Beverlea Tallant, Ph.D., OT (C)

> *In groups people experience life.*
> — S. Leary (1994), *Activities for Personal Growth: A Comprehensive Handbook of Activities for Therapists,* p. 203

Operational Learning Objectives

By the end of this chapter, the learner will:

1. Be aware of the history and current use of groups in psychosocial occupational therapy.
2. Discuss the type and purpose of various therapeutic groups in psychosocial occupational therapy.
3. Identify nine factors that contribute to the curative factor in group therapy.
4. Discuss eight factors to be considered in the development of a therapeutic group in occupational therapy.
5. Identify and explain the current use of screening and group behavioral scales in occupational therapy.
6. Discuss current research on therapeutic groups in psychosocial occupational therapy.

When thinking about human beings and groups, we might also say: In life people experience groups! From birth, human beings become part of a group process that helps the individual to develop and evolve as a person as he or she moves through various stages of his or her life. The majority of human beings encounter their first group experience in their immediate family. From this they move on to peer groups through childhood play and school and enter into powerful friendship groups as adolescents. Throughout these years specific tasks such as team sports, debating teams, drama groups, and so on, help individuals develop the physical, social, and group skills necessary for entering the workforce in late adolescence and early adulthood. As human beings mature, individuals, in turn, apply their group knowledge and experiences to their own families. Many individuals also become involved in volunteer work and community service through charitable, religious, neighborhood, and political organizations. With time, as the demands of their families change, individuals often transfer their group needs to task-oriented interest groups, increase their involvement in work, and/or become more involved in community service that relates to their age and stage in life such as senior citizen organizations.

The group process is an integral part of normal growth and development in all cultures. Therefore, it is little wonder that the "group process" was recognized as early as the 1920s (Howe & Schwartzberg, 1995; Stein & Tallant, 1988a) to have "curative" or "therapeutic" potential, particularly for individuals who for physical or psychological reasons felt rejected, isolated, and abandoned by society. The idea of using a group experience for therapy was embraced by psychiatrists, psychologists, and educational counselors. To this day, these health professionals still value the "group," particularly the importance of "talking" through problems and relationships in a group setting (Kaplan, Sadock, & Grebb, 1994). The specific group therapy process may take varying forms, depending on the clinician's theoretical frame of reference, that is, psychoanalytical, behavioral, gestalt, and/or the specific needs of the clients.

Occupational therapists, concerned with helping an individual to lead normal, healthy, functional lives, introduced the idea of using activities in small group settings in the early 1900s, "to control mischievous behavior, decrease boredom and increase socialization" (Stein & Tallant, 1988a, p. 16). Although, over

time, the purpose of these activity groups became more theoretically defined, goal-oriented or client-centered, the notion of using some form of task or activity remains inherent to the occupational therapy group process (Bruce & Borg, 1993; Cole, 1998; Creek, 1990; Posthuma, 1989).

This chapter acquaints the reader with the historical and current use of group activities in psychosocial occupational therapy and the application of group therapy principles and procedures in the occupational therapy setting.

HISTORICAL AND CURRENT USE OF GROUP ACTIVITIES IN PSYCHOSOCIAL OCCUPATIONAL THERAPY

Activity Groups

In the early 1920s, patients were encouraged to work on individual projects within a collective or group setting (Howe & Schwartzberg, 1995). There were no specific treatment goals and no emphasis on group interaction. Patients were simply asked to work on their own projects in the company of others somewhat similar to the developmental concept of parallel play (Mosey, 1970, 1973). The activities used were individual crafts, such as basketry, weaving, and bookbinding, or work-related activities in the institution such as laundry, housecleaning, sewing, farming, and gardening. By the early 1930s occupational therapists began to recognize the therapeutic value of patients working in a group and, therefore, introduced the idea of a group project. Patients worked together on a common task such as quilt-making, games, or work (Howe & Schwartzberg, 1995). The focus or goal of these groups depended on the activity; for example, quilt-making was used to encourage socialization and communication, games to encourage socialization and an acceptable outlet for aggression and work activities to develop feelings of pride, self, and group worth.

Fidler and Fidler (1963) renamed the process of Task Groups. The goal was to provide the patient with an opportunity for "exploration and learning in the here and now" (Fidler & Fidler, 1963, p. 43). The patient was to learn a task, to learn how he or she and others approached a task, and how he or she got along with others. The task groups were considered to be "learning labs" in which individuals developed skills for life and the work world through task group experiences (Fidler, 1969). The occupational therapist's role was to help clients explore their feelings, reactions, and behavior toward each other and the task and to see alternate ways of functioning. It was felt that participation in this type of group led to ego growth and improved function. Mosey (1973) emphasized the importance of the activity or task group in helping an individual to develop age-specific skills through both the task and the interpersonal interactions generated by the activity. Howe and Schwartzberg (1995) further emphasized the benefits of the Task or Functional Group by pointing out the importance of purposeful activities in influencing health and adaptation, the here and now focus, and experiential learning leading to increased independence in work, play, and self-maintenance.

Gradually, the emphasis shifted from activity used to control behavior and fill time to utilizing the task for individuals to understand themselves in the context of a group setting. The group members demonstrate their problems as they perform the task and the group leader assists them to reflect on their feelings, behavior, and interactions and how they impact on performance. In addition, the therapist helps the patient to focus on conflict resolution or problem solving (Cole, 1998). Task group activities have been well described by various group theorists (Breines, 1995; Cole, 1998; Drake, 1999; Dynes, 1990; Leary, 1994; Posthuma, 1989; Rider & Gramblin, 1987). Currently, the Activity, Task, or Project Group is still one of the primary occupational therapy interventions (Cole, 1998).

Self-Awareness Groups

The influence of the Fidlers (Fidler & Fidler, 1954) and the Azimas (Azima & Azima, 1959a) in the 1950s was considerable. They introduced the concept of object-relations to the occupational therapy setting, recognizing the dynamic use of objects by patients on an individual basis. Unstructured creative activities were used with a group of patients as a form of group psychotherapy (Azima & Azima, 1959b). The assumption was that, through free creation, free association, and discussions, individuals could work through their ego defense mechanisms, psychological drives, conflicts, and transference issues to gain insight into their feelings and behaviors. The created object was viewed as an essential catalyst in the group process (Azima & Azima, 1959b).

Occupational therapists have used this type of group, often called a projective group, employing art, music, poetry, clay, and role-playing to help patients project, confront, and gain insight into their inner conflicts and feelings (Blair, 1975; Monroe & Herron, 1980). The use of the "creative arts'" as a therapeutic tool has recently gained renewed interest (Lloyd & Chandler, 1999; Thompson & Blair, 1998).

Specific themes may be selected and introduced by the occupational therapist to provide the patient with opportunities to explore and confront his or her emotions and reactions to personal issues (Centoni & Tallant, 1986; Posthuma, 1989). In the psychoeducational course of therapy, patients may be asked to imagine, illustrate, and/or enact how they might alter their lives or environment in the future. The role of the occupational therapist is considered critical as the therapist provides the stimulation for the therapeutic experience, facilitates expression within the group, and guides and helps patients to confront, interpret, and support each other within the group setting (Posthuma, 1989). In the projective group, the clients' explanation of their productions, whether drawings, poems, clay figures, or other creative products serve as the basis for insight and learning (Cole, 1998).

Many therapists prepare self-awareness groups at different levels, depending on the patient's needs (Leary, 1994). Selected topics help the patient to become aware of themselves ("Who am I" activities) and others ("How I see you"), build self-esteem ("Caring about each other"), or interpret and confront the issues that affect them personally ("My Problem Is," "Myself in the Future"). The depth of the therapeutic experience is determined by the overall treatment objectives, client variables, and the clinical expertise of the occupational therapy group leader. Well-phrased open-ended questions and statements, skilled observation, confrontation, summarization and interpretation techniques to facilitate expression, reflection, and self-awareness are essential skills for the group leader. This process helps patients gain awareness into their current reactions and fears in relation to other members of the group and then to relate this insight to real-life group experiences with their immediate families, and in work and social settings (Leary, 1994).

While projective groups have traditionally been identified with the objects-relations frame of reference, the concepts, methodology and process now form the basis for self-awareness group activities with other frames of reference as well. The volition subsystem of the Model of Human Occupation (Kielhofner, 1995) can be readily explored through activities such as the

"Personal Coat of Arms" (Stein & Tallant, 1988b). Developmental issues, for instance, the need for intimacy, can be examined through an activity such as "Ideal Woman/Ideal Man" as described by Marilyn B. Cole (1998). Other self-awareness group activities have been well described by others (Campbell, 1993; Jennings, 1986; Leary, 1994; Posthuma, 1989; Remocker & Sherwood, 1998; Sunderland & Engleheart, 1993).

Reality-Oriented Groups

The 1960s saw an increased emphasis on the therapeutic milieu (Jones, 1953) and the impact of the environment or community on the individual and vice-versa (Barris, Kielhofner, & Watts, 1988). The focus of these groups was on "reality, responsibility, and right-and-wrong" (Barris et al., 1988, p. 100). Group activities usually consisted of an educational/lecture component, discussion, and a practical experience to try out the new knowledge. Topics addressed everyday activities such as parenting, management of time, relationships, and current events (Howe & Schwartzberg, 1995). Clients would then participate in activities relevant to the topic in their home, community, or employment (Watson & Thomes, 1983). The occupational therapist served as a problem-solving teacher who helped patients make responsible decisions, organize, and plan in a warm, nonpunishing environment that de-emphasized failure. The aim of the group was to help clients move toward reality and away from dysfunction (Posthuma, 1989) by engaging in activities very closely related to daily reality (Simmons & Mullins, 1981), such as the routine of an army soldier (Watson & Thomes, 1983).

More recently, occupational therapists have expanded their use of reality-oriented groups to clients with various types of organic mental disease, including dementia, substance-induced disorders, and brain injury (Bruce & Borg, 1993; Willson, 1987). An example of a reality-oriented group format for a geriatric program may be found in Stein and Tallant (1988b, p. 48).

Role-Oriented Groups

Mary Reilly (1974) emphasized the importance of roles in life such as worker, parent, friend, or spouse. This led occupational therapists to develop group activities to help patients develop the skills necessary for healthy functioning within a given role. Some group activities might focus on the roles associated with gender (Pezzuti, 1979), on relationship roles, or on work roles (Furner, 1978). In some cases the treatment approach could be educational, consisting of information sessions followed by discussion (Pezzuti, 1979); in other cases the object of the group activity might be to help the individual learn the skills or tasks needed to function within specific roles, for example, parenting sessions for single-teenage mothers or new mothers with postpartum depression, specific work skills (Furner, 1978), or skills necessary for a worker to obtain employment, such as interview strategies or simulated work situations (Simmons & Mullins, 1981; Solberg & Chueh, 1976).

Kielhofner (1995) stressed the importance of habituation in the occupational performance of roles and habits as very integral to the individual and almost automatic. Individuals who are less confident about themselves in various life roles could benefit from discussions and practice sessions or by trying out new roles in a supportive environment, such as a therapeutic group. Another example of a role-oriented group is in the area of wellness. Jackson and her colleagues developed an occupational therapy program that focused on health, wellness, and prevention, successfully used mental, physical, social, leisure, and lifestyle redesign group activities to foster and develop a "well elder"' versus "sick, declining elder" role in a well elderly population in California (Jackson, Carlson, Mandel, Zemke, & Clark, 1998).

Developmental Groups

The developmental frame of reference was described by Anne Cronin-Mosey (1970, 1973, 1986) as a viable treatment approach in occupational therapy for psychiatric patients. The development of Group Interaction Skills, Adaptive Skill 4, was considered to be an essential component of maturation. Mosey (1970) delineated the ages and sequence in which these group skills would normally develop. The skills ranged from parallel group activity (18 months to 2 years), as seen in children's sandbox play, to mature group participation by 15 to 18 years of age. Donohue (1999), in a recent analysis of Mosey's group interaction skills, notes that most people interact at two adjacent age levels. Further, the mature group members are able to take on several group membership roles and adapt their group interaction skills depending on the satisfaction they seek (friendship versus mentorship) or the requirements of the task itself (team sports versus adjacent office workstations).

The occupational therapist needs a good understanding of the normal development of individuals across the lifespan (Bruce & Borg, 1993) to be able to select group activities that are age- and skill-specific but also meet the level of functioning of the patient. For example, a young male with schizophrenia chronologically might be in the mature group category but developmentally be barely able to tolerate working in the presence of others, which would be at the parallel (2-year-old) group level. The object of the therapeutic group is to match the task or group format to the developmental level of the client(s) and then to expose slowly and facilitate growth in the individual(s) through higher level groups until they acquire the appropriate group interaction skills for their chronological age (Broekema, Danz, & Schloemer, 1975). Cole (1998) described examples of developmental group activities used to evaluate midlife (e.g., "Times of Your Life" collage) or to assist with the transition to late adulthood ("Fabric of Life").

Behavioral Groups

Behavioral techniques, such as the systematic use of positive and negative reinforcement, extinction, shaping, modelling, behavioral rehearsal, and feedback, have been used with clients with both chronic (Overbaugh & Bucher, 1970) and acute (Schell & Giles, 1985; Willson, 1988) disorders. Basic skills of daily living, such as grooming, cooking, and work habits, have been taught, shaped, and reinforced by a token economy system (Kaye, Mackie, & Hitzing, 1970; Schell & Giles, 1985). Social skills training has been used to help adolescents control delinquent behaviors (Schell & Giles, 1985), to develop listening and communication skills in patients with chronic illness (Drouet, 1986; Hewitt, Wishart, & Lambert, 1981; Willson, 1987), and to help patients overcome acute anxiety in social or friendship situations in a resocialization group (Davis & Keene, 1983; Leary, 1994). Social skills training could involve discussion and/or activities on such topics as nonverbal communication and expression, verbal expression (simple social greetings to complex conversations), work situations (worker conversations, interviewee behaviors), expressing feelings, group interaction, initiating friendships, and sexual behavior (Willson, 1988).

Competency training for a group of hospitalized soldiers included education classes plus opportunities to practice skills related to work, socialization, leisure-time management, and self-care (Thomes & Bajema, 1983). Appropriate assertiveness has been developed in anxious, underassertive clients through a combination of lectures, assertive techniques, role-playing, homework, and feedback from the group (Bruce & Borg, 1993; Leary, 1994; Prior, 1998; Simmons & Mullins, 1981; Temple & Robson, 1991).

Human Occupation Groups

The Model of Human Occupation (Kielhofner, 1980, 1995) views the human being as an integrated system made up of subsystems concerned with volition, habituation, and performance. In this theory, the higher levels govern the lower ones, so that one's values or interests can help overcome environmental, physical, or psychological obstacles. Conversely, dysfunction at the lower level (performance) could impede the higher levels. For example, a pianist with a physical disability may no longer be able to play the piano and, therefore, must seek other means to use his or her knowledge and interest in music.

Clients are assessed for each subsystem and intervention is directed at the dysfunction at each level. If an individual has good performance and habit skills but no desire to use them, he or she might participate in a group activity directed toward values clarification (e.g., "Personal Coat of Arms"). However, if a client has performance deficits, treatment might focus on basic skills such as perceptual-motor, communication, socialization, and interaction skills through a highly structured, directive group process (Kaplan, 1988).

The Model of Human Occupation addresses the needs of the whole person so that whatever the primary source of dysfunction, the treatment process, including appropriate group activities, can include the dysfunction itself, the ramifications of the dysfunction on the individual's aspirations and attitudes toward him or herself. Examples of this blend or interaction between the physical and psychological needs of the client (Kielhofner, 1995) are reported by the clinical cases of (a) Kim (Baron, 1995) where group activities focused on performance and task skills, adolescent socialization, and "healthy roles;" (b) Mike (Sullivan, 1995) where group activities focused on work-related skills, employee interactions, and roles of worker and home maintainer; and (c) Sally (Furst & Stabenow, 1995) where group activities focused on values, education/information and prevention of injury skills for her physical condition, and leisure interests.

In this frame of reference, sharing and processing feelings and information are not necessary for each group session because the activity or task is considered to be therapeutic in and of itself. Consequently, group sessions are longer and more frequent. Therapists focus on the nature of the activity or occupational role over several treatment sessions (Cole, 1998). Planning and preparing for a special event such as a Valentine's Day party would involve preparing invitations, making decorations, cooking, and providing entertainment. In the groups, therapists assist clients to form good habits by (a) assessing which self-care habits need to be developed, (b) teaching the client to perform and sequence the required tasks, and (c) providing group structure for peers to give feedback until the habits are maintained at an appropriate and automatic level (Cole, 1998).

Cognitive Dysfunction Groups

Recent advances in the neuroscientific understanding of brain function, the impact of brain damage, and the restorative or compensatory mechanisms of the brain (Held, 1993) helps us to better understand the role that cognitive dysfunction plays in limiting functional behavior.

Claudia Allen (1985) proposed that careful assessment of a patient's cognitive disabilities permits placement in activities that can be accurately matched to their level of function. The six levels of cognitive dysfunction (further described in Chapter 4) can be used to place the client in an appropriate group.

The treatment approach is directed toward reducing symptoms of stress associated with cognitive dysfunction, assisting the patient with his or her cognitive impairments while natural healing occurs (e.g., early and later stages following a brain injury), and providing activities that strengthen his or her present cognitive abilities (Bruce & Borg, 1993; Cole, 1998; Kielhofner, 1992). Once the condition is stable, the approach is to provide environmental compensation; that is, the environment may be adapted to compensate for the individual's dysfunction. In the case of short-term memory loss, a memory jog such as a note on the apartment door saying what time the mail is delivered may prevent the client from wandering repeatedly in and out of the apartment.

Earhart (1985) described nine occupational therapy groups that may be used to treat the six levels of cognitive dysfunction. The groups range from simple movement (Level 2), grooming and basic crafts (Levels 3 and 4), and basic educational skills (Level 4) to groups that involve higher levels of organization such as cooking and work evaluation (Levels 5 and 6). She included recommendations for the ideal number and type of patients as well as specific activities for each group. Reminiscence sessions may be used to discuss topics that will help retain remote memory; reactivate past interests, for example, reading the paper, cooking, being interested in current events, watching sports, or listening to music in the present; and maintaining verbal communication and listening skills as well as appropriate affective responses.

Treatment activities to encourage attention, concentration, and spatial planning such as "Find the Way" (Leary, 1994) can be utilized, as well as current affairs topics to encourage awareness of and involvement in real-life events. Games such as Trivia Pursuit or Twenty Questions may be used to reawaken interests and maintain prior knowledge. Other familiar practice activities to improve or maintain memory for objects as well as rules and organization include Kim's game, I Spy (Leary, 1994), card games like Fish, Hearts, and checkers, Chinese checkers, Scrabble, chess, dominoes, and bingo. A group activity that engages clients in making spring hats may be used for Levels 5 and 6 for exploratory and planned actions. The various components of the activity (a) stimulate the senses; (b) improve organization and sequencing, divergent thinking, and safety practices; and (c) prepare the client for life activities in the house and garden. Another benefit of the activity is to provide opportunities for the client to reminisce (Cole, 1998).

Gregory (1996) described a memory maintenance group program held in a community mental health facility for people in the early stages of dementia (mild) still living in their homes. Group activities included current events, reminiscence, quizzes, word games, snooker, darts, music, and simple craft activities in a routine, structured format. Group membership was nine at a time. The majority were 70 to 80 years of age, female, and evenly divided between those who lived alone or with a caretaker. The average length of stay in the group was 5 to 6 months with the majority discharged to continuing day care. The primary purposes of the group were for memory maintenance, to provide a relatively stress-free and safe environment, to introduce people to the idea of accepting activity outside the home, to provide a sense of self-affirmation, and to discuss their reactions to the experience of losing their memory. In addition, the program provided psychological support, encouragement, and some respite for the caretakers.

CURRENT USE OF GROUPS IN PSYCHOSOCIAL OCCUPATIONAL THERAPY

Three studies compared the use of groups in occupational therapy between 1984 and 1994 (Duncombe & Howe, 1985, 1995; Stein & Brintnell, 1986). The populations studied and types of clinical settings were not identical in each case. Stein and Brintnell (1986) surveyed the use of groups in psychiatric settings, and, although, an attempt was made to replicate Duncombe and Howe's earlier study (1985), it was not always possible to collect data from the same facilities as in the original study (Duncombe & Howe, 1995).

When comparing the findings of these studies, we can see that the percentage use of groups for small general hospitals, community programs, and community mental health centers remains approximately the same over the 10-year time span. There has, however, been a decrease in the use of groups by occupational therapists in large general hospitals, nursing homes, psychiatric hospitals and other settings (Table 8–1). This change may be due to the changing role of occupational therapy from a treatment-based practice to the more recent primary focus on assessment in acute care hospital settings. It is difficult though to understand why there would be a decreased use of groups in the other facilities. Some explanations might include an increase in one-on-one treatment; unsuitability of client population; lack of knowledge of group theory, process, and activities for specific populations; problems of reimbursement; and/or a shortage of occupational

Table 8–1. A Comparison of Three Studies Indicating the Occupational Therapy Settings that Used Group Activities, 1985–1995

Facility	Duncombe & Howe, 1985	Stein & Brintnell, 1986[a]	Duncombe & Howe, 1995[b]
	N = 120	N = 34	N = 200
Large General Hospitals	52%		45%
Small General Hospitals	88%		86%
Rehabilitation Centers	44%		61%
Psychiatric Hospitals	100%	100%	83%
Nursing Homes	40%		33%
Community Programs	50%		50%
Community Mental Health Centers	100%		100%
Schools	45%		65%
Mental Retardation Institutions	50%		missing data
Pre-school	not surveyed		75%
Other	50%		28%

[a]Psychiatric settings only in Milwaukee, Montreal, and Alberta, Canada.

[b]Not the same facilities as in 1985, fewer psychiatric settings.

therapists in certain settings (Duncombe & Howe, 1995).

The increased use of group activities in rehabilitation centers may well reflect the expansion of the occupational therapist's role from strictly physical medicine interventions to include the psychosocial rehabilitation of the client as well. The increased use of groups in school systems could be influenced by an increase in referrals. Or, as children who have received earlier treatment mature and reach adolescence, it is developmentally appropriate to learn and interact in group activities, therefore making this a more age-appropriate approach to use.

When comparing these three studies, we find that, although clinicians might not have used exactly the same titles for the groups, there is some consensus on the purpose of the groups used in occupational therapy. Areas that are commonly addressed through group activities include exercise, activities of daily living, leisure interests, self-expression, and values clarification (Table 8–2). Duncombe and Howe (1995) reported that sensorimotor and sensory integration groups (29 percent) as well as educational groups (11 percent) are employed frequently. This may be a reflection of the number of school settings that reported using groups. As expected, the Stein and Brintnell (1986) study, which only looked at psychiatric settings, showed a preponderance of psychological or psychosocial group activities such as cognitive, social skills and assertiveness training groups, stress management, and prevocational training.

Table 8–2. A Comparison of Three Studies on the Type of Psychosocial Group Activities Used by Occupational Therapists, 1985–1995[a]

Duncombe & Howe, 1985 N = 8[b]		Stein & Brintnell, 1986 N = 10		Duncombe & Howe, 1995 N = 8	
Exercise		Exercise	71%	Exercise	15%
Activities of Daily Living	17%	Independent Living Skills	91%	Activities of Daily Living	11%
Arts and Crafts		Leisure Time	88%	Arts and Crafts	7%
Self-Expression		Expressive/Creative	23%	Self-Expressive	5%
Feeling-Oriented Discussions		Values Clarification	65%	Feeling-Oriented Discussions	1%
Reality-Oriented Discussions				Reality-Oriented Discussions	1%
Sensorimotor & Sensory Integration				Sensorimotor & Sensory Integration	29%
Educational				Educational	11%
		Prevocational Training	47%		
		Cognitive Training	12%		
		Social Skills Training	94%		
		Stress Management	79%		
		Assertiveness Training	59%		
				Task	12%
				Other	1%

[a]The titles for the types of groups are those reported by the respective authors.
[b]Except for "Activities of Daily Living Groups," no percentage use for types of groups was reported in this study.

A comparison of the type of group process used (Duncombe & Howe, 1985, 1995) indicated an overall increase in the use of activity-only groups, a decrease in the use of verbal-only groups, and a slight increase in the use of groups that combined both activity and verbal tasks (Table 8–3). The difference between using activity versus verbal versus combination groups was statistically significant within each study with the majority of occupational therapists continuing to use activity or a combination of both activity and verbal group processes.

Although the criteria for examining the size of the group was not the same for each study, we can see an overall increase in the percentage use of small groups (76 to 87 percent) and a decrease in the number of large groups with 10 or more clients (24 to 13 percent). In the 1995 study, Duncombe and Howe defined the size of the groups more specifically and found that the use of groups with 1 to 3 clients was 17 percent; 4 to 6 clients, 43 percent; 7 to 9 clients, 27 percent, and groups with more than 10 clients, 13 percent of the time. As previously noted in Table 8–2, more occupational therapists are using groups within the school system. Because groups for children have traditionally been smaller in size (1 to 3), this may partially account for the increased use of small groups. Overall the majority of occupational therapists

Table 8–3. A Comparison of Two Studies on the Group Process and Size of Groups Used in Psychosocial Occupational Therapy

Group Characteristics	Duncombe & Howe (1985)	Duncombe & Howe (1995)
Type of group		
Activity	54%	63%
Verbal	24%	11%
Both	22%	26%
Size of Group		
Small[a] (1–9)	76%	87%[b]
Large (10+)	24%	13%

[a]Majority had 6 to 9 group members.

[b]Majority had 4 to 9 group members.

conducted small group activities with approximately six clients per group (60 percent). This is the size indicated by most group theoreticians to be most appropriate for satisfactory outcome in the areas of communication and socialization (Howe & Schwartzberg, 1995; Posthuma, 1996; Yalom, 1995).

In addition, the Duncombe and Howe study (1995) informed us that the format of the group, that is, open or closed, is relatively the same in each case, as is the preferred length of a group treatment session (long–53 percent; short–45 percent). Further, the study reported that the majority of clients treated are adults (43 percent), children (37 percent), and adolescents (14 percent). These categories are very broad and do not indicate, for example, in the adult category, which portion of clients might fall into the elderly or young adult range.

In more recent years occupational therapists have developed and/or refined group treatment activities such as integrative group therapy, directive group therapy, and cognitive-behavioral group therapy, including the psychoeducational group. (See Chapter 10.)

Integrative Group Therapy

Mildred Ross (1991) has developed a structured five-stage approach based on neurophysiological principles. This method may be used with clients with special needs across the lifespan. These individuals require considerable cues and assistance from their environment for their central nervous system to become organized enough to respond and to function appropriately. The neurophysiological approach has been used with clients of all ages who have

▶ developmental disabilities

▶ severe physical disabilities

▶ profound retardation

▶ mild mental retardation

▶ psychosocial disabilities while institutionalized

▶ mild dementia or Alzheimer's disease

▶ hemiparesis due to a stroke (Bruce & Borg, 1993; Ross, 1997).

The five stages, sequentially programmed in each session, provide structure, routine, stimulation, cues, and assistance to help the individual achieve the appropriate, organized sensory, motor, affective, or cognitive response. *Stage I* involves sensory stimulation to maximally arouse and welcome the members to the group. Short mixer activities are used, which involve touch, sound, and visual stimulation. In *Stage II*, movement is emphasized through gross motor activities and objects, such as streamers on wands to calm or to stimulate the individual. All the movements or bodily responses involve both sensory stimulation and integration. In *Stage III*, visual motor and perceptual activities, such as games that involve throwing an object or races where an object is moved from one spot to another, are used. The activities provide an opportunity for sensory information to be modified and become meaningful as an adaptive response. In *Stage IV*, activities are used that facilitate organized thought, behavior, and communication through cognitive stimulation. Cortical integration is enhanced through activities, such as creative storytelling, memory games, slide presentations and discussion, or sharing of feelings. Familiar closing activities, which may be calming, stimulating, or simply maintain the energy level and mood attained by the group, are used in Stage V to end the group session on a positive note. These activities provide an opportunity to encourage appropriate leave-taking, handclasps, and plans for the next session. This stage engenders group trust.

Ross (1991) describes each stage and its hypothesized impact on the individual's central nervous system along with numerous examples of stage-appropriate activities and approaches to the client and group. Other examples of group tasks include parachute games, basketball exercises, and sensory stimulating activities such as classification of smells, balloon catch, color matching, and group sway to music (Cole, 1998). A group session may last 20 minutes, 40 minutes, or an hour, depending on the group members and their tolerance for group activity (Ross, 1991).

In addition, Ross (1991) has developed an assessment, the *Smaga and Ross Integration Battery* (SARIB), which is used to screen individuals for the groups as well as to assess the outcome after several sessions. The main impact of this approach lies in the improvement of the quality of life of the group members and maintenance of their sensory-motor abilities. At present, there is no evidence-based research to quantify the outcome of this intervention, considering the extraneous variables in medications inhibiting motor behavior and/or controlling behavior, or in the carryover of treatment effects once treatment ends. In addition, occupational therapists using this approach should be well versed in the impact of neurophysiological procedures so that they do not overdo spinning or stimulation, because this could lead to negative, if not harmful, effects (Bruce & Borg, 1993; Cole, 1998; Ross, 1997).

Directive Group Therapy

The purpose, assessment, method, process, activities, and therapist's role in directive group therapy have been developed and described by Kathy Kaplan (1988). The theoretical framework for this type of group is the Model of Human Occupation (Kielhofner, 1985). The purpose of the therapeutic group is to provide an environment in which clients may structure their feelings and thoughts, interact with others, take risks in new behaviors, and develop insight into their interests and values. The specific goal is to help the individual reorganize his or her behavior to a more functional level. In this model, it is presumed that clients have a continuum of functional and dysfunctional behavior. In therapy, the client, with the help of the therapist, overcomes helplessness, incompetence, and inefficacy by developing basic skills, good habits, and self-awareness (Kaplan, 1988).

Clients selected for directive group therapy are usually unable to tolerate a more traditional, insight-oriented, group psychotherapy situation. This model targets clients with severe psychosocial dysfunctions who have difficulties with organizing and controlling their thoughts, moods, and behaviors. Group therapy is usually held for one week for approximately an hour daily. The format of the group session consists of five activities presented in a structured manner: reality-based orientation, introduction, warm-up, selected, and wrap-up activities. Kaplan (1988) has listed 131 activity ideas and has discussed which activities are most appropriate for each phase of the group session. All patients are assessed on a Baseline Assessment Form prior to entering the group and again at the end of the week.

The adaptation of this method for a geriatric mental health setting (Trace & Howell, 1991) has been found useful to preserve autonomy, enhance integrity, and increase personal and community safety. Directive group therapy has been used to focus on purposeful activity, life roles, lack of pleasure, memory maintenance, environmental adaptations, medication management, and side effects of medication. Trace and Howell felt that the group approach maximized their contact with clients. They also noted that, due to the population involved, maintenance rather than improvement was the main treatment objective.

Cognitive-Behavioral Groups

The cognitive-behavior therapist believes that a person's cognitive function can mediate or influence his or her affect and behavior (Bruce & Borg, 1993; Cole, 1998). For many individuals with psychosocial dysfunction, this means helping them to undo faulty negative attitudes about themselves and the world. Through the treatment process they are taught how to restructure their thinking to replace their unreasonable beliefs with more rational logical beliefs. This eventually leads to a decrease in the extent of their depressed and anxious thoughts and maladaptive emotions and behavior (Yakobina, Yakobina, & Tallant, 1997). Clients most appropriate for this approach are individuals who are depressed, anxious, and unhappy but not severely cognitively disabled.

Clients are taught to recognize, analyze, and evaluate their negative thoughts, and then to incorporate new thoughts and behaviors in group activities. The initial sessions take a more didactic form with the occupational therapist assuming the role of educator/facilitator by modeling an objective attitude through questioning generalizations and modeling more appropriate responses (Bruce & Borg, 1993). Frequently, role-playing is used to increase awareness about the client's thoughts and/or to provide opportunities to rehearse and practice alternative thinking styles and behaviors. Other group members provide feedback and help the clients change their thinking and behavior.

Homework assignments have been found to maximize the treatment process by engaging clients to work on problem-solving, to promote self-awareness and self-control, to increase motivation, and to maintain treatment effects (Luboshitzky & Gaber, 2000). In many programs, each session ends with a homework assignment, such as keeping a daily log of negative thoughts, activity scheduling, initiating dyadic interactions, practicing conversations and behaviors in vivo, using self-talk, and/or reading relevant literature. The next session begins with a review of the homework (Luboshitzky & Gaber, 2000; Yakobina et al., 1997).

The types of group activities used will vary with the specific needs of the client group; however, movies, TV programs, and videos provide an excellent means for patients to observe negative thinking styles in others and to relate it to themselves. Daily living activities such as cooking can be used to help clients become more aware of the pervasiveness of their negative thoughts about their competencies and how to counteract them. With time, the cooking activities learned in the group may be conducted by each group member at home. The food dishes made would then be brought in to share with the group, thus providing an opportunity for the individual to gain support and to increase self-esteem and self-confidence. Task group projects, such as a group project in which a miniature village for a children's hospital ward is built, provide an opportunity for individuals to weigh their actual abilities against their negative self-perception. Eventually, clients are encouraged to plan pleasurable individual projects in their homes or communities and to share the outcome of these experiences in subsequent sessions (Yakobina et al., 1997).

Social skills training with patients with long-term mental illness has helped individuals to develop verbal and nonverbal communication skills and to generalize them (Salo-Chydenius, 1996). These individuals had difficulties with receiving and interpreting communication and with sending or imparting communication to others. The group sessions focused on these areas and taught clients to assess their communication styles, coached them in alternate modes of communication, and provided feedback on their performance. The group activities progressed through developmental stages from parallel to mature group interactions in 12 sessions. Activities used to foster these social skills were drawing, music, social games, role-playing, and verbal discussion of their reactions. Clients assessed their performance on the *Group-Interaction Skills Survey* after each session and

by observing a video of themselves in a social situation. The occupational therapist used this outcome information to plan the tasks for the next treatment session.

Occupational therapists use psychoeducational methods when working in a psychiatric setting to teach social skills and promote functional abilities and self-esteem (Wright, Thase, Ludgate, & Beck, 1993). Psychoeducational groups have been conducted with individuals with chronic psychiatric conditions such as schizophrenia, major mood disorders, and personality disorders (Haertlein & Bloggett, 1994). Careful assessment was made of functional impairment in the self-care, leisure, and work areas. Patients were then placed in groups where they were instructed in self-care management techniques, whether the goal was to improve their personal hygiene, develop a shopping list and shop, budget, or to learn to cope with crowds on a community outing. Educational methods were used to establish group learning objectives, to instruct, to provide feedback, and to reevaluate progress.

A short-term anxiety management psychoeducational course was conducted with patients experiencing anxiety in a day hospital setting (Prior, 1998). The psychoeducational course content included anxiety management, methods for personal stress and coping, relaxation techniques, cognitive recognition of negative thoughts, assertiveness techniques, and problem-solving homework activities. Scripts and audiotapes for group relaxation sessions were readily available (Fairburn & Fairburn, 1979; Harlowe & Yu, 1997). In this model, the therapist, as a precaution, informs the group members of the content of the script since the suggested imagery may be positive for some clients, but noxious for others. In the latter case, the clients might, as a group activity, write their own script for the relaxation sessions.

A group of patients with dual diagnoses (chronic psychosis and substance abuse) (Harrison & Precin, 1996) were studied using the *Neurobehavioral Cognitive Status Examination* (NCSE) and found to have serious cognitive impairment that interfered with their learning capacities, social skills, and retention of new learning. The results of this study led to the development of a remedial treatment approach using structured task groups. The *Progress-Living Skills for Recovery Curriculum*, a 12-step model, which is currently part of the treatment program for this dual diagnosis clinic, was adapted to become a living skills acquisitional training program that focused on social skills, stress and time management, and activities of daily living. Examples of psychoeducational modules on leisure time, parenting, employment, money or time management and discharge preparation can be found in Bruce and Borg (1993), Cole, (1998), and Simmons and Mullins (1981).

Several British occupational therapists (Bender, Waugh, & Orchard, 1997) questioned whether a group of caretakers for individuals with Alzheimer's disease required therapy or education/training. An assessment was made of the level of distress of the caretakers and they were then offered counseling/therapy or career education/training. The education program consisted of information about Alzheimer's disease and its course; behaviors to expect; support services in the community, such as cleaning and Meals on Wheels, to help with the home situation; and anxiety management training sessions for their personal use in times of stress. Eight 1-hour sessions were given. This type of intervention deals with the needs of the caretakers for support, release, and encouragement; prevents serious mental stress; and possibly prevents an abusive situation from arising in relation to the individual with Alzheimer's disease.

A MODEL FOR A THERAPEUTIC GROUP IN PSYCHOSOCIAL OCCUPATIONAL THERAPY

Prior to initiating a therapeutic group in occupational therapy it is important for the therapist to plan the structure of the group and/or series of sessions in advance. The occupational therapist must consider the primary purpose of the group, the group's goals versus individual goals for the client or patient, how to begin the group, the number and method of selecting the group members, and what leadership style to adopt. Further, the therapist needs to anticipate what management strategies might be required for specific populations to develop group cohesiveness or enhance the group's effectiveness. Finally, as an occupational therapist, one must determine which activities will best help to achieve the goals of the group and how to measure the outcome or effectiveness of the occupational therapy group intervention. Table 8–4 identifies some factors that are important in initiating a therapeutic group in occupational therapy (adapted from Stein & Tallant, 1988b).

Establishment of Group Goals

Yalom (1995) identified a number of factors that contribute to the curative factors in group therapy. These factors are also relevant to occupational therapy.

▶ *Instillation of hope in the client or patient.* The therapist must convey the positive benefits to be derived from group therapy. As Yalom points out, the success of self-help groups such as Alcoholics Anonymous and Recovery, Inc. are based on the strong conviction and faith that the method works. Group occupational therapy has been identified as an effective method to

Table 8–4. Factors to Consider for a Therapeutic Group in Psychosocial Occupational Therapy

Group Goals	Group Structure	Contracts	Patient Selection
• self-awareness	• open-ended	• administrative	• age, gender
• instillation of hope	• close-ended	• therapeutic	• diagnoses
• shared experiences	• number of clients		• education
• coping with depression	• number of sessions		• personal goals
• social skills	• length of sessions		• functional level
• vocational preparation	• environment		• motivation
			• assessment

Leadership Style	Group Methodology	Media	Group Effectiveness
• democratic	• didactic	• audio-visual	• operational goals
• laissez-faire	• self-awareness	• expressive	• outcome measures
• directive	• reality-oriented	• crafts	• self-reports
• advisory	• role-oriented	• prevocational	• family and staff
• combination	• developmental	• value clarification	• evaluation
	• behavioral	• ADL	
	• cognitive dysfunction	• role-playing	
	• sensory-integrative	• movement	
	• cognitive-behavioral		

help the client develop self-esteem, interpersonal skills, consensual validation, and social competencies (Posthuma, 1989).

▶ *Universality of sharing experiences.* The group experience conveys to the patient that his or her experiences are not unique. The patient may be comforted knowing that others with similar problems have improved. The patient feels less isolated and begins to disclose feelings of which he or she may have previously felt ashamed or guilty. Sharing feelings in a nonjudgmental milieu is therapeutic. Group members can be supportive, confrontive, empathic, and understanding, thus providing valuable feedback regarding how others see him or her and helping the client to gain insight (Azima & Azima, 1959).

▶ *Imparting of information.* The group is an excellent vehicle for imparting information to the clients using methods of lecture, seminar discussions, and role playing. Psychoeducational groups establish mini-courses targeted for vulnerable groups such as widows, individuals with drug and alcohol addiction, young people with psychosis (Parlato, Lloyd, & Bassett, 1999), and single parents in community settings, as well as for inpatients in a psychiatric setting for specified periods of time (Gracegirdle, 1982; Lindsay, 1983). The use of guest speakers, films, field trips, and topics such as re-entering the job market, holistic health, accident prevention in the home, parent effectiveness, and interpersonal skills can be incorporated into the mini-course organized by the occupational therapist (German, 1964). The occupational therapist can skillfully establish therapeutic groups that are content-oriented and create a supportive climate that allows for individual development.

▶ *Altruism.* A basic premise of any therapeutic group is that the members will help each other (Posthuma, 1989). Indeed, the occupational therapist facilitates and encourages this type of interaction. For example, in a task group such as a ward newspaper, the occupational therapist would help the patients to assign individual components of the project based on each person's skills. Many patients suffer from low self-esteem. Establishing in the group that they are worthy of help and also worthy and capable of helping others is a very ego-enhancing experience. The trust and cohesion in the group permits sharing, feedback, reassurance, suggestions, and often caring for newly developed friendships (Lloyd, Bassett, & Samra, 2000).

▶ *Simulate family structure.* Many psychiatric patients have had unhappy, if not traumatic, family experiences. The therapeutic group provides them with an opportunity to reenact some of their feelings in relation to other group members who may resemble and/or react to them similar to their past experiences. Frequently, the occupational therapist may have the group use role playing, family drawings (Burns, 1982), building figures of families in clay (Cole, 1998), and values clarification exercises (Corey, 1985) in enacting and working through some of their negative attitudes and feelings. Within the "group family" patients are often able to discuss and work through issues from their primary family such as conflicts with parents and

sibling rivalries (Posthuma, 1989). The group process enables them to learn new ways to interact and react with their real families.

▶ *Redevelopment of basic social skills.* Occupational therapists have long been interested in the development of social skills because it is such a basic prerequisite for individuals to perform and communicate in their life roles. The development of social skills may start with activities of daily living regarding personal hygiene or appearance. Behavioral or psychoeducational methods may be the means to develop these skills. Role-playing of social situations, observation and analysis of social interactions through activities such as the Soap Opera Group (Falk-Kessler & Froschauer, 1978), or videotaped rehearsals of social behaviors (Berger, 1983; Holm, 1983) are means to achieve this objective.

▶ *Imitative behavior.* The group provides opportunities for participants to imitate the behavior of the occupational therapist or co-leader as well as other group members. Sometimes this means they will try out negative behaviors as well as positive ones. However, the reaction of the group members provides them with feedback so that they can modify or perfect their new responses (Posthuma, 1989). This is particularly noticeable with adolescents, who even in "normal" situations tend to idolize and model their behavior after the current popular heroes or heroines as they strive to establish their own identities. For patients who are introverted, quite fixed in their responses, or lack identity, this can be a learning experience.

▶ *Interpersonal learning.* In therapeutic groups people express their feelings and share life experiences and their thoughts about them. They also listen and reflect on what they have heard and, in turn, respond to other group members. Engaging in discussion, sharing mutual feelings, and developing memories of shared struggles and good times are ways for individuals to learn that being involved in relationships can be a rewarding experience.

▶ *Catharsis.* Often the group provides a place where people can express their strongest emotions, usually ones they have previously been too ashamed or frightened to divulge. The emotional release can be exhausting for the individual or the group; however, for many it provides such a release of stored-up conflicts and anger that they are able to move forward in their personal development. Activities such as psychodrama (Sacks, 1983), family sculpture, finger painting, and so on can facilitate the cathartic process. The occupational therapist must be able to help the individual regain control while supporting and encouraging the other group members in their support and tolerance of the individual.

Structure of the Identified Group

The occupational therapist must first determine the need for the group by reviewing the case histories of individual patients, overall goals of the treatment ward or program, consultation with the team, and availability of resources such as personnel, patients, space, and supplies. Decisions must be made as to whether the group will be an open-ended group with a constant in and out flow of clients or a closed group. Open groups are often used to help patients become used to the group process prior to graduating to a closed group. A closed group usually deals with a specific set of problems or

population of patients who become involved for a predetermined number of treatment sessions (Howe & Schwartzberg, 1995; Cole, 1998). For a closed group, one must consider what selection criteria will determine group membership: Age? Gender? Diagnosis? Symptomatology? Interpersonal difficulties? Social state? Crisis issue-death, divorce, abuse? Chronicity? How to assess the capability of the patient to function within a given group context must also be determined.

The environment for the group sessions, that is, the room, seating arrangement, type of stimuli in the room, ventilation, privacy, and so on will all play an important role in the cohesiveness of the group. The length of time for each group activity should be determined by the purpose of the group and the nature of the task, as well as the functional level of the group members. The frequency of sessions, that is, daily, weekly, or biweekly must be decided as well as the period of time over which the group will operate.

The occupational therapist must decide whether he or she will run the group alone or with a co-leader, possibly another member of the health care team (Cole, 1998). He or she must consider what type of leadership skills, experience, and knowledge are required to lead a specific type of group. The style of leadership may be influenced by such factors as the therapist's personality, training, skills, a theoretical frame of reference of the group, and/or the type of group to be led. Record keeping of the group sessions must be determined in advance. Will it be observation and recall? Video? Recordings? Sociogram? Assessment scales? Self-assessments completed by the group members? Or a combination of these methods? The choice will be determined by the desired outcomes for the group sessions. Therapeutic outcomes may include symptom reduction, changes in attitude, productivity, behaviors and habits, increased self-esteem. The client population, group treatment goals, and chosen theoretical frame of reference are factors that influence the selection procedures used to assess the outcome of the group.

The establishment or development of group cohesiveness is crucial to the success of any group therapy approach. Group cohesiveness is defined (Cartwright & Zander, 1968) as the resultant of all the forces acting on all members to remain in the group. Group cohesiveness is a positive factor in the group related to an individual's desire to participate and share experiences with others. It provides the basis for social interactions and interpersonal learning. It also promotes attendance to the group and a willingness for group members to share in group decisions. Groups that fail to establish cohesiveness are less likely to succeed (Bednar & Kaul, 1978). Attendance declines, patients become apathetic, and the group dissolves itself. Group cohesiveness is, therefore, an important indicator for the occupational therapist when evaluating the group's effectiveness. When this is reached, the group begins to function as a positive environment for personal growth.

Administrative and Therapeutic Contracts

Administrative contracts may be established between the occupational therapist and the department, program, or agency in which the group is to be conducted. The contract will usually cover issues related to personnel, space, supplies, safety, clients, and reimbursement.

Therapeutic contracts or group treatment protocols (Cole, 1998) may be established between the therapist and group members prior to starting the therapy sessions. The contracts may stipulate the purpose of the group, tasks to be used, outcomes to be expected, responsibilities and functions of the group members in

terms of attendance, behavior, participation, and tasks such as clean-up, coffee making, and so on, in addition to reimbursement (when relevant). In some cases, the therapists and clients/patients develop contracts together regarding specific therapeutic goals the group wishes to attain within a particular amount of time (Posthuma, 1989).

Selection of Patients

In the selection of patients for a group, the therapist considers the size and composition of the group as well as screening criteria for group inclusion (Yalom, 1995). Most researchers stipulate 5 to 15 members with 6 to 8 (Battegay, 1974; Cole, 1998; Howe & Schwartzberg, 1995) considered the ideal number. Group size for younger children usually does not exceed three to four at a time. If the group is too large, individuals will not expose their feelings and are reluctant to participate. If a group is too small, the group lacks variety and patients may become bored with each other. Six to eight means the group members can establish interpersonal relationships and remain interested in each other.

In considering the composition of the occupational therapy group, the therapist determines if the group will be homogeneous with regard to sex, age, and education or not. Yalom (1995) recommends that groups be composed of heterogeneous groups when there is conflict, and homogeneous groups to build ego strength. This means that a variety of diagnoses may be mixed together to create curiosity in group members about each other. However, members should be equal in their abilities to protect their egos, accept criticism, and cope with the dynamics of the group process. The occupational therapist should be aware of members who cannot identify with the majority, who may become isolated and cut off from the group, or who may be destructive to the group process. In selecting members for the group, the therapist considers whether an individual will benefit from the group process. Not everyone is able to become a group member.

Screening and Outcome Measures

Occupational therapists have developed specific assessments to screen potential members and also to serve as a pre-therapeutic group baseline from which to determine the therapeutic outcome for the individual and for the group activity itself. *The Comprehensive Occupational Therapy Evaluation Scale* (COTES; Brayman, Kirby, Misenheimer, & Short, 1976) includes a lengthy list of items that apply to a task group setting; however, it is cumbersome to use, and has not been extensively validated.

The *Bay Area Functional Performance Evaluation* (BaFPE; Bloomer & Williams, 1982; Houston, Williams, Bloomer, & Mann, 1989; Williams & Bloomer, 1987) includes a Social Interaction Scale, a behavioral scale, that assesses an individual's performance in a group activity. The assessment has been well-validated; however, it is time-consuming to administer. The *Group-Interaction Skills Survey* (Salo-Chydenius, 1996) was developed as a screening and ongoing outcome measure for a social skills training program based on a cognitive-behavioral approach for individuals with long-term mental illness. The scale rates the behavior of the individual in different developmental groups. The author also developed a self-evaluation form consisting of 10 items for the patient to complete prior to and after each group session. To my knowledge, to date, neither of these scales has been psychometrically evaluated for validity nor inter-rater reliability.

The *Occupational Therapy Task Observation Scale* (OTTOS; Margolis, Harrison, Robinson, & Jayaram, 1996) was developed as a simple, quan-

titative, and rapid method of evaluating task group performance. It consists of a 10-item task behavior section and a 5-item general behavior section. Each item is rated on a scale from 0 (dysfunctional) to 10 (functional). It serves as a means for reporting client performance to other members of the team and to identify areas of performance that require greater attention. The correlation for inter-rater reliability was .92 for total scores, and the correlation between OTTOS and other rating instruments ranged from .88 (COTES) on task behavior to .34 (BaFPE) on general behavior. Test-retest reliability studies are in progress. It is most effective for gauging progress in activities requiring high functional capacity such as cooking, typing, and individualized projects related to academic studies or employment. Although it is used mainly to record client progress, it has the potential to be used for screening subjects prior to entering a group.

The *Assessment of Communication and Interaction Skills* (ACIS; Forsyth, Lai, & Kielhofner, 1999) is an experimental observational rating scale designed to evaluate a person's social interactional ability in a natural setting. Clients are observed in two of four recommended social situations: (a) an unstructured situation, (b) a parallel group, (c) a cooperative group or (d) dyadic interaction. Preliminary research showed evidence that the instrument could discriminate between different skill levels across diagnostic groups in a clinically relevant manner. The ACIS can be administered and scored in 20 minutes and the information obtained can be readily used in clinical practice.

Leadership Styles

The literature on leadership roles in groups differentiates between democratic (facilitative), laissez-faire, directive (authoritarian), advisory, or combination leadership styles (Cole, 1998; White & Lippitt, 1968). The styles imply levels of control by the occupational therapist in the group. In the democratic group, decisions are made by the total group, who tend to feel enthusiastic about the task or activity, are motivated to complete the task, and feel a strong sense of unity (Posthuma, 1989). This approach is not recommended for clients functioning at a low cognitive level (Cole, 1998). In the laissez-faire situation, the group is virtually leaderless, which means that patients may feel confused and frustrated with the task, productivity is low, members are not unified and show little interest in working together. In the directive style, the occupational therapist plans the goals for the group, guides the group's progress, and makes all final decisions. This often leads to compliance with the tasks, frequent absenteeism, low cooperation, irritability, and participation dependent on leader prodding (Posthuma, 1989). The advisory leader is the most passive, providing expertise as needed but no group structure or goals. This style is most useful with high functioning groups who are working on problem-solving, attitude change, or specific issues such as wellness and health maintenance (Cole, 1998). In reality, most occupational therapists use a combination of these leadership styles, often altering their role depending on the needs of the group for direction or permitting the group to take the lead themselves. The amount of control the therapist assumes in the group, however, has an important effect on the success of the group (Cartwright & Zander, 1968).

Co-leadership offers the advantages of mutual support, increased objectivity, knowledge and skills, opportunity to learn from each other and to take different roles, in the group (Cole, 1998). However, co-leaders must strive to work together as a team for group development, avoid competition, and contribute equally in order to avoid splitting the group, establishing a "dysfunctional family" group, or developing resentment toward each other.

Group Methodology

Occupational therapy group methods can be divided into five major areas:

▶ *Didactic group.* In this type of group the occupational therapist uses lectures, audio-visual aids, and other learning techniques to develop various skills or knowledge.

▶ *Self-awareness group.* Creative media such as drawing, sculpture, puppetry, collage, and so on are used to help the patient project and communicate feelings and ideas to others. The therapist encourages free expression both through the media and verbally. The occupational therapist stimulates the group by suggesting themes that are relevant to the group member's problems and/or to create the type of mood or discussion they need to explore.

▶ *Simulated group.* Groups that explore areas such as work interview and social skills through role-playing and individual life enactment activities fit this category. Specific role-focused group models may be used, for example, a parenting group, social skills development, or a group for leisure interest development in the elderly.

▶ *Task-oriented group.* Here the main focus is to learn about energy attachment, problem solving, success, work habits, group interactions, and play behaviors through building a product. Examples are a cooking group, redecorating an area, planning and carrying out a social event, fund-raising, or producing a film.

▶ *Sensory awareness group.* In this type of group the focus is on bodily sensations and experiences. Activities can be directed at increasing sensory awareness, refining gross or fine motor skills, or engaging in socially acceptable integrated physical activities such as sports, games, dancing. It could also include learning how to recognize the signs of stress in the body and learning to counteract stress through relaxation and stress management activities.

Selection of Therapeutic Media

Therapeutic media are utilized in groups to facilitate group goals. Some activities have characteristics that are more appropriate for meeting the specific needs of the patient or of meeting the concepts inherent to the theoretical frame of reference. The occupational therapist's knowledge of analyzing and grading activities is essential when selecting activities to meet the goals and objectives of the therapeutic group. The selection of activities will depend on the age, education, dysfunction, motivation, physical setting, and ego strength of the clients, as well as interests of the group. Often, the skills, knowledge, and interest of the occupational therapist are a factor in the choice! It is important, however, to try to select activities that will be meaningful to the group members as a means to solve their life problems.

Recently, there has been a resurgence of professional interest in therapeutic activity or occupation, the essence of occupational therapy, and, as a result, several excellent publications have become available as group activity resources (Allen, 1985; Breines, 1995; Campbell, 1993; Cole, 1998; Drake, 1999; Dynes, 1990; Jennings, 1986; Kaplan, 1988; Leary, 1994; Posthuma, 1989; Remocker & Sherwood, 1988; Rider & Gramblin, 1987; Ross, 1991; Sunderland & Engleheart, 1993). Education

libraries are also a good source of activity ideas for children and adolescents. The Internet has become another resource (Reed & Cunningham, 1997). (See Appendix D for useful websites.)

Evaluation of a Group's Effectiveness

Finlay (1993) described eight reasons for occupational therapists to keep a record of the group sessions: (a) for legal reasons, (b) for a debriefing opportunity to clarify feelings and thoughts, (c) to improve our understanding of group dynamics, (d) to sharpen our skills of observation and critical thinking, (e) to monitor progress of clients, (f) to plan subsequent sessions, (g) to form the basis of progress notes, and (h) to provide data for clinical research.

Outcome measures of therapeutic group intervention are necessary to help us to provide the best and most efficacious form of occupational therapy treatment for our clients. It is important for occupational therapists to determine the outcomes they hope to achieve prior to beginning the therapeutic group. With the introduction of various new assessment instruments (Forsyth et al., 1999; Margolis et al., 1996; Salo-Chydenius, 1996), it will be easier for therapists to observe, record, and quantify the progress a client makes through participation in therapeutic psychosocial groups in occupational therapy. Methods such as videocassette and audio recordings can assist in documenting the group process thus allowing later evaluation of individual and group behaviors.

In addition, outcome measures of the efficacy of intervention are crucial to the profession in terms of advancing knowledge and understanding of the components of occupational therapy practice. The *Canadian Occupational Performance Measure* (COPM) is an individualized measure designed for use by occupational therapists to detect subtle changes in a client's self-perception of occupational performance over time (Law et al., 1994). With the current emphasis on client-centered practice and quality of life issues, this measure provides important information from the individuals whom we are attempting to help. No matter how much improvement the therapist sees, if the client is unaware of it or disappointed in his or her progress, treatment will not have achieved its ultimate goal of helping the individual attain a more functional and meaningful life.

Further, if occupational therapists are unable to design intervention programs that consider the real needs, goals, and desired outcomes of their clients, then, once again, treatment will not have served its purpose. A qualitative research approach using focus group discussions with a diverse group of individuals diagnosed with schizophrenia (N = 35) examined their perspective of the meaning of quality of life and factors they considered to be important to quality of life (Laliberte-Rudman, Yu, Scott, & Pajouhandeh, 2000). Seven major factors were identified: (a) activity, (b) social interaction, (c) time, (d) disclosure, (e) "being normal," (f) finances, and (g) management of illness. These factors related to three overall themes of time management, connecting and belonging, and making choices and maintaining control. The subjects provided detailed information on how impairment in these areas directly affected their quality of life. The authors concluded that this client-centered approach provided essential information for the development of occupational therapy programs that include meaningful treatment goals and occupations.

Good outcome measures to assess client-relevant programs will also help occupational therapy retain and expand its position as a significant contributing health profession that is recognized by other members of the health care team and the general public.

RESEARCH ON THERAPEUTIC GROUPS IN PSYCHOSOCIAL OCCUPATIONAL THERAPY

Research on therapeutic groups in psychosocial occupational therapy has focused primarily on comparisons between different types of group processes, the client's perception of a group, and pre- and postcomparisons for an individual group member's behavior, self-esteem, or some outcome measure based on the purpose of the therapeutic group. Recent studies have seen these methodologies used to assess the effectiveness of psychosocial group occupational therapy programs with less traditional populations such as the well elderly (Jackson et al., 1998) and chronic pain patients (Martensson, Marklund, & Fridlund, 1999). Further, a retrospective approach has been used to review and analyze the theoretical underpinnings of theoretical frames of reference commonly used in occupational therapy practice (Donohue, 1999). In one case, the group process was used as the primary research tool to examine quality of life issues with persons with schizophrenia (Laliberte-Rudman et al., 2000).

Instrument Development

Research has been hampered by the lack of appropriate instruments to measure group interaction skills. Recently, several occupational therapists have attempted to overcome this problem by developing various instruments that can serve as screening criteria, outcome measures, or self-ratings by the clients (Forsyth et al., 1999; Law et al., 1994; Margolis et al., 1996; Salo-Chydenius, 1996). As previously mentioned, these instruments either need psychometric validation, or research is currently being conducted on reliability and validity issues. Donohue (1999) plans to use the results of her retrospective study of Mosey's developmental theory to develop a new instrument to measure group interaction skills.

Group Format

McDermott (1988) conducted a study that compared the group format for a task group, a verbal group, and a combination verbal/activity group. Results indicated that patients in the task group showed greater communication, compassion, emotions, and member-to-member interactions but scored lower in expressing feelings and leadership roles. Patients in the verbal or combination group were not significantly different in their communication. The authors concluded that group format does affect interaction patterns. However, it should be noted that the group members were not matched for diagnosis, age, and so on in the different groups, which may have affected the results.

Individuals with a diagnosis of psychosis or borderline personality patients were randomly assigned to either an unstructured psychotherapy or a structured task group in occupational therapy (Cole & Greene, 1988). A six-item semantic differential scale was used to assess the patient's attitude toward the group, the group leaders, and other group members during the eight treatment sessions. The results indicated that both types of patients preferred the occupational therapy task group, rating it as more potent, active, and the group leader as more valuable, potent, and active. These results were significant at the .05 level. Clients with borderline personality viewed themselves more positively in terms of their participation (p < .01) in the psychotherapy group. As participation, attendance, and cohesiveness are important components of any group, it is necessary to know how patients perceive their treatment program.

A study by Eklund (1999) compared 20 patients who participated in a group-based psychosocial outpatient occupational therapy program (task and verbal groups) with a matched group that only received weekly individual verbal therapy. Pre-post comparisons for the occupational therapy group showed statistically significant improvement in relation to psychiatric symptoms (p <.001), global mental health (p <.001), and occupational functioning in the areas of volition (p <.001), habituation (p <.001), and communication and interpersonal skills (p <.005), but no improvement on quality of life measures. A between-group comparison found the occupational therapy group to show significant improvement on the *Global Assessment Scale* (p <.05), but not on the Strauss-Carpenter criteria of social contacts, psychiatric symptoms, hospitalizations and employment. Qualitative analysis of the standard interviews determined specific areas of improvement for 13 of the 20 clients in the treatment group. Generalization of the results will depend on further studies on the effectiveness of this program with other populations having psychosocial disorders.

Therapeutic Outcomes

A mime group activity was conducted daily over a 3-day period with 35 chronic adult patients with chronic psychosocial in a community-based day program (Probst & Howe, 1988). Pre- and postgroup measures included the *Goodenough Human Figure Drawing, Rosenberg Self-Esteem Scale*, and a movement concept scale developed for the study. Eighteen clients completed the study. The results indicated that only body image and proportionality in the Human Figure Drawing were affected significantly by the mime activity. No differences were found for body movement and communication skills. Three sessions may be too short a time for any real changes to occur in these areas.

A social skills training program using the cognitive-behavioral approach with a group of individuals with chronic mental illness (Salo-Chydenius, 1996) found on the *Group-Interaction Skills Survey* that patients had improved in both verbal and nonverbal communication skills. Self-evaluation forms completed before and after each session indicated that the patients also felt they had improved.

In another study, 37 clients of varying diagnoses with major anxiety symptoms participated in a 6-week anxiety management psychoeducational course over a 10-month period (Prior, 1998). The *Hospital Anxiety and Depression Scale* (HAD), the *Spielberger Questionnaire* (state and trait) and the *Fear Questionnaire*, were administered prior to, at the beginning, and at the end of the psychoeducational course, and at two months posttreatment. A cross-over design was used so that the clients on the waiting list for the psychoeducational course could form the control group. Clients showed a significant decrease in symptoms by the end of the psycho-educational course on the HAD scale (p <.05), and a reduction in symptoms on the state section of the *Spielberger Questionnaire*. Clients with the highest depression scores did not reduce their symptoms during the psychoeducational course and client's phobias were not treated by this psychoeducational course. A client satisfaction survey found that clients valued the psychoeducational course overall, liked the group approach, and preferred the cognitive session. No statistically significant changes were seen for the control group. Future research should exclude patients with severe depression and include more patients with severe anxiety in order to assess the effectiveness of this approach further.

Interpersonal problem-solving skills were developed in a group of individuals with a diagnosis of chronic schizophrenia using an occupational therapy intervention based on Siegel and Spivack's problem-solving therapy (Jao & Lu, 1999). When compared with a control group, the treatment group showed significant improvement on the *Means-Ends Problem-Solving Procedure* (p < .007). No statistically significant correlation was found between the acquisition of problem-solving skills and self-esteem. Gender differences were noted in relation to the self-esteem questionnaire; however, the sample size was very small (M5; F5). Future research needs to determine whether the length of the program was sufficient for these clients to be able to generalize their abilities to real social situations and whether the age of onset and chronicity of schizophrenia impeded the acquisition of problem-solving skills.

Nontraditional Populations

An innovative preventive occupational therapy program based on occupational science frame of reference was developed for the well elderly for a 9-month period (Jackson et al., 1998). A large-scale randomized effectiveness study found the program to be very successful in improving the mental and physical health, occupational functioning, and life-satisfaction of a multicultural group of community-dwelling elders (mean age 74.4 years) in comparison with a group receiving only social activities and an untreated group. Content areas such as the usefulness of occupations, aging and occupation, transportation, safety, social relationships, cultural awareness, and finances were covered. The program was delivered through lectures, discussions, direct experience, and personal exploration. Future research might consider replicating this occupational therapy program using populations such as the frail elderly or the middle-aged preretirement adult.

A biopsychosocial rehabilitation program was conducted (Martensson et al., 1999) in primary health care for 70 patients with chronic pain (myalgia, fibromyalgia, tension pain, low back pain, arthrosis, and radiating pain). A 6-week psychoeducational course, based on ego-strengthening psychotherapy, was led by an occupational therapist and a physical therapist. Themes were concerned with thoughts, knowledge and application through group discussions, ego-enhancing exercises, experiential activities, didactic presentations, relaxation training, and applied ergonomics. A *Visual Analogue Scale* (VAS) to measure pain intensity and the *Personality-Physical-Cognitive Questionnaire* (PPC) to assess the influence of the intervention and perceived change due to treatment was given prior to, immediately following, and between 6 and 48 months after treatment. Overall, the results were positive, as clients showed a significant increase in general well-being, ability to influence symptoms, demonstrated increased self-confidence, changed their habits of living, decreased their complaints, improved sleep habits, and reduced their fear of pain. No change in pain management ability was seen posttreatment; however, their ability to manage pain increased significantly at follow-up. The authors concluded that this was an effective, readily available, and cost-efficient intervention for this population.

These studies are encouraging as occupational therapists attempt to understand and determine what group formats and activities best match with specific patient populations. Recent emphasis on the value of qualitative research is extremely useful for observing and quantifying what actually transpires in the therapeutic group process in psychosocial occupational therapy.

CONCLUSION

In this chapter, the historical and current use of therapeutic groups in psychosocial occupational therapy have been reviewed. The purpose and various methodologies used in task, self-awareness, reality-oriented, developmental, behavioral, cognitive dysfunction, and more recently, integrative, direct, cognitive-behavioral, psychoeducational, and preventative groups were outlined. Factors relevant to the development of a group (e.g., group goals, structure of the group, contracts, patient selection, leadership styles, group methodology, selection of activities, and evaluation) of a group's effectiveness were presented. Where possible, research evidence for these practices was included.

The future for the use of the therapeutic group in psychosocial occupational therapy is promising. Indeed, we can see that many occupational therapists are now using frames of references in leading groups with various clients. With the availability of audiovisual and computer technology, we can anticipate an increase in research that will examine the occupational therapy group process more fully.

REFERENCES

Allen, C. (1985). *Occupational therapy for psychiatric diseases: Measurement and management of cognitive disabilities.* Boston: Little, Brown.

Azima, H., & Azima, F. (1959a). Outline of a dynamic theory of occupational therapy. *American Journal of Occupational Therapy, 13,* 215–221.

Azima, H., & Azima, F. (1959b). Projective group therapy. *International Journal of Group Psychotherapy, 9,* 176–183.

Baron, K. (1995). Kim: From running away to joining life. In G. Kielhofner (Ed.), *A model of human occupation: Theory and application* (2nd ed., pp. 305–314). Baltimore: Williams & Wilkins.

Barris, R., Kielhofner, G., & Watts, J. (1988). *Bodies of knowledge in psychosocial practice.* Thorofare, NJ: SLACK.

Battegay, R. (1974). Group psychotherapy as a method of treatment in a psychiatric hospital. In S. de Schill (Ed.), *The challenge for group psychotherapy* (pp. 173–230). New York: University Press.

Bednar, R., & Kaul, T. (1978). Experiential group research: Current perspectives. In S. Garfield & A. Bergin (Eds.), *Handbook of psychotherapy and behavior change* (2nd ed.; pp. 769–815). New York: John Wiley & Sons.

Bender, M., Waugh, M., & Orchard, C. (1997). Are you sure it is therapy your client needs and not education or training? *British Journal of Occupational Therapy, 60,* 23–25.

Berger, M. M. (1983). Use of the video in group psychotherapy. In H. Kaplan & B. Saddock (Eds.), *Comprehensive group psychotherapy* (2nd ed.; pp. 335–362). Baltimore: Williams & Wilkins.

Blair, A. (1975). P*rojective techniques: Their application within a group psychotherapy situation.* Proceedings of the 6th International Congress, World Federation of Occupational Therapists, Vancouver, B.C., Canada (pp. 365–379). Vancouver, BC: World Federation of Occupational Therapists.

Bloomer, J., & Williams, S. (1982). The Bay Area Functional Performance Evaluation (BaFPE). In B. J. Hemphill (Ed.), *The evaluative process in psychiatric occupational therapy* (pp. 255–308). Thorofare, NJ: SLACK.

Brayman, S., Kirby, T., Misenheimer, A., & Short, M. (1976). Comprehensive Occupational Therapy Evaluation Scale. *American Journal of Occupational Therapy, 30,* 94–100.

Breines, E. (1995). *Occupational therapy activities from clay to computers: Theory and practice.* Philadelphia: F. A. Davis.

Broekema, M., Danz, K., & Schloemer, C. (1975). Occupational therapy in a community after care program. *American Journal of Occupational Therapy, 29,* 22–27.

Bruce, M. A., & Borg, B. (1993). *Psychosocial occupational therapy: Frames of reference for intervention* (2nd ed.). Thorofare, NJ: SLACK.

Burns, R. (1982). Self-growth in families: Kinetic family drawings (K-F-D): *Research and application.* New York: Brunner/Mazel.

Campbell, J. (1993). *Creative art in groupwork.* Bicester, Oxon, UK: Winslow Press.

Cartwright, D., & Zander, A. (1968). *Group dynamics: Research and theory.* New York: Harper and Row.

Centoni, M., & Tallant, B. (1986). The projective use of drawings as a treatment technique with the depressed unemployed male. *Canadian Journal of Occupational Therapy, 53,* 81–87.

Cole, M. B. (1998). *Group dynamics in occupational therapy: The theoretical basis and practice application of group treatment* (2nd ed.), Thorofare, NJ: SLACK.

Cole, M., & Greene, L. (1988). A preference for activity: A comparative study of psychotherapy groups vs. occupational therapy groups for psychotic and borderline inpatients. *Occupational Therapy in Mental Health, 8*(3), 53–67.

Corey, G. (1985). *Theory and practice of group counseling* (2nd ed). Monterey, CA: Brooks/Cole.

Creek, J. (Ed.). (1990). *Occupational therapy and mental health: Principles, skills and practice.* Edinburgh: Churchill Livingstone.

Davis, S., & Keene, N. (1983). Making social skills work with outpatients. *Occupational Therapy, 46,* 257–259.

Donohue, M. V. (1999). Theoretical bases of Mosey's group interaction skills. *Occupational Therapy International, 6,* 35–51.

Drake, M. (1999). *Crafts: Therapy and rehabilitation* (2nd ed.). Thorofare, NJ: SLACK.

Drouet, V. (1986). Individual behavioural programme planning with long-stay schizophrenic patients. Part 2: Social skills training. *Occupational Therapy, 49,* 229–231.

Duncombe, L., & Howe, M. (1985). Group work in occupational therapy: A survey of practice. *American Journal of Occupational Therapy, 39,* 163–170.

Duncombe, L., & Howe, M. (1995). Group treatment: Goals, tasks, and economic implications. *American Journal of Occupational Therapy, 49,* 199–205.

Dynes, R. (1990). *Creative games in groupwork.* Bicester, Oxon, UK: Winslow Press.

Earhart, C. (1985). Occupational therapy groups. In C. Allen (Ed.), *Occupational therapy for psychiatric diseases: Measurement and management of cognitive disabilities* (pp. 235–264). Boston: Little, Brown.

Eklund, M. (1999). Outcome of occupational therapy in a psychiatric day care unit for long-term mentally ill patients. *Occupational Therapy in Mental Health, 14*(4), 21–45.

Fairburn, C. & Fairburn, S. (1979). Relaxation training in psychiatric admission units. *Occupational Therapy, 42,* 280–282.

Falk-Kessler, J., & Froschauer, K. (1978). The soap opera: A dynamic group approach for psychiatric patients. *American Journal of Occupational Therapy, 32,* 317–319.

Fidler, G. (1969). The task-oriented group as a context for treatment. *American Journal of Occupational Therapy, 23,* 43–48.

Fidler, G., & Fidler, J. (1954). *Introduction to psychiatric occupational therapy.* New York: Macmillan.

Fidler, G., & Fidler, J. (1963). *A communication process in psychiatry-occupational therapy.* New York: Macmillan.

Finlay, L. (1993). *Groupwork in occupational therapy.* London: Chapman & Hall.

Forsyth, K., Lai, J-S., & Kielhofner, G. (1999). The Assessment of Communication and Interaction Skills (ACIS): Measurement properties. *British Journal of Occupational Therapy, 62,* 69–74.

Furner, L. (1978). Work training groups. *Occupational Therapy, 41,* 232–233.

Furst, G., & Stabenow, C. (1995). Sally: Choosing and organizing life occupations. In G. Kielhofner (Ed.), *A model of human occupation: Theory and application* (2nd ed., pp. 333–341). Baltimore: Williams and Wilkins.

German, S. (1964). A group approach to rehabilitation occupational therapy in a psychiatric setting. *American Journal of Occupational Therapy, 18,* 209–214.

Gracegirdle, H. (1982). A group for depressed mothers and their children. *Occupational Therapy, 45,* 20–21.

Gregory, S. (1996). Memory maintenance groups in the community. *British Journal of Occupational Therapy, 59,* 25–26.

Haertlein, C., & Bloggett, M. (1994). Self-care strategies in intervention for psychosocial considerations. In. C. Christiansen (Ed.), *Ways of living: Self-care strategies for special needs* (pp. 357–377). Rockville, MD: American Occupational Therapy Association.

Harlowe, D. & Yu, P. (1997). *The ROM dance: A range of motion exercise and relaxation program* (2nd ed.). Madison, WI: Uncharted Country Publishing.

Harrison, T., & Precin, P. (1996). Cognitive impairments in clients with dual diagnosis (chronic psychotic disorders and substance abuse): Considerations for treatment. *Occupational Therapy International, 3,* 122–141.

Held, G. (1993). Recovery after damage. In H. Cohen (Ed.), *Neuroscience for rehabilitation* (pp. 388–405). Philadelphia: J. B. Lippincott.

Hewitt, K., Wishart, C., & Lambert, R. (1981). Social skills training with chronic psychiatric patients. *Occupational Therapy, 44,* 284–285.

Holm, M. (1983). Video as a medium in occupational therapy. *American Journal of Occupational Therapy, 37,* 531–534.

Houston, D., Williams, S. L., Bloomer, J., & Mann, W. D. (1989). The Bay Area Functional Performance Evaluation: Development and standardization (BaFPE). *American Journal of Occupational Therapy, 43,* 170–182.

Howe, M., & Schwartzberg, S. (1986). *A functional approach to group work in occupational therapy.* Philadelphia: J. B. Lippincott.

Howe, M., & Schwartzberg, S. (1995). *A functional approach to group work in occupational therapy* (2nd ed.). Philadelphia: J. B. Lippincott.

Jackson, J., Carlson, M., Mandel, D., Zemke, R., & Clark, F. (1998). Occupation in lifestyle redesign: The Well Elderly Study Occupational Therapy Program. *The American Journal of Occupational Therapy, 52,* 326–336.

Jao, H-P., & Lu, S-J. (1999). The acquisition of problem-solving skills through the instruction in Siegel and Spivack's problem-solving therapy for the chronic schizophrenic. *Occupational Therapy in Mental Health, 14*(4), 47–61.

Jennings, S. (1986). *Creative drama in groupwork.* Bicester, Oxon, UK: Winslow Press.

Jones, M. (1953). *The therapeutic community: A new treatment method in psychiatry*. New York: Basic Books.

Kaplan, H., Sadock, B., & Grebb, J. (1994). *Kaplan and Sadock's synopsis of psychiatry behavioral sciences/clinical psychiatry* (7th ed.). Philadelphia: Williams & Wilkins.

Kaplan, K. (1988). *Directive group therapy: Innovative mental health treatment*. Thorofare, NJ: SLACK.

Kaye, J., Mackie, V., & Hitzing, E. (1970). Contingency management in a workshop setting: Innovation in occupational therapy. *American Journal of Occupational Therapy, 34*, 572–581.

Kielhofner, G. (1980). A model of human occupation. Part 1: Conceptual framework and content. *American Journal of Occupational Therapy, 34*, 572–581.

Kielhofner, G. (Ed.). (1985). *A model of human occupation: Theory and application*. Baltimore: Williams & Wilkins.

Kielhofner, G. (1992). *Conceptual foundations of occupational therapy*. Philadelphia: F. A. Davis.

Kielhofner, G. (1995). *A model of human occupation: Theory and application* (2nd ed.) Baltimore: Williams & Wilkins.

Laliberte-Rudman, D., Yu, B., Scott, E., & Pajouhandeh, P. (2000). Exploration of the perspectives of persons with schizophrenia regarding quality of life. *American Journal of Occupational Therapy, 54*, 137–147.

Law, M., Baptiste, S., Carswell, A., McColl, M. A., Polatajko, H., & Pollock, N. (1994). *Canadian Occupational Performance Measure* (COPM; 2nd ed). Toronto, Ontario: CAOT Publications ACE.

Leary, S. (1994). *Activities for personal growth: A comprehensive handbook of activities for therapists*. Sydney: MacLennan & Petty.

Lindsay, W. (1983). The role of the occupational therapist in the treatment of alcoholism. *American Journal of Occupational Therapy, 37*, 36–43.

Lloyd, C., Bassett, J., & Samra, P. (2000). Rehabilitation programmes for early psychosis. *British Journal of Occupational Therapy, 63*, 76–82.

Lloyd, C., & Chandler, L. (1999). Girrebala and the arts in mental health rehabilitation. *British Journal of Therapy and Rehabilitation, 6*, 164–170.

Luboshitzky, D. & Gaber, L. (2000). Collaborative therapeutic homework model in occupational therapy. *Occupational Therapy in Mental Health, 15*(1), 43–60.

Margolis, R., Harrison, S., Robinson, H., & Jayaram, G. (1996). Occupational Therapy Task Observation Scale (OTTOS)®: A rapid method for rating task group function of psychiatric patients. *American Journal of Occupational Therapy, 50*, 380–385.

Martensson, L., Marklund, B., & Fridlund, B. (1999). Evaluation of a biopsychosocial rehabilitation programme in primary healthcare for chronic pain patients. *Scandinavian Journal of Occupational Therapy, 6*, 157–165.

McDermott, A. (1988). The effect of three group formats on group interaction patterns. *Occupational Therapy in Mental Health, 8*(3), 69–89.

Monroe, C., & Herron, S. (1980). Projective art used as an integral part of an intensive group therapy experience. *Occupational Therapy, 43*, 21–24.

Mosey, A. (1970). *Three frames of references for mental health*. Thorofare, NJ: SLACK.

Mosey, A. (1973). *Activities therapy*. New York: Raven Press.

Mosey, A. (1986). *Psychosocial components of occupational therapy*. New York: Raven Press.

Overbaugh, T., & Bucher, B. (1970). Use of operant conditioning to improve behavior of a severely deteriorated psychotic. *American Journal of Occupational Therapy, 24*, 423–427.

Parlato, L., Lloyd, C., & Bassett, J. (1999). Young Occupations Unlimited: An early intervention programme for young people with psychosis. *British Journal of Occupational Therapy, 62*, 113–116.

Pezzuti, L. (1979). An exploration of adolescent feminine and occupational behavior development. *American Journal of Occupational Therapy, 33*, 84–91.

Posthuma, B. (1989). *Small groups in therapy settings: Process and leadership*. Boston: College-Hill Press.

Posthuma, B. (1996). *Small groups in counseling and therapy* (2nd ed.). Needham Heights, MD: Allyn & Bacon.

Prior, S. (1998). Determining the effectiveness of a short-term anxiety management course. *British Journal of Occupational Therapy, 61*, 207–213.

Probst, D., & Howe, M. (1988). The effect of a mime group on chronic adult psychiatric clients' body-image, self-esteem, and movement-concept. *Occupational Therapy in Mental Health, 8*(3), 135–153.

Reilly, M. (1974). *Play as exploratory learning.* Beverly Hills, CA: Sage.

Reed, K., & Cunningham, S. (1997). *Internet guide for rehabilitation professionals.* New York: Lippincott-Raven Publishers.

Remocker, A., & Sherwood, E. T. (1998). *Action speaks louder: A handbook of nonverbal group techniques* (6th ed.). London: Churchill Livingstone.

Rider, B. & Gramblin, T. (1987). *The activity card file.* [Available from Barbara Rider, Occupational Therapy Department, Western Michigan University, Kalamazoo, MI, 49004.]

Ross, M. (1991). *Integrative group therapy: The structured five-stage approach* (2nd ed.). Thorofare, NJ: SLACK.

Ross, M. (1997). *Integrative group therapy: Mobilizing coping abilities with the five stage group.* Baltimore: American Occupational Therapy Association.

Sacks, J. M. (1983). Psychodrama. In H. Kaplan & B. Saddock (Eds.), *Comprehensive group psychotherapy* (2nd ed.; pp. 214–228). Baltimore: Williams & Wilkins.

Salo-Chydenius, S. (1996). Changing helplessness to coping: An exploratory study of social skills training with individuals with long-term illness. *Occupational Therapy International, 3,* 174–189.

Schell, D., & Giles, G. (1985). Behaviour modification with disturbed adolescents: The role of the occupational therapist. *Occupational Therapy, 48,* 172–178.

Simmons, I., & Mullins, L. (1981). *Acute psychiatric care: An occupational therapy guide to exercises in daily living skills.* Thorofare, NJ: SLACK.

Solberg, N., & Chueh, W. (1976). Performance in occupational theapy as a predictor of successful prevocational training. *American Journal of Occupational Therapy, 30,* 481–486.

Stein, F., & Brintnell, E. S. (1986). *Survey of thirty-four occupational therapy programs located in psychiatric facilities in Wisconsin, Alberta and Quebec.* Unpublished study.

Stein, F., & Tallant, B. (1988a). Applying the group process to psychiatric occupational therapy. Part 1: Historical and current use. *Occupational Therapy in Mental Health, 8*(3), 9–28.

Stein, F., & Tallant, B. (1988b). Applying the group process to psychiatric occupational therapy. Part 2: A model for a therapeutic group in psychiatric occupational therapy. *Occupational Therapy in Mental Health, 8*(3), 29–51.

Sullivan, L. (1995). Mike: Making a successful occupational choice for transition to the worker role. In G. Kielhofner (Ed.), *A model of human occupation: Theory and application* (2nd ed., pp. 314–323). Baltimore: Williams & Wilkins.

Sunderland, M., & Engleheart, P. (1993) *Draw on your emotions: Creative ways to explore, express and understand important feelings.* Bicester, Oxon, UK: Winslow Press.

Temple, S., & Robson, P. (1991). The effect of assertiveness training on self-esteem. *British Journal of Occupational Therapy, 54,* 329–332.

Thomes, L., & Bajema, S. (1983). The Life Skills Development Program: A history, overview and update. *Occupational Therapy in Mental Health, 3*(2), 35–48.

Thompson, M., & Blair, S. (1998). Creative arts in occupational therapy: Ancient history or contemporary practice? *Occupational Therapy International, 5,* 49–65.

Trace, S., & Howell, T. (1991). Occupational therapy in geriatric mental health. *The American Journal of Occupational Therapy, 45*(9), 833–838.

Watson, M., & Thomes, L. (1983). Project ABLE: A model for management of stress in the army soldier. *Occupational Therapy in Mental Health, 3*(2), 55–61.

White, R., & Lippitt, R. (1968). Leader behavior and member reaction in three "social climates." In D. Cartwright & A. Zander (Eds.), *Group dynamics research and theory* (3rd ed., pp. 318–335). New York: Harper and Row.

Williams, S., & Bloomer, J. (1987). *Bay Area Functional Performance Evaluation* (BaFPE 2nd ed.). Novato, CA: Consulting Psychologists Press.

Willson, M. (1987). *Occupational therapy in long-term psychiatry* (2nd ed.). London: Churchill Livingstone.

Willson, M. (1988). *Occupational therapy in short-term psychiatry* (2nd ed.). London: Churchill Livingstone.

Wright, J., Thase, M., Ludgate, J., & Beck, A. (1993). The cognitive milieu: Structure and process. In J. Wright, M. Thase, & A. Beck (Eds.), *Cognitive therapy with inpatients* (pp. 61–87). New York: The Guilford Press.

Yakobina, S., Yakobina, S., & Tallant, B. (1997). I came, I thought, I conquered: Cognitive behavior approach applied in occupational therapy for the treatment of depressed (dysthymic) females. *Occupational Therapy in Mental Health, 13,* 59–73.

Yalom, I. (1995). *The theory and practice of group psychotherapy* (4th ed.). New York: Basic Books.

CHAPTER

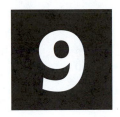

Vocational Exploration and Employment and Psychosocial Disabilities

Joyce Tryssenaar, M.Ed., O.T. (C)

> *Employment is nature's best physician and is essential to human happiness.*
>
> — Galen, 172 A.D.
>
> *Having a job is of exceptional importance in our society. Our public identity is drawn directly from what we do—our occupation. Some occupations are more highly valued than others, but few areas of social status seem so distasteful to our success oriented society as unemployment. Since most individuals are interested in social acceptance and approval and since self-esteem is directly related to visible achievement and accomplishment, unemployment can be a devastating condition for any individual. For people already struggling with the social stigma and self-image problems brought on by mental illness, it is especially undesirable.*
>
> — J. F. Campbell (1989), *Employment Programs for People with a Psychiatric Disability: An Overview, Community Support Network News*, 6(2), 1.

Operational Learning Objectives

By the end of this chapter, the learner will:

1. Identify similarities and differences between theories of career development.

2. Define principles of work and rehabilitation.

3. Discuss a range of conceptual models which are or have been used with persons with psychiatric disabilities.

4. Explore service delivery models of vocational rehabilitation in light of the consumer movement.

5. Define a variety of work programs and work preparation activities available for persons with psychiatric disabilities.

6. Describe role of balance and the impact of a serious mental illness in developing work awareness.

7. Analyze personal and environmental components integral to effective vocational rehabilitation.

8. Identify a variety of assessment tools and strategies.

9. Develop an understanding of advocacy and reasonable accommodation.

10. Consider effective vocational rehabilitation programs and the role of the occupational therapist.

The ability to love and to work has been considered as evidence of mental health since the time of Freud (1953). By the same token, occupational therapy philosophy suggests that people have an occupational nature and for their survival and well-being they require participation in work, play, and daily living tasks; and that engaging persons in meaningful occupations is beneficial to their health (American Occupational Therapy Association [AOTA], 1994; Canadian Association of Occupational Therapists [CAOT], 1997). The entire spectrum of daily occupations related to productivity is within the domain of occupational therapy practice.

There is often a surprising gap between occupational therapy programs and vocational rehabilitation and mental health services. Each profession appears to be working in isolation with little crossover between them (Rabin & Jeong, 1991). Barker (1994) remarks that many mental health professionals see employment at best as a therapeutic tool, at worst as a cause of stress, and not as a goal for most clients. The gap between the medical professions and vocational rehabilitation is counterproductive as there is evidence that effective vocational programs are those which are integrated among service areas (Lang & Cara, 1989; Drake, 1998).

Consumers consistently identify employment as having paramount importance in their ability to live normal and healthy lives (Bailey, 1998; Capponi, 1997; Deegan, 1988). This is not surprising given the value contemporary society places on productivity. Employment is related to improved health and well-being, whereas unemployment increases the risk of physical and mental health problems (Ekdawi & Conning, 1994). Furthermore, for persons with mental illness, work has a stabilizing effect and reduces the chance of relapse (Lloyd, 1995). People with serious mental illness need and want to make their own vocational choices and this necessitates ownership of the process of vocational rehabilitation. Positive vocational outcomes may be a result of the degree to which consumers, significant others, employers, and health/social service providers have an enthusiastic partnership in the process.

The concepts of *productivity*, *work*, and *employment* are all used in the occupational therapy literature. AOTA (1994) defines *work and productive activities* as, "purposeful activities for self-development, social contribution, and livelihood" (p. 1052). Vocational activities, a subset of this section, include vocational exploration, job acquisition, work or job performance, retirement planning, and volunteer participation (AOTA, 1994). CAOT (1997) broadly defines *productivity* as, "occupations that make a social or economic contribution, or that provide economic sustenance. Examples include play in infancy and childhood, school work, employment, homemaking, parenting, and community volunteering" (p. 37). Jacobs (1991) states that *work* "includes all forms of productive activity regardless of whether they are reimbursed" (p. 17). Morgan (1993) suggests that *employment* "is used more narrowly to refer specifically to work activity, but may include sheltered or voluntary work" (p. 166). Perhaps the process of occupational therapy involvement in vocational rehabilitation is directed toward employment, whereas the outcome may be in the broad area of productivity.

This chapter describes the theoretical foundations of vocational rehabilitation with persons with psychiatric disabilities. Principles of work and rehabilitation guide intervention as do practice models. The rise of the consumer movement and the influence of client-centered practice have also had an impact on the development of vocational rehabilitation services. Within these broad parameters, occupational therapy has a unique contribution to make based on knowledge of a balance of work, rest, and play; an understanding of the person/environment/occupation fit; the ability to analyze task and job requirements; and awareness of skills and support needs of all key stakeholders.

THEORIES OF CAREER DEVELOPMENT

How do we choose our careers? What are the variables that might be part of making a suitable or realistic vocational choice? What theory will best explain the vocational choice process? France (1985) suggested that theories come in and out of fashion, and many assumptions behind the different theories are tentative and only partly research based. The following major theories related to career development as reviewed by France, are briefly summarized:

▶ *The Trait-Factor Career Theory*: The matching of people to jobs is the main tenet of this theory. It assumes people differ in development and growth and therefore job opportunities must be matched with interests and abilities. Interest and aptitude testing are an essential component of this concept.

▶ *Developmental Theories*: Career choices follow certain age-specific developmental stages, beginning with fantasy where anything is possible, then becoming more tentative as some choices are discarded, and finally reaching the realistic stage where career choices are based on compromises among job requirements, skills, and values. Although the person has a measure of control and choice, the environment plays a significant role.

▶ *Psychoanalytical Theories*: These theories emphasize "internal" factors related to early life experiences as primary in career choice while minimizing external factors. Work gratifies childhood needs.

▶ *Sociological Theories*: Economic and social factors have a significant impact on work life stages. These theories suggest work choice is related to socioeconomic status and family life conditions. However, it can also be influenced by personality development and availability of job opportunities.

▶ *Decision-Making Theories*: Work choices are based on personal values. Decisions are driven by information, or knowledge, and desired results about work choices.

▶ *Need Theories*: People choose the occupations that they believe will best meet their needs. Personality as well shapes career behaviors initially; later, the career itself impacts on personality. Job satisfaction is a result of how closely the job meets the individual's needs.

All theories identify the complexity of vocational choices; they recognize the influence of the environment, and the individual's wishes, needs, and values. The idea of development and change over time is inherent to all theories. Occupational choice is not a singular event but a process. It is often related to life experiences, maturity issues, and self-concept (France, 1985) and therefore can be significantly influenced by the functional sequelae of mental illness.

PRINCIPLES OF WORK AND REHABILITATION

Mental health professionals should not expect more of individuals with mental illness than they do of themselves. If professionals in this field permit themselves the flexibility to alter their aspirations and change jobs, to have some days that are less "productive" than others, and to view employment as but one of several areas of accomplishment, they must do no less for those who suffer from mental illnesses (Bachrach, 1991).

Mental illness can have a serious impact on occupational performance, particularly in the area of productivity. Until recently, this meant persons with mental illness were seen as marginally employable or unemployable and this was reflected in extremely low employment rates. Baron (1995) states that the 85 percent unemployment rate for persons with mental illness still remains valid.

In the past decade much more emphasis has been placed on helping people return to work or enhance their productivity. Psychosocial rehabilitation principles identify work and vocational rehabilitation as central to the rehabilitation process. Because of its integrating and regenerative effect on clients, work is considered the main focus of the rehabilitation process. The emphasis on employment directs clients to constructive activities so that they can take their roles in society and attain income gains, status, and self-esteem (Cnaan, Blankertz, Messinger, & Gardner, 1990). Bachrach (1991) suggested using the following principles to guide practice for effective vocational rehabilitation for persons with mental illness.

▶ *Access to Treatment Concomitantly with Rehabilitation*: Work opportunities for the individuals with chronic mental illness must not be pursued in a vacuum. Services for nonwork needs must also be provided.

▶ *Diversity*: There is a need for an adequate array of vocational options for individuals with mental illness, who, like other people, possess a variety of skills, wishes, and talents.

▶ *Support and Back-up*: Finding ways to adjust to the realities of the illness is an essential part of vocational rehabilitation. Ongoing support by peers, family, and mental health workers is necessary.

▶ *Realistic Expectations*: We should not expect either too much or too little of the patients. A variety of opportunities ranging from leisure activities to competitive employment should be available.

▶ *Adequate Compensation*: Pay is important to everyone. We need to facilitate ease of movement between competitive work earnings and the social security system for individuals with disabilities.

▶ *Economic and Political Awareness*: The success of vocational interventions depends to some extent on external economic and political conditions that cannot be controlled. These circumstances must be acknowledged.

The 1990s are distinguished by the Americans with Disabilities Act (ADA, 1990) and its guarantee of the employment rights of people with disabilities. The role of the rehabilitation professional has expanded to not only serve persons with disabilities but to provide assistance directly to employers to hire persons with disabilities (Mullins, Rumrill, & Roessler, 1996). Furthermore, the employment plight of those with mental illness, coupled with the demands of the ADA and its accompanying regulations, provides weight behind an effort to do better in response to the employment needs of persons with mental illness (Akabas,1994). When occupational therapists are thoroughly acquainted with the power and conditions of the law, they will be able to invoke it where appropriate, propose reasonable accommodations, and challenge employers who appear reluctant to comply with the law on behalf of clients.

The 21st century will be influenced by federal disability policy, The *Ticket-to-Work and Work Incentives Improvement Act of 1999*, which reduces barriers to work for people with disabilities. The act gives people with disabilities, including mental illnesses, the opportunity to move into employment and reduce their dependency on benefits and other assistance. The Ticket-to-Work provision modernizes the employment services system by supporting persons on SSI or SSDI to go to any public or private provider for job-related support services. The legislation also enhances health care coverage for beneficiaries and eliminates some disincentives to work. The Ticket-to-Work program starts in 2001 and will be phased in over 3 years.

WORK AS TREATMENT

Work has been identified not just as an outcome of effective intervention, but as an intervention itself in the course of mental illness. Strauss, Harding, Silverman, Eichler, and Lieberman (1988) identified nine treatment models that include or exclude work as a treatment activity for persons with mental illness. The first five models either exclude or minimally include the role of work as a treatment modality.

▶ *Natural History Model:* Few factors other than the disease itself have an impact on the natural history of the disorder and work is seen as irrelevant to treatment.

▶ *Diathesis-Stress Model*: There is a biological vulnerability for a disease that is affected by stress. The disease can be triggered by a environmental stressor. Work may or may not be a stressor depending on the individual's vulnerability.

▶ *Stimulus Window Model*: Illness restricts stimulation above or below a certain point. Some kinds of work might be helpful depending on the individual's "window."

▶ *Deficit Model*: The individual has a basic defect or lacks some capacity. Work would not change the disorder but reasonable accommodation might allow the client to work. This model is similar to the Cognitive Disabilities Model described by Allen (1985). She suggests persons with serious mental illness are not able to change their level of cognition. Therefore, treatment by the occupational therapist is primarily directed toward modifying the person's environment.

▶ *Conflict Model*: The meaning of the work situation could generate conflict for the person, for example, a fear of success. The kind of work chosen may need to avoid conflict issues.

▶ *Social Learning Model*: Work success provides rewards for competent behavior or work failure is punishment for incompetent behavior. Rewards from successful work behavior may counteract any secondary "rewards" from psychiatric symptoms.

▶ *Psychiatric Rehabilitation Model*: The illness is an entity that may result in disability and/or handicap. Clients learn skills and use supports to be successful and satisfied in the work environment.

▶ *Person-Environment Fit Model*: Optimal functioning is determined by interactions between the person and the environment and the specific characteristics of both can be defined in ways that allow for optimal "fit."

▶ *Interactive-Developmental Model*: The main focus of this model is on the interactions between the person, illness, and environment. Changes in any component impact on all other components.

Strauss et al. (1988) recommend that the clinical, rehabilitation, and industrial psychology arenas need to be integrated to improve work as a treatment in psychiatric disorders.

An extension of the person-environment fit model to include occupation has been developed by Law et al. (1996). The *Person/ Environment/Occupation Model* is a dynamic clinical practice model that employs a transactive approach, rather than a static approach, to the interactions among person, environment, and occupation. Each component influences the others and changes throughout the lifespan. The outcome of occupational performance can be clearly identified as the fit between person, environment, and occupation.

SERVICE DELIVERY

How do theories, principles, and conceptual models become operationalized? The consumer movement has resulted in significant expansion of vocational approaches and options. Work is now seen as everyone's right rather than something only aspired to by those who are least ill. Nevertheless this concept is still not applied universally, and concerns regarding "creaming" the population by exclusionary programs continue to be raised (West & Parent, 1995). The consumer's voice emphasizes real jobs for real money (Consumer/Survivor Business Council of Ontario, 1995) and states that how work/rehabilitation occurs is as important as why it occurs. Chamberlin (1978), a consumer activist, suggested the following service delivery paradigms:

▶ *Traditional Treatment*: Professionals provide vocational rehabilitation and clients receive it.

▶ *Partnership*: Professionals and nonprofessionals work together to provide services. The recipients are told that they, too, are partners in the service. However, the distinction between those who give help and those who receive it remains clearly defined.

▶ *Supportive*: Membership is open to all people who want to use the service. Everyone is equal and capable of helping each other. Professionals are excluded from this model, except in external roles, because they use a different model of helping, which separates those who give from those who receive help.

▶ *Separatist*: Ex-patients provide the support and run the service. Nonpatients and professionals are excluded from the service.

In current vocational rehabilitation practice there is a range and variety of vocational programs based on different service delivery approaches, philosophies, and principles.

VOCATIONAL OUTCOMES

Volunteer Work

A person with mental illness may work in the volunteer sector. Some advantages of this type of productivity are that the client can choose the hours and types of activity. Volunteering also provides an avenue to be altruistic and contribute to society. However, clients do not have any increase in income and may incur added expenses such as transportation and clothing. Woodside (1995), an occupational therapist, has developed, in collaboration with consumers and volunteer agencies, an educational pamphlet for agencies that outlines steps to successful, effective volunteer placements for persons with schizophrenia. These steps include (a) taking time to match the person to the volunteer job, (b) educating the volunteer agency about schizophrenia, (c) supporting the person with schizophrenia as a volunteer, and (d) making accommodations at the volunteer site. Many volunteer agencies have programs for persons with special needs. Volunteering can result in positive effects on self-perception, sense of identity, personal development, and quality of life for both volunteers with serious mental illness and the clients they serve (Armstrong, Korba, & Emard, 1995; Woodside & Luis, 1997).

Sheltered Work

Sheltered workshops typically solicit factory contract work that is carried out in a protected environment. Sheltered employment is usually part of an institution or work-training site. Yip

and Ng (1999) state sheltered workshops are a way to provide meaningful occupation for persons with serious mental illnesses who are not able to enter competitive employment and the controlled environment accommodates the limitations of their mental illness. Traditional hospital-based sheltered workshops have been criticized for inadequate remuneration and for creating dependency (Trainor & Tremblay, 1991). Furthermore, the use of menial tasks leaves no opportunity to develop capacities, self-esteem, and job skills directly applicable for client's participation in the labor force (Hartl, 1992). Although there is little evidence that this type of employment results in more normalized work experiences, Black (1992) has voiced concern with the shift to supported employment and suggested that we may yet find sheltered work is necessary for many persons with serious mental illness.

Cooperatives

A cooperative is an organization run by consumers that develops contracts for a variety of tasks, such as maintenance, gardening, or courier service, requiring both skilled and unskilled labor. Individual clients can work and receive wages when they are able to participate in the contract, and the contracts can be maintained because there is a group/pool of employees. A modification of this type of program was described by Lang and Cara (1989). Occupational therapists helped develop a model for all clients based on the existing structure of the mental health system in San Francisco, the need to employ clients, and the functional levels of the clients in the system. This nonprofit organization, Community Vocational Enterprises (CVE), develops and maintains contracts with employers that are completed by clients in day treatment programs. CVE also acquires contracts for mobile work crews and work enclaves with a range of support and supervision available.

Affirmative Businesses/Social Firms

An affirmative business is a consumer-driven business working in partnership with service providers and community and business representatives. Affirmative businesses redefine the relationship of the individual to the employment setting as a consequence of the enterprise being run and often owned by former psychiatric clients. They provide opportunities for flexible employment in a realistic work environment. These businesses represent not only a change in the client's physical environment by being community based, but also in the social/interpersonal environment with adjustments in expectations and requirements of consumer/provider roles. Their nature is complimentary to rehabilitation values and beliefs in using a client-centered empowering approach with a meaningful activity focus. Affirmative businesses represent an environmental intervention with the potential to make a significant difference in clients' occupational performance. However, their effectiveness is difficult to determine given the many different compositions of affirmative businesses. Kremer's (1991) preliminary report described many organizational and developmental pitfalls encountered by six Ohio consumer-operated services/businesses, yet he concluded that persons diagnosed with mental illness can operate their own services if given the opportunity and funding. Descriptions of consumer-run businesses by Mowbray, Chamberlain, Jennings, and Reed (1988) reported high turnovers ascribed to interpersonal demands on consumer staff that exceeded their capacity. However, the results reported in a retrospective survey conducted on five Ontario programs indicated that involvement in affirmative businesses significantly reduced use of formal mental health services, as reflected in number of admissions to hospital, inpatient days, and contacts with crisis services (Trainor & Tremblay, 1991). Kakutani (1998) describes a consumer-run coffee shop business that has made a significant difference in the lives of the participating consumers.

Home Employment

An in-home employment program is a cottage industry that employs people working in their own homes, at their own pace. Participants are paid at a piece work rate. Kates, Nikalaou, Baillie, and Hess (1997) found that persons involved in a home employment program demonstrated significant improvement in self-esteem, and that participation in the program increased the likelihood of further involvement in other work programs. This program was developed to meet the needs of people with mental illness who were no longer seen as candidates for existing local vocational programs. Work tasks are brought to the individuals' homes and completed at their own rate. Every 2 weeks new material is supplied, completed tasks are picked up, and clients are paid. It is a flexible program that may be easily adaptable to different locations, and can be run in a cost-efficient manner. The occupational therapist affiliated with the program develops personalized vocational goals with each client through an initial assessment conducted in the client's home. Ongoing review of the individual's work goals and linking the client with community resources are also included in the occupational therapist's role.

Jacobs' (1991) description of home employment included any paid competitive work done at home. She suggested that technology has significantly expanded the number of persons who can work at home and that this type of employment now allows persons with disabilities who cannot leave home to do meaningful, productive work from their homes. Although few occupational therapists are involved in home employment programs in the United States, the skill and knowledge base of occupational therapy makes it a natural fit. Therapists can assess both the environment and worker skills, develop suitable supports and thereby improve the quality of the person's life (Breen, Clark, & Moran, 1991).

Transitional Employment

Transitional employment (TE) was developed through the clubhouse movement. The clubhouse model of psychiatric rehabilitation argues that work is the medium out of which relationships are created and through which, in mutually dependent tasks, members gain self-respect and respect for the work of others (Jackson, 1992). A work-ordered day encourages the development of prevocational and vocational skills related to specific clubhouse activity units. Clubhouse members are then able to move to similar community-based entry-level positions for a time limited period. TE is seen as nonpermanent and a stepping stone to permanent employability. The sponsoring agency develops the placement and trains and orients clients. They also guarantee replacement workers if clients are absent. Dulay and Steichen (1982) described the development and implementation of a TE program by an occupational therapist. Three key elements of the program are job development with the business community, developing criteria for involvement in the TE, and linking the TE workers with ongoing support. The occupational therapist completes a task analysis of each developed job site and an assessment of each worker to find the best person for the job.

Supported Employment (SE)

This option is currently very popular in the psychosocial rehabilitation field. The philosophy of SE is that all people can do meaningful work in normal work environments if they wish and if they have the necessary supports. The goal of SE is permanent competitive employment. There is minimal screening for employability and prevocational training is avoided. Training occurs after individualized job placement and is driven by client choice. Job coaches provide support indefinitely to the client and/or employer. Bond, Drake, Mueser, and Becker (1997) suggested the following principles of SE: (a) clients need direct assistance in finding and keeping jobs because general approaches do not lead to vocational outcomes that clients want; (b) the integration of vocational and clinical approaches is more effective than brokered approaches; (c) clients who obtain jobs in their preferred area retain their jobs twice as long as those who do not; and (d) there is a need for long-term support, especially in the area of social skills training. Research shows 58 percent of clients achieved competitive employment with accelerated placement into supported jobs compared to 21 percent of clients with prevocational training (Bond et al., 1997).

Casual Employment

Clients apply and register with a temporary labor agency or engage in intermittent employment such as delivering flyers, picking fruit, or seasonal rush jobs. This provides them with additional income and allows them to make short-term work commitments when they are well. Day labor is one of the most frequent forms of employment of men who are homeless, although the majority of these men indicate a preference for other types of employment (Balkin, 1992).

Self-Employment

Becoming an entrepreneur is described by many consumers as an employment option. It has advantages similar to home employment and allows for self-regulating of time and energy by the entrepreneur. The Canadian Mental Health Association (CMHA, 1996) developed a brochure, as part of the Access to Real Work campaign, with resources and guidelines to entrepreneurship for consumer/survivors.

Part-Time Competitive Employment

This work option is often chosen because of economic restrictions and potential loss of disability pension. It allows a person to work up to the maximum allowable hours of their disability pension without being penalized. Some clients find it less stressful than full-time employment. Buckley (1981) described the development of a partial employment program for persons with serious mental illness that not only resulted in maintaining people in the community but facilitated their social integration.

Full-Time Competitive Employment

People choosing this option are capable and willing to work in full-time work situations. They can do this at home in some instances (see "Home Employment") or at the job site. This work option is less likely to be considered by many persons with serious mental illness because of concerns related to the episodic nature of the illness. However, Evans (1997) has argued that it is often

the mental health professionals who implicitly suggest that even motivated consumers will fail at working full-time by advising a gradual entry into work. She noted that persons who are interested in full-time employment need optimum support, encouragement, and resources to reach their full potential.

WORK PREPARATION AND SUPPORT OPTIONS

Vocational Assessment Tools

There are many standardized and unstandardized methods of vocational assessment. These can focus on work choices, behaviors, skills, and competencies. Some common tools are described.

▶ *Interest Inventories*: These tests can be pictorial (e.g., *Wide Range Interest and Opinion Test* [WRIOT; Jastak & Jastak, 1979]) or written (e.g., *Ashland Interest Inventory*; Jackson & Marshall, 1997). They typically contain a list of questions or a set of drawings/pictures pertaining to work activities. Individuals select the activities in which they are most interested or those in which they are least interested or a combination of both. These inventories provide information about a client's likes and dislikes.

▶ *Aptitude Tests*: The most widely used test batteries are the *General Aptitude Test Battery* (GATB; U.S. Department of Labor, 1970) and the Differential Aptitude Tests (DAT; Bennett, Seashore, & Wesman, 1982). These batteries provide information on a person's ability in a specific area such as mechanical or clerical as well as in more general areas such as verbal or numerical. These scores can be related to the

Dictionary of Occupational Titles (DOT; U.S. Department of Labor, Employment and Training, 1991) to ascertain fit between a person's known aptitudes and the aptitudes required for specific jobs.

▶ *Work Samples*: Work samples are actual or simulated samples of real work. Their purpose is to assess the client's potential for a range of occupational areas. They incorporate the physical and mental requirements of a job but lack the environmental and psychological conditions of real work. Work samples can be "homemade" specific to individual job components or they can be commercial systems. Commercial systems can be evaluated across a number of parameters. These include the target group, theoretical or organizational principles behind the development of the system, organization of the system, packaging of the samples, availability of the manual, process, administration, scoring, norms, client observation requirements, reporting, utility, training required, and technical considerations (Pruitt, 1977). Very few commercial work samples have been developed for persons with mental illnesses. However, components of a sample may be helpful in ascertaining job specific-skills. Micro–TOWER, Valpar, and Singer are all examples of commercial work sample systems. Descriptions and evaluations of these systems are available in *Vocational Evaluation Systems and Software: A Consumer's Guide* by Brown, McDaniel, Couch, and McClanahan (1994).

▶ *Situational Assessment*: This approach can be defined as a *systematic* procedure for observing, recording, and interpreting work behavior. Pruitt (1977) suggests that the effectiveness of this approach depends almost entirely on the sensitivity and skill of the observer. The client is evaluated in real or simulated job situations. Common tools used to assist in evaluating situational assessment are behavior rating scales and adjective checklists.

▶ *Job Shadowing*: This approach assists in developing job awareness for clients and is especially helpful with persons who are job naive or unaware of job requirements. The client follows a worker doing a specific job for a length of time suitable for him or her to understand the major components of the job. Job shadowing is often used in conjunction with interest testing.

Work Adjustment Training

This process uses work or work-related activities to create an understanding of and appreciation for the meaning of work, values, and demands of work; it assists in developing or modifying appropriate attitudes, personal characteristics, and work behaviors and may develop functional capacities as required to enable individuals to reach their full vocational potentials.

Work Hardening

Clients participate in a gradual exposure to a real or simulated job. With increasing time spent in a work setting, clients improve their physical and mental tolerance of work demands. On the job, work hardening may be the ideal setting and means for maximizing return to work. Work hardening through simulation is superior to traditional clinic activities.

Supported Education

Using principles similar to those described under supported employment, students are assisted in entry and re-entry into the education system.

Career Counseling Programs

Clients learn about the world of work and the way their own interests, skills, and values impact on job success.

Career Placement Programs

This type of program assists clients in locating and securing permanent full- or part-time paid employment through agency connections and professional knowledge of the job market.

Job Clubs

The primary emphasis of this type of program is to provide training in job seeking skills and support during job search (Jacobs, 1988). Solving Community Obstacles and Restoring Employment (SCORE) is a training program developed by an occupational therapist that covers the essential component of job search skills and is delivered in a group format (Kramer, 1984). It has been used successfully in clinical practice (Wassink, 1988).

Employment Support or Follow Along

Postemployment supports, both group and individual, help clients retain jobs by providing regular opportunities to share problems and offer resolutions to them. *Follow along* allows monitoring of performance and functioning and ongoing career guidance. It should be long-term and include regular contact with employers. Often success at work can result in increased needs in the work or other rehabilitation areas

(Russert & Frey, 1994). Follow along is a vital, yet often overlooked, component of the vocational rehabilitation process.

THE OCCUPATIONAL THERAPY PROCESS

An effective vocational process for persons with serious mental illness is (a) driven by desire first, (b) is educational and experiential in nature and includes all essential stakeholders, (c) takes into account the complexity of vocational rehabilitation, and (d) is usually long-term. The CAOT (1988) position paper on the role of occupational therapy in vocational rehabilitation indicates that occupational therapists are most frequently involved in the evaluation or assessment and skill-building components of the vocational rehabilitation process. Their knowledge and skills in therapeutic interactions and the demands of work and the workplace allow them to fill a number of roles. One example of an expanded role is that of a case manager who reintegrates persons who are disabled into the workplace.

Occupational therapy's historical/traditional approach to the work process is sequential in nature. The ladder or step method includes assessment, planning, treatment and programming, termination, and follow-up care (Jacobs, 1988; Lloyd, 1995). The bulk of occupational therapy intervention tends to be in the prevocational assessment and vocational evaluation phases with the assessment process predicting current and future employment potential (Hume, 1990). Some exceptions to this have been identified under vocational options.

This type of approach is gradually changing with the consumer movement. From a hierarchical approach based on a "train and place" model, there is a shift to client choice through an insight gaining process where assessment is geared toward that choice. The model more closely approximates a "place and train" model. The consumer should be able to enter and re-enter the system at any time and to be involved in only those aspects of vocational rehabilitation they require. Otherwise we are doing a great deal of irrelevant job preparation and intervention.

This evolving model appears to be more helpful for persons with serious mental illnesses. The client group often presents with a long involvement with mental health systems and many attempts at vocational rehabilitation through traditional avenues with little success. Often a typical vocational history includes a number of short-term entry-level jobs such as dishwasher, security guard, or parking lot attendant. In this group there is little evidence that skills learned are generalizable from one setting to another (Hayes & Halford, 1993) and vocational testing does not predict work success (Anthony & Jansen, 1984). Often vocational assessment suggests that skills and habits are generalizable and equates an inability to keep to a day hospital program as an indication that a person is not work ready. However, assumptions cannot be made about a person's vocational capacity based on his or her daily nonvocational capacity. In fact, we know very little about who will be successful. In part this may be because of the idiosyncratic effects of the illnesses. Serious mental illnesses are often heterogenic in nature and can be further compromised by substance abuse. Anthony and Jansen (1984) identified psychiatric symptomatology and diagnosis as poor predictors of vocational capacity, whereas prior employment history and performance in actual or simulated work settings are good predictors of future potential. However, much needs to be done to clarify which patients with schizophrenia, for example,

will benefit from the various models of vocational rehabilitation (Bond, 1994).

Persons with serious mental illness have much to fear and little to hope for in terms of vocational rehabilitation (Rabin & Jeong, 1991). They may associate vocational rehabilitation with rejections and failure, resulting in low self-esteem and associate previous job loss with relapse. Because serious mental illnesses often emerge in the teenage years, clients may not have learned the basic requirements of working, job seeking, or job behaviors. They are often job naive and have little information with which to make job choices. Because each person is uniquely affected by the illness, the matching of the person's strengths and needs to the job become of paramount importance. At the same time employers may be reluctant to hire persons with serious mental illness because of a stigma attached to the illness. They may lack knowledge about mental illness, have had prior unsuccessful experiences, or not understand how to provide reasonable accommodations for persons with mental illness.

Many consumers identify having a job as their most important goal and also indicate that employment is helpful to their mental health (Vostanis, 1990). In part this may be a result of societal expectations or family hopes, but it is also their own innate drive to engage in occupations. Jobs are seen as important to their self-esteem, financial independence, and reflect their contribution to society. Consumers also note that rehabilitation counselors offer little range of job opportunity with limited options (Evans, 1997).

The journey toward a successful vocational outcome is a shared educational process where the occupational therapist and the client work together in a therapeutic alliance. The optimal rehabilitation for any particular client will be discovered in the context of a personal relationship with that client. The occupational therapist learns what the client's individual experiences are with work and the illness. The client learns or relearns the tasks of a being a worker, a student, a volunteer. Most people do not think about what being a worker means until they experience a vocational disruption such as changing jobs or returning to school when they have to deal with different or new requirements. When clients have no work experiences or a number of unsuccessful experiences, understanding that becoming a worker is something one can learn is very powerful.

Toward a Conceptual Approach

In the following quote, Marshall (1985) cited a program description from the 1930s: "Work assignments were matched with experience, aptitude, and interest of the patient. Each patient's needs were considered, the job was analyzed, and supervised occupation was the method of treatment" (p. 297). The spirit of the quote remains relevant today.

To facilitate collaboration, all essential stakeholders need to learn a common language and acquire information about vocational rehabilitation and employment. The approach that follows is based on the occupational therapy philosophy that a balance of work, rest, play, and engagement in meaningful activity is essential for maintaining health. This approach also provides an opportunity for personal growth and life satisfaction. Using an educational model that incorporates this approach has been helpful in engaging clients in a therapeutic partnership. This conceptual approach can be used concurrently in educating service provider agencies, employers, and families. When all parties have a common understanding of both the complexity of vocational rehabilitation and the potential for consumer success and satisfaction, the ensuing collaboration can be more effective.

Reilly (1962) stated that the philosophical and operational base of occupational therapy could be found in the understanding of the human organization as a balance between work, rest/sleep, and play. Being able to look after oneself is integral to an optimal balance. Christiansen (1994) has suggested that balance cannot be used in the time-budgeting sense, but is unique to each individual. For example, he has observed that some people by nature are "high active" people in all areas of their lives and others are less so. Personal experiences of satisfaction or fulfillment are strongly linked to the organization of time throughout life and in the ideal world time is organized so that people can enjoy life, contribute to the social and economic fabric of their communities, and look after themselves (CAOT, 1997).

However, one must also add the impact of the illness, which is unique to the individual in how it affects the balance. Braitman et al. (1995) found that the effects of mental illness were perceived as a significant barrier to success for both employed and unemployed clients. If, for example, someone's sleep is disturbed by ongoing symptomatology, it is quite possible that the ability to work full-time will be compromised. If an individual is not able to complete basic self-care tasks related to personal hygiene, it may affect his or her vocational success. For many clients, particularly in beginning a vocational path/program/course, a gradual or part-time entry allows them to maintain balance among these areas and therefore may assist them in the recovery process.

THE VOCATIONAL PROCESS

Along with access to vocational opportunities, persons with psychiatric disabilities often need assistance in choosing, getting, and keeping a job. This process is a component of the psychiatric rehabilitation technology developed by Anthony, Cohen, and Farkas (1990).

Case Scenario

Daniel is a 38-year-old man who has had a schizo-affective disorder over a 20-year period. He completed a Masters degree in English as a part-time student 6 years ago. He has tried many short term full-time jobs, such as research assistant, insurance salesperson, and various clerical types of work. However, he experiences increasing affective symptoms with the stress of work and resigns or elapses within 2 to 3 months. He is involved in an assertive case management program and has been referred to Occupational Therapy to assist him with his vocational pursuits. Daniel is living in his own apartment and sees few people other than his widowed mother twice a week and his case manager.

---

reports that he is able to maintain his apartment in preparing meals, buying groceries, cleaning his apartment, paying bills, and banking. However, it takes him a long time to complete these activities. He is interested and motivated (a) in returning to work in order to supplement his income, (b) to have more structure to his day, and (c) to be more involved in the community. When he considers his ability to balance all his activities, he comes to the conclusion that he would prefer to work part-time so that he can maintain his apartment. This would prevent him from having overwhelming stress. He recognizes it is difficult to get started in the mornings because of depression. He sees work as a possible means of expanding his friendships and social network.

The occupational therapist has met with Daniel's mother and has discussed the vocational rehabilitation path. She would very much like to see Daniel in a white collar job where he uses his education. She is supportive of Daniel and the occupational therapy goals of helping him to obtain a job and be involved in meaningful activities.

Step One: Setting the Scene

The therapist discusses the individual's balance of work, rest, and play with the client. He or she explores how the illness uniquely affects the client and his or her perceived optimum balance. Simultaneously, significant others acquire knowledge about balance and the illness, explore the vocational process, and develop an understanding of the long-term nature of vocational rehabilitation.

Case Example: Step One

Daniel identifies his difficulties with sleeping through the night, waking up slowly, and feeling depressed in the morning. He spends a great deal of time in solitary passive leisure activities, such as reading and watching documentaries on specialty cable channels. He

---

Step Two: Gathering Information

Taking a work history can be diminishing, discouraging, and defeating if approached from the perspective of "tell me about your jobs and why you left them." This type of interview often increases defensiveness and decreases openness because the person is talking from a position of risk and often has a history of job failures. In this tentative vocational journey we need to build in as many affirming strategies as possible. The occupational therapist must develop an understanding of the meaning and values attributed to previous work experience by the client. One way to do this is to have the client describe what he or she particularly liked and disliked about the job with lots of detail. The therapist needs to experience the job demands from the client's perspective. Not only does this approach leave the client's self-esteem intact, it often allows the interviewer to know what particular tasks or interactions led to job failure or loss and also increases connectedness and rapport with the client. Effective vocational rehabilitation encourages individuals to explore their potential, discover what work suits them, and make choices based on compromises, self-awareness, and availability of work.

Case Example: Step Two

Daniel reports his last job was as a dispatcher for a courier company. He liked going to work because it gave him a reason to get up and provided extra money. He liked working with his supervisor. He did not like feeling responsible for meeting deadlines and found it very stressful dealing with disappointed or irate customers. This caused him to lie awake at night worrying and, as his sleep patterns deteriorated, his ability to attend and concentrate at work also decreased. He resigned after talking it over with his supervisor.

Daniel described a number of jobs with similar patterns—he found dealing with the public or with a number of people's demands very stressful, and he did not like feeling responsible. He did like having a place to go, the extra money, and developing individual relationships.

Step Three: Evaluating Personal Variables

Personal variables are the unique components the client brings to the vocational partnership. They include interests, aptitudes, and tolerances. They are grounded in the client's personal value system.

▶ *Interests.* What types of work has the client been interested in? How did the client find out about different types of jobs? Why does a client choose a specific job?

We know that if someone is not interested in an area (based on values and knowledge) he or she will be neither happy nor motivated. Psychosocial rehabilitation is most effective when the goals are determined primarily by the consumer. The occupational therapy process begins with the development of client-articulated goals. A person may be interested in vocational rehabilitation but not yet ready. Readiness, a concept defined and explicated by the psychiatric rehabilitation approach, includes recognition of how choices have been made in the past, closeness with the therapist, and self and environmental awareness.

Assessment in this area is related to how well-informed the client's job choice is and should be directed toward helping the client choose a specific career path rather than generalized to all types of work. Intervention includes values clarification tasks, interest inventories, information about job demands (people, data, things, plants and animals), and job shadowing.

Case Example: Interests

Daniel completed an interest inventory and reviewed a great deal of written information on different types of jobs and careers. He felt most comfortable working with things or data, in a quiet setting, with no responsibility for deadlines. Because of his previous degree and passive leisure interests, we narrowed down his interests to the family of jobs relating to information and education. *What type of work can you think of that might suit Daniel?*

▶ *Aptitudes.* Are there some aptitudes the client has which are stronger than others? What jobs could the client not do because of weaker aptitude levels?

Aptitudes are potential abilities that are innate and/or acquired. Certain jobs require specific levels of aptitudes. If someone has a limited aptitude in a specific area, jobs requiring a higher level of competence would be difficult for them. For example, someone who has difficulty with fine motor tasks could not be a jeweler. Intervention includes aptitude testing as well as exploring the requirements of different jobs. The *Dictionary of Occupational Titles* (DOT; U.S. Department of Labor, Employment and Training, 1991) and *Canadian Classification and Dictionary of Occupations* (CCDO; Ministry of Supply and Services, 1989) identify the minimum aptitudes necessary for all jobs listed.

Case Example: Aptitudes

Daniel completed a self report on various aptitudes and scored high in general knowledge, verbal and numerical knowledge, and clerical abilities. He did not score well on mechanical and spatial ability. When we compared his scores to the job family he was interested in, we found he was compatible with many of the jobs.

▶ *Tolerances.* What tolerance does the client have for the physical and mental demands of a job?

  ▶ *Physical*: Medication side-effects, sleep deprivation, fatigue, dry mouth, and competing symptoms can all affect physical capacity. Often persons with serious mental illness are not physically fit (Byrne, Isaacs, & Voorberg 1991)

  ▶ *Mental*: Mental tolerance reflects the mental demands of a job or the meaning ascribed to work by the client. The idea of work plus the responsibility it entails, can become stressful. Self-efficacy expectations are a person's expectation that he or she is capable of performing the tasks or set of behaviors to produce a desired outcome. If self-efficacy is to be maintained, it is necessary to experience success performing a particular task. Certain types of jobs may also require a degree of mental attention or multitasking, which may challenge some persons with mental illness or, conversely, some jobs may not be challenging enough or be seen as demeaning.

Physical and mental tolerances can be evaluated through situational assessments and some work sample components. Intervention can also be directed toward helping employers make reasonable accommodations. For example, screens can be provided to reduce auditory and visual stimulation. Clients can also be encouraged to explore choices within a similarly defined family of jobs so that they can switch to a less physically or mentally demanding job or to a more mentally challenging job.

Case Example: Tolerances

Because Daniel was fatigued in the morning, he preferred an afternoon start time, as well as access to a water fountain because of medication side effects. He was not physically strong so he needed work that required light physical demands. Daniel recognized that full-time work had been too stressful for him in the past and compromised his ability to maintain his apartment. Although he liked a job with mental stimulation he did not want to feel he was key to other people's work success.

Case Example: Step Three

Daniel narrowed his work choices down to four:

1. Magazine or newspaper clipping service
2. Library assistant
3. Using word processing to edit student essays
4. Working in the museum archives gathering data

He then needed to compare the job requirements to his aptitudes and expectations.

Step Four: Evaluating Environmental Requirements

What does the workplace expect from the worker? One way of explaining workplace expectations is the concept of press. *Press* is defined as an expectation for certain kinds of behaviors (Palmer & Gatti, 1985) or as the match between environmental demands for performance and the systems ability to perform (Barris, 1992). The evaluation of the environmental requirements for Daniel is described in Figure 9–1.

Case Example: Step Four

Daniel decided he wanted to work as a **Library Assistant**. The occupational therapist met with the public library staff and discussed potential work arrangements. Daniel would work 3 days per week, in the afternoons. Every 2 weeks, the O.T. would meet with the library staff supervisor and Daniel and review how things were going. She was also invited to do an information seminar on vocational rehabilitation and persons with mental illness.

Basic workplace expectations encompass three areas: work habits, work skills, and work personality.

▶ *Work Habits.* The routines required by the job site usually include attendance, punctuality, and reliability. Intervention can be directed at the skill or resource deficits. For example, if a client was typically late for work because he or she did not own an alarm clock, that would be a lack of a resource. If he or she was late because of not knowing the shortest bus route, that would be a skill deficit.

Case Example: Work Habits

Daniel worked from 1:00–4:00 p.m. Monday, Wednesday, Friday. He had no problems with attendance, punctuality, reliability. His grooming and appearance were acceptable.

▶ *Work Skills.* These are the skills required by the specific job. For example, clerical jobs require computer skills, construction jobs require physical strength, and courier jobs may require the ability to drive a vehicle. If the client does not have a required skill, he or she may need further education or retraining through supported education.

Case Example: Work Skills

Daniel was able to use a computer, he understood the library MIS, and had vast general knowledge so could use these skills in his assigned tasks.

▶ *Work Personality.* This can be defined as a reasonable response to social cues. These can be most difficult to learn as they often reflect implicit rather than explicit norms in the workplace. Social skills and awareness of social etiquette are an integral part of work success for every employee (Pruitt, 1977). Persons without disability often are

	Daniel's Work Choices			
Personal Variables	Clipping Service	Library Assistant	Word Processing and Editing Student Essays	Museum Archives
Information/Education Job Family	x[1]	x	x	x
Low Physical Demands	x	. . . x	. . . x	x
High Mental Stimulation	possible	possible	possible	possible
Work at Own Pace	x	x	no	x
Quiet Setting	sometimes	mostly	. . .x	x
Afternoon Start/Part-Time	no	x	x	possible
Fewer People	x	x	x	x
Some Ability to Control Amount of Interactions with Co-workers	no	. . . x	no	x
Water Fountain	x	x	x	x
Paid Employment	possible	x	x	not to start

[1]x = yes. When there is a . . . preceeding the x, it means that some information in some components is more complex but is not included because of space.

Figure 9–1. Evaluation of the environmental requirements for employment. The environmental demands of the job and the personal needs of the client need to match.

asked to leave jobs because their social skills are poor (Mueller, 1988). In the field of developmental disability, a lack of social skills has been identified as a significant factor in job loss and independent living (Wilgosh & Covassi, 1988). Mueller and Wilgosh (1991) also found that job loss is related to perceived deficits of employee character or social awareness, while job success is related to the quality and quantity of work performance. Because persons with serious mental illness have difficulty interpreting subtle social nuances, social skills have a significant effect on employability and maintaining employability (Lloyd, 1995). Furthermore, Lysaker et al. (1993) suggested clients with mental illness

had trouble relating effectively to other workers on the job. Specifically, interpersonal problems included interpreting the behavior of their co-workers, figuring out how personal their work relationships should be, and recognizing the impact of their own behaviors. Watts (1976) found that client enthusiasm, social relationships, and response to supervision are more important than task performance for successful employment. We cannot ignore the importance to the whole process of matching clients to agencies and employers across all aspects. Akabas (1994) maintains that the key to success is making the fit between the individual and the employer/workplace. The therapist must make an attempt to clarify, identify, and match cultures not only at the physical demands level but at the more subtle, social and emotional levels. The process itself encourages awareness and realism.

Case Example: Work Personality

Initially there were only minor issues related to learning a new job. However, although the library appeared to be a quiet setting, it became apparent that Daniel's immediate supervisor was very talkative. She tended to chat incessantly all day long. Although well meaning, she made many inquiries regarding his personal life, which increased his paranoid symptoms. Daniel found this extremely stressful and became more withdrawn at work. As a consequence the supervisor became increasingly voluble. Finally, Daniel told his case manager he wanted to quit. When the issue was explored, we first suggested some changes at the worksite. For example, we tried having him work on a different floor of the library. However, he continued to feel sensitive to co-workers and struggled with benign routine social questions, such as "How was your weekend?" We then explored the possibility of transfer to another library in the system. His supervisor at this library was also a quiet person. With the change in setting and different supervisor this became a successful return to work for Daniel.

Step Five: Keeping the Job

Reasonable Accommodation and Advocacy. A study of reasonable accommodation for workers with serious mental illness undertaken at a community-supported employment program in the United States found that 231 accommodations at the worksite were identified for these individuals, for an average of 5.1 accommodations per job (Fabian, Waterworth, & Ripke, 1993). The most frequently identified accommodation was orientation and training of supervisors to provide necessary assistance, followed by modifications of the nonphysical work environment, and modifications to work hours and schedules. Furthermore, the number of job accommodations was positively associated with employment tenure. Persons with psychiatric disabilities interested in employment opportunities may require a broader range of services and supports than do persons with other disabilities (Rutman, 1994).

Mancuso (1990) found that most accommodations for workers with psychiatric disabilities are not costly (<$500) or free; for example, flexible work schedules, time off for therapy, or job restructuring to eliminate or exchange nonessential job functions that increase pressure for the worker. However, it is important to be aware that the ongoing nature of these accommodations can represent significant indirect costs. For example, increasing the intensity and frequency of supervisory time is a "hidden" management cost that is not an out-of-pocket expense, but may be a significant expenditure in company resources. Employers tend to underestimate the use of nonphysical accommodations, because associated expenditures were not out-of-pocket expenses and the resources expended, such as additional supervisory time, are more difficult to calculate (Collignon,1986).

The role of the occupational therapist includes employer education regarding mental illness and marketing the client appropriately. One method of assessing workplace culture is to use a tool such as the *Work Environment Scale* (Moos, 1994). Employers who maintain positive work environments for persons without mental illness will probably provide the same positive environment for persons with mental illness. A positive work environment encourages productivity and a sense of community (Tilson, 1996). The provision of support in the workplace, social skills training, environmental assessment and modification, and education of co-workers will assist clients in ongoing vocational success.

In addition to the roles currently assumed by occupational therapists in the area of reasonable accommodation, there is potential for even more. Knowledge is power, and providing information to clients is an essential aspect of empowerment. A key challenge for occupational therapists is to shift toward partnerships by involving clients in advocacy roles. CAOT (1993) suggests occupational therapists need to become more visible in working with groups, agencies, and organizations to reduce injustices that both contribute to and perpetuate mental disorders and mental health problems. The consumer/survivor perspective underlines the importance of allowing employees with psychiatric disabilities to maintain full control over what accommodations are applied to them, and how they use those accommodations (Howie the Harp, 1994). Client education about the ADA provides an understanding not only of the employer's rights and responsibilities specifically related to the employment process, but of the client's responsibility in that process. Ideally, occupational therapists should be less willing to accept individual explanations for problems that are essentially economic, social, or political and become more involved in advocacy with persons with disabilities (Jongbloed & Crichton, 1990).

Case Example: Step Five

Regular meetings were scheduled with Daniel, the library staff, his mother, and his case manager. Daniel was also involved in a support and education group for consumers who were employed. The occupational therapist gradually withdrew involvement until she saw Daniel in the support group only, while any issues related to his work were dealt with by his case manager. However, she was available if he wanted or needed to make changes in the job or for future career planning.

The occupational therapist needs to play an active role in advocacy. The mental health system has only recently begun to employ consumers as providers of service (Mowbray, Moxley, Howell, & Jasper, 1997). Not only should we advocate for employment in mental health agencies, but also in our own social network, and at the places we do business. We need to talk to service clubs, local business groups, and municipalities. Furthermore, we can use our success experiences to help new employers consider hiring persons with mental illness by exposing them to employers who do hire persons with mental illnesses.

ADDITIONAL CASE STUDIES
Case Study #1: Sally

Step One

Sally is a 40-year-old single, Caucasian female with a 24-year history of serious mental illness. She has a developmental delay due to birth trauma. Her mother wants her to do more than smoke cigarettes and drink coffee all day.

> *What is most important for you to accomplish in Step One?*
>
> *What are the issues?*

Step Two

Sally has not worked competitively since she was 17. She has had some unsuccessful and unsatisfying involvement with sheltered work at various times since then.

What further questions do you need to ask Sally? And/or her parents?

What kind of information do you need about Sally's experiences?

Step Three

Interests: Sally says she would like to be a professional figure skater. She was involved in figure skating as a child and in early adolescence and longs for that time before she became ill.

> *Using a client-centered approach, how would you use this information to explore Sally's interests?*

Aptitudes: Look up the aptitudes required to be a figure skater in the Dictionary of Occupational Titles.

> *Where else might you find similar information?*

> *Write <u>word for word</u> what you would say to Sally when you both have explored this information.*

Tolerances: Sally has had problems with her right knee following an anterior cruciate ligament tear. She is also underweight and becomes tired easily.

> *What would Sally have to be able to do if she was going to become a skater?*

> *How would you assess the physical demands?*

> *What meaning does figure skating have for Sally?*

> *Does she (and do you) understand the requirements?*

Consider what you might do to help Sally understand the process thus far.

Synopsis

Sally is depressed and discouraged about not being able to fulfill this dream. Identify the counseling skills required by the therapist to help Sally through this time. You review her values and explore her knowledge of jobs with similar values. Develop a list of possibilities you and she can explore.

Complete Step Four Using Four Different Work Sites.

Choose the most appropriate site. What did you come up with? What would you put into place to help Sally keep her job? (* Sally became a Wal-Mart greeter.)

Case Study #2: Lorraine

Lorraine is a 32-year-old, single Hispanic woman with a diagnosis of bipolar affective disorder. She is currently living with her parents although has lived independently in the past. She is a lawyer. She has not been working for 14 months. She is starting to feel better. Her mood is stable, and she has more energy. Lorraine is referred to you for vocational assessment and re-integration. Use the vocational process to help her reach any of the following outcomes:

1. She changes occupations altogether.

2. She returns to law as a part-time lawyer (private practice).

3. She returns to law as a full-time lawyer (law firm).

4. She teaches law at a local community college.

5. She volunteers at Legal Aid.

SUMMARY

In summary, talking with clients, families, agencies, and employers using these paradigms can encourage vocational partnerships in which everyone is reasonably satisfied with outcomes. It is a long process that needs to be repeated and supported in all aspects of the clients' care. There are a variety of avenues ranging from the individual level to the larger system where acting in an advocacy role can further the development and maintenance of opportunities throughout the vocational area.

"I have . . . a job at the College of San Mateo . . . I enjoy every minute of it and it constitutes a challenge for me that brings a sense of worth back into my life that glitters beyond gold and shines like silver" (Knight, 1994, p. 143).

REFERENCES

Akabas, S. H. (1994). Workplace responsiveness: Key employer characteristics in support of job maintenance for people with mental illness. *Psychosocial Rehabilitation Journal, 17*(3), 91–101.

Allen, C. K. (1985). *Occupational therapy for psychiatric diseases: Measurement and management of cognitive disabilities.* Boston: Little, Brown.

American Occupational Therapy Association. (1994). Uniform terminology for occupational therapy—Third edition. *American Journal of Occupational Therapy, 48,* 1047–1059.

Americans with Disabilities Act of 1990, Pub. L. No. 101–336, §2,104 Stat.327. (1990).

Anthony, W. A., Cohen, M. R., & Farkas, M. D. (1990). *Psychiatric rehabilitation.* Boston, MA: Boston University, Center for Psychiatric Rehabilitation.

Anthony, W. A., & Jansen, M. A. (1984). Predicting the vocational capacity of the chronically mentally ill: Research and policy implications. *American Psychologist, 39,* 537–544.

Armstrong, M. L., Korba, A. M., & Emard, R. (1995). Of mutual benefit: The reciprocal relationship between consumer volunteers and the clients they serve. *Psychiatric Rehabilitation Journal, 19,* 45–49.

Bachrach, L. L. (1991). Perspectives on work and rehabilitation. *Hospital and Community Psychiatry, 42,* 890–891.

Bailey, J. (1998). I'm just an ordinary person. *Psychiatric Rehabilitation Journal, 22*(1), 8–11.

Balkin, S. (1992). Entrepreneurial activities of homeless men. *Journal of Sociology and Social Welfare,19*(4), 129–148.

Barker, L. T. (1994). Community-based models of employment services for people with psychiatric disabilities. *Psychosocial Rehabilitation Journal, 17,* 55–65.

Baron, R. (1995). Establishing employment services as a priority for persons with long-term mental illness. *American Rehabilitation, 21,* 32–35.

Barris, R. (1992). Environmental interactions: An extension of the model of occupation. *American Journal of Occupational Therapy, 36,* 637–656.

Bennett, G. K., Seashore, H. G., & Wesman, A. G. (1982). *Differential Aptitude Tests* (DAT). New York: Psychological Corp.

Black, B. J. (1992). A kind word for sheltered work. *Psychosocial Rehabilitation Journal, 15*(4), 86–89.

Bond, G. R. (1994). Supported work as a modification of the transitional employment model for clients with psychiatric disabilities. In The Publications Committee of the IAPSRS (Eds.), *An introduction to psychiatric rehabilitation* (pp. 215–229). Columbia, MD: The Publications Committee of the International Association of Psychosocial Rehabilitation Services (IAPSRS).

Bond, G. R., Drake, R. E., Mueser, K. T., Becker, D. R. (1997). An update on supported employment for people with severe mental illness. *Psychiatric Services, 48,* 335–346.

Braitman, A., Counts, P., Davenport, B., Zurlinden, B., Rogers, M., Clauss, J., Kulkarni, A., Kymla, J., & Montgomery, L. (1995). Comparison of barriers to employment for unemployed and employed clients in a case management program: An exploratory study. *Psychiatric Rehabilitation Journal, 19*(1), 3–8.

Breen, T. L., Clarke, K. A., & Moran, M. (1991). Home-based employment. In K. Jacobs (Ed.), *Occupational therapy: Work related programs and assessments* (2nd ed., pp. 383—391). Boston: Little Brown.

Brown, C., McDaniel, R., Couch, R., & McClanahan, M. (1994). *Vocational evaluation systems and software: A consumer's guide.* Menomonie, WI: Stout

Vocational Rehabilitation Institute, University of Wisconsin–Stout.

Buckley, L. R. (1981, December). Partial employment for persons with chronic mental illness. *Canada's Mental Health, 29*(4), 10–12.

Byrne, C., Isaacs, S. & Voorberg, N. (1991). Assessment of the physical health needs of people with chronic mental illness: One focus for health promotion. *Canada's Mental Health, 39*(1), 7–12.

Campbell, J. F. (1989). Employment programs for people with a psychiatric disability: An overview. *Community Support Network News, 6*(2), 1, 11.

Canadian Association of Occupational Therapists. (1988). Position paper on occupational therapist's role in work related therapy. *Canadian Journal of Occupational Therapy, 55*(4), 1–4.

Canadian Association of Occupational Therapists. (1993). *Occupational therapy guidelines for client-centred practice.* Toronto: Author.

Canadian Association of Occupational Therapists. (1997). *Enabling occupation: An occupational therapy perspective.* Ottawa, Ontario: Canadian Association of Occupational Therapy Publications.

Canadian Mental Health Association. (1996). *How to become self-employed: Entrepreneurship for consumer/survivors.* [Brochure]. Toronto: Author.

Capponi, P. (1997). *Dispatches from the poverty line.* Toronto: Penguin.

Chamberlin, J. (1978). *On our own: Patient controlled alternatives to the mental health system.* New York: Hawthorne.

Christiansen, C. H. (1994). Three perspectives on balance in occupation. In R. Zemke & F. Clark (Eds.), *Occupational science: The evolving discipline* (pp. 431–451). Philadelphia: F. A. Davis.

Cnaan, R. A., Blankertz, L., Messinger, K. W., & Gardner, J. R. (1990). Experts' assessment of psychosocial rehabilitation principles. *Psychosocial Rehabilitation Journal, 13*(3), 59–73.

Collignon, F. C. (1986). The role of reasonable accommodation in employment of disabled persons in private industry. In M. Berkowitz & M. A. Hill (Eds.), *Disability and the labour market.* Ithaca, NY: ILR Press.

Consumer/Survivor Business Council of Ontario. (1995). *Yes we can! . . . promote economic opportunity and choice through community businesses.* Toronto: Author.

Deegan, P. (1988). Recovery: The lived experience of rehabilitation. *Psychosocial Rehabilitation Journal, 11*(4), 11–19.

Drake, R. K. (1998). A brief history of the individual placement and support model. *Psychiatric Rehabilitation Journal, 22*(1), 3–7.

Dulay, J. F., & Steichen, M. (1982). Transitional employment for the chronically mentally ill. *Occupational Therapy in Mental Health, 2*(3), 65–77.

Ekdawi, M. Y., & Conning, A. M. (1994). *Psychiatric rehabilitation: A practical guide.* London: Chapman & Hall.

Evans, C. (1997). Do mental health consumers have the right to fail? *PSR Connection Newsletter, 1,* 7.

Fabian, E. S., Waterworth, A., & Ripke, B. (1993). Reasonable accommodation for workers with serious mental illness: Type, frequency, and associated outcomes. *Psychosocial Rehabilitation Journal, 17,* 163–172.

France, M. H. (1985). Vocational education. *Canadian Vocational Journal, 21*(2), 36–39.

Freud, S. (1953). *Civilization and its discontents.* London: Hogarth.

Hartl, K. (1992). *A-Way Express: A way to empowerment through competitive employment.* Unpublished manuscript. (Available from A-Way Express, 320 Danforth Ave., Toronto, ON, M4K 1N8.)

Hayes, R., & Halford, W. (1993). Generalization of occupational therapy effects in psychiatric rehabilitation. *American Journal of Occupational Therapy, 47,* 161–167.

Howie, the Harp. (1994). Empowerment of mental health consumers in vocational rehabilitation. *Psychosocial Rehabilitation Journal, 17*(3), 83–89.

Hume, C. A. (1990). Rehabilitation. In J. Creek (Ed.), *Occupational therapy and mental health: Principles, skills & practice* (pp. 333–348). London: Churchill Livingstone.

Jackson, D. N., & Marshall, C. W. (1997). *Ashland Interest Assessment.* London, Ontario: Research Psychologists Press.

Jackson, R. (1992). How work works. *Psychosocial Rehabilitation Journal, 16*(2), 63–67.

Jacobs, H. E. (1988). Vocational rehabilitation. In R. P. Liberman (Ed.), *Psychiatric rehabilitation of the chronic mental patient* (pp. 245–284). Washington, DC: American Psychiatric Association.

Jacobs, K. (1991). *Occupational therapy: Work-related programs and assessments* (2nd ed.). Boston: Little, Brown.

Jastak, J. F., & Jastak, K. S. (1979). *Wide Range Interest—Opinion Test* (WRIOT). Wilmington, DE: Jastak Assessment Systems.

Jongbloed, L., & Crichton, A. (1990). A new definition of disability: Implications for rehabilitation practice and social policy. *Canadian Journal of Occupational Therapy, 57*(1), 32–37.

Kakutani, K. (1998). New life espresso: Report on a business run by people with psychiatric disabilities. *Psychiatric Rehabilitation Journal, 22*(2), 111–116.

Kates, N., Nikalaou, L., Baillie, B., & Hess, J. (1997). An in-home employment program for people with mental illness. *Psychiatric Rehabilitation Journal, 20*(4), 56–60.

Knight, H. (1994). The invisible client. In The Publications Committee of IAPSRS (Eds.) *An introduction to psychiatric rehabilitation* (pp. 137–144). Columbia, MD: International Association of Psychosocial Rehabilitation Services (IAPSRS).

Kramer, L. W. (1984). SCORE: Solving community obstacles and restoring employment. *Occupational Therapy of Mental Health, 4*(1), 1–134.

Kremer, K. B. (1991). *Six Ohio consumer-operated services and businesses.* Formative Evaluation Report. Columbus: Ohio Department of Mental Health, Office of Program Evaluation and Research.

Lang, S. K., & Cara, E. (1989). Vocational integration of the psychiatrically disabled. *Hospital and Community Psychiatry, 40*, 890–892.

Law, M., Cooper, B., Strong, S., Stewart, D., Rigby, P., & Letts, L. (1996). The Person-Environment-Occupational Model: A transactive approach to occupational performance. *Canadian Journal of Occupational Therapy, 63*, 9–23.

Lloyd, C. (1995). *Forensic psychiatry for health professionals.* London: Chapman & Hall.

Lysaker, P., Bell, M., Milstein, R., Bryson, G., Shestopal, A., & Goulet, J. B. (1993). Work capacity in schizophrenia. *Hospital and Community Psychiatry, 44*(3), 278–280.

Mancuso, L. L. (1990). Reasonable accommodation for workers with psychiatric disabilities. *Psychosocial Rehabilitation Journal, 14*(2), 3–19.

Marshall, E. M. (1985). Looking back. *American Journal of Occupational Therapy, 39*, 297–300.

Ministry of Supply and Services. (1989). *Canadian classification and dictionary of occupations* (9th ed.). Ottawa: Author.

Moos, R. H. (1994). *Work environment scale manual* (3rd ed.). Palo Alto, CA: Consulting Psychologists Press.

Morgan, S. (1993). *Community mental health; practical approaches to long-term problems.* London: Chapman & Hall.

Mowbray, C. T., Chamberlain, P., Jennings, M., & Reed, C. (1988). Results from five demonstration projects. *Community Mental Health Journal, 24*, 151–156.

Mowbray, C., Moxley, D., Howell, L., & Jasper, C. (1997). *Consumers as providers in psychiatric rehabilitation.* Columbia, MD: International Association of Psychosocial Rehabilitation Services (IAPSRS).

Mueller, H. H. (1988). Employers' reasons for terminating the employment of workers in entry-level jobs: Implications for workers with mental disabilities. *Canadian Journal of Rehabilitation, 1*, 233–240.

Mueller, H. H., & Wilgosh, L. (1991). Employment survival skills: Frequency and seriousness of skill depict occurrences for job loss. *Canadian Journal of Rehabilitation, 4*(4), 213–228.

Mullins, J. A., Rumrill, P. D., & Roessler, R. T. (1996). The role of the rehabilitation placement professional in the ADA era. *Work, 6*, 3–10.

Palmer, F., & Gatti, D. (1985). Vocational treatment model. *Occupational Therapy in Mental Health, 5*(1), 41–58.

Pruitt, W. A. (1977). *Vocational (work) evaluation.* Menomonie, WI: Walter Pruitt Associates.

Rabin, J., & Jeong, G. (1991). Work programs for adults with psychosocial problems. In K. Jacobs (Ed.), *Occupational therapy: Work-related pro-*

grams and assessments (2nd ed., pp. 197–254). Boston: Little, Brown.

Reilly, M. (1962). Occupational therapy can be one of the great ideas of 20th century medicine. *American Journal of Occupational Therapy, 16,* 1–9.

Russert, M. G., & Frey, J. L. (1994). The PACT vocational model. A step into the future. In W. Anthony & L. Spaniol (Eds.), *Readings in psychiatric rehabilitation* (pp. 339–354). Boston: Center for Psychiatric Rehabilitation.

Rutman, I. D. (1994). How psychiatric disability expresses itself as a barrier to employment. *Psychosocial Rehabilitation Journal, 17*(3), 15–35.

Strauss, J. S., Harding, C. M., Silverman, M., Eichler, A., & Lieberman, M. (1988). Work as treatment for psychiatric disorders: A puzzle in pieces. In J. A. Ciardiello & M. D. Bell (Eds.), *Vocational rehabilitation of persons with prolonged psychiatric disorders* (pp. 47–55). Baltimore: John Hopkins University Press.

Tilson, G. (1996). Building relationships with employers by applying solid customer service principles. *Journal of Vocational Rehabilitation, 6,* 77–82.

Trainor, J., & Tremblay, M. (1991). *Consumer/survivor businesses in Ontario: Challenging the rehabilitation model.* Unpublished report.

U.S. Department of Labor, Employment and Training Administration. (1970). *Manual for the USES General Aptitude Test Battery* (GATB). Washington, DC: Government Printing Office.

U.S. Department of Labor, Employment and Training Administration. (1991). *Dictionary of occupational titles* (4th ed., rev. ed.). Washington, DC: Government Printing Office.

Vostanis, P. (1990). The role of work in psychiatric rehabilitation: A review of the literature. *British Journal of Occupational Therapy, 53*(1), 24–28.

Wassink, K. E. (1988). Job search skills for unemployed psychiatric patients. *Occupational Therapy in Health Care, 2/3,* 149–158.

Watts, F. N. (1976). Modification of the employment handicaps of psychiatric patients by behavioural methods. *American Journal of Occupational Therapy, 30,* 487–490.

West, M. D., & Parent, W. S. (1995). Community and workplace supports for individuals with severe mental illness in supported employment. *Psychosocial Rehabilitation Journal, 18,* 13–24.

Wilgosh, L., & Covassi, S. (1988). A long term follow up of vocational trainees with mental handicaps. *Canadian Journal of Rehabilitation, 1,* 177–181.

Woodside, H. (1995). *Making the difference: On site support for volunteers with schizophrenia.* [Brochure]. (Available from Hamilton Program for Schizophrenia, Hamilton, ON.)

Woodside, H. & Luis, F. (1997). Supported volunteering. *Psychiatric Rehabilitation Journal, 21*(1), 70–74.

Yip, K-S., & Ng, Y-N. (1999). The dilemma of productivity-oriented management versus treatment-oriented management in sheltered workshops in Hong Kong. *Psychiatric Rehabilitation Journal, 22*(4), 390–398.

CHAPTER

10

Stress Management, Biofeedback, and Relaxation Techniques

> *Life is largely a process of adaptation to the circumstances in which we exist. A perennial give-and-take has been going on between living matter and its inanimate surroundings, between one living being and another, ever since the dawn of life in the prehistoric oceans. The secret of health and happiness lies in successful adjustment to the every–changing conditions on this globe; the penalties for failure in this great process of adaptation are disease and unhappiness.*
>
> — H. Selye, 1956, *The Stress of Life*, p. vii.

Operational Learning Objectives

By the end of this chapter, the learner will:

1. Define stress and eustress.

2. Understand the difference between stress and distress.

3. Understand the components of stress from a biological, psychological, and physiological aspect.

4. Understand the relationship between stress and the autonomic nervous system.

5. Understand stress as a precipitating factor in the development of mental illness.

6. Describe the protocol in setting up a stress management program.

7. Understand the use of the *Stress Management Questionnaire* (Stein, 1986b) in the qualitative measurement of stress.

8. Describe how to set up a stress management compliance program for clients.

9. Identify relaxation techniques and apply them to a stress management program.

KEY QUESTIONS FOR STUDENTS

▶ What is stress?

▶ What is the different between stress and distress?

▶ What is the physiology of stress?

▶ What are the bio-psycho-social components of stress?

▶ What are the symptoms of stress?

▶ What are the everyday stressors and hassles in life?

▶ What are the everyday copers that help individuals reduce stress?

▶ How can we reduce the effects of stress?

▶ Can we condition the body to be able to handle stress more effectively?

▶ Is insight into (a) causes of stress, (b) symptoms of stress, and (c) activities to reduce stress helpful in managing stress?

▶ How can we measure an individual's ability to manage stress?

▶ How can we measure the effectiveness of a stress management program?

▶ Can individuals inoculate themselves from stress?

▶ Are some people more vulnerable to stress than others?

▶ How can we effectively teach stress management techniques to individuals who are vulnerable?

▶ What is the relationship between stressful life events and the precipitation of illness?

▶ What are the components of a stress management program?

▶ What is the relationship between stress and the onset of mental illness (e.g., schizophrenia or depression and drug and alcohol addiction)?

▶ What are the results of research studies on the relationships between stress management and mental health?

▶ What are effective relaxation techniques?

▶ How can we integrate biofeedback into a stress management program?

▶ What can we learn from the research on longevity to reduce the effects of stress?

▶ What are some relaxation exercises to counteract stress and to build up our resources?

▶ How can we develop a stress management protocol that can be easily replicated in a psychosocial occupational therapy program?

STRESS AND ITS RELATIONSHIP TO MENTAL ILLNESS

Definition

The understanding of the effects of stress on the causes of mental illness is a fairly recent event. Prior to the 1950s stress was not considered a factor in the onset of a psychiatric illness except for unusual situations such as at a time of disaster or during a war. Currently, there is much interest by investigators in the relationship of stress to the onset of psychological illness. Stress as a variable has been implicated in many diseases—heart attacks, strokes, cancer, and arthritis. The relationship between stress and illness is shown in Figure 10-1.

Hans Selye (1993), an endocrinologist, defined stress as "the *nonspecific* (that is, common) *result of any demand upon the body, be the effect mental or somatic*" (p. 7). By nonspecific, Selye meant that the body responds to all stressors with a common reaction. The response to any stressor creates a change in the autonomic nervous system producing an arousal reaction.

A more technical definition of stress is proposed by Stoyva and Carlson (1993):

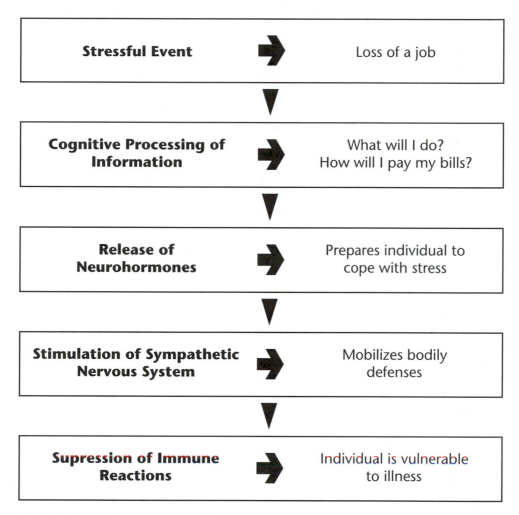

Figure 10–1. The linkage between stress and illness.

[P]sychosocial stress centrally refers to a situation in which the challenges or threats facing the individual exceeds his or her estimated coping resources. The individual perceives a gap between the challenge and the physical and psychological resources he or she judges to be available. The perception of this discrepancy sets off a coordinated pattern of physiological, behavioral, and psychological reactions. (p. 729)

Selye (1974) proposed that there are two types of stress: *eustress* and *distress*. Both eustress and distress arouse the autonomic nervous system and are experienced the same physiologically. However, the outcomes of stress and eustress are different. Distress is considered to be a threat to health and a precipitating factor in disease and mental illness. Lazarus (1993) proposed that distress centers on the negative emotions, such as anger, fright, anxiety, shame, guilt, sadness, envy, jealously, and disgust. On the other hand, eustress is seen as positive emotion, "one designed to achieve the pleasant stress of fulfillment" (Selye, 1993, p. 16). According to Selye (1993), *eustress* is derived from the Greek prefix *eu*, meaning good, as in the terms "euphremia" and "euphoria." Eustress motivates individuals, sets standards on the performance of an individual, and helps the individual to organize goals. Individuals who state that they work better under stress are more accurately stating that they work better under eustress.

Causes of Stress

Stress is caused by a "stressor" and "stress reactivity." A stressor is a stimulus that can trigger the fight-flight-flight response. Walter Cannon (1939), was the first to identify the fight-or-flight response.

In the medical field, stress is considered the rate of wear and tear on the body. The body's response to the stress will always be the same regardless of the stimulus. It is the degree of response that varies, and this depends on the amount of adjustment that is needed by the body. Therefore, it will not matter whether the factor causing the stress is pleasant or unpleasant. There are a variety of situations that are capable of producing stress—not one can be singled out as *the* cause of the reaction. The relationship between stress and physiological dimensions are shown in Table 10–1.

Table 10–1. Simplified Sequential Outline of the Physiology of Stress

1. Agent or stressor in the environment disrupts the body's internal homeostasis
    - death of family member
    - loss of job
    - school failure
    - disappointment

2. Hypothalamus (major CNS control for ANS) is stimulated, changing
    - body temperature
    - endocrinal function
    - cardiovascular response
    - body fluid capacity
    - eye function (mechanical)
    - emotional and rage responses
    - hunger and thirst needs

3. Chemical messenger is released (CRF: corticotrophine releasing factor)

4. Anterior pituitary is stimulated and tropic hormones are secreted

5. Discharge of adrenocorticotropic (ACTH) hormone from the pituitary

6. Adrenal gland is stimulated triggering corticoids

7. Through gluconeogenesis, these compounds supply a ready source of energy (glucose) and fatty acids for the adaptive reactions (fight, fright, or flight)
    - facilitate enzyme response in the sympathetic nervous system
    - suppress immune reactions and inflammations in the parasympathetic responses

Stress as a Precipitating Factor in Mental Illness

Dohrenwend and Dohrenwend (1981) proposed the vulnerability (diathesis–stress model) hypothesis, suggesting that stress triggers an episode of an illness in individuals who have a vulnerability such as migraine headaches, back pain, depression, or schizophrenia. Sources of vulnerability include developmental or genetic factors that lead to a predisposition such as in mental illness. For example, a person who has a genetic marker for bipolar depression (manic-depression) experiences a family environment that includes such dysfunctional factors as inconsistency in parenting, discouragement of self-esteem, and lack of opportunity to express feelings. In the presence of severe stressors such as the pressure to achieve from the family, the lack of appropriate peer interactions and an inability to be productive, the individual may experience a depressive episode. The severity of the depression will depend on the individual's personal and environmental resources. Intelligence, presence of a support group, and opportunity for individual and group counseling are individual resources that can mitigate one against the depression. If the individual had come from a more supportive family, it is possible that even in the presence of severe stressors, the individual would not have experienced an episode of depression. This model is depicted in Figure 10–2. Responses (cognitive, physiological, emotional, and behavioral) are interrelated. While in a depressed state, the person with bipolar depression may sleep too long and not feel like eating, have stomach pains, and be preoccupied with suicidal ideation. When in the manic state, the individual may not sleep, may eat constantly, may also have stomach pains, and have poor judgment with regard to money matters.

Sapolsky (1998), a neuroscientist, supports the diathesis–stress model. In his book, *Why Zebras Don't Get Ulcers: An Updated Guide to Stress, Stress-related Diseases, and Coping*, he discusses the relationship between stress and depression.

> The first stress-depression link is an obvious one. Statistically, stress and the onset of depression tend to go together. People who are undergoing a lot of significant life stressors are more likely than average to succumb to a major depression, and people sunk in their first major depression are more likely than average to have undergone a recent and significant stressor. However, as noted, some people have the grave misfortune of suffering from repeated depressive episodes, ones that can take on a rhythmic pattern stretching over years. When considering the case histories of those people, stressors emerge as triggers for only the first few depressions. Somewhere around the fourth depression or so, a mad clockwork takes over, and the depressive waves crash, regardless of what is going on in the outside world. (p. 247)

In this view, Sapolsky links depression and stress through a neurobiological model. In the first episode of depression, the stressor is predominant; however, in later episodes, individual neurobiological factors come into play and trigger depression.

Symptoms of Stress

Theoretical Assumptions Underlying Research in Stress in Mental Illness

▶ Stress is a precipitating factor in individuals with a vulnerability toward mental illness (diathesis-stress hypothesis; see Figure 10–1). For example, Russo, Vitaliano, Brewer, Katon, and Becker (1995) found that the stress of caregiving precipitated a recurrence of psychiatric illness in individuals with a psychiatric history.

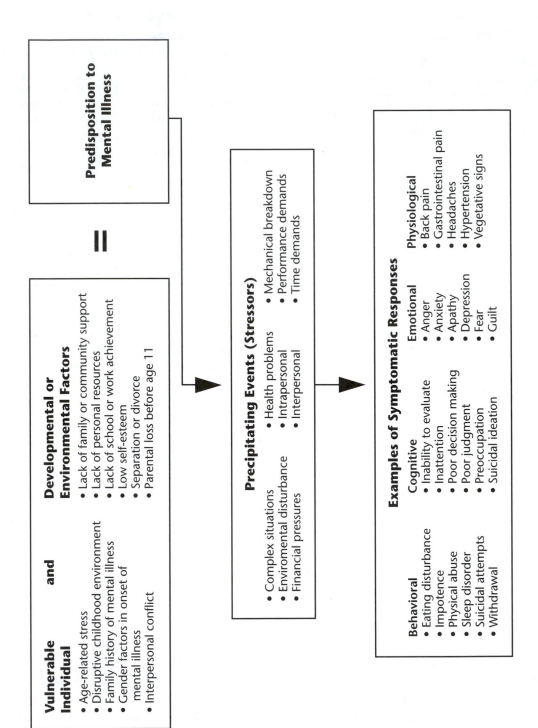

Figure 10–2. Diathesis-Stress Model. Precipitating factors leading to symptoms of mental illness.

▶ Psychophysiogical mechanisms based on genetic coding impact on neurotransmitters such as dopamine and serotonin to affect the etiology of mental illness (vulnerability hypothesis) (Dohrenwend & Dohrenwend, 1981).

▶ Stress impacts on psychophysiological mechanisms (neurotransmitters) affecting the amount or availability of serotonin and dopamine (Anisman & Zacharko, 1992) in a review article concluded that:

> Stressful events cause various neurochemical changes, which have similarities with those associated with depression. It is proposed that stressors cause various neurochemical changes, which have similarities with those associated with depression. It is proposed that stressors cause neurochemical changes which may be of adaptive value. On initial exposure to a stressor, NE (norepinephrine, DA (dopamine), and 5-HT (serotonin) may be released and their synthesis increased. If the stressor is sufficiently severe, and particularly if it is uncontrollable, then release may exceed synthesis, so that levels decline. (p. 41)

▶ Neuroleptic and psychotropic drugs are effective in controlling symptoms in schizophrenia and depression because they impact on reuptake, availability, and depletion of neurotransmitters.

▶ Individuals can learn to self-regulate symptoms through cognitive-behavioral methods emphasizing exercise, relaxation therapy, self-monitoring and daily compliance (Blumenthal et al., 1999; Engel & Rapoff, 1990; Hollon & Beck, 1979; Konkol & Schneider, 1988; Kwako, 1980; Stein & Nikolic, 1989; Stein & Smith, 1989; Stockwell, Duncan, & Levens, 1988; Turk, Meichenbaum, & Genest, 1983).

▶ Psychoeducational methods are effective in teaching patients to self-regulate symptoms (Crist, 1986; Lillie & Armstrong, 1982).

ASSESSMENT OF STRESS

The *Stress Management Questionnaire* (SMQ; Stein, 1986b) is a self-administered paper and pencil test that was developed in 1986 by Stein, at the University of Wisconsin-Milwaukee. The SMQ consists of 158 questions. The questionnaire uses a forced choice format for each item listed and a section for ranking the top 10 symptoms, stressors, or copers covered in each section.

The major purposes of the SMQ are to identify the (a) symptoms and problems precipitated by stress, (b) stressors in the individual's life that cause a stress response, and (c) coping activities that the individual currently uses to manage or alleviate stress. The SMQ can be used clinically to help the therapist and patient to develop an individualized stress management program and as a qualitative outcome measure to evaluate the patient's improvement in managing stress.

Conceptual Definition of Stress as Defined by the SMQ

Stress is defined in the SMQ, as the personal responses or symptoms that are the results of daily situations or thoughts that make life difficult and/or create discomfort. The intensity of the stress reaction will depend on the individual's perceived ability to cope and his or her available resources (copers). Symptoms result from the individual's inability to deal successfully with the stressors. Within the individual's life space, stressors are defined as external, while stressors that are generated by an individual, such as anticipatory anxiety, are internal. In this context stress is depicted as an effect or consequence. On a healthy level, mild or moderate degrees of stress (eustress) can be a motivating force in the individual such as meeting time demands and in public performances.

The Components of the SMQ

The questionnaire has three sections: (a) listing of symptoms, (b) listing of stressors, and (c) listing of coping activities. The SMQ consists of 73 items describing symptoms, 37 items describing stressors, and 48 items describing copers. The questionnaire usually takes about 10 minutes to complete. Individuals completing the questionnaire are asked to check yes or no to (a) a list of symptoms and problems resulting from stress, (b) everyday stressors that precipitate the stress response, and (c) the coping activities that manage or reduce stress. They are then asked to list and rank in order each symptom, stressor, and coper identified. There is also space for individuals to list other items in each of the three categories.

The *symptoms* and problems resulting from stress were generated from four factors:

▶ *Physiological*: such as headaches, tremors, neck/low back pain

▶ *Cognitive*: such as difficulty concentrating, remembering, decision-making

▶ *Emotional*: such as feeling angry, hopeless, tense

▶ *Behavioral*: such as difficulty sleeping, eating and speaking

Everyday *stressors* precipitating stress reactions were grouped under nine factors:

▶ *Complex situations*: such as raising a child as a single parent

▶ *Environmental disturbance*: such as excessive noise

▶ *Financial pressures*: such as loss of income

▶ *Health problems*: such as having the flu

▶ *Interpersonal*: such as arguments with family members

▶ *Intrapersonal*: such as low self-esteem

▶ *Time demands*: such as meeting a deadline at work

▶ *Mechanical breakdown*: such as dealing with a broken household appliance

▶ *Performance demands*: such as taking a test

Everyday activities or occupations that manage or reduce stress (*copers*) were organized into nine factors:

▶ *Appreciation*: such as listening to music

▶ *Creative*: such as writing a poem

▶ *Construction or assembly*: such as knitting a sweater

▶ *Exercise*: such as walking

▶ *Plant and animal care*: such as having a pet

▶ *Performance*: such as singing in a choir

▶ *Self-care*: such as taking a bath

▶ *Social*: such as talking to friends

▶ *Sports*: such as swimming

A final section of the questionnaire asks for demographic information and also poses questions concerning the experience of completing the questionnaire itself.

Conceptual Development of the SMQ

In the development of the SMQ, Stein (1986a) conducted two descriptive studies collecting data from 113 subjects in the first pilot study and 639 subjects in the second study. The concurrence of agreement in a test-retest reliability study of 34 normal subjects ranges from .85 to .89. The instrument was later applied in three clinical research studies: Stein and Neville

(1987), Stein and Nikolic (1989), Stein and Smith (1989).

In these studies the SMQ was used to establish the extent and nature of improved stress responses and lowered stress levels following relaxation and biofeedback therapy. In general the SMQ provides a personal stress profile, which helps the individual to identify stressors and to reduce resultant symptoms by incorporating individual copers into one's everyday life. It is envisaged that the SMQ has wide potential for self-monitoring symptoms, stressors, and copers as part of holistic stress management programs. It can serve as a comprehensive interactive measuring instrument for guided self-understanding and healthy lifestyle planning, for example, in health promotion and disease prevention programs in school and work environments.

The instrument takes account of response-based, stimulus-based, and interactional-stress theories (Bentley & Stein, 1994; Stein, Bentley, & Natz, 1999). Response-based theories describe bodily and psychological patterns of response to causes of stress—in terms of symptomatology, emotions, and personal difficulties. Examples of such theories are Cannon's (1939) "Fight or Flight" syndrome and Hans Selye's (1936), "General Adaptation" syndrome. Stimulus theories are concerned with identifying stressors—the situational causes of the effects described in response theories. Familiar examples of these include: *Life Events* as a cause of stress (Holmes & Rahe, 1967) or the accumulated irritations of daily life encapsulated in such measures as the *Daily Hassles* approach (Kanner, Coyne, Schaefer, & Lazarus, 1981; Kohn & MacDonald, 1992). Other self-report measures of stress are discussed by Derogatis and Coons (1993). This approach is reflected in the SMQs section enumerating stressful situations (stressors). Interactional theories, such as that of Lazarus

and Folkman (1984), emphasize the mediating role of coping and adaptive mechanisms in determining overall levels of stress. This approach is reflected in the SMQ section listing coping responses.

The *Stress Management Questionnaire* (SMQ) is reproduced in Figure 10–3. It may be reproduced as necessary for use in clinical studies. Please send results to Dr. Stein at the University of South Dakota.

APPLICATION OF STRESS MANAGEMENT TO OCCUPATIONAL THERAPY PRACTICE

Psychoeducational occupational therapy programs exemplify cognitive-behavior theory (Bruce & Borg, 1987). Such programs assist the client in broadening one's self-concept, fostering a positive self-image, and acquiring self-management skills. Stress management training, a cognitive behavioral strategy, has been used successfully in the following diagnostic groups:

▶ treatment of depression (Hollon & Beck, 1979; Stein & Smith, 1989)

▶ schizophrenia (Stein, 1987; Stein & Nikolic, 1989)

▶ pain (Engel & Rapoff, 1990; Turk et al., 1983)

▶ substance abuse (Konkol & Schneider, 1988; Stockwell, et al., 1988)

▶ attention deficit disorder with hyperactivity (Kwako, 1980)

The ability to cope with stress has also been evaluated in woman who are homeless (Davis & Kutter, 1998) and women with systemic lupus (Da Costa et al., 1999). In a study by Timmerman, Emmelkamp, and Sanderman (1998) stress management training was found to be effective as compared to a control group. The

Stress Management Questionnaire[1]

For the purpose of this questionnaire, stress refers to the personal responses or symptoms that are the result of daily situations or thoughts that make life difficult and/or create discomfort.

I. When I feel stressful, I experience the following symptoms, feelings, or problems. (Circle Yes (Y) or No (N) for each item.)

Y	N	101. Bleeding ulcer	Y	N	115. High blood pressure
Y	N	102. Blushing	Y	N	116. Hot flashes
Y	N	103. Chest pains	Y	N	117. Indigestion
Y	N	104. Cold hands/feet	Y	N	118. Menstrual changes
Y	N	105. Constipation	Y	N	119. Muscle tension
Y	N	106. Diarrhea	Y	N	120. Nausea
Y	N	107. Difficulty swallowing	Y	N	121. Neck/low back pain
Y	N	108. Dizziness	Y	N	122. Rapid heart rate
Y	N	109. Dryness of mouth	Y	N	123. Skin disorder
Y	N	110. Fatigue	Y	N	124. Stomach pain
Y	N	111. Frequent urination	Y	N	125. Sweaty palms
Y	N	112. Grinding teeth	Y	N	126. Tremors
Y	N	113. Headaches	Y	N	127. Trouble breathing
Y	N	114. Heart burn			

Difficulty:

Y	N	128. Concentrating	Y	N	132. Listening
Y	N	129. Reacting	Y	N	133. Remembering
Y	N	130. Decision making	Y	N	134. Problem solving
Y	N	131. Reasoning	Y	N	135. Thinking

Feeling:

Y	N	136. Angry	Y	N	145. Low tolerance/others
Y	N	137. Anxious	Y	N	146. Moody
Y	N	138. Apathetic	Y	N	147. Nervous
Y	N	139. Defensive	Y	N	148. Panicky
Y	N	140. Fearful	Y	N	149. Resentful
Y	N	141. Guilty	Y	N	150. Restless
Y	N	142. Hopeless	Y	N	151. Self-conscious
Y	N	143. Irritable	Y	N	152. Tense
Y	N	144. A loss of control	Y	N	153. Upset

Problems with:

Y	N	154. Being lazy	Y	N	164. Keeping eye contact
Y	N	155. Biting nails	Y	N	165. Relating to others
Y	N	156. Being obnoxious	Y	N	166. Sitting still
Y	N	157. Being sarcastic	Y	N	167. Sleeping
Y	N	158. Changing tone of voice	Y	N	168. Smoking

[1]Copyright © F. Stein, 1987

(continued)

Figure 10–3. Stress Management Questionnaire. This can be reproduced at will; however, the authors would like the results sent to Dr. Stein at the University of South Dakota.

Stress Management Questionnaire (*continued*)

I. Problems with (*continued*)

Y N	159. Complaining	Y N	169. Speaking
Y N	160. Compulsiveness	Y N	170. Spending money
Y N	161. Drinking	Y N	171. Talking excessively
Y N	162. Eating	Y N	172. Twisting hair
Y N	163. Giving compliments	Y N	173. Other: _____

After you have checked all the items you experience, go back to your responses and rank order below from 1–10* with the rank of "1" being the item experienced most often and is the most troublesome.

SYMPTOMS EXPERIENCED   SYMPTOMS EXPERIENCED

1. _____   6. _____

2. _____   7. _____

3. _____   8. _____

4. _____   9. _____

5. _____   10. _____

*Not everyone will have as many as 10 symptoms or problems.

II. What are the everyday situations or thoughts that cause stress for you? (Circle Yes (Y) or No (N) for each item.)

Y N 201. Arguments with (parents, friends, siblings, children, spouse)
Y N 202. Being evaluated for performance
Y N 203. Being in crowds
Y N 204. Criticism by others
Y N 205. Doing new things for the first time
Y N 206. Driving in traffic
Y N 207. Excessive noise
Y N 208. Feeling too much pressure at school or work
Y N 209. Financial situations
Y N 210. Having problems in relationships
Y N 211. Hearing sad or depressing news
Y N 212. Mechanical breakdown (car, appliance, tools, etc.)
Y N 213. Raising children along
Y N 214. "Red tape" (filling out forms, waiting in lines, etc.)
Y N 215. Speaking in front of groups
Y N 216. Taking tests
Y N 217. Being alone
Y N 218. Being bored
Y N 219. Being late for an appointment

(*continued*)

Figure 10–3. Stress Management Questionnaire (*continued*)

Stress Management Questionnaire (*continued*)

II. (*continued*)

Y   N   220.   Being unprepared (date, test, guests, speaking, etc.)
Y   N   221.   Being watched by others
Y   N   222.   Failure to meet goals (expected of you)
Y   N   223.   Feeling guilty for inadequate behavior
Y   N   224.   Feeling frustrated
Y   N   225.   Gaining or losing weight
Y   N   226.   Having no control over a situation
Y   N   227.   Having too many things to do with not enough time
Y   N   228.   Lack of confidence in oneself
Y   N   229.   Misplacing something
Y   N   230.   Meeting deadlines
Y   N   231.   Not having any free time for oneself or friends
Y   N   232.   Not knowing what is expected of you
Y   N   233.   Poor performance on a test
Y   N   234.   Studying for an exam
Y   N   235.   Trying to please people
Y   N   236.   Waiting for expected letter or decision
Y   N   237.   Other (please list): _____

After you have checked all the items you experience, go back to your responses and rank order below from 1–10* with the rank of "1" being the most stressful situation or thought.

SITUATIONS/THOUGHTS   SITUATIONS/THOUGHTS
CAUSING STRESS   CAUSING STRESS

1. _____   6. _____

2. _____   7. _____

3. _____   8. _____

4. _____   9. _____

5. _____   10. _____

*Rank order only those situations or thoughts that apply to you. Not everyone will have 10 items.

III. List the following activities which help you relieve stress, by circling Yes (Y) or No (N) for each item.

Y   N   301.   Analyze situation   Y   N   325.   Needlecraft
Y   N   302.   Avoid situation   Y   N   326.   Painting

(*continued*)

Figure 10–3. Stress Management Questionnaire (*continued*)

Stress Management Questionnaire *(continued)*

III. *(continued)*

Y	N	303.	Be active in social club	Y	N	327.	Play musical instrument
Y	N	304.	Baking	Y	N	328.	Prepare for school/work
Y	N	305.	Being by myself	Y	N	329.	Read for pleasure
Y	N	306.	Being busy	Y	N	330.	Relax (lie down)
Y	N	307.	Bicycling	Y	N	331.	Running long distance
Y	N	308.	Cleaning house	Y	N	332.	Screaming
Y	N	309.	Cooking	Y	N	333.	Sex
Y	N	310.	Crocheting	Y	N	334.	Singing
Y	N	311.	Crying	Y	N	335.	Sleeping
Y	N	312.	Dancing	Y	N	336.	Stretching muscles
Y	N	313.	Deep breathing	Y	N	337.	Swimming
Y	N	314.	Drawing	Y	N	338.	Take a drive in a car
Y	N	315.	Eating	Y	N	339.	Take care of a pet
Y	N	316.	Exercising	Y	N	340.	Talk to a friend
Y	N	317.	Gardening	Y	N	341.	Throw something
Y	N	318.	Go shopping	Y	N	342.	Visit friends
Y	N	319.	Go to dinner	Y	N	343.	Watch TV
Y	N	320.	Go to movie	Y	N	344.	Walking
Y	N	321.	Hot shower/bath	Y	N	345.	Writing letters
Y	N	322.	Jogging	Y	N	346.	Writing poetry
Y	N	323.	Listen to music	Y	N	347.	Writing short stories
Y	N	324.	Meditate or pray	Y	N	348.	Yoga

Please list any other activities which help you relieve stress.

Y   N   349. Other _____

Again rank order your responses 1–10* with the rank of "1" being the activity which most relieves your stress.

ACTIVITIES THAT RELIEVE STRESS   ACTIVITIES THAT RELIEVE STRESS

1. _____   6. _____

2. _____   7. _____

3. _____   8. _____

4. _____   9. _____

5. _____   10. _____

*Rank as many items up to 10 that are appropriate to you.

(continued)

Figure 10–3. Stress Management Questionnaire *(continued)*

Stress Management Questionnaire (*continued*)

Evaluation of Stress Management Questionnaire

We are interested in improving the usefulness and clarity of this questionnaire. Your feedback and reponses will be helpful to us in revising the questionnaire.

Please circle Yes, No, or Unsure.

1.	Was the questionnaire too long?	Yes	No	Unsure
2.	Were the directions clear?	Yes	No	Unsure
3.	Did you find the questionnaire interesting?	Yes	No	Unsure
4.	Did the list of items accurately reflect your feelings?	Yes	No	Unsure
5.	Did the questionnaire help you to become more aware of the stressors in your everyday life?	Yes	No	Unsure
6.	Did you identify from the questionnaire any new methods to manage stress?	Yes	No	Unsure
7.	Do you feel you would benefit from an individualized stress management program?	Yes	No	Unsure
8.	When you are stressful do you use alcohol?	Yes	No	
	When you are stressful do you use drugs?	Yes	No	
	When you are stressful do you use cigarettes?	Yes	No	

422.   GENDER _____

423.   YEAR OF BIRTH _____

424.   OCCUPATION _____

425.   LEVEL OF EDUCATION COMPLETED _____

426.   STUDENT MAJOR IN COLLEGE (if applicable) _____

427.   MARITAL STATUS _____

428.   TODAY'S DATE _____

Figure 10–3. Stress Management Questionnaire *(continued)*

authors reported that the clients in the training group had "less distress, less trait anxiety, less daily hassles, more assertiveness, and more satisfaction with social support at follow-up" (p. 863).

Designing a Stress Management Program

The outline that follows describes the major questions that an occupational therapist will need to answer in designing a stress management program for clients with psychosocial diagnoses.

DESIGNING STRESS MANAGEMENT PROGRAM
IN PSYCHOSOCIAL OCCUPATIONAL THERAPY

1. What is the target population?

    _____ Children   _____ Adolescents   _____ Adults   _____ Elderly

2. What is the diagnostic group?

    _____ Learning Disability   _____ Eating Disorder   _____ Schizophrenia

    _____ Post Traumatic Stress Disorder (PTSD)   _____ Affective Disorders

    _____ Chemical Dependence and Substance Abuse

3. What are the specific therapy goals for the group or the individual?

    _____ increase client's awareness of how stressors cause symptoms

    _____ increase client's awareness of the relationship between activity and the reduction of stress

    _____ increase compliance to stress management program

    _____ learn new way to manage stress through relaxation therapy

    _____ reduce anxiety

    _____ teach clients the psychological mechanisms of stress

    _____ teach intervention techniques as copers of stress

    _____ teach preventative techniques and self-regulation to stress

4. Will stress management be done individually or in group?

5. What is the environment for stress management?

    _____ private, no distractions, quiet

    _____ gymnasium or large exercise room

    _____ other

6. If group sessions, how many clients will be selected? Will clients be selected for specific reasons so as to balance group?

7. How long will group meet (i.e., hours per week, number of sessions)? Will it be open-ended or close-ended group?

8. Will group be co-led?

(continued)

**DESIGNING STRESS MANAGEMENT PROGRAM
IN PSYCHOSOCIAL OCCUPATIONAL THERAPY** *(continued)*

9. Group Methodology: What will be the content and modalities of group sessions?

_____ adapted for needs of client, (e.g., developmental disabilities)

_____ arts and crafts and creative media

_____ biofeedback

_____ creative literary media

_____ dealing with occupational stress

_____ horticulture

_____ nutrition/health awareness

_____ prescriptive exercise

_____ progressive relaxation

_____ relaxation response

_____ role playing

_____ use of *Stress Management Questionnaire* (Stein, 1986b)

_____ visualization

_____ values clarification

10. How will client and therapists evaluate effectiveness of stress management program?

_____ biofeedback measures pre- and posttest individual interventions

_____ client completes daily diary of stress management

_____ qualitative evaluation by ward personnel and or family members

_____ standardized test pre- and posttest first and last session

_____ standardized test, pre- and posttest for every session

_____ subjective evaluation by client

11. What are potential problems that can interfere with the effectiveness of the stress management program?

_____ information and program activities presented are not congruent with client cognitive potential, acute symptoms, severity of disability

_____ lack of attendance, absenteeism

_____ lack of commitment from treatment staff

_____ lack of data in evaluating program

_____ lack of follow-up by client-compliance

_____ poor client interest or motivation

_____ poor environment—creating distractions

(continued)

**DESIGNING STRESS MANAGEMENT PROGRAM
IN PSYCHOSOCIAL OCCUPATIONAL THERAPY** *(continued)*

12. How will clients be followed up to determine:
    A. effectiveness of intervention?
    B. compliance with stress management program?
    C. presenting opportunities for ongoing programs?

13. How can clinical research in occupational therapy be used to objectively evaluate and report results?

Psychoeducational Model[1]

A psychoeducational approach can be incorporated into a cognitive-behavioral therapy. In this approach, the therapist uses educational technology integrating lecture methods, discussion, role playing, behavioral rehearsal, homework, and laboratory experiences. An example of an educational model is described in the following material:

▶ A *course schedule* presented to individuals who have either been hospitalized for depression or have been treated for depression in the community. Participants in the course come from a chapter of the Manic-Depression Society. All participants volunteered to participate in the group after receiving a letter of invitation that described the purposes of the group and the sessions involved. The course description, objectives and outline of the sessions were distributed to the group's 18 members on the first day of the course

▶ *Handouts* on (a) stress management as a critical life skill, (b) getting up in the morning, (c) sleep hygiene, and (d) humor

▶ *Compliance* with stress management program

▶ *Example* of individualized compliance form

---

[1]The material in this section is intended to be incorporated into a psychoeducational program for clients attending a stress management group. It can be used as a handout to clients and as a basis for discussion.

Course Outline

RELAXATION TECHNIQUES TO PREVENT DEPRESSION

Instructor: Frank Stein, PhD, OTR

Description of the Course

This course is intended to help individuals who have experienced severe depression. The course is divided into lectures, discussions and practical demonstrations. The course will meet for eight consecutive weeks for approximately 11/2 hours. The content of the course will be discussions of the causes, symptoms, and treatment of depression; discussions on the effects of stress and coping skills; and practical demonstrations of relaxation techniques.

Specific Objectives of the Course:

By the end of the course the adult learner will:

▶ understand the dynamics of depression as a biopsychosocial illness

▶ understand the symptoms of stress, the stressors that trigger stress, and the copers that are effective in managing stress

▶ incorporate a stress management program into his or her everyday life

▶ learn the Benson Relaxation Response

▶ learn how to do the Jacobson Progressive Relaxation

▶ use visual imagery as a relaxation technique

▶ use behavioral strategies to cope with the symptoms of depression such as insomnia, eating disturbance, difficulty getting up in the morning, sad mood, low energy, low self-esteem, poor concentration, and inability to feel pleasure

▶ understand the use of biofeedback as a technique for self-regulation of anxiety

▶ practice other techniques to prevent and cope with depression

Tentative Schedule for Class

SESSION 1

▶ Introduction and objectives of course

▶ Discussion of depression

▶ Benson Relaxation Response

SESSION 2

▶ Discussion of the relationship between stress and the onset of symptoms

▶ Progressive Relaxation

▶ Getting up in the morning

(continued)

RELAXATION TECHNIQUES TO PREVENT DEPRESSION *(continued)*

SESSION 3

▶ Discussion of the everyday stressors

▶ Visual Imagery

▶ Preventing insomnia

SESSION 4

▶ Discussion of the copers and resources in managing stress

▶ Biofeedback

▶ Exercise as a method to go from sad to glad

SESSION 5

▶ Discussion of pleasant activities in one's life

▶ Role playing stressful situations

▶ The gourmet in you, food as enjoyment

SESSION 6

▶ Setting up an Individualized Stress Management Program

▶ Learning how to control feelings by self-talk

▶ Activities to increase concentration

SESSION 7

▶ Techniques to use to interrupt negative thoughts such as music, concentrating on activity, sports, and others

▶ Paradoxical Intention or consciously producing anxiety and depression so as to control the feelings

SESSION 8

▶ Closure activity: Individual evaluation of the experience

▶ Our reward a picnic or dinner or whatever the group decides

Student Assignments

▶ Complete SMQ

▶ Practice relaxation techniques everyday

▶ Set up daily schedule for toughening self against depression

▶ Keep diary of symptoms, stressors and copers

▶ Write a first person account of illness

Handout on Stress Management

STRESS MANAGEMENT AS A CRITICAL LIFE SKILL

What is stress and what is its relationship to illness? Stress can be defined as either a cause or an effect. As a cause, stress is an everyday event in a person's life. Some examples are the pressure to do well on an examination, the fear of being rejected by a friend, the reaction to a loss of a job, or an anxious thought about the future. These situations are referred to as stressors that trigger a reaction in the individual. The body reacts to these stressors by increasing the response rate such as increasing heart rate, blood pressure, and metabolism. When an individual perceives that he or she is under pressure the body mobilizes as if it is under attack. If the response is intense or prolonged it can lead to symptoms such as headaches, heartburn, blurring of vision, anxiety, or numerous other common problems.

How the individual responds to a stressor is the key to managing stress. For example being able to talk about a stressful event with a friend or good listener will ease the stress. Exercising will help in dissipating the negative buildup of energy of a stressor. Listening to relaxing music, writing letters, cleaning house, doing crossword puzzles, or any number of activities can be used as stress reducers. Managing stress should be a key part in everyone's daily routine just like brushing our teeth and eating regularly.

If we accept the fact that individuals will encounter situations in their daily lives that will cause stress then we should be prepared to deal with stress. One way to help ourselves deal with stress is to toughen ourselves physically and mentally so that we can cope well with the tasks at hand. Toughening oneself means developing the resources within us and in our lives through positive personal relationships and the buildup of our physical strength. For example, building up physical health through exercise and sports can condition the body to handle the symptoms of stress and also increase the potential of the immune system to react. Being in a support group on a continuous basis builds up a network of people resources especially for individuals who are vulnerable in developing symptoms of mental illness. When an individual is under severe stress, the weakest or most sensitive area becomes most at risk.

For example, if an individual is vulnerable to migraine headaches, stress will precipitate this symptom. For a person with a tendency to become depressed under severe pressure a stressful event or thought can trigger an episode of depression. Recent research findings have shown that the major mental illnesses such as depression and schizophrenia are episodic illnesses with periods of intense symptoms and remissions. These symptoms are usually triggered by stress which can be external such as a loss of a job or internal such as harboring negative thoughts about oneself. The ability of an individual to cope with these stressors before they become overwhelming is critical in preventing an episode of mental illness.

Coping effectively with stress means accepting the fact that everyone experiences stress everyday and that we are all at risk in developing symptoms that are related to common illnesses and diseases. We are best able to respond to stress when we are healthy. When we are run down and already ill, stress becomes an additional factor in the onset of disease. Prevention is a better alternative than cure. To prevent episodes of mental illness the individual should develop an everyday strategy that produces maximum health. Activities should be incorporated into an individual's daily life. Time should be set aside everyday for talking to someone you like and trust, listening to relaxing music, exercising, reading, doing a craft activity or engaging in other activities that one finds pleasant or productive. The key is to do the activities on a consistent basis so that it becomes part of one's daily routine. I like to visualize stress management as a toughening exercise that prepares you for the hassles of everyday life.

(continued)

STRESS MANAGEMENT AS A CRITICAL LIFE SKILL *(continued)*

Managing stress effectively starts with developing a systematic strategy by answering three questions: (a) what are the symptoms and problems that occur when I am stressful? (b) what are the everyday hassles that trigger my stress? and (c) what are the best methods or activities that have been effective in the past to cope with my stress? Each individual will answer these questions uniquely. For example the symptoms of stress include four basic areas: (a) *cognitive*, such as difficulty in concentrating or learning; (b) *emotional*, such as feeling anxious; (c) *physiological*, such as neck pain; and (d) *behavioral*, such as difficulty sleeping. The everyday stressors or hassles include having too many things to do and not enough time, arguments with friends and family, and feeling rejected. The copers are the positive activities or behaviors that in the past have been effective in making us feel more relaxed, less anxious, and generally more secure about ourselves. These copers include talking to an empathetic listener, listening to music, taking a long walk, engaging in a craft activity, or playing with your cat. A stress diary is an excellent way to gain insight into what makes us stressful and what we do successfully to manage our stress. By handling our stress effectively we are promoting our own mental health.

The last point in dealing with stress is to put humor into our lives by learning how to laugh at oneself and with other people. A good laugh a day is better than the proverbial apple.

Handout on Sleep Hygiene

SELF-REGULATING RESTFUL SLEEP

▶ Set a specific time for going to bed and getting up in the morning. Give yourself a little leeway on the weekends. As a rule go to bed when you are drowsy. Your body will become conditioned to a specific bedtime.

▶ Do not take afternoon naps. If you feel tired during the day, try meditating for 10 to 15 minutes. This should make you feel more energetic.

▶ Exercise in the morning and early evening such as before dinner is desirable. Do not exercise 2 hours before bedtime. Vigorous exercise will arouse your body.

▶ Maintain a cool temperature in the bedroom. Preferably keep a window open during the times of year when it is possible and the noise isn't disturbing. As a rule use blankets to keep warm rather than overheating the room.

▶ A warm bath before going to bed may make you feel drowsy, especially if the bedroom is cool.

▶ A light snack before going to bed is sometimes helpful. However chocolate or excessive sweets may keep you awake. A glass of low-fat milk and some crackers are sufficient.

▶ Do not drink alcohol within 2 hours of your bedtime. Although alcohol is a depressant and may initially make you feel drowsy, it has a delayed effect that may lead to restlessness during the night. It also may upset your stomach. In addition if you are on medication there may be an interactive effect that could be detrimental.

▶ Coffee, caffeinated tea or soda serve as stimulants and could keep you awake. The effect of caffeine takes about 6 hours to wear off.

▶ Some people actually become drowsy by reading, listening to music, or watching television. Other people need a completely quiet and dark room to fall asleep. Try to find out what is the best environment for you.

▶ Visualization of pleasant experiences, past or future, has been helpful for some individuals in falling asleep especially when feeling tense, stressful, or preoccupied with disturbing thoughts. The individual is encouraged to think of a past scene in one's life that is serene and or pleasurable. The individual then tries to recapture the sensory experiences surrounding the event.

Handout on Humor

HUMOR AS A MEANS TO COUNTERACT DEPRESSION

1. What is humor?

2. What makes us laugh?

3. What is a funny story?

4. Why does humor make us feel good?

5. What are different types of humor?

6. How do you develop a sense of humor?

7. Can we learn how to tell a funny story?

8. Comedy styles
   —The wit, thinks while he is talking
   —Satirist finds humor in the daily news
   —Punster has fun with words
   —Clown exaggerates life
   —Joke teller has a stock of stories
   —Kidder loves to tease
   —Masochist loves to put him- or herself down, a la Rodney Dangerfield

9. Collect funny stories from books, magazines, TV, friends

10. Try to take a philosophical view of life

Handout on Getting Up in the Morning

GETTING UP IN THE MORNING

A morning ritual should be established that arouses the body and activates the individual. This includes:

▶ Getting up at a set time everyday such as 7:15 a.m.

▶ Putting on a bright light as soon as the alarm goes off. The light arouses the neurological system. Research on Seasonal Affective Disorders (SAD) verifies the importance of light in countering depression.

▶ Listening to a melodic music such as Bach's Brandenburg Concerti, Mozart, or Vivaldi, or other individual pieces that are pleasant to listen to and are stimulating. Music is another way to arouse the neurological system.

▶ Taking a warm bath for about 10 to 15 minutes followed by a stimulating shower. Water and heat tone the muscles and joints of the body while reducing muscle tension. The individual is now prepared to do morning exercise.

▶ Morning exercises should be conservative in nature in that they do not put undue stress on the muscles, joints and cardiovascular system. The main purpose of the exercises is to tone the muscles and joints. Exercise is an excellent activity to counteract depression. The morning exercise of about 10 minutes should be seen as preventative with regard to back injuries and as helping to build muscle strength and to maintain range of muscles in the joints. Stress management exercise of tensing and releasing the muscles of the face are good starting activity. Other suggestions are push-ups, modified sit-ups, stretching upper and lower extremities, jogging in place, and leg raises while on your back.

BREAKFAST AND IMPLICATIONS FOR NUTRITION

▶ It is probably a good idea to take a multivitamin every day. This way you are insured of obtaining the essential vitamins that are necessary for sustaining health and preventing disease. This is the most conservative approach. On the other hand, megavitamins or massive doses of vitamins can be detrimental.

▶ Breakfast is probably the most important meal especially for an individual with a tendency toward depression. The suggested breakfast should include a citrus fruit (Vitamin C), grains (Vitamin B), and coffee (stimulant).

Compliance

An important aspect of any stress management program is to help the client comply with the recommendations that were jointly agreed on by the therapist and client. The model below is an example of operationalizing a stress management program by defining the activity to be engaged in, explaining the therapeutic purpose of the activity, and having the client individualize the activity so that it is feasible and meets his or her unique needs. For example, in the first activity in the following compliance tool, therapist and client agree that talking to a personal friend or relative on an ongoing basis will help the client release feelings and be able to analyze a situation as a means of dealing with the stress of everyday life. In the individual response, the client records the specific plan to meet this objective and how he or she monitors the implementation.

COMPLIANCE: INDIVIDUALIZED STRESS MANAGEMENT PROGRAM

1. *Activity* –Talk to personal friend or relative on ongoing basis to discuss the stresses and strains of everyday life.

   Purpose – Release of feelings and opportunity to analyze situations.

   Individual Response – For example: "I will telephone friend 1 time per week."

2. *Activity* – Exercise periods of 5 to 45 minutes every day. For example, 5 minute flexion exercise in morning, 5 minutes Progressive Relaxation after lunch and 2-mile walk after dinner.

   Purpose – Reduce muscular tension and to work out pent up emotions.

   Individual Response – For example: "Before breakfast I will do stretching exercises for 10 minutes and at 5 p.m. I will take a walk in the neighborhood."

3. *Activity* – Engage in ongoing activity that leads to a finished project, such as a home improvement, model, fibers project.

   Purpose – Increase self esteem and feelings of accomplishment.

   Individual Response – For example, "I will crochet 1 hour everyday after dinner."

4. *Activity* – Volunteer in social service agency, school or library.

   Purpose – Provides opportunity to help others and at the same time creates meaning in one's life. Increases responsibility and commitment.

   Individual Response – For example, "I will volunteer in the library on Saturday mornings."

5. *Activity* – Active participation in social support or self-help group such as Recovery Inc., Single People Together, AA and Alliance for the Mentally Ill (AMI).

   Purpose – Provides for ongoing support - especially during periods of crisis.

   Individual Response – For example, "I will attend an AMI meeting 1 time per month."

(continued)

COMPLIANCE: INDIVIDUALIZED STRESS MANAGEMENT PROGRAM *(continued)*

6. *Activity* – Monitoring diet because of a concern with nutrition and input.

   Purpose – Help body cope with physical and psychological effects of stress.

   Individual Response – For example, "I will record daily food I consume and ensure that I eat 5 fruits and vegetables a day."

7. *Activity* – Ongoing concern with body appearance.

   Purpose – Increase self-esteem.

   Individual Response – For example, "I will use cleansing cream on my face before going to bed."

8. *Activity* – Taking responsibility for plant or animal.

   Purpose – Increase opportunity to nurture and make a commitment to life.

   Individual Response – For example, "I will care for a cat."

9. *Activity* – Engage every day in other stress reduction activities, for example, Progressive Relaxation, yoga, quieting response, visualization, meditation, biofeedback.

   Purpose – Inoculate self against negative effects of stress by incorporating relaxation response.

   Individual Response– For example, "I will take a class in Tai Ch'i."

10. *Activity* – Eliminate or reduce: excessive alcohol, reliance on abusive drugs, smoking, excessive caffeine, excessive "junk foods."

    Purpose – Increase body's resistance to stressors.

    Individual Response– For example, "I will drink only one cup of coffee per day and eliminate junk foods from my diet."

Example of an Individualized Compliance Outcome

Outcome Evaluation for Self-regulation of Symptoms								
Put a check mark for each positive activity for everyday								
	Tues	Wed	Thurs	Fri	Sat	Sun	Mon	Tues
SLEEPING BEHAVIOR								
• asleep before 30 minutes in bed	☐	☐	☐	☐	☐	☐	☐	☐
• 6 $^1/_2$ hours of continuous sleep	☐	☐	☐	☐	☐	☐	☐	☐
• awaken in the morning refreshed	☐	☐	☐	☐	☐	☐	☐	☐
EXERCISE								
• 15 minutes of morning routine	☐	☐	☐	☐	☐	☐	☐	☐
• 30 to 45 minutes of aerobics	☐	☐	☐	☐	☐	☐	☐	☐
MEDITATION								
• 10 minutes of Relaxation Response	☐	☐	☐	☐	☐	☐	☐	☐
COMMUNICATION								
• shared worries with supportive listener	☐	☐	☐	☐	☐	☐	☐	☐
• specify below, major concerns	☐	☐	☐	☐	☐	☐	☐	☐
1. _____	☐	☐	☐	☐	☐	☐	☐	☐
2. _____	☐	☐	☐	☐	☐	☐	☐	☐
3. _____	☐	☐	☐	☐	☐	☐	☐	☐
LEARNING NEW ACTIVITY								
• spent time practicing or learning skill (e.g., music, computer, craft)	☐	☐	☐	☐	☐	☐	☐	☐
• specify activity below	☐	☐	☐	☐	☐	☐	☐	☐
1. _____	☐	☐	☐	☐	☐	☐	☐	☐
2. _____	☐	☐	☐	☐	☐	☐	☐	☐
3. _____	☐	☐	☐	☐	☐	☐	☐	☐
READING								
• spent time reading (e.g., fiction, history, biography) for enjoyment	☐	☐	☐	☐	☐	☐	☐	☐
• specify book below	☐	☐	☐	☐	☐	☐	☐	☐
1. _____	☐	☐	☐	☐	☐	☐	☐	☐

Outcome Evaluation for Self-regulation of Symptoms								
Put a check mark for each positive activity for everyday								
	Tues	Wed	Thurs	Fri	Sat	Sun	Mon	Tues
CUISINE								
• selected favorite food for meal	☐	☐	☐	☐	☐	☐	☐	☐
• specify food below	☐	☐	☐	☐	☐	☐	☐	☐
1. _____	☐	☐	☐	☐	☐	☐	☐	☐
2. _____	☐	☐	☐	☐	☐	☐	☐	☐
Total Checks for the Day								

BIOFEEDBACK

Definition of Biofeedback

The term *biofeedback* was officially defined at the first meeting of the Biofeedback Research Society in 1969 as "any technique using instrumentation to give a person immediate and continuing signals in changes in a bodily function that he is not usually conscious of such as fluctuating blood pressure; brain wave activity or muscle tension. The individual is then able to use the information to learn how to control these functions which were in the past automatic and involuntary" (personal communication from the Biofeedback Research Society, Santa Monica, CA, 1969). Barbara Brown (1974, 1977), a psychologist and one of the forerunners in research in biofeedback, defined biofeedback as a nonspecific therapy, that is, a technique for the mastery of psychogenic stress by bringing into awareness certain physiological measures such as change in heart rate, a rise in blood pressure, muscular tension, brain wave activity, or any combination of these. From a medical perspective, Schuster (1977), a physician, defined biofeedback as a technique for training the

mind to control bodily functions. He considered it to be a form of behavioral therapy, whose methodology is based on operant conditioning.

In 1995, Schwartz and Schwartz defined biofeedback in the following way:

As a process, applied biofeedback is:

1. A group of therapeutic procedures that ...
2. uses electronic or electromechanical instruments ...
3. to accurately measure, process, and feed back, to persons *and their therapists* ...
4. information with *educational* and reinforcing properties ...
5. about their neuromuscular and autonomic activity, both normal and abnormal ...
6. in the form of analogue or binary, auditory and/or visual feedback signals.
7. Best achieved with a competent biofeedback professional, the objectives are ...
8. to help persons develop greater awareness *of, confidence in, and an increase in* voluntary control over their physiological processes that are otherwise outside awareness and/or under less voluntary control ...
9. by first controlling the external signal, ...
10. and then with internal psychophysiological *cognitions, and/or by engaging in and*

applying behaviors to prevent symptom onset, stop it, or reduce it soon after onset. (p. 41)

All of these definitions imply that biofeedback is a learned behavioral technique that enables the individual to regulate bodily functions that traditionally have been thought to be automatic and unconscious. Biofeedback as a therapeutic method has primarily been used to reduce the damaging effects of stress that is linked to anxiety (Townsend, House, & Addario, 1975).

Biofeedback also can be potentially useful in helping an individual to decrease habitual self-defeating behavior such as drug and alcohol abuse (Peniston & Kulkosky, 1989) that interfere with social adjustment.

Biofeedback as a Cybernetic Model

In its most elemental form, biofeedback is essentially based on the principle of cybernetics (Weiner, 1948), that is, an input-process-output. Input can represent any cognitive information that precipitates or "triggers off" an internal physiological response. Process represents the internal emotional reactions and physiological changes. The output is the organism's behavioral responses. Information can arouse and change the organism's emotional and physiological state, causing an action response.

For example, a telegram reporting the death of a close relative can produce an emotion of sadness, abdominal pain, and a lessening of physical activities. Diagrammatically, this can be represented by the following:

INPUT	→	PROCESS	→	OUTPUT
External Event		*Internal Reaction:*		*Behavior*
(e.g., telegram reporting death of close relative)		Emotional reactions and physiological changes		(e.g., decreased activity, a symptom of depression)

In analyzing an emotional response Lazarus (1975) stated that: "I define and analyze emotion as a complex disturbance which includes three main components: subjective affect, physiological changes related to species-specific forms of mobilization for adaptive action, and action impulse having both instrumental and expressive qualities" (p. 554). In Lazarus' model the following occurs during the process stage:

INPUT	→	PROCESS	→	OUTPUT

Subjective Affect (e.g., anger)

Physiological Changes (e.g., heightened blood pressure)

Action Impulses (e.g., verbalizations)

having both

Instrumental and Expressive Qualities

In this model Lazarus separated out the impulse to act and the resultant actions. In fact, the actions may be inhibited because of social or internal pressure. However, the external event (*input*) elicited in the individual, emotional, physiological, and cognitive responses. These responses may or may not stimulate the individual to act. In biofeedback therapy this information enables the individual to become aware of his or her own internal responses and, as a result, to be able to control or express these responses.

Biofeedback is a method to enable the individual to be aware of sensations and detect change in his/her internal state of bodily functions (Stoyva & Budzynski, 1993). These sensations, which are unique to each individual, are associated with a bodily function. For example, physical and psychological sensations to the individual can alert us to whether our heart is beating quickly, a headache is impending, or we are experiencing anxiety. Biofeedback is a self-regulating activity that enables the individual to become acutely aware of bodily processes. There are common indicators of internal emotional reactions that are manifested in external signs. For example, individuals who are experiencing anxiety internally may show their anxiety externally by speaking in a high-pitched voice, having a dry mouth, having cold sweaty hands, have a slight hand or knee tremor, having an urgency to urinate, or through a stammer show other signs of fear. The first step in self-regulating behavior is to help the client become aware of the individual symptoms or behaviors that are associated with emotional reactions. This initial training in biofeedback is designed to help the individual become aware of what the body is telling him or her through the psycho-physiological system by using machines such as a heart rate monitor, finger temperature trainer, EMG, or galvanic skin response.

The knowledge that the individual's internal environment is affected by external events was first recognized by the French physiologist Claude Bernard in 1865 (Bernard 1865/1957). A number of researchers since Bernard have demonstrated that a constant internal environment is important in health maintenance. W. B. Cannon (1939) introduced the concept of homeostasis to describe the brain's automatic function in regulating internal visceral responses. The body has a number of physiological mechanisms that serve as biofeedback loops in keeping a constant internal environment. For example, warm body temperature is controlled by sweating, causing water evaporation that produces a cooling effect. When the body is cold, blood vessels constrict, and less of the blood is cooled in the hands, feet, and extremities. The regulation of a constant body temperature is controlled by thermostatic mechanisms that trigger autonomic nervous system responses. The diagram below explains this relationship.

INPUT	→	PROCESS	→	OUTPUT
Body temperature changes	Thermosensors in body	Hypothalamus controls body temperature		Vasomotor responses

▼

Warm responses *vasodilation*

OR

Cold responses *vasoconstriction*

Blood sugar level is another example of thermostatic control in the human body. The mechanism for control is diagrammed below:

INPUT	→	PROCESS	→	OUTPUT
Increased blood glucose level		Glucoreceptors in hypothalamus stimulate islet cells of Langerhans in pancreas		Secretion of insulin to reduce blood glucose level

Other self-regulating mechanisms controlled by the hypothalamus in autonomic reactions follow (Barr & Kiernan, 1993; Gilman & Newman, 1992):

▶ regulation of body temperature
▶ coordination of feeding and drinking with gastrointestinal functions
▶ fluid balance
▶ carbohydrate and fat metabolism
▶ blood pressure
▶ sexual function
▶ sleep
▶ emotional states

Autonomic Nervous

System and Biofeedback

Biofeedback theory is based on the voluntary control of autonomic nervous system responses. The landmark study by Miller (1969) established the possibility that animals could learn to control visceral and glandular responses that were previously thought to be involuntary and autonomic. Although Miller's discovery came as a surprise to many traditional scientists, there was evidence that Indian yogas could voluntarily control blood pressure, pain, heart rate, and respiratory rate by bringing the body into a relaxed, meditative state (Green, Green, & Walters, 1970). An understanding of the effects of the autonomic nervous system (ANS) on visceral organs as listed in Table 10–2 is essential in becoming an effective biofeedback trainer.

> Under ordinary circumstances, the ANS functions at the subconscious level. It acts to regulate the ongoing, reflexively driven activity of smooth muscle, cardiac muscle, and glands, and integrates visceral systems with one another and with somatic motor functions. (Gilman & Newman, 1992, p. 43)

In general, when an individual is highly emotional or under severe stress, sympathetic responses of the autonomic nervous system dominate behavior due to the increased epinephrine or adrenaline. "When the flight-or-flight response is activated, there is a sudden, massive increase in metabolic rate: increased blood pressure and heart rate and the increased blood flow to the heart, brain and muscles" (Preston, O'Neal, & Talaga, 1994, pp. 39, 42). Additionally, these responses include increased activity in the sweat glands, dilation of pupils, and increased glucose for energy. The individual may experience "goose bumps" on the skin. Digestion of food in the gastrointestinal system is interrupted. When the body is at rest or an individual is meditating, the parasympathetic responses dominate behavior. These responses result in a slowed heart rate, decreased blood pressure, normal digestion of food, and increased secretion of thin saliva. The neurotransmitter acetylcholine is implicated in the parasympathetic responses.

Biofeedback Modalities

The biofeedback modalities most commonly used in clinical practice are the following:

Electromyographic (EMG)

EMG biofeedback is used for relaxation training, reduction of tension headaches, muscle re-education, and in conjunction with behavior modification to desensitize the patient for phobias. In EMG biofeedback, the patient first becomes responsive to the state of muscle tension and then later develops control in relaxing specific muscle groupings.

A common body site for EMG biofeedback for relaxation/training is the frontalis muscle located in the forehead. The individual uses auditory and visual output from the EMG to learn how to reduce muscle tension and thereby to increase relaxation. The electrical impulse from the muscle is transmitted by a transducer (surface electrode) to a signal amplifier which magnifies the impulse. The impulse is then transferred by a signal processor to a visual or auditory display, such as a numerical value in microvolts or auditory beep. The individual becomes aware of sensations in the muscle, which telegraphs whether the muscle is tense or relaxed. The individual then consciously tries to produce a relaxed muscle state by using the information provided. EMG biofeedback has been applied successfully with patients experiencing tension headaches (Philips, 1977), anxiety (Townsend et al., 1975), temporomandibular joint disorders ([TMJ], Turk, Zaki, & Rudy,

Table 10–2. Autonomic Nervous System Action

Site	System Division	
	Sympathetic Activity	*Parasympathic Activity*
	Adrenergic: Fight and flight—Organism alert and ready to respond	**Cholinergic:** Rest and digest
Dominant neurotransmitter	Epinephrine or adrenaline	Acetycholine
Eye pupil	dilation	constriction
Lacrimal glands	no response	secretion
Salivary glands	vasoconstriction, secretion of small amounts of thick saliva	dilate vessels increasing salivary secretion (thin saliva)
Lungs (Bronchi)	dilation	constriction
Heart muscle	increased heart rate	decreased heart rate
	increased contractile force	decreased contractile force
Arterioles (Small Arteries)		
Coronary	constriction	no effect observed
Cutaneous	constriction	no effect observed
Skeletal muscle	constriction	no effect observed
Abdominal	constriction	no effect observed
Cerebral	constriction	no effect observed
Pulmonary	constriction	no effect observed
Stomach	interruption of digestion	digestion
Motility and tone	decreased activity	increased activity
Sphincters	contraction	relaxation
Secretion	inhibition	stimulation
Small Intestine		
Mobility and tone	decreased activity	increased activity
Sphincters	contraction	relaxation
Secretion	inhibition	stimulation
Pancreas (Islets)	increased secretion	no effect observed
Liver	release glucose	no effect observed
Gallbladder ducts	relaxation	contraction
Kidneys	resin secretion	no effect observed
Urinary bladder	contraction	relaxation
Ovaries (female)	progesterone synthesis or release	no effect observed
Sex organs (male)	ejaculation	erection
Adrenal medulla	secrete epinepherine	no effect observed
Pineal gland	melatonin synthesis/ secretion	no effect observed
Basal metabolism	increased activity	no effect observed

Source: Adapted from "The Autonomic Nervous System" by J. Dodd & L. W. Role (1991). In *Principles of Neural Science* (3rd ed.) by E. R. Kandel, J. H. Schwartz, & T. M. Jessell, NY: Elsevier; and *Handbook of Clinical Psychopharmacology for Therapists* by J. Preston, J. H. O'Neal, & M. C. Talaga, 1994, Oakland, CA: New Harbinger.

1993), insomnia (Raskin, Johnson, & Rondes-tvedt, 1973), hyperactivity (Braud, 1978), asthma (Peper & Tibbitts, 1992), upper extremity dys-function (Tries, 1989), incontinence (Tries, 1990), and schizophrenia (Acosta, Yamanoto, & Wilcox, 1978).

Skin Temperature Feedback Equipment

The portable skin temperature feedback instru-ment is designed to measure and display changes in skin temperature from a selected body site (Gaarder & Montgomery, 1981). The thermometer usually is used to detect minute changes in skin temperature in the forefinger reflecting blood flow. The purpose of skin tem-perature biofeedback is to help the patient con-sciously be able to raise and lower finger tem-perature. Skin temperature biofeedback has been used successfully with Reynaud's disease, a condition in which there is inadequate blood flow in hands and feet, causing cold extremities (Blanchard & Haynes, 1975; Rose & Carlson, 1987). Migraine headaches have also been the focus of skin temperature biofeedback (Johnson & Turin, 1975; Morrill & Blanchard, 1989). Patients have been taught to increase their finger temperature as a conscious method to control migraine headaches (Blanchard et al., 1990) and blood pressure (McGrady, 1994).

Electroencephalogram (EEG)

The EEG is a record of the electrical activity of the cerebral cortex. It is used routinely by neurol-ogists to detect abnormal brain activity such as present in brain lesions and epilepsy. The EEG can also be used to monitor the waveforms of the normal brain. EEG biofeedback training is used to teach the patient to produce alpha brain waves, which are associated with relaxation and medita-tion. Alpha EEG feedback has been used clinical-ly with patients suffering from anxiety (Glueck & Stroebel, 1975; Stroebel, 1982), chronic pain

(Melzack & Perry, 1975), drug addiction (Cohen, Graham, Fotopoulos, & Cook, 1977; Trudeau, 2000), attention deficit hyperactivity disorders (Lubar, 1991), and migraine headaches (Andreychuk & Skriver, 1975).

Galvanic Skin Response (GSR) Feedback Equipment

"The purpose of portable modular GSR feed-back equipment is to detect and display changes in the skin resistance (or conductance) caused by changes in the subject's emotional state" (Gaarder & Montgomery, 1981, p. 202). The GSR can detect anxiety. Decreases in the GSR are usually associated with increased relaxation. In recording GSR, surface electrodes are attached to the palmar side of two nonadjacent fingers. Arousal, or tension in the autonomic nervous system, causes an increase in the gal-vanic skin response. GSR biofeedback has also been used clinically to diminish phobias (Javel & Denholtz, 1975).

Other Biofeedback Instrumentation

► Electrocardiogram (EKG) is a recording of the electrical activity accompanying the muscular contraction of the heart.

► Blood pressure cuff is used to monitor sys-tolic and diastolic blood pressure (sphyg-momanometer).

► Pulse rate to record heart rate and rhythm.

► Pneumograph is used to record respiratory rate.

Using Biofeedback Technology

Biofeedback is one of the most active research areas in behavioral medicine. It has attracted researchers in the field of psychiatric rehabilita-tion because it presents a treatment model that links physiological changes with emotions. The methodology enables the clinician to work cooperatively with the client in reducing psychophysiological and behavioral symptoms. The clinician can tangibly document changes in the patient's behavior. The patient is an active participant in the treatment process, which is one of the ultimate goals of medical practice. The patient takes responsibility for his or her health by learning to monitor and control physiological responses. Biofeedback is congruent with the treatment philosophy of occupational therapy, which rests on the principles of encouraging independence and self-regulation in the patient (Abildness, 1982). The occupational therapist can incorporate biofeedback technology in the treatment process in conjunction with other therapeutic media.

In using biofeedback technology with psychosocial clients the occupational therapist should have sufficient educational background in the following areas:

▶ *Psychophysiology*: an understanding of the relationship between brain function and autonomic nervous system responses

▶ *Electromyography instrumentation*: psychophysics of muscle potential and equipment methodology

▶ *Cybernetic theory*: an understanding of the feedback loop, thermostatic mechanisms, and homeostasis

▶ *Behavioral therapy*: reinforcement schedules and operant conditioning

Recent evidence has shown that biofeedback is effective with clients with eating disorders (Pop-Jordanova, 2000), attention deficit hyperactivity disorder (Nash, 2000), anxiety disorders (Moore, 2000), alcoholism (Sharp, Hurford, Allison, Sparks, & Cameron, 1997), and schizophrenia (Gruzelier, 2000).

MEDITATION

Meditation is a type of relaxation therapy in which the individual tries to produce a calm body. It is essentially a mental exercise that can beneficially influence the individual's mood (Teasdale, Segal, & Williams, 1995), reduce intrusive or negative thoughts (Fabbro, Muzur, Bellen, Calacione, & Bava, 1999), secretion of endorphins (Elias & Wilson, 1995), T-cell count (Taylor, 1995), heart rate (Telles, Nagarathna, & Nagendra, 1995), anxiety states (Miller, Fletcher, & Kabat-Zinn, 1995), and blood pressure (Wenneberg et al., 1997). Meditation is defined as

> a self-directed practice for relaxing the body and calming the mind. Meditation is a self-discipline skill where we can train ourselves to relax and learn how to concentrate on one thing at a time. The mediator makes a concentrated effort to focus on a single thought—peace, for instance; or a physical experience, such as breathing; or a sound (repeating a word or mantra, such as "one" or a Sanskrit word such as "krim"). The aim is to still the mind's "busyness"—its inclination to mull over the thousand demands and details of daily life. (Workshop on Alternative Medicine, 1994, p. 13)

Meditation is an ancient practice that has roots in the religious traditions in India and Tibet. Meditation or silent prayer has been part of almost every religion in the Eastern and Western cultures such as Judaism, Christianity, Moslem Sufism, Japanese Zen, Chinese Tao, Hinduism, and Buddhism. It has been adapted by modern practitioners and incorporated into stress management and cognitive-behavioral treatment programs (Benson, 1975, 1979; Carrington, 1993; Glueck & Stroebel, 1975; Smith, 1986).

The basic principles of all types of meditation are to sit comfortably in a quiet room, close one's eyes or focus on a specific point, breathe through the abdomen, concentrate on an inner process or visualize a pleasant scene, and repeat an encouraging phrase to oneself (mantra) such as "alert mind, calm body" (Stroebel, 1982). One aspect of meditation is to focus your attention on a calming repetitive phrase or visual object such as a spot on a wall so as to clear your mind of preoccupying worries or fears. Meditation in this case is a type of displacement of thoughts and feelings that are negative, such as anxiety and depression by substituting a calming influence. Meditation can also be used as a way of releasing attitudes to allow one's mind to wander freely. When one's focus is on a point or visual stimulus in a room such as an object or piece of furniture, the individual assumes a nonjudgmental or neutral attitude. Greenberg (1984) gives an example of the process of focusing on an object:

> Now, look at that object for about five seconds. Most likely, you saw and focused upon the object while excluding the other stimuli in your field of vision. Behind the object (in your field of vision) might have been a wall or window, a floor, maybe a poster, a table, or something else. In spite of the presence of these other visual stimuli, you can put them back in the background, ignore them, and focus your attention on one object. The object of focus is called the *figure* and the objects in the background of our field of vision are called the *ground*. (p. 134)

How Does Meditation Work?

Meditation appears to have a profound influence on the autonomic nervous system, producing a calming effect such as slower heart rate, decreased blood pressure, lower oxygen consumption, increased warming of the extremities, slowing of brain waves, and a decrease in muscle tension. What is the connection between meditation and the autonomic nervous system? The autonomic nervous system is in a continual state of dynamic change. When an individual is under extreme stress, the body mobilizes into action and stimulates the secretion of hormones and the release of neurotransmitters that produce strong responses such as increased heart rate, blood pressure, and a heightened state of arousal. This reaction as first identified by Cannon (1939) in the term fight-or-flight response, and by Selye (1956) in the concept of the General Adaptation Response (G.A.S.) outlined the response mechanisms in the body. In Selye's (1956) concept the "G.A.S. consists of three stages: the alarm reaction, the stage of resistance, and the stage of exhaustion" (p. 64). Selye, working with an animal model, found that the pituitary and adrenal glands played an important role in the stress response in triggering the mechanisms that increased the body's arousal. Meditation works as an opposite effect, calming the body by producing parasympathetic responses in lowering heart rate and blood pressure. However, not all of the parasympathetic responses are in synch with the relaxation response. The complexity of the autonomic nervous system and its relationship to stress versus relaxation are the focus of much current research. The empirical research does support the general concept that meditation as a relaxation therapy does have a beneficial affect on the autonomic nervous system in reducing the symptoms of stress (Everly & Benson, 1989). It has also been suggested by a number of animal studies that there is a relationship between chronic stress and the hypothalamic-pituitary axis (Keller et al., 1988). If meditation is effective, it must have an influence on the complex mechanism involving the hypothalamus, adrenal glands, neurotransmitters, and hippocampus in reducing the stress reaction (McEwen & Mendelson, 1993).

The two major meditation programs related to psychological variables that have generated the most research are transcendental meditation and relaxation response. Taylor (1995), in a study of a behavioral stress-management program that included progressive muscle relaxation, biofeedback, meditation, and hypnosis with individuals who were HIV positive, found in a controlled study that an experimental group, compared with a no-treatment group, showed significant improvement in decreasing anxiety and increasing self-esteem and positive mood. T-cell count also improved. The investigators concluded that a stress management program with a meditation component is effective in treating individuals with HIV infection.

Miller et al. (1995) did a 3-year follow-up study of an original group of 22 patients with a diagnosis of anxiety disorders. The patients had taken part in an 8-week outpatient group stress reduction intervention based on meditation training. Follow-up data were obtained on 18 of the 22 subjects. They used standardized tests such as the *Beck Depression Scale* (Beck, Ward, Mendelson, Mock, & Erbaugh, 1961) and the *Hamilton Scale* (Hamilton, 1967) to measure improvement. They concluded that meditation can have a long-term beneficial effect on individuals diagnosed with anxiety disorders and depression.

In a study on stress reduction through meditation, Astin (1997) examined the effects of an 8-week treatment program for volunteer patients who experienced chronic pain. In a controlled study comparing an experimental and randomized, no-treatment, control group of 14 participants in each group, the investigators found the following:

> The techniques of mindfulness meditation, with their emphasis on developing detached observation and awareness of the contents of consciousness, may represent a powerful cognitive behavioral coping strategy for trans-

forming the ways in which we respond to life events. They may also have potential for relapse prevention in affective disorders. (p. 97)

In a review article of 24 studies on transcendental meditation (TM) in the prevention and treatment of individuals with substance abuse, Gelderloos, Walton, Orme-Johnson, and Alexander (1991) found that all of the studies of TM showed positive effects. The effects included long-range improvements in well-being, self-esteem, and personal empowerment.

The Relaxation Response

The relaxation response was developed by Herbert Benson (1975), a cardiologist who had studied transcendental meditation in India. As a cardiologist he was interested in nonpharmacological treatments of hypertension. Benson was also interested in applying a behavioral medicine approach that emphasizes the mind-body relationship.

> The relaxation response is elicited through specific behavioral practices and techniques which have existed for centuries, including certain types of prayers, Eastern meditative techniques and Western relaxation techniques. These practices contain four basic components necessary to elicit the relaxation response. The components are; a comfortable position; a quiet environment; repetition of a prayer, word, sound or phrase; adoption of a passive attitude when other thoughts come into consciousness. The relaxation response, which is elicited by these specific behaviors, is the counterpart of the fight or flight response. (p. 140)

The relaxation response is conceptualized to be a generalized approach to stress reduction that reduces sympathetic arousal and decreases norepinephrine receptor activity.

Recommendations to Clients and Therapists for Using Meditation (Carrington, 1993; Cotton, 1990; Greenberg, 1984)

1. Incorporate meditation into your everyday schedule, such as 10 minutes in the afternoon or 10 to 20 minutes right before dinner. Do not take any stimulants before meditating because they will keep the body aroused, interfering with the affects of relaxation. Think of meditation as a relaxation exercise that becomes part of your healthy schedule of aerobic exercise, nutritious diet, and stress reduction.

2. Select a quiet place to meditate. For example, close your office door during work for 10 minutes, take a meditation break instead of coffee or smoking by finding a quiet place at your job.

3. Meditate in a comfortable chair with your feet on the ground, rest your hands in your lap, and your head in a comfortable position. Do not attempt to fall asleep during meditation. Maintain a passive attitude while you meditate and try to focus on one object, on breathing, or on a point in space. If your mind wanders to obsessive thoughts or anxieties, try to distract it by thinking of pleasant scenes that you have experienced in the past or by counting after each breath.

4. Do a body scan to determine if your muscles are tense or relaxed. Massage with a gentle circular movement the muscles that seem tense.

5. Start a meditation program with as little as 5 minutes and then condition yourself to increase the amount of time to 20 minutes. You will be surprised how long 10 minutes is when you are in a state of relaxation.

6. Meditation is helpful in increasing your energy so it may be beneficial to meditate during the afternoon when most people feel less energetic and somewhat tired.

7. Focus on an internal bodily process, such as visualizing your heart pumping nutrients to your body, or the warmth of your hands and arms as you keep your eyes closed.

8. If an individual wants to keep his or her eyes open during meditation, then that individual can focus on an object in a room while letting go of obsessive or anxious thoughts.

9. Use diaphragmatic breathing. This refers to breathing inward through your nose while expanding your abdomen, holding your breath for a moment, and then letting go by breathing through your mouth while contracting your abdomen. Practice diaphragmatic breathing before meditating and then incorporate it into the relaxation exercise.

10. Use a relaxing and calm subvocal phrase, or mantra, repeatedly while you are meditating, such as "alert mind, calm body," "one, " "my arms are warm and heavy," "I feel happy," or "pleasant scenes."

11. Use visualization exercises such as building a dream house with meditation.

12. Have the client audiotape directions for meditating that can be used at home.

13. Incorporate relaxing music, such as New Age music or Pachelbel's "Canon in D" with meditation sessions. Introduce client to relaxing music tapes or ask the client for his or her personal selections of relaxing music.

14. Some individuals (i.e., Type A individuals) may try too hard to become relaxed and in the process they actually become more tense. It is important to reassure these individuals that relaxation and meditation are effective when an individual does not rush

through the session and try to have instant success. It is better that the individual take the time to learn how to relax and learn how to enjoy meditation.

15. After the meditation session, give your body a chance to readjust by rising gradually from your chair, stretching your muscles by bringing your arms over your head and standing on your tiptoes. Some people may experience dizziness if they stand up too abruptly, because during meditation your blood pressure may actually drop, causing an orthostatic reaction upon standing.

Progressive Relaxation

Edmund Jacobson (1929), a physician, was one of the first scientists to use relaxation exercises in treating patients for anxiety, generalized stress reactions, gastrointestinal disorders, and hypertension. He developed the method based on his observations in clinical practice that patients with clinical symptoms appeared tense. This tension was observed to have a negative effect on the organs of the body. For example, he stated that: "The tenseness in our digestive tracts, then, I believe, is part and parcel of our actions and reactions to the situations and problems when we meet them with excessive effort" (Jacobson, 1957, pp. 42–43). His advice to patients in controlling their tenseness was to learn how to relax. He developed the Progressive Relaxation as a practical method that patients can incorporate into their everyday lives and practice daily. An important assumption underlying his technique is that: "*It is physically impossible to be nervous in any part of your body, if in that part you are completely relaxed*" (Jacobson, 1957, p. 85).

Many clinical research studies have tested the efficacy of Progressive Relaxation. In a survey of the literature on applying an abbreviated form

of Progressive Relaxation Training (Abbreviated Progressive Relaxation Training [APRT]) based on Jacobson's work, Bernstein and Carlson (1993) cited the following articles in relationship between APRT and psychological factors:

▶ depression in adolescents (Reynolds & Coats, 1986)

▶ postpartum depression (Halonen & Passman, 1985)

▶ hypertension (Hoelscher, Lichstein, & Rosenthal, 1986; Southam, Agras, Taylor, & Kraemer, 1982)

▶ low back pain (Turner, 1982)

▶ tension headaches (Blanchard et al., 1991)

▶ anxiety (Borkovec et al., 1987)

▶ aggressive behavior in clients with mental retardation (To & Chan, 2000)

▶ reduction of insomnia in individuals with chronic alcoholism (Greeff & Conradie, 1998)

Applying Progressive Relaxation (PR) in Practice

Following are recommendations for occupational therapists who are using PR in therapy. The client can also use these directions for practicing PR at home.

1. The client should practice PR in a quiet room without distraction. Sometimes it is necessary to use a white noise or headphones to block out distracting noises. One hour should be set aside for the exercise. However, the client will need to build up to that point, and at first 15 to 20 minutes may be appropriate.

2. A comfortable but firm mattress, tatami, or an exercise mat should be used with enough room between mats to spread out one's

arms and legs. If an individual needs bodily support (e.g., because of arthritis or athletic injuries), pillows and thin cushions may be used under knees or the small of the back or the head. Use comfortable loose clothing or shorts. Remove shoes and any hanging jewelry.

3. Practice in the prone position on the back. The best time to practice is before eating.

4. Before starting the exercise, have the client lie quietly, without interruption, on his or her back for 3 or 4 minutes with eyes closed.

5. As a precaution do not contract or flex a muscle that is strained or sprained or is painful. Do not force joints when there is pain. In the beginning use gentle movements and avoid jerky movements.

6. In the first exercise, have the client bend his or her left hand upward at the wrist for a few minutes while his or her arm is supported on the bed or mat. Have the client observe the feeling of tenseness in the upper portions of the forearm.

7. Have the client release the wrist by letting it go. As he or she releases the wrist, have him or her observe the feeling of tenseness that has disappeared or diminished.

8. Repeat the movement at the wrist and again notice the difference between tenseness and relaxation.

9. After feeling comfortable in tensing and relaxing the muscles surrounding the wrist joint, have the client flex and relax in a progressive manner the other joints of the upper extremities starting with the elbow and shoulder. Then have the client flex the muscle groups around the head, face, neck, and shoulders, which frequently are focal areas for stress and express an individual's anger, sadness, anxiety, and fatigue.

10. In the next session, have the client flex and relax the muscles of the lower extremities starting with the ankle, doing dorsiflexion (upward movement of the ankle) and plantarflexion (downward movement). Flex the knee, hip, buttocks, and then have the client go on to the abdominal muscles and chest.

11. In the next session the client learns to flex the muscles around the neck, face, and mouth by wrinkling and frowning around the forehead. Have the client experience the sensation of closing the eyes tightly and then releasing. Have the client look to one side and then look to the other side without moving the head and notice the tenseness in the eyeball muscles. Have the client use his or her eyeball muscles to look at the ceiling and then at the floor while still in the prone position.

12. Learning and practicing progressive relaxation should occur over a period of time so that the client feels comfortable in the process. The individual should not hurry through each muscle group, but should take the time to experience each muscle sensation while flexing and relaxing. In actuality, the client should focus on a few muscle groups during each session.

13. Relaxing music can be incorporated into the sessions with the client and therapist deciding on the specific pieces of music.

14. Have the client approach the relaxation exercises as he or she would in learning a sports technique such as tennis, golf, or swimming. The more one practices, the better one will get at learning how to relax. Have a client use a relaxation exercise every day just as he or she would do in eating and brushing one's teeth.

15. Jacobson (1957) also recommended that progressive relaxation can be done while

seated in a chair. The basic principle is to learn how to relax by feeling the tension and noticing the difference as muscle groups are flexed and relaxed.

16. Another variation of PR is to incorporate contracting, and relaxing while standing and imagining that one is pushing against a brick wall while contracting, and then relaxing the muscles of one's face.

17. PR can also be used on a plane. While seated, one can flex and relax muscles.

18. Have the client become aware of how he or she sits and stands during the day and whether tension is felt in these positions.

19. Have the client evaluate the effectiveness of PR by keeping a daily diary of stress.

Another way to relax is by using a visualization exercise.

VISUALIZATION EXERCISE

Building a Dream House

1. The visualization exercise occurs while the client is in the relaxation response in a quiet, nondistracted environment.

2. The first step, while the client's eyes are closed sitting comfortably in a chair and experiencing the relaxation response in his or her mind, is the building of a dream house.

3. The therapist should explain to the client that the purpose of this exercise is to visualize a dream house in one's mind, which can be used as a mental state of serenity. The visualization exercise can be used to reduce anxiety, increase relaxation, and used as an aid to good sleep basis and a countermeasure against insomnia.

Directions for Building a Dream House

The therapist can read directions to the client or have the client listen to a cassette.

1. Select an area where you would like to build the dream house, such as in a forest, near a lake, along a river, in the mountains, or in a sunny field or prairie.

2. Now build the structure of the house, such as a two-story house, castle, farmhouse, log cabin, or mansion.

3. Now build the house with wood, brick, stone, stucco, or a combination. Visualize the house in your mind so that you can describe it to another person.

4. Open the door of the house and build the living room. Start with comfortable chairs to relax in, chat with friends and family, listen to music, read, and enjoy the sunrises and sunsets. Build the rugs, flooring, and wall decorations. Select paintings and prints or photographs that will make you feel relaxed and secure, such as pictures of the ocean, flowers, clouds and sky, mountains, and other scenes from nature. Picture the living room and firmly plant it in your mind as a familiar place to return to over and over.

(continued)

> ## VISUALIZATION EXERCISE *(continued)*
>
> 5. Now build the kitchen as a place where you can experience cooking and eating the foods that you enjoy. Select the utensils and kitchen gadgets that make work lighter. Visualize firmly in your mind your dream kitchen with the tastes and aromas of your favorite foods.
>
> 6. Now build your bedroom as a place to rest your body and mind and to awake rejuvenated and refreshed in the morning. It is a soft, serene place serving as a refuge from the hustle and bustle of everyday living. Visualize your bed and fix it firmly in your mind so that you can call it up to consciousness when you feel tense.
>
> 7. Now build your workshop where you can build the projects that you enjoy making, creating art, writing poetry, working with clay, or doing woodwork. Furnish the workshop with the machines and tools that you need. Visualize your workshop as a place that brings you happiness, pleasant thoughts, and brings out your creativity.
>
> 8. Now build you recreation, entertainment, and music room where you can watch the television programs you enjoy, listen to the radio, hear the music that makes you happy, and play musical instruments. Furnish the room with the furniture that you need to make your room unique. Now visualize the room clearly so that you can go to the room in your mind when you feel anxious or depressed.
>
> 9. Build any other rooms that will create the serenity, peace, pleasant sensations, and happiness that comes from one's mental impressions. Visualize these rooms firmly in your mind.
>
> 10. Now step outside your dream house and build your garden of flowers and paths amidst rocks and grass or vegetables and herbs. Select the flowers—roses, geraniums, petunias, peonies, lilies, gladiolas, and so on. Visualize your garden as a place of refuge and serenity. Fix it firmly in your mind.
>
> 11. Now go back into your house and visualize the living room, bedroom, kitchen, workplace, and other rooms that you have built. See your house and the rooms and the garden clearly in your mind's eye. Tuck it away so that you can recall it in an instant. Where is the house? How does each room look? What is the garden like?
>
> 12. Now think of the people who you love and admire. Invite them into your house to share in its serenity, peace, and joy.

REFERENCES

Abildness, A. (1982). *Biofeedback strategies.* Rockville, MD: American Occupational Therapy Association.

Acosta, F., Yamanoto, J., & Wilcox, S. (1978). Application of electromyographic feedback to the relaxations of schizophrenic, neurotic and tension headache patients. *Journal of Consulting and Clinical Psychology, 46,* 383–384.

Andreychuk, T., & Skriver, C. (1975). Hypnosis and biofeedback in the treatment of migraine headache. *International Journal of Clinical and Experimental Hypnosis, 23,* 172–183.

Anisman, H., & Zacharko, R. M. (1992). Depression as a consequence of inadequate neurochemical adaptation in response to stressors. *British Journal of Psychiatric, 160*(Suppl. 15), 36–43.

Astin, J. A. (1997). Stress reduction through mindfulness mediation. Effects on psychological symptomatology, sense of control, and spiritual experiences. *Psychotherapy of Psychosomatics, 66,* 97–106.

Barr, M. L., & Kiernan, J. A. (1993). *The human nervous system: An anatomical viewpoint* (6th ed.). Philadelphia: Lippincott.

Beck, A., Ward, C., Mendelson, M., Mock, J., & Erbaugh, J. (1961). An inventory for measuring depression. *Archives of General Psychiatry, 4,* 546–571.

Benson, H. (1975). *The relaxation response.* New York: William Morrow.

Benson, H. (1979). *The mind/body effect: How behavioral medicine can show you the way to better health.* New York: Simon & Schuster.

Bentley, D. E., & Stein, F. (1994, July). *The stress management questionnaire: Development and work in progress.* Paper presented at National Consultation on Career Development (NATCOM), Ontario, Canada.

Bernard, C. (1957). *An introduction to the study of experimental medicine* (H. C. Greene, Trans.). New York: Dover. (Original work published 1865)

Bernstein, D. A., & Carlson, C. R. (1993). Progressive relaxation: Abbreviated methods. In P. M. Lehrer & R. L. Woolfolk (Eds.), *Principles and practice of stress management* (2nd ed., pp. 53–88). New York: Guilford.

Blanchard, E. B., Applebaum, K. A., Radnitz, C. L., Morill, B., Michultka, D., Kirsch, C. L., Guarnieri, P., Hillhouse, J., Evans, D. D., Jaccard, J., & Barron, K. D. (1990). A controlled evaluation of thermal biofeedback and thermal biofeedback with cognitive therapy in the treatment of vascular headache. *Journal of Consulting and Clinical Psychology, 58,* 216–224.

Blanchard, E., & Haynes, M. (1975). Biofeedback treatment of a case of Raynaud's disease. *Journal of Behavior Therapy and Experimental Psychiatry, 6,* 230–234.

Blanchard, E. B., Nicholson, N. L., Taylor, A. E., Steffek, B. D., Radnitz, C. L., & Appelbaum, K. A. (1991). The role of regular home practice in the relaxation treatment of tension headache. *Journal of Consulting and Clinical Psychology, 59,* 467–470.

Blumenthal, J. A., Babyak, M. A., Moore, K. A., Craighead, W. E., Herman, S., Khatri, P., Waugh, R., Napolitano, M. A., Forman, L. M., Appelbaum, M., Doraiswamy, P. M., & Krisnan, K. R. (1999). Effects of exercise training on older paints with major depression. *Archives of Internal Medicine, 159,* 2349–2356.

Borkovec, T. D., Mathews, A. M., Chambers, A., Ebrahimi, S., Lytle, R., & Nelson, R. (1987). The effects of relaxation training with cognitive or nondirective therapy and the role of relaxation-induced anxiety in the treatment of generalized anxiety. *Journal of Consulting and Clinical Psychology, 55,* 883–888.

Braud, L. (1978). The effects of frontalis EMG biofeedback and progressive relaxation upon hyperactivity and its behavioral concomitants. *Biofeedback and Self-Regulation, 3,* 69–89.

Brown, B. (1974). *New mind, new body and biofeedback: New directions for the mind.* New York: Harper & Row.

Brown, B. (1977). *Stress and the art of biofeedback.* New York: Harper & Row.

Bruce, M. A., & Borg, B. (1987). *Frames of reference in psychosocial occupational therapy.* Thorofare, NJ: SLACK.

Cannon, W. B. (1939). *The wisdom of the body.* New York: Norton.

Carrington, P. (1993). Modern forms of meditation. In P. M. Lehrer & R. L. Woolfolk (Eds.), *Principles and practice of stress management* (2nd ed., pp. 139–168). New York: Guilford.

Cohen, H. D., Graham, C. Fotopoulos, S. S., & Cook, M. R. (1977). A double-blind methodology for biofeedback research. *Psychophysiology, 14,* 603–608.

Cotton, D. H. G. (1990). *Stress management; Integrated approach to therapy.* New York: Brunner/Mazel.

Crist, P. H. (1986). Community living skills: A psychoeducational community-based program. *Occupational Therapy in Mental Health, 6*(2), 51–64.

Da Costa, D., Dobkin, P. L., Pinard, L., Fortin, P. R., Danoff, D. S., Esdaile, J. M., & Clarke, A. E. (1999). The role of stress in functional disability among women with systemic lupus erythematosus: A prospective study. *Arthritis Care and Research, 12,* 112–119.

Davis, J., & Kutter, C. J. (1998). Independent living skills in posttraumatic stress disorder in women who are homeless: Implication for future practice. *The American Journal of Occupational Therapy, 52,* 39–44.

Derogatis, L. R., & Coons, H. L. (1993). Self-report measures of stress: In L. Goldberger, & S. Breznitz (Eds.), *Handbook of stress theoretical and clinical aspects*, (2nd ed., pp. 200–233). New York: Free Press.

Dodd, J., & Role, L. W. (1991). The autonomic nervous system. In E. R. Kandel, J. H. Schwartz, & T. M. Jessell (Eds.), *Principles of neural science* (3rd ed., pp. 761–775). New York: Elsevier.

Dohrenwend, B. S., & Dohrenwend, B. P. (1981). Life stress and illness: Formulation of the issues. In B. S. Dohrenwend & B. P. Dohrenwend (Eds.), *Stressful life events and their contexts* (pp. 1–27). New York: Prodist.

Elias, A. N., & Wilson, A. F. (1995). Serum hormonal concentrations following transcendental meditation–potential role of gamma aminobutyric acid. *Medical Hypotheses, 44*, 287–291.

Engel, J. M., & Rapoff, M. A. (1990). Biofeedback-assisted relaxation training for adult and pediatric headache disorders. *Occupational Therapy Journal of Research, 10*, 283–299.

Everly, G. S., & Benson, H. (1989). Disorders of arousal and the relaxation response: Speculations on the nature and treatment of stress-related diseases. *International Journal of Psychosomatics 36*, 15–21.

Fabbro, F., Muzur, A., Bellen, R., Calacione, R., & Bava, A. (1999). Effects of praying and a working memory task in participants trained in meditation and controls on the occurrence of spontaneous thoughts. *Perceptual Motor Skills, 88*(3, Pt 1), 767–770.

Gaarder, K., & Montgomery, P. (1981). *Clinical biofeedback: A procedural manual* (2nd ed.). Baltimore: Williams and Wilkins.

Gelderloos, P., Walton, K. G., Orme-Johnson, D. W., & Alexander, C. N. (1991). Effectiveness of the Transcendental Meditation program in preventing and treating substance abuse. *International Journal of Addiction, 26*, 293–325.

Gilman, S., & Newman, S. W. (1992). *Manter and Gatz's essentials of clinical neuroanatomy and neurophysiology* (8th ed.). Philadelphia: F. A. Davis.

Glueck, B., & Stroebel, C. (1975). Biofeedback and meditation in the treatment of psychiatric illness. *Comprehensive Psychiatry, 16*, 303–321.

Greeff, A. P., & Conradie, W. S. (1998). Use of progressive relaxation training for chronic alcoholics with insomnia. *Psychological Reports, 82*, 407–12.

Green, E., Green, A., & Walters, E. (1970). Voluntary control of internal states: Psychological and physiological. *Journal of Transpersonal Psychology, 2*, 1–25.

Greenberg, J. S. (1984). *Managing stress: A personal guide.* Dubuque, IA: William C. Brown.

Gruzelier, J. (2000). Self-regulation of electrocortical activity in schizophrenia and schizotypy: A review. *Clinical Electroencephalography, 31*, 23–29.

Halonen, J. S., & Passman, R. H. (1985). Relaxation training and expectation in the treatment of post-partum distress. *Journal of Consulting and Clinical Psychology, 53*, 839–845.

Hamilton, M. (1967). Development of a rating scale for primary depressive illness. *British Journal of Social Clinical Psychology, 26*, 99–103.

Hoelscher, T. J., Lichstein, K. L., & Rosenthal, T. L. (1986). Home relaxation practice in hypertension treatment: Objective assessment and compliance induction. *Journal of Consulting and Clinical Psychology, 54*, 217–221.

Hollon, S. D., & Beck, A. T. (1979). Cognitive therapy of depression. In P. C. Kendall & S. D. Hollon (Eds.), *Cognitive-behavioral interventions* (pp. 153–203). New York: Academic.

Holmes, T. H., & Rahe, R. H. (1967). The Social Readjustment Rating Scale. *Journal of Psychosomatic Research, 11*, 213–218.

Jacobson, E. (1929). *Progressive relaxation.* Chicago: University of Chicago.

Jacobson, E. (1957). *You must relax.* New York: McGraw–Hill.

Javel, A., & Denholtz, M. (1975). Audible GSR feedback and systematic desensitization: A case report. *Behavior Therapy, 6*, 251–253.

Johnson, W., & Turin, A. (1975). Biofeedback treatment of migraine headache: A systematic case study. *Behavior Therapy, 6*, 394–397.

Kanner, A. D., Coyne, J. C., Schaefer, C., & Lazarus, R. S. (1981). Comparison of two modes of stress measurement: Daily hassles and uplifts versus major life events. *Journal of Behavioral Medicine, 4*, 1–39.

Keller, S. E., Schleifer, S. J., Liotta, A. S., Bond, R. N., Farhoody, N., & Stein, M. (1988). Stress induced alterations of immunity in hypophysectomized rats. *Proceedings of the National Academy of Science, 85*, 577–566.

Kohn, P. M., & MacDonald, J. E.(1992). The survey of recent life experiences: A decontaminated hassles scale for adults. *Journal of Behavioral Medicine, 15*, 221–236.

Konkol, B., & Schneider, M. J. (1988). Treatment of substance abuse and alcoholism. In D. W. Scott & N. Katz (Eds.), *Occupational therapy in mental health: Principles in practice* (pp. 196–205). London: Taylor & Francis.

Kwako, R. (1980). Relaxation as therapy for hyperactive children. *Occupational Therapy in Mental Health, 1*(3), 29–45.

Lazarus, R. S. (1975). A cognitively oriented psychologist looks at biofeedback. *American Psychologist, 30*, 553–561.

Lazarus, R. S. (1993). Why we should think of stress as a subset of emotion. In L. Goldberger & S. Breznitz (Eds.), *Handbook of stress: Theoretical and clinical aspects* (2nd ed., pp. 21–39). New York: Free Press.

Lazarus, R. S., & Folkman, S. (1984). *Stress, appraisal and coping.* New York: Springer.

Lillie, M. D., & Armstrong, H. E. (1982). Contributions to the development of psychoeducational approaches to mental health service. *American Journal of Occupational Therapy, 36*, 438–443.

Lubar, J. F. (1991). Discourse on the development of EEG diagnostics and biofeedback treatment for attention-deficit/hyperactivity disorders. *Biofeedback and Self-Regulation, 16*, 201–225.

McEwen, B. S., & Mendelson, S. (1993). Effects of stress on the neurochemistry and morphology of the brain: Counterregulation versus damage. In L. Goldberger & S. Breznitz (Eds.), *Handbook of stress: Theoretical and clinical aspects* (2nd ed., pp. 101–126). New York: Free Press.

McGrady, A. V. (1994). Effects of group relaxation training and thermal biofeedback on blood pressure and related psychophysiological variables in essential hypertension. *Biofeedback and Self-Regulation, 19*(1), 51–66.

Melzack, R., & Perry, C. (1975). Self-regulation of pain: The use of alpha-feedback and hypnotic training for the control of chronic pain. *Experimental Neurology, 46*, 452–469.

Miller, N. (1969). Learning of visceral and glandular responses. *Science, 163*, 434–445.

Miller, J. J., Fletcher, K., & Kabat–Zinn, J. (1995). Three-year follow-up and clinical implications of a mindfulness meditation-based stress reduction intervention in the treatment of anxiety disorders. *General Hospital Psychiatry, 17*, 192–200.

Moore, N. C. (2000). A review of EEG biofeedback treatment of anxiety disorders. *Clinical Electroencephalography, 31*, 1–6.

Morrill, B., & Blanchard, E. B. (1989). Two studies of the potential mechanisms of action in the thermal biofeedback treatment of vascular headache. *Headache, 29*, 169–176.

Nash, J. K. (2000). Treatment of attention deficit hyperactivity disorder with neurotherapy. *Clinical Electroencephalography, 31*, 30–37.

Peniston, E. G., & Kulkosky, P. J. (1989). Alpha-theta brainwave training and beta endorphin levels in alcoholics. *Alcoholism: Clinical and Experimental Research, 13*, 271–279.

Peper, E., & Tibbitts, V. (1992). Fifteen-month follow-up with asthmatics utilizing EMG/Incentive Inspirometer feedback. *Biofeedback and Self-Regulation, 17*, 143–151.

Philips, C. (1977). The modification of tension headache pain using EMG biofeedback. *Behavior Research and Therapy, 15*, 119–129.

Pop-Jordanova, N. (2000). Psychological characteristics and biofeedback mitigation in preadolescents with eating disorders. *Pediatric International, 42*, 76–81.

Preston, J., O'Neal, J. H., & Talaga, M. C. (1994). *Handbook of clinical psychopharmacology for therapists.* Oakland, CA: New Harbinger.

Raskin, M., Johnson, G., & Rondestvedt, J. W. (1973). Chronic anxiety treated by feedback-induced muscle relaxation. *Archives of General Psychiatry, 28*, 263–267.

Reynolds, W. M., & Coats, K. I. (1986). A comparison of cognitive-behavioral therapy and relaxation training for the treatment of depression in adolescents. *Journal of Consulting and Clinical Psychology, 54*, 653–660.

Rose, G. D., & Carlson, J. G. (1987). The behavioral treatment of Raynaud's disease: A review. *Biofeedback and Self-Regulation, 12*, 257–272.

Russo, J., Vitaliano, P. P., Brewer, D. D., Katon, W., & Becker, J. (1995). Psychiatric disorders in spouse caregivers of care recipients with Alzheimer's disease and match controls: A diathesis-stress model of psychopathology. *Journal of Abnormal Psychology, 104*, 197–204.

Sapolsky, R. M. (1998). *Why zebras don't get ulcers: An updated guide to stress, stress- related diseases, and coping. New York: Freeman.*

Schuster, M. (1977). Biofeedback treatment of gastrointestinal disorders. *Modern Clinics of North America, 61*, 907–912.

Schwartz, N. M., & Schwartz, M. S. (1995). Definitions of biofeedback and applied psychophysiology. In M. S. Schwartz and Associates, *Biofeedback: A practitioner's guide* (2nd ed., pp. 32–42). New York: Guilford.

Selye, H. (1936). A syndrome produced by diverse nocuous agents. *Nature, 138*, 32.

Selye, H. (1956). *The stress of life.* New York: McGraw–Hill.

Selye, H. (1974). *Stress without distress.* Philadelphia: Lippincott.

Selye, H. (1993). History of the stress concept. In L. Goldberger & S. Breznitz (Eds.), *Handbook of stress: Theoretical and clinical aspects* (2nd ed., pp. 7–17). New York: Free Press.

Sharp, C., Hurford, D. P., Allison, J., Sparks, R., & Cameron, B. P. (1997). Facilitation of internal locus of control in adolescent alcoholics through a brief biofeedback-assisted autogenic relaxation training procedure. *Journal of Substance Abuse Treatment, 14*, 55–60.

Smith, J. C. (1986). *Meditation: A sensible guide to a timeless discipline.* Champaign, IL: Research Press.

Southam, M. A., Agras, W. S., Taylor, C. B., & Kraemer, H. D. (1982). Relaxation training: Blood pressure lowering during the working day. *Archives of General Psychiatry, 39*, 715–717.

Stein, F. (1986a). *Reliability and validity of the Stress Management Questionnaire.* Unpublished manuscript, University of Wisconsin-Milwaukee.

Stein, F. (1986b). *Stress management questionnaire.* (Available through F. Stein, University of South Dakota, Department of Occupational Therapy, 414 E. Clark, Vermillion, SD 57069.)

Stein, F. (1987). *Stress and schizophrenia.* Alberta Psychology, 16, 10–11.

Stein, F., Bentley, D. E., & Natz, M. (1999). Computerized assessment: The Stress Management Questionnaire. In B. J. Hemphill-Pearson, *Assessments in occupational therapy mental health: An integrative approach* (pp. 321–337). Thorofare, NJ: SLACK.

Stein, F., & Neville, S. A. (1987). *Biofeedback, locus of control and reduction of anxiety in alcohol dependent adults.* Unpublished manuscript, University of Wisconsin-Milwaukee.

Stein, F., & Nikolic, S. (1989). Teaching stress management techniques to a schizophrenic patient. *American Journal of Occupational Therapy, 43*, 162–169.

Stein, F., & Smith, J. (1989). Short-term stress management programme with acutely depressed inpatients. *Canadian Journal of Occupational Therapy, 56*, 185–192.

Stockwell R., Duncan, S., & Levens, M. (1988). Occupational therapy with eating disorders. In D. W. Scott & N. Katz (Eds.), *Occupational therapy in mental health: Principles in practice* (pp. 206–218). London: Taylor & Francis.

Stoyva, J. M., & Budzynski, T. H. (1993). Biofeedback methods in the treatment of anxiety and stress disorders. In P. M. Lehrer & R. L. Woolfolk (Eds.), *Principles and practice of stress management* (2nd ed., pp. 263–300). New York: Free Press.

Stoyva, J. M., & Carlson, J. G. (1993). A coping/rest model of relaxation and stress management. In L. Goldberger & S. Breznitz (Eds.), *Handbook of stress: Theoretical and clinical aspects* (2nd ed., pp. 724–756). New York: Free Press.

Stroebel, C. F. (1982). *QR: The quieting reflex.* New York: G. P. Putnam.

Taylor, D. N. (1995). Effects of a behavioral stress-management program ion anxiety, mood, self-esteem, and T-cell count in HIV positive men. *Psychological Reports, 76*, 451–457.

Teasdale, J. D., Segal, Z., & Williams, J. M. (1995). How does cognitive therapy prevent depressive relapse and why should attentional control (mindfulness) training help? *Behavioral Research Therapy, 33*, 25–39.

Telles, S., Nagarathna, R., & Nagendra, H. R. (1995). Autonomic changes during "OM" meditation. *Indian Journal of Physiological Pharmacology, 39*, 418–420.

Timmerman, I. G., Emmelkamp, P. M., & Sanderman, R. (1998). The effects of a stress-management training program in individuals at risk in the community at large. *Behavioral Research Therapy, 36*, 863–875.

To, M. Y., & Chan, S. (2000). Evaluating the effectiveness of progressive muscle relaxation in reducing the aggressive behaviors of mentally handicapped patients. *Archives of Psychiatric Nursing, 14*, 39–46.

Townsend, R. E., House, J. F., & Addario, D. (1975). A comparison of biofeedback-medicated relaxation and group therapy in the treatment of chronic anxiety. *American Journal of Psychiatry, 132*, 598–601.

Tries, J. (1989). EMG feedback for the treatment of upper–extremity dysfunction: Can it be effective? *Biofeedback and Self-Regulation, 14*, 21–53.

Tries, J. (1990). The use of biofeedback in the treatment of incontinence due to head injury. *Journal of Head Trauma Rehabilitation, 5*, 91–100.

Trudeau, D. L. (2000). The treatment of addictive disorders by brain wave biofeedback: A review and suggestions for future research. *Clinical Electroencephalogy, 31*, 13–22.

Turk, D. C., Meichenbaum, D., & Genest, M. (1983). *Pain and behavioral medicine.* New York: Guilford Press.

Turk, D., Zaki, H., & Rudy, T. (1993). Effects of intra-oral appliance and biofeedback/stress management alone and in combination in treating pain and depression in patients with temporomandibular disorders. *Journal of Prosthetic Dentistry, 70*, 158–164.

Turner, J. A. (1982). Comparison of group progressive-relaxation training and cognitive-behavioral group therapy for chronic low back pain. *Journal of Consulting and Clinical Psychology, 50*, 757–765.

Weiner, N. (1948). *Cybernetics or control and communication in the animal and the machine.* New York: John Wiley.

Wenneberg, S. R., Schneider, R. H., Walton, K. G., Maclean, C. R., Levitsky, D. K., Salerno, J. W., Wallace, R. K., Mandarino, J. V., Rainforth, M. V., & Waziri, R. (1997). A controlled study of the effects of the Transcendental Meditation program on cardiovascular reactivity and ambulatory blood pressure. *International Journal of Neuroscience, 89*, 15—28.

Workshop on Alternative Medicine. (1994). *Alternative medicine: Expanding medical horizons.* (NIH Publication No. 94-066). Washington, DC: Government Printing Office.

CHAPTER

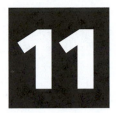

Leisure-time Occupations, Self-care, and Social Skills Training

> *Leisure consists of a number of occupations in which the individual may indulge of his own free will—either to rest, to amuse himself, to add to his knowledge or improve his skills disinterestedly or to increase his voluntary participation in the life of the community after discharging his professional, family and social duties.*
>
> — J. Dumazedier (1960), "Current Problems of the Sociology of Leisure," *International Social Science Journal # 4*, cited in Parker, S. R. (1972), *The Future of Work and Leisure*, London: Paladin, p. 22.

Operational Learning Objectives

At the end of this chapter, the learner will:

1. Define and distinguish between leisure, work, play, and free time within the framework of occupation.

2. Identify the major categories and specific leisure activities of a client.

3. Identify measures of leisure activity, self-care, or social skills and incorporate findings from the evaluation or assessment into a treatment plan.

4. Define self-care activities.

5. Identify performance areas and performance components within self-care.

6. Develop an activity analysis for subdomains in self-care.

7. Identify barriers that prevent the client with psychosocial illness from completing self-care tasks.

8. Define social skills.

9. Identify ways to teach social skills or self-care skills.

LEISURE SKILLS

Focusing Questions

▶ How is leisure defined?

▶ What is the difference between leisure and free time?

▶ How can leisure activities be systematically categorized?

▶ How can we help our clients to develop leisure activities?

▶ How do we analyze leisure activities?

▶ How do we evaluate interests in specific leisure activities?

▶ How do we justify the incorporation of leisure activities in a therapeutic program?

▶ What factors should be considered in developing a leisure program?

▶ How do we teach leisure-time activities effectively?

▶ How do we evaluate the needs of an individual in areas of leisure and play?

▶ How can we teach leisure skills in community mental health centers (CMHCs)?

▶ How can we use community resources to enable an individual to use leisure time?

▶ What are the purposes of leisure for an individual?

The *Uniform Terminology, Application to Practice for Occupational Therapy*, Third Edition (AOTA, 1994) identifies Play or Leisure Activities as one of three important Performance Areas for occupational therapy intervention. The other two areas are Activities of Daily Living and Work and Productive Activities. Foley (1967), a psychiatrist, discussed the value of leisure in a community mental health program:

> It is important that special attention be given to the understanding and effective utilization of leisure time, including an educative aspect

and a practical aspect. The educative aspect should be directed toward study and discussion of leisure time, its meaning, usefulness, and applicability to various age groups, with emphasis on the need for meaningful patterns of leisure time activities. The practical aspect might concern exploring possibilities for constructive leisure time use in light of the specific needs of various age groups and current cultural trends. . . . The comprehensive program of the community mental health center, with its strong emphasis on consultation, education, and research, seems an appropriate model from which to pattern a program designed to explore the concept of leisure time and to promote specific recommendations for its effective utilization. (p. 101)

Definitions of Leisure and Play

Knox (1993) defined work, leisure, and play as follows:

> To summarize, **work** can be defined as activity done for production or reward as well as non-salaried activity that contributes to subsistence or reproduction. It usually is constrained by time, space, or task, and it derives meaning through satisfaction, providing a livelihood and goal achievement. Work is usually driven by external motivation. **Leisure** usually occurs outside the obligations of one's work and provides opportunities for enjoyment, relaxation, recreation, personal growth, and goal achievement. Leisure is driven by internal motivation, implies freedom of choice, and is not usually constrained. **Play** is a developmental phenomenon, a type of activity and a way children interact with their environment. Play is the way children learn about the world through exploration, experimentation, and repetition. Play is spontaneous, intrinsically motivated, fun, totally absorbing, and performed for its own sake. (pp. 261–262, italcs and bold added.)

A study group defined leisure as:

> the hours when a man is not working primarily for money. Those hours have to include

many things; household duties, rest, relaxation, social contact, family life, voluntary work, sport and hobbies and an opportunity for a man's mind and mood and whole being to move in a different world from the world of work and production. (Hunter, 1961, p. 16)

Parker (1972) stated:

One of the chief problems of defining leisure is that it is very difficult to take an objective approach to the subject. Perhaps even more than in the case of work, the way in which someone defines leisure tends to be determined by his view of what it ought to be. (p. 20)

In contrast to leisure, which is free time, the purpose of play is to teach and reinforce skills. According to Fagan (1976):

The two basic tenets of this view of play [contrast between leisure and play] are that the organism is building or modifying an internal model of itself or of its environment and that it must perform motor or manipulative "experiments" in order to produce the necessary information. (p. 98)

Assumptions Underlying Leisure Activities

▶ Leisure can enhance an individual's quality of life such as in the areas of physical, mental, social, developmental activities, and psychological well-being (Barry & Crosby, 1996; Felce & Perry, 1996; Fine, 1996).

▶ In psychosocial occupational therapy, leisure activities are an important aspect of an individual's life and should be incorporated into a comprehensive, holistic treatment program (Fasting, 1982). The other areas are work, self-care, and social skills.

▶ A definition of leisure depends on the individual's view of what leisure is. In other words, each individual has his or her own concept of what leisure is.

▶ Where work ends and leisure begins can be subjective. For example, some individuals extend their work into leisure activities (e.g., people who use computers in their employment and also enjoy working with computers in their free or leisure time).

▶ Leisure can be viewed in terms of time, such as "free time" spent relaxing during the day. Leisure can also be viewed as an attitude toward life. For example, an individual can use leisure time to learn a new activity, or to take part in spiritual or self-reflection activities.

▶ Leisure can also be organized around daily chores, such as farmers, who during leisure time continue to engage in necessary daily or seasonal tasks.

▶ Many times, leisure activities are discontinued when an individual has a mental disability (Parker, Gladman, & Drummond, 1997). In other words, the occurrence of major symptoms, such as in depression or schizophrenia, interfere with the individual's ability to take part in leisure activities (Barry & Crosby, 1996; Sullivan & Poertner, 1989).

▶ Many individuals with mental illness or other disabilities can benefit from direct instruction in initiating and incorporating leisure activities into their everyday life (Menks, Sittler, Weaver, & Yanow, 1997).

▶ Activities can be classified into meaningful categories (Table 11–1).

Identifying Client Interests

The *Leisure Occupations Interest Inventory* (LOII; Stein & Cutler, 1997) is a tool that can be used with clients to identify leisure occupations of interest and to develop a feasible plan for clients to use in scheduling leisure activities in

Table 11–1. Categories of Leisure Activities

ACTIVITY	EXAMPLES
ANIMAL CARE:	caring for cats, dogs, rodents, fish
ARTS AND CRAFTS:	constructing objects with wood, fiber, ceramics, metal
COMPUTERS:	designing web pages, playing games, repairing hardware
CULINARY:	going to restaurants, preparing gourmet meals
CREATIVE COMPOSING:	creating poetry, art, drama, room designs
DANCE:	performing ballet, modern dance, ballroom
EXERCISE:	aerobic (e.g., running), isometric (e.g., lifting weights)
HOBBIES:	collecting stamps, Barbie dolls, coins, antiques
HORTICULTURE:	growing plants, arranging flowers
MIND GAMES:	playing chess, completing crossword puzzles
MUSIC:	playing musical instrument
RELAXATION EXERCISES:	meditating or doing yoga or tai ch'i'
REPAIRING OBJECTS:	repairing appliances, cars, household objects
SELF-CARE:	grooming, dressing, cooking
SHOPPING:	window, personal, or household shopping
SOCIAL:	participating in clubs, family activities, support groups
SPECTATOR ACTIVITIES:	attending events (e.g., sports, music), watching TV
SPORTS:	engaging in competitive, noncompetitive activities
TRAVEL:	taking trips to local, state, national, international places
VOLUNTEER WORK:	volunteering in library, nursing home, hospital, community organizations, League of Women Voters

their everyday lives. This scale is reproduced in Figure 11–1.

A quick way for the therapist to find out about the client's interest is the use of the *Leisure Occupations Sentence Completion* (Stein, 1993), which follows. Use of this tool allows the thera-pist to gain additional information about the client's specific areas of interest. Comparison of this task and the LOII allows the therapist to val-idate and reinforce the client's responses on the LOII.

Leisure Occupations Interest Inventory (LOII)
(A tool to help client identify leisure activities in which to engage)

Directions:

1. The therapist should go through the list of categories with the client to identify which activities the client enjoys or has enjoyed in the past.

2. The client should identify the level of current interest (e.g., high, medium, or low) for each leisure occupation. High interest means that a person would like to, or does, incorporate the activity into a daily or weekly schedule. Medium interest means that the individual enjoys the activity and would or does engage in the activity when he or she has time. Low interest means that an individual either has no interest or engages in the activity occasionally, such as 1–2 times a year.

3. The therapist and client together should identify a goal for participation in the leisure occupation. The goal should include the specific type of activity and the amount of time spent either daily or weekly. Example of a targeted goal: gardening, including pruning, cultivating, and planting, 1 hour daily before breakfast.

Category and Examples of Specific Activities	Degree of Interest			Targeted Goal, including • *specific activity* • *time spent (daily, weekly)* • *time of day spent*
	H	**M**	**L**	
HORTICULTURE • working in garden • growing plants • identifying different plants • arranging flowers	x			Working in the garden, 1 hour daily before breakfast
SPECTATOR ACTIVITIES • watching live sports			x	Attending football game once a year
SPORTS • engaging in competitive and noncompetitive sports		x		Playing tennis once a month
MUSIC • listening to music • playing an instrument				

Figure 11–1. The *Leisure Occupations Interest Inventory* (LOII; Stein & Cutler, 1997) can be used to assess leisure skills for clients with psychosocial deficits. This may be reproduced at will providing the authors are given credit. Please send comments regarding this form to Dr. Frank Stein, Occupational Therapy Department, University of South Dakota, 414 E. Clark St., Vermillion, SD 57069.

Category and Examples of Specific Activities	Degree of Interest			Targeted Goal, including • *specific activity* • *time spent (daily, weekly)* • *time of day spent*
	H	M	L	
COMPUTER ACTIVITIES • interactive games • "surfing" for information on Internet or the Web • word processing • analyzing data				
READING • books • magazines • newspapers				
ARTS AND CRAFTS • woodworking • sewing • hand crafts				
CREATIVE ACTIVITIES • composing, creating, or designing: oil painting, poetry, musical composition, furniture, weaving				
SOCIAL • being a member or participant in a club, church group, or organizational support group				
EXERCISE • relaxation or aerobic exercises for health and wellness, such as stretching, walking, yoga, Tai Ch'i				
ANIMAL CARE • caring for and bonding with animals and pets such as cats, horses, and dogs				
TABLE OR MIND GAMES • chess • crossword puzzles • card games				
DANCE • ballroom • disco • square dancing				

Category and Examples of Specific Activities	Degree of Interest			Targeted Goal, including • *specific activity* • *time spent (daily, weekly)* • *time of day spent*
	H	**M**	**L**	
COLLECTING OBJECTS • stamps • thimbles • coins • dolls • cards				
SELF-CARE • hair restyling • taking a bath • grooming • planning wardrobe				
TELEVISION OR RADIO • watching or listening to favorite programs				
VOLUNTEERING • engage in altruistic or philanthropic activities such as community service in library, hospital, or school				
SHOPPING • window shopping • gifts • clothes • books or CDs • household items				
CULTURAL ACTIVITIES • visiting museums and art galleries • travel • attending symphonies, concerts, theater, lectures				
CULINARY ACTIVITIES • restaurants • gourmet cooking				

Category and Examples of Specific Activities	Degree of Interest			Targeted Goal, including • *specific activity* • *time spent (daily, weekly)* • *time of day spent*
	H	**M**	**L**	
REPAIRING AND REFINISHING OBJECTS • car repair • household repair • refinishing furniture • painting rooms • sorting closets • cleaning				

©Stein & Cutler, 1997

Leisure Occupations Sentence Completion

1. My favorite composer or musical group is . . .

2. The best movie I saw this year was . . .

3. My favorite author or book I enjoyed is . . .

4. If I had to watch only one television show a week it would be . . .

5. My favorite sport that I like to watch is . . .

6. When I have time to exercise or play a sport I . . .

7. My favorite painting or artist is. . .

8. The individual I admire the most living or dead is . . .

9. If I could travel to any place in the world I would like to go to . . .

10. When I am alone I like to . . .

Copyright © 1993, F. Stein

Purposes of Leisure Occupations

What goals are met by specific leisure occupations? Both the specific activity and the therapeutic goal need to be considered when developing a treatment plan with the client. Therapeutic goals to be considered include cognitive, emotional, social or interpersonal, physical, moral or ethical, neuromuscular movements, work adjustment, developmental tasks, encouragement of creative expression, cultural awareness, perceptual/motor stimulation, and sensory processing. The therapist will want to ask and answer the following questions when analyzing the leisure occupation considered for the treatment plan.

▶ Does the activity or occupation involve relationships with people (e.g., active participation in social clubs)?

▶ Is the activity primarily working with an object (e.g., computers or woodworking)?

▶ Is there an emotional component to the activity (e.g., competitive sports)?

▶ Does the activity develop work habits (e.g., volunteer work in a library)?

▶ Does the activity encourage creative expression (e.g., composing poetry)?

▶ Does the activity fulfill the need for exercise (e.g., biking)?

▶ Does the activity increase self-esteem (e.g., completing an arts and crafts project)?

▶ Does the activity increase relaxation (e.g., Tai Ch'i)?

▶ Does the activity stimulate cognitive function (e.g., playing chess)?

▶ Does the activity increase self-image (e.g., grooming and dressing)?

▶ Does the activity stimulate nurturance in an individual (e.g., animal care)?

SELF-CARE ACTIVITIES

Focusing Questions

▶ What is the difference between ADLs and IADLs for the client with a psychosocial disability?

▶ What are the areas in which the client demonstrates independence?

▶ What are the assessment tools used to evaluate the client's self-care skills?

▶ How does a psychosocial disability affect self-care skills?

▶ How can a therapist help a client to improve his or her self-care skills?

▶ How can we analyze the self-care skills using a task analysis (Watson, 1997)?

Definition

Self-care activities are part of the activities of daily living. The *AOTA Uniform Terminology for Occupational Therapy* (AOTA, 1994) refers to activities of daily living as self-maintenance tasks such as grooming, oral hygiene, bathing/showering, toilet hygiene, personal device care, dressing, feeding and eating, medication routine, health maintenance, socialization, functional communication, functional mobility, community mobility, emergency response, and sexual expression. More complex tasks that are needed to maintain independent living are termed Instrumental ADLs (IADLs; Duke University Center for the Study of Aging and Human Development, 1978). These include safety procedures, care giving, and home management (e.g., clothing care, cleaning, shopping, money management, meal preparation) (Spector, Katz, Murphy, & Fulton, 1987).

Teaching Self-Care

The components of an effective self-care program for individuals with psychosocial disabilities include the following:

▶ *Assessment* of the client's ability to perform the self-care or ADL tasks, using an ADL scale (e.g., the *Kohlman Evaluation of Living Skills* (KELS; Thomson, 1992), or *Milwaukee Evaluation of Daily Living Skills* (MEDLS; Leonardelli, 1988)

▶ *Motivation of the client* so that he or she has the volition or will to perform the task.

▶ *Target goals* that are set by the client and therapist.

▶ *A task analysis* that breaks the targeted goal into the smallest components, so that each component can be taught separately. Backward or forward chaining can be used in the process of teaching self-care skills.

▶ *Use of the teaching model* of demonstration, guided or behavioral practice, and independent practice. (See section on social skills for a more complete description of the model.)

▶ *Periodic evaluation* of the client's ability to perform the task both in the clinic and at home.

The following areas should be considered in a holistic psychosocial treatment program. The occupational therapist should evaluate the client's ability to perform the following tasks.

Personal Care. Skills Necessary for Independent Living

▶ *Hygiene*
  ▶ Washing hands and face at appropriate times before meals
  ▶ Bathing and showering safely, use of side rails
  ▶ Brushing teeth and flossing, using toothbrush correctly
  ▶ Shaving face with either electric shaver or razor
  ▶ Hair care and shampooing periodically, massaging scalp
  ▶ Toiletry and caring for bodily areas in healthy ways
  ▶ Medical care and being able to apply simple first aid for cuts, bruises, and sprains
  ▶ Trimming finger and toe nails
  ▶ Engaging in safe sex and knowing how to use prophylactics

▶ *Eating*
  ▶ Preparing and cooking meals
  ▶ Cleaning up after meal preparation
  ▶ Using kitchen appliances in meal preparation, cooking, and clean up
  ▶ Organizing kitchen storage so that foods are easily accessible
  ▶ Appropriate eating behavior and table etiquette
  ▶ Shopping and ability to plan for week's meals using good nutritional information and being budget wise
  ▶ Dining out and ability to select restaurants that serve favorite foods that are within budget

▶ *Dressing and grooming*
  ▶ Caring for clothing and use of laundromat and hand washing
  ▶ Selecting clothing for everyday and special occasions
  ▶ Purchasing clothing using good judgment in wearability and budget
  ▶ Using cosmetics in an appropriate way and considering budget
  ▶ Using deodorants, lotions, and perfumes that enhance appearance and are safe.

Communication Aids

▶ Using telephones and communicating clearly, seeking appropriate support from friends and relatives

▶ Using telephone directories and locating telephone numbers and addresses

▶ Obtaining help in emergency situations by dialing 911 or hospital

▶ Writing letters for information, to social networks, and for business affairs

▶ Using a computer for communication and leisure pursuits

Medical Management

▶ Compliance with medical prescriptions and rehabilitation program

▶ Understanding purposes of medication and reporting side effects to physician

▶ Renewing prescriptions and relating to pharmacist or physician any changes in symptoms or interactions of medication

▶ Stopping medications without severe effects and withdrawal symptoms and communicating with physician about problems with medications

▶ Controlling for side effects of medications by notifying pharmacist, physician, and therapist of adverse symptoms

▶ Dosages and understanding how many pills to take a day and at the proper times

▶ Discussion with physicians on any problems relating to medications, side effects, symptoms, remissions, or exacerbation

Transportation

▶ Using public transportation and reading maps correctly

▶ Pedestrian travel

▶ Driving and abiding by traffic safety rules

▶ Bicycling

Money Management

▶ Budgeting expenses and keeping records

▶ Using bank accounts for checking and saving

▶ Paying bills in a timely way using checks and money orders

▶ Using good judgment in money decisions

▶ Using credit cards appropriately and reducing interest payments

▶ Filing tax returns and seeking help as available from IRS and volunteers in community

▶ Organizing receipts and documents using a filing system.

Apartment and Home Maintenance

▶ Cleaning and dusting areas on a weekly basis

▶ Vacuuming and proper maintenance of a vacuum cleaner

▶ Maintaining proper indoor temperatures and lighting by controlling thermostat

▶ Repairing minor problems in residence (e.g., changing light bulbs)

▶ Calling and engaging repair person when needed

Prevention of Disease and Maintenance of Health

▶ Buying and using appropriate over-the-counter medications

▶ Knowing first aid (see medical management)

▶ Exercising daily and understanding the benefits of a regular exercise program

▶ Taking a daily multivitamin

▶ Knowing how to get medical assistance when needed

▶ Learning how to get restful sleep by exercising, relaxation, and proper food

▶ Knowing how to maintain good hygiene by keeping skin clean, avoiding infections

▶ Managing stress by exercising, relaxation therapy, using Tai Ch'i and yoga

▶ Obtaining emergency help when needed

Leisure

▶ Identifying leisure activities that are satisfying

▶ Scheduling daily leisure activities into daily or weekly schedule

▶ Using community recreational facilities

▶ Using library and developing interest in reading books and magazines

▶ Exploring and extending new leisure activities by joining special groups

▶ Volunteering in community services such as Meals-on-Wheels

▶ Participating and watching sports, cultural events, and television, and listening to radio and stereophonic music

▶ Engaging in ongoing crafts that can be done every day or weekly

▶ Initiating or continuing in hobbies for enjoyment

▶ Maintaining friendships through correspondences, telephone calls, lunch dates, and social activities

Validation of the Individual's Competencies in Self-Care

Validation of competencies can be done in a number of ways.

▶ *Interview of the client*: First, the therapist will want to interview the client. Client interviews are (a) quick, (b) easy to obtain,

and (c) easily administered. However, there are disadvantages. First, the information the client reports may be difficult to confirm. Second, the client's response may not be accurate if he or she cannot understand all the steps in the task. Validity or confirmation of the client's ability to perform the self-care task can be improved by asking the individual to (a) explain in detail how he or she performs the task or (b) demonstrate the task.

▶ *Interview of the family*: Validation can also be obtained by interviewing family members, caregivers, or others living with the client. This type of validation is quick and easy to obtain and administer. The disadvantages are that (a) the interviewee may not be objective in evaluating the family member's accomplishments and (b) response may not be accurate if the interviewee does not understand all the steps in the task. Validation can be improved by asking the interviewee to (a) give examples of when and where task is performed by the client without assistance or (b) using a second family member to consensually validate the information.

▶ *Simulated situation*: A third way to obtain information about a client's ability to perform a task is to arrange a simulated task where the individual performs an ADL task observed by the therapist. An advantage in this method is direct observation of the client's behavior by the therapist. For example, the therapist can observe the client as he or she prepares a meal. On the other hand, the client may not be motivated to complete the task, or the facilities in the clinic may be different than facilities at home. This method can be improved by (a) asking client how facilities differ from facilities at home, and accommodating for differences, and (b) getting the client to verbalize the task while doing it.

▶ *Standardized tests*: Standardized tests have been developed to assess self-care skills, for example, the *Bay Area Functional Performance Inventory* (BaFPE; Bloomer & Lang, 1991), *Street Survival Skills Questionnaire* (SSSQ; Linkenhoker & McCarron, 1979, 1993), *Kohlman Evaluation of Living Skills* (KELS; Thomson, 1992), *Independent Living Skills* (ILS; Johnson, Vinnicombe, & Merrill, 1981), or the *Milwaukee Evaluation of Daily Living Skills* (MEDLS; Leonardelli, 1988). (See Chapter 7 for further information regarding standardized tests.) Advantages of using standardized tests include: (a) standardized norms are established for what is expected in terms of behavior, outcome, and all steps of the task and (b) tasks or questions are hierarchically sequenced. There are some disadvantages, however: (a) the test might not be administered in standardized fashion; (b) the environment may not be conducive in obtaining accurate results; (c) the test may not be exhaustive in measuring all areas of self-care; (c) the test may not have adequate reliability or validity; and (d) the individual may know how to do the task on a test, but not able to do it in a real-life situation. Administering a standardized test can be improved by (a) establishing rapport with client before administering test; (b) providing a secure environment for testing free of distractions; (c) having all test materials available and ready to use; (d) being familiar with the purposes and the administration of test; (e) giving the client an opportunity to ask questions before beginning to administer the test; (f) carefully observing instructions for administering test and following directions verbatim; and (g) scoring according to norms, but using clinical judgment in interpreting results.

▶ *In vivo observations*: Clinical observations (in vivo) are obtained by occupational therapists as the client performs ADL tasks in independent living arrangements, the home, hospital, clinic, sheltered workshop, or school. Some advantages of obtaining data using this method include: (a) the assessment is authentic because the client is being evaluated actually doing the task; (b) the task is not contrived or simulated; (c) assessment is done in a place or natural setting that is familiar to the client; and (d) the client can demonstrate accommodations in the setting that enable him or her to do task. Disadvantages include: (a) the assessment takes longer and is more expensive than a test or interview; (b) the assessment requires time for scheduling of a field visit and expenditures on part of therapist; (c) the presence of the observer may affect the performance of client; and (d) what is observed may not be representative of the client's capabilities. In vivo observation may be improved by having the therapist (a) establish rapport with client before observing; (b) use a checklist of self-care items while observing the client's performance; and (c) sit or observe at a distance in an unobtrusive manner so that the therapist does not interfere with the activity.

How do we determine the client's level of independence in self-care? The following six levels will be helpful in determining the client's degree of independence. It also will be important to determine if the individual is motivated to perform the activity. The client may be able to perform the activity independently but may not be motivated to do so.

Level I: The client is unable to do task even with assistance: For example, an individual who is chronically mentally ill is unable to cook dinner or assist in food preparation even with assistance from family member.

Level II: The client can do part of the activity with manual assistance or accommodations. For example, the individual follows simple directions to assist in preparing the meal, such as peeling the potatoes.

Level III: The client can do part of the activity with verbal or visual prompts. For example, the client can take a telephone message with reminders of appropriate questions written on a card next to the telephone.

Level IV: The client can do part of the activity without assistance. For example, the individual is not able to do laundry independently, but can sort laundry into colored clothing and whites before it is washed.

Level V: The client can do the entire activity with accommodation or verbal prompts. For example, the client can travel on bus and ask the bus driver to announce the stop where he or she is getting off.

Level VI: The client is independent and motivated to perform activity. At this level, for example, the individual can perform all the tasks required in laundering without assistance or cues.

Assessment in a performance area requires a task analysis of the skill. First, the ADL performance area must be operationally defined so that measurement is possible, for example: the individual will prepare for and take a bath or shower independently. Second, the therapist must identify possible barriers that prevent the client from accomplishing the task. For example, (a) the presence of symptoms of mental illness, such as apathy, delusions and phobia, interfere with task activities; (b) lack of motivation to perform the task; (c) cognitive deficits interfering with task completion, such as difficulty sequencing tasks in the activity, poor memory or inattention, or difficulty in decision-making; (d) sensory or motor deficits, such as tardive dyskinesia, blindness, or hearing impairment that interfere with task completion; or (e) social deprivation, such as no instruction or no opportunity to learn the task. Third, the therapist identifies the preskills or performance components necessary for accomplishing self-care task (AOTA, 1994):

Sensory Motor Components

► *Sensory*: awareness and processing: visual, auditory, tactile, proprioceptive, gustatory, olfactory

► *Perceptual processing*: interpretation of information

► *Neuromusculoskeletal*: range of motion, muscle tone, strength, endurance

► *Gross and fine motor*: laterality, bilateral integration, praxis

Cognitive Integration and Cognitive Components

► Arousal, orientation, and attention span

► Memory, sequencing, spatial organization, categorization

► Problem-solving, learning, generalization

Psychosocial Skills and Psychological Components

► *Psychological*: values, self-concept, interests

► *Social: social* conduct, interpersonal skills

► *Self-management skills*: coping skills, time management, self-control

Finally, the therapist must assess the client's ability to do an ADL task in the context of time and the environment (i.e., performance contexts) (AOTA, 1994). Time refers to chronology, developmental, life-cycle aspects, and disability status, while the environment refers to the physical, social, and cultural aspects of the task.

An example of assessment in a specific performance area of ADL, personal hygiene, is given in Figure 11–2. This figure provides a model for evaluating the client's ability to perform a specific self-care task and can be used by therapists in evaluating the client's level of independence for other areas of self-care.

SOCIAL SKILLS

Focusing Questions

▶ What are social skills?

▶ How is social skills training defined?

▶ How can a therapist teach social skills to a client with a psychosocial disability?

▶ What are the components of social skills training?

▶ How can a therapist incorporate a social skills training program into a group format?

▶ What are some of the findings from recent research studies evaluating the effectiveness of social skills training?

PERSONAL HYGIENE
(washing, bathing, shaving, brushing teeth, washing hair, cutting/cleaning nails, etc.)

Validation of information (Circle method)

a.   Interview with client

b.   Interview with family or care givers

c.   Simulated task where individual performs ADL task with therapist

d.   Results from a standardized test

e.   Observation by nurse, aide, therapist, or special educator, of individual performing ADL task in independent living arrangements, client's home, hospital, sheltered workshop, or school

Determine the level of independence in self-care (Score each task from 1 to 6 and record in the section below)

1.   Unable to do activity even with assistance

2.   Can do part of the activity with manual assistance or accommodations

3.   Can do part of the activity with verbal or visual prompts

4.   Can do part of the activity without assistance

5.   Can do the entire activity with accommodation or verbal prompts

6.   Independent and motivated to perform activity

Skills: Can the individual. . . (e.g., shave)	Date Evaluated	Level of Independence
• Regulate frequency of task (e.g., 1x/day)	(enter date)	(e.g., 1–6)
• Regulate water temperature (hot and cold) for each task		
• Collect supplies before task (e.g., soap, gel, towels, washcloths, electric razor)		
• Return supplies to proper place		

© Stein & Cutler, 1997

Figure 11–2. Example of an assessment of ADL task. This example can be used with all other performance areas in self-care. The form may be reproduced as needed, provided credit is given to the authors.

Definition of Social Skills

Social skills are comprised of skills in (a) attending and listening, (b) conversation, (c) supporting others, (d) problem-solving, and (e) self-control. These areas are outlined in Figures 11–3 and 11–4.

Liberman et al. (1984) included the following dimensions under social skills. One includes discrete nonverbal behaviors that constitute person-to-person communications: eye contact, facial expression, posture, gestures, loudness, tone of voice, pacing or speed of speech, latency, duration of responding, and fluency of speech. A second dimension includes the content of speech or conversation: requesting something of another person; praising, thanking, or complimenting other person; saying "no" to an unreasonable request; going through a job interview; reacting appropriately to criticism; and managing other daily instrumental and affectional encounters. A third dimension involves reciprocity in communicating: giving reinforcement to another to maintain conversation, initiating conversation, terminating conversations, and timing one's entry and exit from social groups.

Rinn and Markle (1979) categorized social skills of children into a taxonomy of four areas:

1. Self-Expressive Skills

   a. Expression of feeling (sadness, jealousy, anger, disappointment, or happiness)

   b. Expression of opinion (judgment, belief, or point of view)

   c. Accepting compliments (ability to be objective about oneself)

   d. Stating positives about oneself (ability to have insight into one's behavior)

2. Other Enhancing Skills

   a. Stating positives about a best friend (ability to judge others objectively)

   b. Stating genuine agreement with another's opinion (ability to be congruent)

   c. Praising others (ability to communicate positive thoughts)

3. Assertive Skills (ability to express feelings)

   a. Making simple requests

   b. Disagreeing with another's opinion

   c. Denying unreasonable requests

4. Communication Skills

   a. Conversing

   b. Interpersonal problem solving

SOCIAL SKILLS TRAINING

Definition

Hersen, Bellack, and Himmelhoch (1982) defined social skills training as

> a structured learning therapy. It is designed to develop the specific skills necessary to perform effectively in interpersonal situations. By "perform effectively," we mean the maximization of positive reinforcement, while keeping social punishment at a minimum. This conception presumes that the individual may reap some negative consequences from others in the process of standing up for personal rights and maintaining a healthy adjustment. (p. 167)

Goldsmith and McFall (1975) defined social skills training as

> A general therapy approach aimed at increasing performance competence in critical life situations. In contrast to the therapies aimed primarily at the elimination of maladaptive behaviors, skills training emphasizes the positive educational aspects of treatment. It assumes that each individual always does the best he can, given his physical limitations and unique learning history in every situation. Thus, when an individual's best effort is judged to be maladaptive, this indicates the presence of a situation specific skill deficit in the indi-

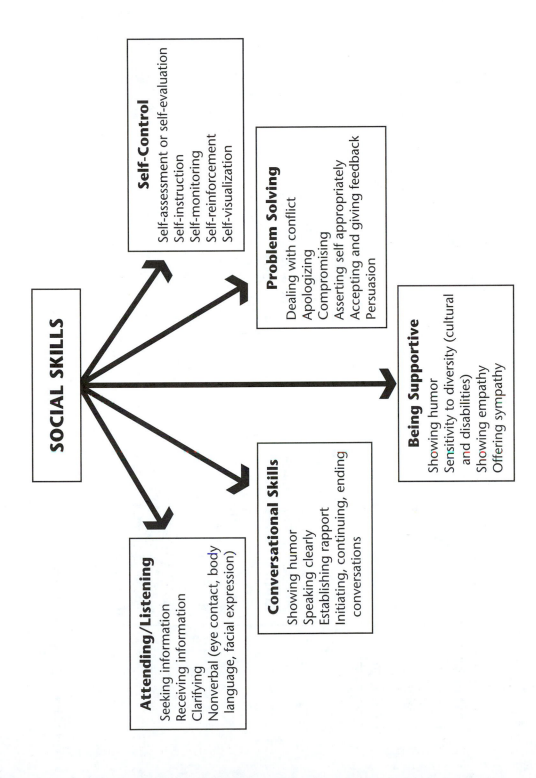

Figure 11–3. The major areas of social skills.

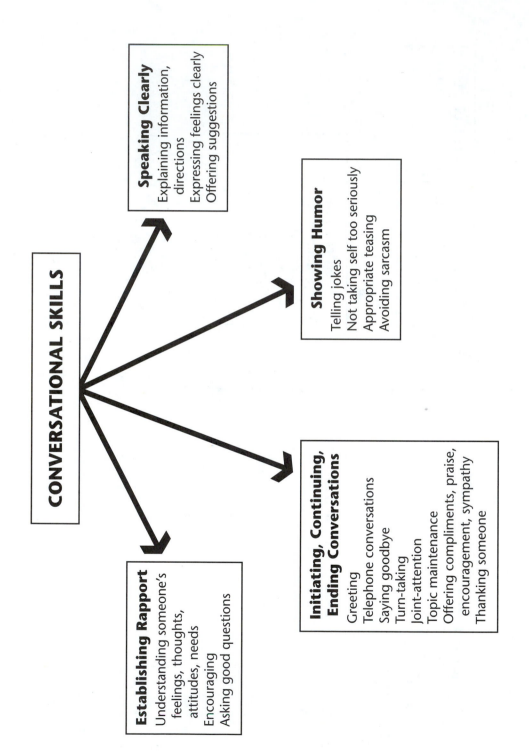

Figure 11–4. Conversational skills are one area of social skills. The major components of conversation skills are outlined in this figure.

vidual's repertoire. . . . Whatever the origin of this deficit (e.g., lack of experience, faulty learning, biological dysfunction), it often may be overcome or partially compensated through appropriate training in more skillful response alternatives. (p. 51)

This approach emphasizes the positive aspects of behavior where the therapist introduces a new social skill or works with the client in improving social behavior. For example, Wehman and Marchant (1978) examined the effects of a behavioral training program on improving free play and motor skills of four children with severe and profound mental retardation as a model for occupational therapists working in school settings. The free play and motor skills training included (a) selection of reactive toys such as stacking blocks, Slinky, and music box that produce an effect when played with; (b) demonstration to the child on how to use the toy in a one-to-one relationship; and (c) verbal praise and physical affection. Social skills training represents a general approach to a broad list of human behaviors that can be directly introduced, developed, or improved in the client. In this example, play is considered an important social skill for children with mental retardation that is essential in personal interactions.

Social skills training is an important component of every psychosocial rehabilitation program. It is based on the assumption that individuals with a psychosocial disability have a deficit in social skills (Corrigan, Schade, & Liberman, 1992). For example, Hersen et al. (1982) described three types of social skills that can be helpful for women with depression: (a) positive assertion, (b) negative assertion, and (c) conversational skills. Positive assertion refers to giving compliments to others, expression of affection to others, offering approval and praise to others, and making apologies. Negative assertion includes refusing unreasonable requests from others, asking someone to change his or her behavior, compromising and negotiating with others, and expressing disapproval and annoyance at someone's behavior. The third target area, conversational skills, refers to the ability to initiate, maintain, and terminate conversations.

Need

Social skills training is a key component of a holistic psychosocial treatment program. The lack of social and self-care skills in individuals with psychosocial disabilities has been described by many clinicians and investigators. Sylph, Ross, and Kedward (1978) presented the following observations in a study of 147 individuals with chronic mental illness:

> One third of the patients had distasteful table manners. Almost all could dress and undress, but without supervision many would attract unfavorable attention in the community. About half were unkempt, were inappropriately attired or groomed, or would go about dirty unless reminded to wash. A slightly smaller proportion could not take a bath unaided, and 30% were unable to wash their hands and face adequately. A quarter wet or soiled themselves at least occasionally, and about 20% needed help at the toilet. Over three-quarters could not manage money satisfactorily, 57% had difficulties with public transportation, and almost half were unable to use the telephone or find their way about outside the hospital.
>
> Impairment of work capacity was marked. Poor performance of domestic chores was universal, and only a third of the patients managed other types of work. Common types of work failure are suggested by the prevalence of slow and sluggish movements and lack of initiative, perseverance, and organizing capacity among 58%–75% and unreliability in carrying out assignments in 96%.

Between 10% and 30% of the patients had defects of sight, hearing, mobility, or manual control, and the body balance of 79% was rated as impaired. Language and communication handicaps were common. 10% of the patients were mute or unintelligible and a third had blocked or unclear speech. Vocabulary and sentence construction were severely limited in 60%–75%. One-third could not understand complex instructions, and twice as many had difficulty reading. (pp. 1391–1392)

Assessment

The social skills training model is based on the assumption that mental illness impairs an individual's ability to function independently. Treatment and rehabilitation of an individual with mental illness primarily involves teaching specific social and self-care skills that will enable the individual to be adaptive. This approach is congruent with occupational therapy's role in psychosocial rehabilitation. The effectiveness of the social skills model depends on the therapist selecting key areas in the client's life that interfere with adjustment and then setting up a psychoeducational or behavioral treatment program that provides adaptive skills. Trower (1979) stated that:

Goal achievement is dependent on skilled behavior which involves a continuous cycle of monitoring and modifying performance in the light of feedback. Failure in skill is defined as a breakdown or impairment at some point in the cycle, which results in failure to achieve targets, leading to negative outcomes and abnormal behavior pattern. (p. 4)

Social skills training is a goal-directed approach toward having the client learn practical skills that counteract abnormal behavior patterns.

Initiating a Social Skills Training Program

The first step in social skills training is assessment of the individual's behavior. Bellack (1979) suggested the specific focus of assessment in the following questions, which are used to guide the therapist in setting up target behaviors:

▶ *"Does the individual manifest some dysfunctional interpersonal behavior"?* (p. 77) This question elicits specific descriptions of the individual's interpersonal behavior. For example, does the individual have difficulty in the following areas?

   ▶ initiating conversations
   ▶ contributing to discussions
   ▶ engaging in group activities
   ▶ listening and understanding others
   ▶ showing appropriate feelings expressed when interacting with others
   ▶ following through in relationships
   ▶ maintaining eye contact when relating to others

▶ *"What are the specific circumstances (i.e., situations) in which the dysfunction is manifested"?* (p. 78). For example, does the individual find it difficult to relate to other family members, co-workers, members of the other sex, strangers, people in authority, specific ethnic groups, neighborhood friends, casual acquaintances, and storekeepers? Does the individual experience stress or anxiety in some general or specific situations? The therapist would try to assess individual areas of dysfunction.

▶ *"What is the (probable) source of the dysfunction"?* (p. 78). The therapist and the patient work together in trying to determine the internal factors that precipitate the individual's dysfunctional interpersonal behavior. Is the primary problem anticipatory anxiety such that the individual is overwhelmed by fear of failure or rejection and becomes immobilized in an interpersonal situation? Do distortions in perception and cognition interfere with interpersonal relationships? Is the failure in behavior due to faulty learning in childhood or a paucity of positive experiences with others?

Assessment

Bellack (1979) identified a number of strategies that can be used or modified by the therapist for assessing an individual's behavior.

▶ *Initial Interview:* The occupational therapist can use a formal structured interview, which identifies the individual's specific dysfunctional behaviors and situations that are extremely anxiety provoking. The therapist can gather a historical perspective into the client's interpersonal history. Areas such as personal interactions at work, friendship patterns, ability to deal with interpersonal problems in the family, participation in social activities and social organizations, and responding to one's feelings of anger and frustration can be explored. The occupational therapist can incorporate these areas into a social skills training program.

▶ *Self-report Inventories:* In this behavioral assessment technique the therapist provides the client with the opportunity to assess his or her own behavior by identifying descriptions or statements that accurately relate to him or her. The self-report inventory can be open-ended or directed. For example, the therapist can ask the client to describe situations that are anxiety provoking. The therapist can also ask the client to use creative media such as art, clay, or poetry to portray these social situations. The self-report inventory can also be used to assess the client's progress. Does the client feel confident or comfortable with members of the opposite sex? For example, the following questions can be posed: Can I listen with understanding toward others? Do I feel confident in playing a competitive sport with others? Do I enjoy having coffee and sharing my inner feelings with others? A self-report inventory is limited by nature by its subjective format. However, it can provide additional information that can be used in following the client's progress.

▶ *Self-monitoring:* This is one of the most widely used behavioral assessment procedures. It is one of the methods used in Rational Emotive Therapy (Ellis, 1970). The client records his or her behavior in a diary or log. For example, the client can keep a record of when he or she feels depressed or elated, anxious or relaxed, inferior or confident, tired or energetic. The client can note what events precipitated a negative emotion, how it influenced interpersonal behavior, and how long it lasted. The individual can also record in what situations or with what people he or she feels most comfortable. The individual can gain insight into the activities he or she enjoys while being with others. Self-monitoring is an effective method in reducing weight, controlling smoking, reducing alcoholic intake, and managing stress.

▶ *Behavioral Observation:* This is the method most frequently used by occupational therapists in assessing a client's social skills. While the client engages in an activity in a group situation, the occupational therapist evaluates the client's interactions with others. The occupational therapist can also simulate social situations through role-playing, for example, where the client telephones a friend, interviews for a job, tells a joke, asks for a date, expresses a feeling, or tells a group a story from his or her childhood. The therapist can make home visits to observe a client with family members and to gain insight in a natural environment.

▶ *Ratings by Peers and Significant Others*: This method is used frequently in family therapy to help the client gain insight into his or her social interactions by asking family members and friends to evaluate the client's progress. Is there congruity in how the client feels he or she is relating in comparison to the reports of his or her family and friends? Consensual validation and congruence between the client and others are important in establishing the baseline of behavior. The client may be underestimating or overestimating his or her behavioral dysfunctions. The perceptual reality can be reinforced by the evaluations of others. Many times the clients think their behavior is more bizarre than others have noticed. This is important feedback for the client. For even though the client may feel anxious, unconcerned with others and self-centered, his or her friends may simply note that he is just quieter than others.

▶ *Physiological Assessment*: The introduction of physiological measurements such as electromyograph, temperature trainer, heart rate monitors, and other biofeedback tools have been helpful in providing clients with concrete parameters that parallel psychological states. The symptoms of stress-related behavior such as feelings of anxiety, back pain, headache, gastrointestinal pain, and excessive sweating can be verified by physiological assessments used in biofeedback training.

Teaching Methods

After assessing the individual's dysfunction in social skills, a training program incorporated within a treatment model can be implemented. Therapists can use methods of *direct instruction* in teaching the client through demonstrations and discussions to use nonverbal and verbal responses effectively in interacting with another client. For example, the client can be taught to be positive in interactions with others and to maintain eye contact. *Behavior rehearsal* is another approach in which the therapist coaches the client through practice in a simulated situation or through role-playing positive behavioral techniques and positive interpersonal reactions. The client can role-play past situations that were stressful or upcoming events such as applying for a job. *Modeling* is another approach in social skills training in which the therapist helps the client to acquire a targeted behavior through demonstration of positive interactions with others. The therapist can also use films or videotapes to demonstrate successful interactions. For example, O'Connor (1969) successfully used a 23-minute sound-color film with nursery school children who were socially withdrawn. The film showed positive interrelationships that the children could imitate and model in their interactions. In a clinical study Cermak, Stein, and Abelson (1973) demonstrated how occupational therapists can create an environment for facilitating positive change through a group activity model using behavioral rehearsal in a group situation with children diagnosed with hyperactivity.

As a systematic approach to the field of psychiatric rehabilitation, behavior therapy has made significant progress in the last 60 years. Currently, the major trends in applying behavior therapy have been in the areas of social skills training (Liberman, 1992) and stress reduction (Meichenbaum, 1993). Occupational therapists in psychosocial settings have much in common with behavior therapists. Both fields emphasize the development of practical skills in coping with environmental adaptation. Behavior therapy is an excellent model for the psychosocial occupational therapist to use in teaching social skills and in managing stress.

Psychosocial Training

There are four steps in teaching any social skill: *psychoeducational instruction, demonstration and modeling, guided practice, and independent activities.* These four steps can be used sequentially with any social skill being taught. Only when the individual is able to perform the social skill independently in the community or at home, is the skill considered to be incorporated into the client's everyday life situation. Effective behavioral techniques are used in the following methods when teaching social skills:

▶ *Psychoeducational teaching* is verbal instruction using a variety of instructional techniques. Audiovisual aids, such as videotapes, blackboards, and overheads, can be used to illustrate the social skill to be taught. Handouts, readings, and homework reinforce the lectures or class discussions. Task analysis is used to break a given social skill into smaller components. The individual learns the components of the social skills, so that they can be practiced in role playing at a later stage of training.

▶ *Modeling* is a means of teaching a consumer or client to imitate a desired way to perform a social skill. A single social skill is modeled by the therapist who uses explicit directions

and directly demonstrates the skill. The therapist teaches the components of the skill. The client watches a therapist perform the activity and then imitates the behavior. The therapist explains the behavior being taught and why that behavior is important. Videotapes can be used to demonstrate a specific skill or to videotape a consumer role-playing a specific social skill so that other members can evaluate performance on the tape while the client can objectively evaluate his or her social skill.

▶ *Guided practice* involves having the client perform an actual social skill under the watchful eye of the therapist and other members of the group. Guided practice "offers clients a unique opportunity to practice new skills, to receive constructive criticisms in areas of potential improvement, and to receive social praise for using these skills" (Monti, Corriveau, & Curran, 1982, p. 191). One purpose of guided practice is to shape the behavior of individual by allowing him or her to practice a particular social skill in a safe environment. During this period, the client performs behavior while the therapist coaches as necessary. Verbal, physical, and visual prompts are used as needed.

Several techniques are used in guided practice.

▶ *Role-playing or behavioral rehearsal*: The client has an opportunity to participate in a situation such as initiating a conversation, applying for a job, speaking to a family member, or providing constructive feedback. The therapist and client can select the social skill to be used in the role-playing.

▶ *Role reversal*: The client takes the role of another individual in a social situation, such as the employer in a job interview. This gives the client an opportunity to experience the feelings of another individual.

▶ *Paradoxical intention* (Frankl, 1963, 1965; Walker, 1975): Paradoxical intention is based on the theory that anticipatory anxiety leads to fears and tensions. Therapists using this technique ask clients to create a negative emotion or situation by thinking of something they fear most. In so doing, the client will begin to gain control over the situation. For example, the client who is fearful about making a mistake, is told to think about or intentionally make a mistake. By doing this, the anticipatory anxiety is lessened and the client begins learning how to control the anticipatory anxiety. This technique can be used in conjunction with "systematic desensitization" (Wolpe, 1969).

▶ *Homework*: Homework or assignments are given to the individual to practice a social skill in the community. The use of homework reinforces the academic learning of the social skill and role-playing and enables the client to learn the skill more quickly (Ellis, 1970).

▶ *Independent Practice and Generalization.* After the client has an opportunity to learn the social skill and receive feedback from the therapist and members of the group, the client needs to practice the social skills in vivo. In vivo practice means that the behavior occurs in actual living situations. Examples of in vivo practice include the community, a social setting, school, on the job, at home, when shopping, or when engaging in daily interactions with others. During this time, training structure and supervision are gradually terminated

("faded"). Clients are taught to use self-management techniques during this period.

Generalization involves the ability to use a social skill learned in one situation and apply it to other situations. In general, generalization occurs when there are changes in the situation in which the social skill is being used, when the social skill is directed toward another individual, or when the social skill involves materials not included in the original situation. There are several techniques to help with generalization.

▶ *Overlearning*: A client will master the learning of a specific social skill so that when an occasion to use that skill arises, he or she will perform it automatically. In addition, the client will master more information or performance skills than would necessarily be needed in a given situation.

▶ *Use of natural reinforcers and caregivers*: This has to do with practicing techniques in the home where caregivers or family members can help the individual in a supportive environment. The caregiver or family member must be taught how to help the client. Reinforcers occur spontaneously, rather than being contrived. For example, a client fixes dinner for the rest of the family and the family members praise him or her in a natural manner, rather than giving points, taking him or her out to dinner, or buying a gift. Reinforcement may be intermittent, that is, not given each time the behavior occurs.

▶ *Accepting personal criticism*: The therapist must help the client be objective in accepting criticism from others about his or her behavior. Likewise, the client must learn to separate the criticism about one's behavior from criticism of oneself. For example, a client with a cognitive style of field dependency (i.e., responsive to personal and verbal criticism) needs to learn to be more objective in therapy in order to become more field independent (i.e., responsive to objects in the environment). The therapist must teach the client to moderate his or her cognitive style, because neither extreme is healthy in interpersonal communication.

▶ *Problem-solving strategy:* This technique teaches the client to use problem-solving skills in everyday situations. The steps in problem-solving include: (a) identifying the problem clearly, (b) generating as many solutions as possible, (c) identifying pros and cons of each solution, (d) determining consequences for each solution, (e) choosing and applying a solution to the situation, and (f) evaluating the effectiveness of the solution.

Self-Regulation

Another aspect of social skills training involves self-regulation. One aspect of self-regulation is the development of self-control. Workman and Katz (1995) have provided definitions and guidelines for helping a client improve these skills.

▶ *Self-control:* the ability of a client to assess, monitor, and regulate feelings, thoughts, behaviors, and symptoms.

▶ *Self-assessment or self-evaluation:* the ability to systematically assess or evaluate one's behavior so (a) that it can be changed and improved or (b) to affirm appropriate behavior. Individuals can assess their feelings, thoughts, behaviors, and symptoms

through a diary or log. (See examples in Chapter 10, including compliance management and the Outcome Evaluation for Self-regulation of Symptoms.)

▶ *Self-instruction training:* using self-talk with clients to teach them to give verbal cues to themselves in order to perform a task in a particular way and then to provide verbal feedback to themselves about their performance. This can include writing tasks (e.g., essays, poems, journals) to evaluate their behavior, or participation in role-play, acting out their own behavior.

▶ *Self-monitoring of symptoms, thoughts, feelings, behavior:* self-charting of one's behavior through, for example, recording of duration, frequency, or severity of behaviors to evaluate and possibly change the behavior. For example, an individual on a job could record how many times he or she speaks to a colleague in a friendly manner and receives positive reinforcement for his or her behavior.

▶ *Self-reinforcement of positive behavior:* the use of positive reinforcements, such as verbal affirmation (e.g., "I did a good job today."), primary reinforcers (e.g., eating a favorite food or going to a favorite restaurant), or secondary reinforcers (e.g., watching a film, going to the theater, listening to music, spending time with a friend).

▶ *Self-visualization:* instances when the individual visualizes or anticipates a successful outcome or positive exchange in a future event, for example, going for a job interview, taking a test, meeting a new person, or anticipating the first day on a job. This can also occur when an individual visualizes the steps needed to get to that future event.

Assertiveness Training

One of the most important areas of social skills training is teaching assertive behavior. Assertive behavior includes helping and empowering clients to make choices for themselves, make independent decisions, request information or help, defend oneself from being taking advantage of, giving constructive criticism. King, Liberman, Roberts, and Bryan (1977) gave examples of hierarchies of assertive behavior for three community situations:

Department store

▶ Ask where to buy something that store does not have

▶ Ask for information about some product without buying

▶ Try on clothes without buying

▶ Return item with receipt for credit

▶ Return item with receipt for cash

▶ Return item without receipt for credit

▶ Return item without receipt for cash

▶ Ask to use the phone

▶ Ask where the restroom is

▶ Bargain with sales person on price

Service stations

▶ Without buying gas, ask for directions

▶ Without buying gas, ask for key to restroom

▶ Without buying gas, ask for free map

▶ Ask for estimate on repairs

▶ When buying gas, ask attendant to check oil, water, tire pressure and wash windows

▶ Go to unknown station and ask for advice about doing own repairs

▶ Ask to borrow tools

▶ Buy $5.00 worth of gas and write a check for it

▶ Buy $5.00 worth of gas and charge it

▶ Without buying gas, ask attendant to check oil, water, tire pressure, and wash windows

Restaurants

▶ Compliment waitress on service

▶ Request substitutions on menu

▶ Request special preparation of food

▶ Request bill at time of being served

▶ Ask for a separate check

▶ Change mind about order right after waitress had taken it

▶ Request order be hurried

▶ Question a bill

▶ Send food back to be recooked or warmed

▶ Criticize waitress on service

A treatment program similar to the social skills model as related to emotions was used as part of a psychiatric occupational therapy group in a general hospital (Angel, 1981). Group sessions involving 24 patients for 1 1/2 hour sessions were used for the expressed purpose of looking at different emotions, such as sadness, shyness, loneliness, anger, love, inferiority, anticipation, kindness, fear, jealousy, and happiness. Patients were encouraged to identify these emotions in poetry, music, art, drama, and role-playing. Finally, activities were incorporated into the session "that move the patient closer to experiencing and/or expressing ownership of some grade of the specific emotion under discussion" (p. 259). The author concluded that "Emotions identification defined as an individual's awareness of effective responses that occur during varied daily object interactions . . . as a skill that occupational therapy can help patients develop" (p. 262).

Developing a Social Skills Program

The development of social skills training is an integral part of a holistic psychosocial occupational therapy program. It is recommended that social skills be taught as part of a group experience. Following are guidelines for establishing a social skills training group in a CMHC.

▶ Establish 6 to 10 sessions in a group format, with the number of clients in a group ranging from 8 to 15.

▶ Select clients who can benefit from social skills training. Clients in the group should have similar cognitive levels (Allen, 1985), rather than having some clients with average cognitive abilities and others with moderate to severe cognitive delays.

▶ A psychoeducational model stating the themes of each session should be established in advance. For example, in a social skills training program emphasizing communication skills and interpersonal relationships, the following is an example of an 8-week module in a CMHC planned by an occupational therapist.

a. Session 1: Introduce the course and help the clients get to know each other.

b. Session 2: Introduce conversational skills, such as initiating and ending conversations with one another.

c. Session 3: Emphasize listening skills, attending behaviors, and understanding the role of nonverbal behavior in conversations and interpersonal relationships.

d. Session 4: Focus on language and speech patterns (e.g., clarity in speaking, topic maintenance, volume and pitch of speech).

e. Session 5: Focus on giving and receiving positive and negative feedback (e.g., giving of compliments, receiving criticism).

f. Session 6: Discuss the use of humor in interpersonal relationships.

g. Session 7: Practice social skills by videotaping and evaluating the role-play of group members in various social situations.

h. Session 8: Closure, with a potluck meal, involving each member in the cooking, serving, clean-up, and mealtime discussion.

Vary the methods used in the program. These include role-playing, films, videotaping, imitation of gestures, behavioral rehearsal or guided practice, homework, small group (e.g., 2 to 3 individuals) and whole group discussion, and direct instruction. Table 11–2 provides some references that might be helpful for occupational therapists to use in developing a social skills training program in a CMHC.

ANNOTATED BIBLIOGRAPHY OF RECENT STUDIES ON THE EFFECTIVENESS OF SOCIAL SKILLS TRAINING

Schindler, V. P. (1999). Group effectiveness in improving social interaction skills. *Psychiatric Rehabilitation Journal, 22,* 349–354.

ABSTRACT: This study examines the effectiveness of an activity group, structured discussion group, and control group on the social interaction skills of 25 individuals with psychiatric disabilities. Bivariate analysis revealed that the individuals participating in the activity group demonstrated significant improvement in scores in comparison to no significant changes in scores of participants in the structured discussion group or the control group. Findings suggest that activity groups are more conducive to improving social interaction than structured discussion groups or control groups (no treatment) for individuals with severe psychiatric disabilities.

Table 11–2. Helpful References to Use in Developing a Social Skills Training Program

Alberto, P. A., & Troutman, A. C. (1999). *Applied behavioral analysis (5th ed.).* Columbus, OH: Prentice Hall/Merrill.

Becker, R. E., Heimberg, R. G., & Bellack, A. S. (1987). *Social skills training treatment for depression.* Elmsford, NY: Pergamon.

Bellack, A. S., Turner, S. M., Hersen, M., & Luber, R. T. (1984). An examination of the efficacy of social skills training for chronic schizophrenic patients. *Hospital and Community Psychiatry, 35,* 1023–1028.

Cole, J. R., Klarreich, S. H., & Fryatt, M. J. (1982). Teaching interpersonal coping skills to adult psychiatric patients. *Cognitive Therapy and Research, 6,* 105–112.

Collins, J., & Collins, M. (1992). *Social skills training and the professional helper.* Chichester, NY: John Wiley.

Corrigan, P. W., Schade, M. L., & Liberman, R. P. (1992). Social skills training. In R. P. Liberman (Ed.), *Handbook of psychiatric rehabilitation* (pp. 95–126). Boston: Allyn and Bacon.

Curran, J. P., & Monti, P. M. (Eds.). (1982). *Social skills training: A practical handbook for assessment and treatment.* New York: Guilford.

Fecteau, G. W., & Duffy, M. (1986). Social and conversational skills training with long-term psychiatric inpatients. *Psychological Reports, 59,* 1327–1331.

Frisch, M. B., Elliott, C. H., Atsaides, J. P., Salva, D. M., & Denney, D. R. (1982). Social skills and stress management training to enhance patients' interpersonal competencies. *Psychotherapy: Theory, Research and Practice, 19,* 349–358.

Hersen, M., & Bellack, A. S. (Eds.). (1978). *Behavior therapy in the psychiatric setting.* Baltimore: Williams & Wilkins.

Hogarty, G. E., Anderson, C. M., & Reiss, D. J. (1987). Family psychoeducation, social skills training, and medication in schizophrenia: The long and short of it. *Psychopharmacology Bulletin, 23,* 12–13.

Hollin, C. R., & Trower, P. (Eds.). (1986). *Handbook of social skills training: Clinical applications and new directions.* Elmsford, NY: Pergamon.

Karoly, P., & Kanfer, F. H. (Eds.). (1982). *The psychology of self-management: From theory to practice.* Elmsford, NY: Pergamon.

Kendall, P. C., & Hollon, S. D. (Eds.). (1981). *Assessment strategies for cognitive–behavioral interventions.* New York: Academic.

Liberman, R. P. (Ed.). (1992). *Handbook of psychiatric rehabilitation.* Boston: Allyn and Bacon.

Liberman, R. P., DeRisi, W. J., & Mueser, K. T. (1989). *Social skills training for psychiatric patients.* New York: Pergamon

Liberman, R. P., Lillie, F. J., Falloon, I. R. H., Harpin, E. J., Hutchinson, W., & Stoute, B. A. (1984). Social skills training for relapsing schizophrenics: An experimental analysis. *Behavioral Modification, 8,* 155–179

Liberman, R. P., Mueser, K. T., & Wallace, C. J. (1986). Social skills training for schizophrenic individuals at risk for relapse. *American Journal of Psychiatry, 143,* 523–526.

McGinnis, E., & Goldstein, A. P. (1990). *Skillstreaming in early childhood: Teaching prosocial skills to the preschool and kindergarten.* (Available through Research Press Company, 2612 North Mattis Avenue, Champaign, IL 61821)

McGinnis, E., & Goldstein, A. P. (1997a). *Skillstreaming in elementary school: New strategies and perspectives for teaching prosocial skills.* (Available through Research Press Company, 2612 North Mattis Avenue, Champaign, IL 61821)

McGinnis, E., & Goldstein, A. P. (1997b). *Skillstreaming the adolescent: New strategies and perspectives for teaching prosocial skills.* (Available through Research Press Company, 2612 North Mattis Avenue, Champaign, IL 61821)

Rehm, L. P. (1984). Self-management therapy for depression. *Advances in Behavioral Research and Therapy, 6,* 83–94.

Spencer, P. G., Gillespie, C. R., & Ekisa, E. G. (1983). A controlled comparison of the effects of social skills training and remedial drama on the conversational skills of chronic schizophrenic inpatients. *British Journal of Psychiatry, 143,* 165–172.

Trower, P. (Ed.). (1984). *Radical approaches to social skills training.* New York: Methuen.

Wallace, C. J., & Liberman, R. P. (1985). Social skills training for patients with schizophrenia: A controlled clinical trial. *Psychiatry Research, 15,* 239–247.

Kopelowicz, A., Liberman, R. P., Mintz, J., & Zarate, R. (1997). Comparison of efficacy of social skills training for deficit and nondeficit negative symptoms in schizophrenia. *American Journal of Psychiatry, 154,* 424–425.

OBJECTIVE: The purpose of this pilot study was to compare the efficacy of social skills training for individuals with schizophrenia who did or did not have the deficit syndrome. METHOD: Three subjects with the deficit syndrome and three with nondeficit negative symptoms received 12 weeks of social skills training. Social skills and negative symptoms were evaluated before and after training and at 6-month follow-up. RESULTS: Patients with schizophrenia who did not have the deficit syndrome demonstrated significantly better social skills and lower negative symptoms both after training and at follow-up than did those who had the deficit syndrome. CONCLUSIONS: Schizophrenic patients with nondeficit negative symptoms appear amenable to intensive social skills training, but schizophrenic patients with the deficit syndrome may have significant deficits in skill acquisition.

Marder, S. R., Wirshing, W. C., Mintz, J., McKenzie, J., Johnston, K., Eckman, T. A., Lebell, M., Zimmerman, K., & Liberman, R. P. (1996). Two-year outcome of social skills training and group psychotherapy for outpatients with schizophrenia. *American Journal of Psychiatry, 153,* 1585–1592.

OBJECTIVE: The authors evaluated the effectiveness of behaviorally oriented social skills training and supportive group therapy for improving the social adjustment of schizophrenic patients living in the community and for protecting them against psychotic relapse. METHOD: Eighty male outpatients with schizophrenia were stabilized with a low dose of fluphenazine decanoate (5 to 10 mg every 14 days), which was supplemented with oral fluphenazine (5 mg twice daily) or a placebo when they first met criteria for a prodromal period. (Half of the patients did so at some time during the study.) Patients were randomly assigned to receive either social skills training or supportive group therapy twice weekly for 6 months and then weekly for the next 18 months. Rates of psychotic exacerbation were monitored, as were scores on the Social Adjustment Scale II. RESULTS: There were significant main effects favoring social skills training over supportive group therapy on two of the six Social Adjustment Scale II cluster totals examined (personal well-being and total) and significant interactions between psychosocial treatment and drug treatment for three items (external family, social and leisure activities, and total). In each case, these interactions indicated that the advantage of social skills training over supportive group therapy was greatest when it was combined with active drug supplementation. Social skills training did not significantly decrease the risk of psychotic exacerbation in the full group, but an advantage was observed (post hoc) among patients who received placebo supplementation. CONCLUSIONS: These findings suggest that social skills training resulted in greater improvement in certain measures of social adjustment than supportive group therapy. The greatest improvement in social outcomes occurred when social skills training was combined with a pharmacological strategy of active drug supplementation at the time prodromal worsening of psychotic symptoms was first observed. However, these improvements were modest in absolute terms and confined to certain subgroups of patients.

McKay, D., & Neziroglu, F. (1996). Social skills training in a case of obsessive-compulsive disorder with schizotypal personality disorder. *Journal of Behavioral Therapy in Experimental Psychiatry, 27,* 189–194.

The present study illustrates a case of obsessive-compulsive disorder (OCD) with schizotypal personality treated by social skills training. Prior research suggests that OCD with schizotypal personality predicts poor treatment outcome using exposure-based treatments. Following social skills treatment and at 6-month follow-up, the patient had considerable obsessive-compulsive symptom reduction, although he was still symptomatic for OCD, anxiety and depression. Controlled trials are indicated to illuminate the specific contributions of this approach for OCD with schizotypal personality disorder.

Dobson, D. J., McDougall, G., Busheikin, J., & Aldous, J. (1995). Effects of social skills training and social milieu treatment on symptoms of schizophrenia. *Psychiatric Services, 46*, 376–380.

OBJECTIVE: The study compared the effects of social skills training and social milieu treatment on symptoms of schizophrenia, particularly on negative symptoms.

METHODS: Thirty-three patients aged 18 to 55 years with a diagnosis of schizophrenia were randomly assigned to a nine-week program of social skills training or social milieu treatment. Patients were assessed at 3-, 6-, and 9-week intervals during treatment and at follow-up using the *Positive and Negative Syndrome Scale* (PANSS), which measured both positive and negative symptoms of schizophrenia and general psychopathology.

RESULTS: Fifteen patients completed social skills training, and 13 completed social milieu treatment. Comparison of PANSS scores at different assessment times showed that both treatments were effective in reducing symptoms, but social skills training appeared to be more effective in reducing negative symptoms. No differences were found between treatment groups in relapse rates or in symptom measures at 3-month follow-up. However, 6-month follow-up data available only for the social skills training group showed that improvement in negative symptoms had begun to decline.

CONCLUSIONS: Psychosocial approaches are a necessary component in the treatment of patients with schizophrenia, and social skills training appears to be particularly helpful. The gradual decline in improvement in negative symptoms at 6-month follow-up suggests the need for more extended treatment.

Halford, W. K., & Hayes, R. L. (1995). Social skills in schizophrenia: Assessing the relationship between social skills, psychopathology and community functioning. *Social Psychiatry and Psychiatric Epidemiology, 30*, 14–19.

Social skills training (SST) has been widely used in attempts to rehabilitate chronic schizophrenic patients. The key assumption underlying SST is that social skills deficits are important determinants of the social isolation, poor social role functioning, and low quality of life characteristic of schizophrenic patients. To test this assumption, 89 patients meeting DSM-III-R criteria for schizophrenia were assessed on behavioral and self-report measures of social skills. A structured clinical interview, a self-report inventory of distress during social interaction, and self-monitoring of time in social interaction were used to assess social functioning. Positive psychotic symptoms were assessed in a standardized clinical interview. A structural equation modeling analysis showed that observed social skills predicted social functioning, and that this association was statistically independent of severity of psychotic symptoms. This finding is consistent with the hypothesis that social skills are important in the social functioning of patients with schizophrenia.

Albano, A. M., Marten, P. A., Holt, C. S., Heimberg, R. G., & Barlow, D. H. (1995). Cognitive-behavioral group treatment for social phobia in adolescents. A preliminary study. *Journal of Nervous Mental Disorder, 183*, 649–656.

The present study is a preliminary evaluation of the effectiveness of a new cognitive-behavioral group treatment protocol for social phobia in adolescents. Five adolescents with social phobia were treated in a 16-session group treatment program, with parental involvement in selected sessions. Treatment involved skills training (social skills, problem solving, assertiveness), cognitive restructuring, behavioral exposure, and homework. Self-report measures of anxiety and depression, taken throughout treatment, indicated significant improvements over a 1-year follow-up period.

Behavior test measures also indicated a decrease in subjective anxiety ratings after treatment which was maintained at follow-up. Structured diagnostic interviews 1 year after treatment confirmed full remission of social phobia for four subjects, with one subject's phobia in partial remission. Overall, the present findings support the continued evaluation of this protocol for social phobic adolescents.

Halford, W. K., Harrison, C., Kalyansundaram, Moutrey, C., & Simpson, S. (1995). Preliminary results from a psychoeducational program to rehabilitate chronic patients. *Psychiatric Services, 46,* 1189–1191.

Twenty-two chronic psychiatric patients enrolled in a psychoeducational rehabilitation program were assessed before and after the program to determine whether participation decreased severity of psychopathology and improved community functioning and quality of life. The program consisted of five 14-week modules that provided training in five skill areas: medication and symptom self-management, coping with anxiety and depression, social skills, living skills, and leisure skills. Most patients experienced significantly reduced psychopathology and negative symptoms and improved quality of life and community functioning. The program appears helpful to clients, and a controlled trial to further evaluate its effects is underway.

Smith, T . E., Hull, J. W., MacKain, S. J., Wallace, C. J., Rattenni, L. A., Goodman, M., Anthony, D. T., & Kentros, M. K. (1996). Training hospitalized patients with schizophrenia in community reintegration skills. *Psychiatry Services, 47,* 1099–1103.

OBJECTIVE: The study examined the effectiveness of the Community Re-Entry Program, a brief, time-limited skills training module designed to help acutely ill inpatients become engaged in community-based treatment programs.

METHODS: Of 84 consecutive admissions to a chronic psychotic disorders unit, 44 completed assessments and attended the Community Re-Entry Program. The program consists of 16 daily small-group therapy sessions that engage the patient in efforts to define discharge readiness, identify symptoms and medication effects, and assist with discharge planning. Skill levels and positive and negative symptoms were assessed on admission and on completion of training, and a sub-sample of patients received two-week post-discharge follow-up assessments.

RESULTS: From admission to discharge, positive symptoms diminished substantially, negative symptoms diminished to a lesser but statistically significant degree, and skill levels increased significantly. Post-training skill level was predicted by pretraining skill level and level of participation in the skills training module. Patients' symptom levels did not predict participation in the program or skill acquisition. Skill level at discharge was also more predictive of two-week postdischarge community adjustment than were symptom levels.

CONCLUSIONS: Although further controlled studies are required to fully establish the efficacy of the Community Re-Entry Program, these data suggest that brief, focused skills training may play an important role in augmenting optimal pharmacotherapy for hospitalized patients with chronic psychotic disorders.

REFERENCES

Albano, A. M., Marten, P. A., Holt, C. S., Heimberg, R. G., & Barlow, D. H. (1995). Cognitive-behavioral group treatment for social phobia in adolescents. A preliminary study. *Journal of Nervous Mental Disorder, 183,* 649–656.

Allen, C. K. (1985). *Occupational therapy for psychiatric diseases: Measurement and management of cognitive disabilities.* Boston: Little, Brown.

American Occupational Therapy Association. (1994). Uniform terminology for occupational therapy—Third edition. *American Journal of Occupational Therapy, 48,* 1047–1059.

Angel, S. (1981). The emotion identification group. *American Journal of Occupational Therapy, 35,* 256–262.

Barry, M. M., & Crosby, C. (1996). Quality of life as an evaluative measure in assessing the impact of community care on people with long-term psychiatric disorders. *Birmingham Journal of Psychiatry, 8*(2), 210–216.

Bellack, A. S. (1979). A critical appraisal of strategies for assessing social skill. *Behavior Assessment, 1,* 157–176.

Bloomer, J. S., & Lang, S. (1991). *Bay Area Functional Performance Inventory* (BaFPE). Pequannock, NJ: Maddak.

Cermak, S., Stein, F., & Abelson, C. (1973). Hyperactive children and an activity group therapy model. *American Journal of Occupational Therapy, 26,* 311–315.

Corrigan, P. W., Schade, M. L., & Liberman, R. P. (1992). Social skills training. In R. P. Liberman (Ed.), *Handbook of psychiatric rehabilitation* (pp. 95–126). Boston: Allyn & Bacon.

Dobson, D. J., McDougall, G., Busheikin, J., & Aldous, J. (1995). Effects of social skills training and social milieu treatment on symptoms of schizophrenia. *Psychiatric Services, 46,* 376–380.

Duke University Center for the Study of Aging and Human Development. (1978). *Multidimensional Functional Assessment Questionnaire* (2nd ed.). Greensboro, NC: Author.

Dumazedier, J. (1960). Current problems of the sociology of leisure. *International Social Science Journal, 4.*

Ellis, A. (1970). *The essence of rational psychotherapy: A comprehensive approach to treatment.* New York: Institute for Rational Living.

Fagan, J. (1976). Modeling how and why play works. In J. S. Bruner, A. Jolly, & K. Sylva (Eds.), *Play: Its role in development and evolution* (pp. 96–115). New York: Basic Books.

Fasting, K. (1982). Leisure time, physical activity and some indices of mental health. *Scandinavian Journal of Social Medicine, 29*(Suppl.), 113–119.

Felce, D., & Perry, J. (1996). Exploring current conceptions of quality of life: A model for people with and without disabilities. In R. Renwick, I. Brown, & M. Nagler (Eds.), *Quality of life in health, promotion and rehabilitation: Conceptual approaches, issues, and applications* (pp. 51–62). Thousand Oaks, CA: Sage.

Fine, A. H. (1996). Leisure, living and quality of life. In R. Renwick, I. Brown, & M. Nagler (Eds.), *Quality of life in health, promotion and rehabilita-tion: Conceptual approaches, issues, and applications* (pp. 342–354). Thousand Oaks, CA: Sage.

Foley, A. R. (1967). Community psychiatry: A model for the study of leisure time activities. Committee on Leisure Time and Its Uses. *Leisure and mental health: A psychiatric viewpoint* (pp. 93–103). Washington, DC: American Psychiatric Association.

Frankl, V. (1963). *Man's search for meaning.* New York: Washington Square.

Frankl, V. (1965). *The doctor and the soul: From psychotherapy to logotherapy.* New York: Bantam.

Goldsmith, J., & McFall, R. (1975). Development and evaluation of an interpersonal skill-training program for psychiatric patients. *Journal of Abnormal Psychology, 84,* 51–58.

Halford, W. K., Harrison, C., Kalyansundaram, Moutrey, C., & Simpson, S. (1995). Preliminary results from a psychoeducational program to rehabilitate chronic patients. *Psychiatric Services, 46,* 1189–1191.

Halford, W. K., & Hayes, R. L. (1995). Social skills in schizophrenia: Assessing the relationship between social skills, psychopathology and community functioning. *Social Psychiatry and Psychiatric Epidemiology, 30,* 14–19.

Hersen, M., Bellack, A. S., & Himmelhoch, J. M. (1982). Skills training with unipolar depressed women. In J. P. Curran & P. M. Monti (Eds.), *Social skills training: A practical handbook for assessment and treatment* (pp. 159–184). New York: Guilford.

Hunter, G. (1961). *Work and leisure.* London: Central Committee of Study Groups.

Johnson, T. P., Vinnicombe, B. J., & Merrill, G. W. (1981). Independent living skills, (ILS). *Occupational Therapy in Mental Health, 1*(2), 5–18.

King, L. W., Liberman, R. P., Roberts, J., & Bryan, E. (1977). Personal effectiveness: A structured therapy for improving social and emotional skills. *European Journal of Behavioral Analysis, 2,* 82–91.

Knox, S. H. (1993). Play and leisure. In H. L. Hopkins & H. D. Smith (Eds.), *Willard and Spackman's occupational therapy* (8th ed., pp. 260–268). Philadelphia: J. B. Lippincott.

Kopelowicz, A., Liberman, R. P., Mintz, J., & Zarate, R. (1997). Comparison of efficacy of social skills training for deficit and nondeficit negative symptoms in schizophrenia. *American Journal of Psychiatry, 154,* 424–425.

Leonardelli, C. A. (1988). *Milwaukee Evaluation of Daily Living Skills* (MEDLS). Thorofare, NJ: SLACK.

Liberman, R. P. (Ed.). (1992). *Handbook of psychiatric rehabilitation.* Boston: Allyn & Bacon.

Liberman, R. P., Lillie, F. J., Falloon, I. R. H., Harpin, E. J., Hutchinson, W., & Stoute, B. A. (1984). Social skills training for relapsing schizophrenics: An experimental analysis. *Behavior Modification, 8,* 155–179.

Linkenhoker, D., & McCarron, L. T. (1979). *Adaptive behaviors: Street Survival Skills Questionnaire* (SSSQ). (Available from McCarron-Dial Systems, P. O. Box 45628, Dallas, TX 75245)

Linkenhoker, D., & McCarron, L. T. (1993). *Adaptive behaviors: Street Survival Skills Questionnaire* (SSSQ; Rev. ed.). (Available from McCarron-Dial Systems, P.O. Box 45628, Dallas, TX 75245)

Marder, S. R., Wirshing, W. C., Mintz, J., McKenzie, J., Johnston, K., Eckman, T. A., Lebell, M., Zimmerman, K., & Liberman, R. P. (1996). Two-year outcome of social skills training and group psychotherapy for outpatients with schizophrenia. *American Journal of Psychiatry, 153,* 1585–1592.

McGinnis, E., & Goldstein, A. P. (1990). *Skillstreaming in early childhood: Teaching prosocial skills to the preschool and kindergarten.* Champaign, IL: Research Press.

McGinnis, E., & Goldstein, A. P. (1997a). *Skillstreaming in elementary school: New strategies and perspectives for teaching prosocial skills.* Champaign, IL: Research Press.

McGinnis, E., & Goldstein, A. P. (1997b). *Skillstreaming the adolescent: New strategies and perspectives for teaching prosocial skills.* Champaign, IL: Research Press.

McKay, D., & Neziroglu, F. (1996). Social skills training in a case of obsessive-compulsive disorder with schizotypal personality disorder. *Journal of Behavioral Therapy in Experimental Psychiatry, 27,* 189–194.

Meichenbaum, D. (1993). Stress inoculation training: A 20 year update. In P. M. Lehrer & R. L. Woolfolk (Eds.), *Principles of stress management* (pp. 373–406). New York: Guilford.

Menks, F., Sittler, S., Weaver, D., & Yanow, B. (1997). A psychogeriatric activity group in a rural community. *American Journal of Occupational Therapy, 6,* 376, 381–384.

Monti, P. M., Corriveau, D. P., & Curran, J. P. (1982). Social skills training for psychiatric patients: Treatment and outcome. In J. P. Curran & P. M. Monti (Eds.), *Social skills training: A practical handbook for assessment and treatment* (pp. 185–223). New York: Guilford.

O'Connor, R. D. (1969). Modification of social withdrawal through symbolic modeling. *Journal of Applied Behavioral Analysis, 2,* 15–27.

Parker, C. J., Gladman, J. R., & Drummond, A. E. (1997). The role of leisure in stroke rehabilitation. *Disability Rehabilitation, 19,* 1–5.

Parker, S. (1972). *The future of work and leisure.* London: Paladin.

Rinn, R. C., & Markle, A. (1979). Modification of social skill deficits in children. In A. S. Bellack & M. Hersen (Eds.), *Research and practice in social skills training* (pp. 107–129). New York: Plenum.

Schindler, V. P. (1999). Group effectiveness in improving social interaction skills. *Psychiatric Rehabilitation Journal, 22,* 349–354.

Smith, T. E., Hull, J. W., MacKain, S. J., Wallace, C. J., Rattenni, L. A., Goodman, M., Anthony, D. T., & Kentros, M. K. (1996). Training hospitalized patients with schizophrenia in community reintegration skills. *Psychiatry Services, 47,* 1099–1103.

Spector, W. D., Katz, S., Murphy, J. B., & Fulton, J. P. (1987). The hierarchial relationship between activities of daily living and instrumental activities of daily living. *Journal of Chronic Disabilities, 40,* 481–489.

Stein, F. (1993). *Leisure Occupations Sentence Completion.* Unpublished instrument. (Available from F. Stein, Department of Occupational Therapy, University of South Dakota, 414 E. Clark St., Vermillion, SD 57069)

Stein, F., & Cutler, S. K. (1997). *Leisure Occupations Interest Inventory* (LOII). Unpublished instrument. (Available from F. Stein, Department of

Occupational Therapy, University of South Dakota, 414 E. Clark St., Vermillion, SD 57069)

Sullivan, W. P., & Poertner, J. (1989). Social support and life stress: A mental health consumers prospective. *Community Mental Health, 25*(1), 21–32.

Sylph, J. A., Ross, H. E., & Kedward, H. B. (1978). Social disability in chronic psychiatric patients. *American Journal of Psychiatry, 134*, 1391–1394.

Thomson, L. K. (1992). *Kohlman Evaluation of Living Skills*, (KELS; 3rd ed.). Rockville, MD: American Occupational Therapy Association.

Trower, P. (1979). Fundamentals of interpersonal behavior: A social-psychological perspective. In A. S. Bellack & M. Hersen (Eds.), *Research and practice in social skills training*, (pp. 3–40). New York: Plenum.

Walker, C. E. (1975). *Learn to relax: Thirteen ways to reduce tension.* Englewood Cliffs, NJ: Prentice-Hall.

Watson, D. E. (1997). *Task analysis: An occupational performance approach.* Bethesda, MD: The American Occupational Therapy Association.

Wehman, P., & Marchant, J. (1978). Improving free play skills of severely retarded children. *American Journal of Occupational Therapy, 32*, 100–104.

Wolpe, J. (1969). *The practice of behavior therapy.* New York: Pergaman.

Workman, E. A., & Katz, A. M. (1995). *Teaching behavioral self-control to students* (2nd ed.). Austin, TX: Pro-Ed.

CHAPTER

12

Exercise, Nutrition, and Alternative Treatment Techniques

> *The ancient belief in the healing power of nature, Hippocrates' Naturae vis Medicatrix, is an expression of the faith that the integrated organism can respond in an adaptive manner to environmental insults. But this large philosophical concept of biology will not become part of scientific medicine until precise knowledge is available of the physiological, immunological, and psychological mechanisms through which the healing power operates.*
>
> — R. Dubos, 1979, *Medicine Evolving*, p. 30.
>
> *The growing popularity of alternative medicine, despite all the accomplishments of medical science in this century, is the direct result of the many questions relating to health, well-being, and survival that remain unanswered. In the words of one great physician, Sir William Osler, "Medicine is a science of uncertainty and an art of probability."*
>
> — I. Rosenfeld, 1996, *Dr. Rosenfeld's Guide to Alternative Medicine: What Works, What Doesn't—and What's Right for You*, p. xvi.

Operational Learning Objectives

By the end of this chapter, the learner will:

1. Define exercise, nutrition, and alternative medicine.

2. Understand the classifications of exercise.

3. Describe the research evidence regarding the beneficial effects of exercise, nutrition, and alternative medicine on general health.

4. Discuss the relationship of exercise and nutrition to mental health.

5. Identify the benefits of alternative medicine on mental health.

6. Design a prescriptive exercise program or a nutritional program for a patient taking into consideration individual factors.

EXERCISE

Focusing Questions

▶ What is exercise and how can exercise be classified?

▶ How does exercise fit into an occupational therapy program?

▶ What is the relationship between exercise and physical and mental health?

▶ What is the biological and neurological evidence that demonstrates how physical exercise reduces depression?

▶ What are the components of an exercise program?

▶ What is the relationship between type, frequency, intensity, duration, and compliance in exercise?

▶ How do we help clients to be compliant in an exercise program?

Definition of Exercise

Exercise can be defined as any physical activity that is "planned, structured, repetitive and purposeful" (McArdle, Katch, & Katch, 1991, p. 698). Exercise has been shown to have beneficial effects on many conditions and diseases:

▶ to prevent an injury, such as in performing stretching exercises before playing a game of tennis (Etnyre & Abraham, 1986)

▶ to increase muscle strength in muscles that have atrophied because of a joint being immobilized when it is put in a splint

▶ to lose weight (Jeffery, 1995)

▶ to condition the heart so that resting heart rate or blood pressure is reduced (Green, Jones, & Painter, 1990)

▶ to increase strength in muscles to compensate for loss such as in increasing the muscles of the upper extremity in individuals who have weakness or paralysis in the lower extremities (Davis, 1993)

▶ to relax the individual (Ross & Hayes, 1988)

▶ to reduce blood sugar in those with mild diabetes (Björntorp & Krotkiewski, 1985)

▶ to reduce cholesterol (Stefanic & Wood, 1994)

▶ to prevent osteoporosis (Drinkwater, 1993)

▶ to counteract the effects of depression (Callen, 1983).

In general, exercise potentially can have a positive effect on the musculoskeletal, cardiovascular, endocrine, and nervous systems. The type of exercise, duration of exercise program, intensity of the exercise, frequency of exercise, compliance to exercise prescription, and interest of client will all affect the benefits of the exercise program. An individual's degree of physical fitness is an indication of his or her ability to engage in physical exercise. Physical fitness is defined "as the ability to carry out daily tasks with vigor and alertness, without undue fatigue, and with ample energy to enjoy leisure-time pursuits" (President's Council on Physical Fitness and Sports, 1996, p. 20). Engaging in aerobic exercise increases one's physical fitness. Table 12–1 describes the 15 most favorite exercises in the United States in 1996.

Table 12–1. Fifteen Favorite Exercise Activities

Sport/Activity	*Total Number of Participants (in millions)*
exercise walking	73.3
swimming	60.2
bicycle riding	53.3
exercising with equipment	47.8
fishing	45.6
camping	44.7
bowling	42.9
billiards/pool	34.5
basketball	33.3
boating, motor/power	28.8
hiking	26.5
inline skating	25.5
aerobic exercise	24.1
golf	23.1
running/jogging	22.2

Source: Adapted from *Snowboarding Leads 1996 Sport Growth While Exercise Walking Remains America's Favorite Activity* by the National Sporting Goods Association, 1997. Retrieved August 29, 1997 from the World Wide Web: http://www.fitnesslink.com/features/stats.htm

Types or Classifications of Exercise

Exercise can be grouped into aerobic and anaerobic exercises:

▶ *Aerobic exercises* are physical activities where oxygen is consumed and metabolized by the body and heart rate is increased. Aerobic exercise increases blood flow to all the organs of the body, including the brain and heart. Physical activities that involve continuous movement such as walking, biking, swimming, and jogging are examples of aerobic exercises. These types of exercises increase endurance, which is the ability of the body to perform an activity without becoming excessively fatigued. These exercises also increase the aerobic capacity of an individual, which

means that the individual is able to utilize oxygen efficiently (Smith, 1991). The beneficial effects of aerobic exercises will depend on the intensity of the exercise, whether it is mild, moderate, or intense. For example, a healthy individual walking at 4 miles an hour will use up less energy or calories than when he or she is walking at 6 to 8 miles an hour. This is the *intensity* of the exercise. How long the individual walks every day (*duration*) and the *frequency* of the exercise, such as three or five times a week, will affect the benefits gained from the exercise.

▶ *Anaerobic exercises* are usually exercises of high intensity and low duration, for example, in weight lifting, tennis, football, or sprinting in which the individual does short spurts of physical activities. These types of exercises improve muscle strength and endurance, flexibility, and coordination (Martinsen, 1994). In contrast, in aerobic exercises, the blood supply cannot keep up with the muscle's demand for oxygen and subsequently causes fatigue in the individual. Fatigue occurs in anaerobic activities if the activities are at a high intensity level.

Another way to group exercises is to determine whether they are isometric, isotonic, or isokinetic.

▶ *Isometric exercises* are active exercises performed against stable resistance, without change in the length of the muscle nor joint movement. An example of an isometric exercise is flexing muscles in place by pressing against an immovable object. Progressive muscle relaxation (Jacobson, 1929), which involves flexing muscles without moving the joints, is an example of an isometric exercise.

▶ *Isokinetic exercises* combine isometric exercises with weight training. It is usually done on a mechanical device that provides resistance to a muscle. Isokinetic exercises are used by athletes to build up muscles that are important in a specific sport, for example, strengthening the quadriceps in preparing for football.

▶ *Isotonic exercises* are active exercises in which the muscle contracts without resistance. Most movements such as walking and running are examples of isotonic exercises. Joint mobility, muscle strength, and muscle tone are improved by isotonic exercises. Relaxation exercises such as Tai Ch'i and yoga are other examples.

▶ *Stretching exercises* are used consistently by athletes to improve joint mobility and to reduce the risks of joint sprains and strains. The muscles that are stretched are related to the specific muscles that are at risk when an athlete engages in a sport. For example, it is recommended that tennis players stretch the hamstrings, quadriceps, back muscles, and shoulder flexors. Stretching muscles is especially recommended for morning exercises after warming the joints with a bath or shower. For individuals who are vulnerable to back pain, morning stretching exercises such as flexion and extension of the back muscles have been shown to be beneficial.

▶ *Relaxation exercises* such as Tai Ch'i, yoga, progressive relaxation, range of motion dance (ROM dance), and the relaxation response are active exercise techniques that the individual learns and then incorporates into his or her everyday schedule. The exercises usually involve cognitive control where the participant moves his or her joints in slow circular movements, such as in Tai Ch'i and ROM dance, or flexes muscles without joint movement, such as in progressive relaxation, or uses breathing, posture and visualization, such as in yoga and the relaxation response.

▶ *Passive exercises* are repetitive exercises that are applied to an individual's muscles, such as massage, rolfing, passive range of motion, or by externally controlled through machines or water.

Exercise as Part of an Occupational Therapy Program

Brollier, Hamrick, and Jacobson (1994), in a research study investigating the effects of aerobic exercise in reducing depression symptomatology in adolescents, concluded that

[i]f occupational therapy programs are to be client driven, a variety of potentially meaningful occupations which promote wellness need to be provided. An aerobic exercise group seems to address many principles central to occupational therapy and appears to be particularly appropriate for adolescent boys with depression. (p. 27)

The authors cited the Model of Human Occupation (Kielhofner, 1985) as guiding the program design. The authors discussed the concepts of volition, habituation, and performance in analyzing aerobic exercise. Exercise can also fit into the cognitive-behavioral frame of reference. Fillingim and Blumenthal (1993), in a review article, concluded that "there is growing evidence to suggest that physical exercise may reduce psychophysiological stress response" (p. 457).

The link between exercise and the reduction of stress has been examined by a number of investigators (Blumenthal et al., 1990, 1991; Cox, Evans, & Jamieson, 1979; Crews & Landers, 1987; Roth & Holmes, 1985). Cotton (1990) stated, "This evidence suggests that aerobically fit individuals are more resistant to the physiological and psychological effects of stress, and that aerobically fit individuals may recover more quickly from stress" (p. 171).

Aerobic exercise is a purposeful activity that is meaningful to the individual. When the individual with depression is active and is motivated to increase his or her fitness, exercise can reduce the negative effects of stress and the symptoms of depression. It can be considered a performance component related to sensorimotor stimulation, cognitive control, and mastery of psychological skills in self-regulating depression. This relationship between exercise as a purposeful activity is shown in Figure 12–1.

Kaplan, Mendelson, and Dubroff (1983) described an exercise program for individuals with diagnoses of depression, schizophrenia, and substance abuse. The sessions were led by occupational therapists in an inpatient psychiatric unit of a hospital. The study conducted over an 8-week period included jogging sessions, three times weekly for 90-minute sessions. The researchers concluded that "the results indicated that beneficial changes in symptoms of depression occurred in the young adult patients who believed that exercise was important and were able to practice jogging for several weeks" (p. 175).

Beneficial Effects of Exercise

Exercise has been a recommended activity for maintaining one's health for centuries, but it was not until the latter half of the 20th century that scientific evidence has demonstrated the benefits (President's Council on Physical Fitness and Sports, 1996). The following examples from the research literature demonstrate the effects of exercise on various conditions.

Cardiovascular disease

▶ Individuals who are physically active have an overall lower risk of coronary disease (Mittleman et al., 1993).

▶ Exercise training when combined with a cholesterol-lowering diet, hypertension reduction, or other risk factor reduction activities can help prevent the progression of or reduction in severity of coronary atherosclerosis (Hambrecht et al., 1993; Haskell et al., 1994; Niebauer et al., 1995; Ornish et al., 1990).

Colon cancer

▶ Increased physical exercise and decreased body weight result in less risk for development of colon cancer in women (Martinez et al., 1997).

Purposeful Activity (AOTA, 1993)
- Goal-directed behavior
- Individual is active
- Meaningful to individual

Characteristics of Aerobic Exercise
- Goal-directed toward increasing fitness, reducing stress, reducing depression
- Individual is active in incorporating exercise into everyday schedule
- Activity is meaningful

Performance Components
(AOTA, Uniform Terminology, 1994)
Developmental mastery of skills in:
- Sensorimotor
- Cognitive
- Psychosocial

Characteristics of Aerobic Exercise
- Stimulate sensorimotor components
- Cognitive control in intensity, frequency, and duration of aerobics
- Psychosocial
- Self-regulation of depression

Figure 12–1. The relationship of aerobic exercise, occupational therapy, and purposeful activity.

Hypertension

▶ Studies have shown significant reductions in blood pressure after endurance exercise training (American College of Sports Medicine, 1978; Fagard et al., 1990; Fagard & Tipton, 1994; Towner & Blumenthal, 1993).

Immune system

▶ Individuals who were serious marathoners had greater natural killer cell activity than did a control group of nonexercisers (Mongeau, Blier, & de Montigny, 1997).

Cancer

▶ Regular, daily exercise significantly reduces the number of individuals who are at risk of dying from cancer or heart disease (Blair et al., 1989).

Osteoarthritis

▶ On completion of an exercise program, 40 individuals with osteoarthritis of the knee demonstrated significant improvement in their ambulation and gait, including reduced pain and physical function, without increasing medication or the use of walking aids (Fransen, Margiotta, Crosbie, & Edmonds, 1997).

Osteoporosis

▶ Women who were involved in high-intensity weight training showed an increase in bone mineral content, reducing their risk for osteoporosis, when compared to a group of nonexercisers (Nelson, Fisher, Dilmanian, Dallal, & Evans, 1991).

Pain

▶ Sixty-four percent of patients with low back pain reported a substantial reduction in pain after an exercise therapy program, compared to 12 percent who reported no change in pain and 3 percent who reported worse pain. Twenty-one percent reported a change, but the change was not significant (Nelson et al., 1995).

Quality of life

▶ Improved daily function and psychological well-being has been noted when individuals whose physical function is compromised by heart disease and arthritis are involved in physical activity (Ewart, 1989; Fisher et al., 1933).

Weight management

▶ When a regular high-volume, low-intensity prolonged physical activity occurs (e.g., purposeful walking for 30 to 60 minutes daily), energy expenditure is substantially increased and body weight and fat are reduced (Bouchard, Deprés, & Tremblay, 1993; DiPietro, 1995; Ewbank, Darga, & Lucas, 1995).

Self-esteem

▶ After a 20-week exercise program, "significant improvements in self-esteem at all levels were discovered with global esteem, physical self-worth, and perceptions of physical condition and attractive body increasing" (McAuley, Mihalko, & Bane, 1997, p. 67).

Enhanced mood

▶ Higher positive mood was noted in persons reporting higher levels of daily leisure-time expenditures than those reporting lower levels of daily leisure-time expenditures (Stephens & Craig, 1990).

▶ Individuals with no physical exercise were three times more likely to be depressed than those who were regular exercisers (Weyerer, 1992)

Depression

▶ Individuals who are highly active showed significantly fewer symptoms of depression than those who are moderately active or not active at all (Brown et al., 1995).

Relationship of Exercise to Mental Health

In Table 12–2 clinical research evidence demonstrates the effectiveness of exercise on depression. In general, both aerobic and weight training are effective.

Research on Effects of Exercise on Depression

1. Research with animals has shown that exercise increases the serotonin in the system (Dey, 1994; Dey, Singh, & Dey, 1992; Jacobs, 1994).

2. Individuals with depression have been shown to have less serotonin available in their bodies (Jacobs, 1994).

3. Forty women having a diagnosis of major or minor depression took part in a study that demonstrated that both running and weight lifting were effective in reducing depression (Doyne et al., 1987).

4. Twenty-four women and men who were hospitalized for depression participated in a controlled study in which half the group were in a running treatment group that ran 45 minutes three times a day for 8 weeks. This group showed significant progress (Bosscher, 1993).

5. Doyne, Chambless, and Beutler (1983) demonstrated the positive effects of aerobic exercise as a treatment method for four women diagnosed with major depression.

6. Greist et al. (1979) showed that running was more effective than psychotherapy with 13 men and 15 women who were diagnosed with depression.

7. Martinsen, Medhus, and Sandvik (1985) found no significant difference between medication and exercise in the treatment of depression.

8. In a major analysis of the literature in 1990, North, McCullagh, and Tran found the following results:

   ▶ all types of exercise are effective to some extent in reducing depression

   ▶ the longest exercise programs showed the greatest effects

   ▶ a combination of exercise and psychotherapy are significantly more effective than medication in reducing depression

   ▶ exercise significantly reduces depression across all ages and for both sexes

   ▶ exercise is beneficial in single session, multisessional, and follow-up exercise treatments

   ▶ exercises are more effective at decreasing depression than relaxation and pleasant activities and are just as effective as psychotherapy

Biological and Neurological Evidence Related to Exercise and Reduction of Depression

Meeusen and De Meirleir (1995), in a review of the literature on physical exercises on the dopaminergic, noradrenergic, and serotonergic systems, found that there is significant "evidence in favor of changes in synthesis and metabolism of monamines during exercise" (p. 160) and that the "release of most neurotransmitters is influenced by exercise" (p. 160). Lechin et al. (1995), in examining the relationship between neurotransmitters and exercise in individuals with major depression, concluded that both the neuronal sympathetic and cholinergic mechanisms are involved in major depression. In another study, Soares, Naffah-Mazzacoratti, and Cavalheiro (1994) found that serotonin levels were increased by exercise training in normal subjects. Animal studies have also supported the claim that physical exercise stimulates serotonin. Dey et al. (1992) found that acute exercise

Table 12–2. Effects of Exercise on Depression

Study	Subjects	Treatment Technique	Outcome Measures	Results
Blue, R. F. (1979). Aerobic running as a treatment of moderate depression.	2 adult patients with chronic depression	Aerobic running program 3 times per week, for 9 weeks	*Zung Self-Rating Depression Scale* (SDS; Zung, 1965)	Significant reduction of depression
Bosscher (1993). Running and mixed physical exercises with depressed psychiatric patients.	24 men and women diagnosed with depression and hospitalized in psychiatric hospital	E[a]: short-term running therapy, 3 times a week for 8 weeks C: mixed physical and relaxation exercises, 3 times a week for 8 weeks	*Zung Self-Rating Depression Scale* (SDS; Zung, 1965)	Significant improvement for running group; no significant improvement for mixed physical and exercise group
Brollier et al. (1994). Aerobic exercises: A potential occupational therapy modality for adolescents with depression.	4 adolescent boys from a private psychiatric hospital with diagnosis of depression	Brisk walking and running 3 times a week for 1 hour over a 65-day period	*Beck Depression Inventory* (BDI; Beck et al., 1961)	General decrease in depression scores of all subjects
Doyne, et al. (1983). Aerobic exercise as a treatment for depression in women.	4 women with major depressive disorder (MDD)	Aerobic exercise for 6 weeks	*Beck Depression Inventory* (BDI; Beck et al., 1961) *Depression Adjective Checklists* (DACL; Lubin, 1981)	Significant reduction in depression scores compared with pre-exercise screening phase
Doyne, et al. (1987). Running versus weight lifting in the treatment of depression.	40 women diagnosed with depression	E$_1$: walked/ran on indoor track in 7-minute intervals for 8 weeks E$_2$: used weight-lifting machine for 8 weeks C: no treatment	*Beck Depression Inventory* (BDI; Beck et al., 1961) *Hamilton Rating Scale for Depression* (HRSD; Hamilton, 1960) *Depression Adjective Checklists* (DACL; Lubin, 1981)	Both aerobic and weight-lifting groups showed significant improvement in depression; no change in control group
Greist et al. (1979). Running as a treatment for depression.	13 men, 15 women, aged 18 to 30	E: 10 patients ran 3 to 4 times/ week C: 18 in psychotherapy	*Response Symptom Checklist* (Greist et al., 1979)	Running as treatment for moderate depression was as effective as psychotherapy
Kaplan et al. (1983) The effect of a jogging program on psychiatric inpatients with symptoms of depression.	12 women, 6 men, aged 15 to 38, patients in acute care psychiatric ward	Warm-up and cool-down exercises; 20 minutes of graded walking/jogging on indoor track; short discussion of exercise and health-related topics	Self-report questionnaire (5-point Likert scale); observation by co-leaders	Decreased sleep disturbances and increased self-esteem

Table 12–2. Effects of Exercise on Depression

Study	Subjects	Method	Measures	Results
Martinsen et al. (1985). Effects of aerobic exercise on depression: A controlled study.	43 subjects, ages 17 to 60, with MDD	E_1: 9 patients receiving tricyclic antidepressants (TCAs) and aerobic exercise for 1 hour, 3 times a week for 9 weeks E_2: 15 patients receiving aerobic exercise but no TCAs C_1: 14 patients receiving TCAs and OT 3 times a week for 9 weeks C_2: 5 patients receiving OT but not TCAs	*Comprehensive Psychopathological Rating Scale* (CPRS; Åsberg et al., 1987) *Beck Depression Inventory* (BDI; Beck et al., 1961)	Significantly lower depression scores for those participating in aerobic exercises than others; maximum oxygen uptake noted in aerobic training groups resulted in greater antidepressive effects
Martinsen et al. (1989) Comparing aerobic with nonaerobic forms of exercise in the treatment of clinical depression: A randomized trial.	90 inpatients of a psychiatric hospital with diagnosis of depression	E: 43 patients, brisk walks and jogging 3 times a week for 8 weeks C: 47 patients; muscular strength, flexibility, and relaxation exercises 3 times a week for 8 weeks	*Beck Depression Inventory* (BDI; Beck et al., 1961) *Montgomery and Åsberg Depression Rating Scale* (MADRS; Montgomery & Åsberg, 1979)	Depressed scores in both groups were reduced significantly, but no significant difference between groups
Rape, R. N. (1987). Running and depression.	21 Caucasian males running 15 or more miles per week; 21 Caucasian males, nonexercisers	Matched two-group design comparing runners with nonexercisers	*Beck Depression Inventory* (BDI; Beck et al., 1961)	Runners were significantly less depressed than were nonexercisers

[a]Note: "E" refers to the experimental group. "C" refers to the control group.

in rats significantly increased the synthesis and metabolism of 5HT (serotonin) in the brain stem. Jacobs (1994), in a review of his 10-year research at Princeton University studying the factors that controlled the activity of serotonin using animals models, suggested that "regular motor activity may be important in the treatment of affective disorders" (p. 462). Furthermore, he suggested that "some form of repetitive motor task, such as riding a bicycle or jogging, may help to relieve the depression" (p. 462). He based this conclusion on his studies of cats in which he observed that serotonin neurons increased their activity when an animal engaged in any of a variety of repetitive behaviors, such as chewing food or running on a treadmill. The evidence from human and other animal studies demonstrates that physical exercise increases the synthesis and metabolism of serotonin. There is also much evidence that exercise increases the levels of endorphins in animals (Rape, 1987).

Components of an Exercise Program

Present Level of Physical Fitness

The first component to consider is one's present level of physical fitness (President's Counsel on Physical Fitness and Sports, 1997). The client should have a physical examination to rule out any limitations in exercising (e.g., cardiovascular state). Identify the client's resting heart rate by counting the number of heart beats for 20 seconds and multiplying by three to obtain beats per minute. The average adult heart rate is 72 beats per minute. Establish the client's blood pressure in resting condition. The average blood pressure is 80:120::diastolic:systolic.

Current Physical Activities

Obtain from the client the physical activities in which he or she participates. For example, the client may state that he or she walks two to three times a week, plays golf once a week, and walks up three flights of stairs every day.

Physical Expenditure of Activity

The therapist should determine the total calories expended by the total activities. A good reference for this is McArdle et al. (1996). Appendix E provides a list of typical activities and the calories expended per minute.

Selection of New Activities

The client and the therapist together should develop a list of new activities to be considered. In the selection of this activity, consider the interest of the client, the purposefulness of the activity, the affordability of the activity, time availability for the activity, and whether the activity can be engaged in throughout the entire year. Activities that are not tied to changes in the weather, availability, or friends are best. For example, walking, biking, and calisthenics can occur both indoors and outdoors. Skiing, on the other hand, can only be done in the winter when there is snow, and tennis involves the availability of another person. Goal setting is important when selecting the new activity. For example, the client may wish to reduce his or her resting heart rate, blood pressure, anxiety or depression, or weight. By setting goals, the client will, in general, be more compliant, especially if he or she sees results from the activity.

Social and Emotional Needs of the Activity

The client is most apt to comply if the activity meets his or her social or emotional needs. For example, if the activity provides friendly group interaction, relaxation, skill development, or mental stimulation, and these are valued by the client, the client's motivation and compliance will increase.

Achievability

The activity should be able to be rated in terms of duration, frequency, and intensity. For example, walking can be increased from 20 to 30 minutes per day, from 3 to 5 days a week, or from slow to fast walking. Additionally, the success of the activity may depend on the client's physical fitness status, his or her body composition, motor abilities, and prior activity experiences. For example, asking a person to play tennis when he or she has difficulty tracking the ball or moving quickly ensures failure.

Incorporation of Activity into One's Schedule

It is important to stress that the client must incorporate this activity into his or her daily or weekly schedule and keep a log of the times in which he or she performs the activity.

Factors to Be Considered

When designing an exercise program, there are a number of factors to consider (Table 12–3). These factors are:

▶ The *purpose and goals of the exercise program*, for example, to reduce depression, increase cardiovascular function, reduce weight, increase relaxation, reduce anxiety, or increase self-esteem

▶ The *type of exercise program* such as aerobic (e.g., walking, jogging, biking, swimming); stretching (e.g., Range of Motion Dance [Van Deusen, & Harlowe, 1987]); Tai Ch'i,

yoga); isometric weight lifting (e.g., barbells, dumbbells, or weight machine); relaxation therapy (e.g., relaxation response, progression relaxation)

▶ *Frequency of exercise program*, such as three times per week or daily

▶ *Duration of exercise program*, such as 8 weeks or continuous

▶ *Intensity of exercise program*, such as light walking (3.6 calories/minute), moderate (e.g., mowing the lawn at 7.7 calories/minute), or heavy (e.g., running up stairs at 16.2 calories/minute)

Compliance and Motivation to Adhere to the Exercise Program

The benefits of exercise on the cardiovascular system and the psychological well-being of the individual have been widely cited and advocated by the Surgeon General (President's Council on Physical Fitness and Sports, 1996) and by other individuals in the public health section. In spite of this, few Americans exercise regularly.

> At any given time about 40% of Americans do not exercise during leisure time, another 40% are active at levels probably too low and infrequent for fitness and health gains, while just 20% exercise regularly and intensely enough (Stephens, Jacobs, & White, 1985) to meet current guidelines for fitness (American College of Sports Medicine, 1978) or reduced risk for several chronic diseases and premature death (Paffenbarger, Hyde, Wing, & Hsieh, 1986; Powell, Spain, Christenson, & Mollenkamp, 1986). (Dishman, 1988, p. 1)

A client, therefore, needs to be motivated and to apply self-discipline in order to comply with the program.

> Individuals with minor mood disorders usually lack the self-confidence, and clinically depressed subjects will undoubtedly lack the

Table 12–3. Factors in Setting up a Therapeutic Exercise Program

Type of Exercise	Client Interest (Examples)	Duration: Time Interval	Methods to Increase Compliance	Intensity	Frequency
AEROBIC	• biking • jogging • hiking/ backpacking • swimming • walking	• 5–15 minutes • 15–30 minutes • 1/2–1 hour • 1–2 hours	• diary/monitoring • external reinforcement • self-reinforcement • weekly goal setting	• Mild • Moderate • Intense	• daily • 2–3 times per week • weekly
ANAEROBIC	• gardening • golf • raking leaves • weight-lifting				
STRETCHING	• extension exercises • flexion				
RELAXATION	• meditation • progressive relaxation • relaxation response • Tai Ch'i • yoga				

motivation to commence an exercise programme on their own. Therefore a patient will initially nearly always require the support and training of a health professional. (de Coverley Veale, 1987, p. 118)

Self-motivation in exercise adherence is conceptualized by Dishman and Gettman (1980) "as a generalized, nonspecific tendency to persist in the absence of extrinsic reinforcement and is thus largely independent of situational influence" (p. 297). Figure 12–2 is an example of an exercise compliance program that can be used with clients.

NUTRITION

Focusing Questions

▶ How does nutrition fit into a holistic program?

▶ What does a therapist need to know about exercise and nutrition to help patients?

▶ How does nutrition affect one's health?

▶ What is a healthy diet?

▶ How can we fit nutrition into an occupational therapy program?

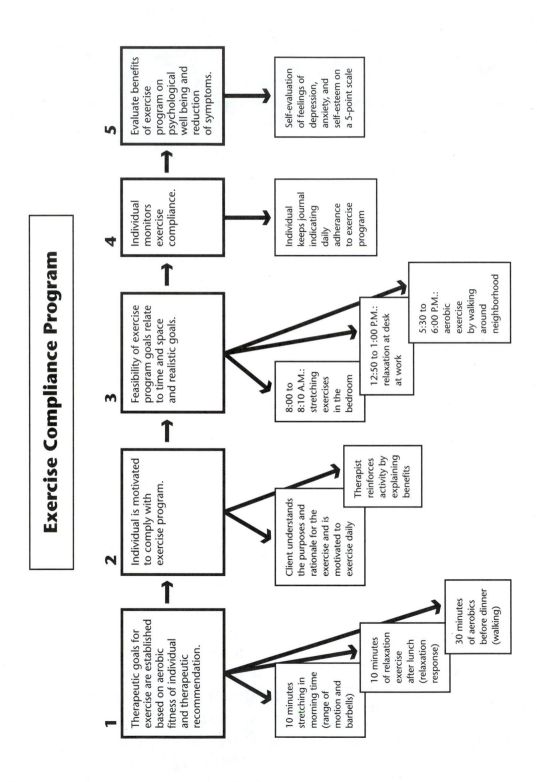

Figure 12-2. Exercise compliance program.

Role of Nutrition in a Holistic Program

The idea of using nutritional therapy in a holistic program has been promoted for over 2,500 years. Hippocrates, who was known as the "Father of Medicine," told his students "Let thy food be thy medicine and thy medicine be thy food." Later, Moses Maimonides, a physician in the 12th century, echoed Hippocrates stating "No illness which can be treated by diet should be treated by any other means." To be effective, a psychosocial occupational therapist who uses a holistic approach in treatment should be familiar with the essential aspects of nutrition.

> Diet has always had a vital influence on health. Until as recently as the 1940s, diseases such as rickets, pellagra, scurvy, beriberi, xerophthalmia, and goiter (caused by lack of adequate dietary vitamins D, niacin, vitamin C, thiamin, vitamin A, and iodine, respectively) were prevalent in this country and throughout the world. (U.S. Department of Health and Human Services, Public Health Services, 1988, p. 4)

Assumptions

▶ Nutrition is an essential part of being healthy.

▶ Individuals who are mentally ill should have a healthy diet to counteract the illness and the effects of medication.

▶ Many patients who are mentally ill often have poor or inadequate diets. For example, they may have diets that are high in fats, salt, and sugar, and low in grains, carbohydrates, fruits, and vegetables.

▶ People who are mentally ill tend to be obese because of the high-fat diets.

▶ The inadequate diet and lack of exercise interacts with the mental illness in an individual causing a vicious cycle of continued poor diet, further breakdown in health, further depression or anxiety, and lack of motivation to exercise.

▶ Nutrients affect moods; therefore, what we eat can affect our mood state. If we do not have enough of the right nutrients, the symptoms of depression or schizophrenia (e.g., anxiety, fatigue, insomnia, hyperirritability) can occur.

▶ "The foods we eat can influence your brain chemistry, to the extent that it produces high concentrations of the neurotransmitter-precursor nutrients in an available form" (Whitney & Cataldo, 1983, p. 164).

> The neurotransmitter serotonin is made in the brain from the essential amino acid tryptophan. The amount of serotonin made normally varies with the amount of tryptophan that is available. Tryptophan availability, in turn, depends on what is eaten (remember, an essential amino acid can't be made in the body). And a lack of tryptophan flowing into the brain can manifest itself in wakefulness, enhanced sensitivity to pain, and possibly depression. (Whitney & Cataldo, 1983, p. 166)

Nutrients and Their Classes

A *nutrient* is "a substance obtained from food using the body to promote growth, maintenance, and or repair" (Whitney & Cataldo, 1983, p. 4). Nutrients can be classified into carbohydrates, fats, proteins, vitamins, minerals, and water.

Carbohydrates

Carbohydrates are "one of a group of chemical substances, including sugars, glycogen, starches, dextrins, and celluloses" (*Taber's Cyclopedic*

Medical Dictionary, 1997, p. 302). Carbohydrates can be divided into simple carbohydrates (monosaccharides and oligosaccharides) and complex carbohydrates (polysacchrides). Simple carbohydrates are made up of sugars, such as those found in fruits and refined sugars made from sugar cane or sugar beets. Carbohydrates serve as the energy fuel for the body and are essential for the proper functioning of the central nervous system. Adequate intake of carbohydrates aids proteins in maintaining and repairing body tissue. If glucose, a carbohydrate, is reduced in the blood, it can cause weakness, hunger, and dizziness and, eventually brain damage (McArdle et al., 1991). The two common forms of plant polysaccharides are known as starch and fiber. The Surgeon General (U.S.

Department of Health and Human Services, Public Health Services, 1988), using research studies, recommends that 50 to 60 percent of the daily calories in one's diet come from carbohydrates (Table 12–4).

Proteins

Proteins are one class of complex nitrogenous compounds "composed of carbon, hydrogen, oxygen, nitrogen and arranged into amino acids linked in a chain" (Whitney & Cataldo, 1983, p. 95). The important functions of proteins include growth and repair of all body tissues and the formation of antibodies, hormones, and enzymes. A complete protein contains all of the amino acids necessary for tissue growth and repair. Sources of complete protein are eggs, milk, meat, fish, and

Table 12–4. Carbohydrates

CLASSIFICATION	FOODS
Monosaccharides	
• *Glucose or dextrose*	natural sugar in food
• *Fructose:* works directly in blood from digestive tract, then converted to glucose in liver	fruits and honey
• *Galactose:* converted to glucose in the body	from lactating animals, mammary glands: milk sugar
Oligosaccharides: double sugars (formed from two monosaccharides); simple sugars	
• *Sucrose*	beet or cane sugar, brown sugar, maple sugar, and honey
• *Lactose*	artificially processed dairy products (milk sugar)
• *Maltose*	malt products and germinating products (e.g., wheat germ or beer)
Polysacchrides, complex carbohydrates	
• *Starches*	corn, various grains, peas, beans, roots, bread, cereal, spaghetti, pastry, potatoes, beets
• *Dietary fibers or cellulose*[a]	leafy green vegetables, stems, roots, seed, fruit skins

Source: Information obtained from *Exercise Physiology: Energy, Nutrition and Human Performance* (4th ed.), by W. D. McArdle, F. I. Katch, & V. L. Katch, 1996, Philadelphia: Lea & Febiger.

[a]Ingestion of dietary fibers or cellulose is associated with lower occurrence of obesity, diabetes, intestinal disorders, heart disease, and may also lower cholesterol.

poultry. Incomplete proteins, on the other hand, lack one or more of the essential amino acids. "Diets containing predominately incomplete protein may eventually result in protein malnutrition, even though they are adequate in caloric value and protein quantity" (McArdle et al., 1991, p. 30). Foods containing incomplete proteins include lentils, dry beans, peas, nuts, and cereals. The average adult should get 20 to 25 percent of his or her daily calories from protein (U.S. Department of Health and Human Services, Public Health Services, 1988).

Vegetarians typically do not eat meat, although they may eat fish or shellfish. In spite of this, they still can have a balanced nutritional meal. This is because a healthy diet will contain all of the essential amino acids if the individual uses a variety of grains, fruits, and vegetables (McArdle et al., 1991, 1996).

Fats

Fats, or lipids, are a family of compounds that insulate the body against temperature changes, protect the heart, kidney, liver, brain, and spinal cord against trauma (McArdle et al., 1991, 1996), and provide the necessary vehicle for fat-soluble vitamins. Thus, vitamins that are not water-soluble (e.g., vitamin A, D, E, and K) can be stored in the body. Fats can be classified as saturated or unsaturated.

Saturated fats are generally solid at room temperature. These are found in red meat, pork, chicken, egg yolks, dairy products, coconut and palm oil, vegetable shortening, and hydrogenated margarine. In general these fats raise the total blood cholesterol, especially the very low density lipoprotein (VLDL), producing plaques on the inner lining of the arteries and eventually leading to atherosclerosis, which is the narrowing and blockage of the arteries. Sources of high cholesterol in foods include egg yolk, red meat,

liver, kidneys, brains, shellfish, and dairy products (e.g., ice cream or cheese). Cholesterol is not present in any food of plant origin, however. Thus, coconut and palm oil, vegetable shortening, and hydrogenated margarine do not contain any cholesterol. Cholesterol rich, low-density lipids (LDL) have been implicated in heart disease (Martin et al., 1986).

Unsaturated fats are divided into monounsaturated and polyunsaturated fats, both of which are usually liquid at room temperature. Monounsaturated fats, such as olive oil, canola, or peanut oil, tend to increase the concentration of high density lipoprotein (HDLs), which are beneficial and considered to be the "good" part of blood cholesterol. Unlike VLDLs or LDLs, HDLs do not cause plaques. Polyunsaturated fats lower the overall blood cholesterol, including HDLs. Thus, although polyunsaturated fats are better than saturated fats, they are not as good as monounsaturated fats in protecting against heart disease and stroke. Examples of polyunsaturated fats include sunflower, safflower, soybean, and corn oil (McArdle et al., 1991, 1996). During light and moderate exercise, fat provides 50 percent of the body's energy needs. As exercise continues, fat becomes more important, and may provide up to 80 percent of the energy needed for the activity (McArdle et al., 1991, 1996).

Vitamins

Vitamins are noncaloric, organic substances that are essential for normal metabolism, growth, and development. There are two types of vitamins: water-soluble and fat-soluble. A list of the vitamins, their sources, and results of deficiencies are listed in Table 12–5. Many vitamins, especially the B-vitamins, are adversely affected by alcohol, excessive coffee, oral contraceptives, stress, drugs, and smoking.

Table 12–5. Vitamins

Vitamin	Nutritional Sources	Results of Deficiency
A (fat-soluble)	• dark green, deep orange, or other richly colored fruits and vegetables (e.g., squash, carrots, spinach, yams) • beef liver • dairy products • pink grapefruit	• visual disturbances, especially night blindness • skin problems • infections in respiratory, gastrointestinal, or urinary tract • retarded bone growth • dental problems • severe problems to the nervous system
B_1 (water-soluble; Thiamine)	• meat • whole grain breads and cereals • legumes • nuts • dairy products • rice • many vegetables	• beriberi • disturbance in nervous system, muscles, and cardiovascular system (e.g., mental confusion, muscle weakness, atrophy) • poor memory or concentration • tingling hands and prickly legs
B_2 (water-soluble; Riboflavin)	• vegetables • fish • dairy products • milk • red meat • enriched breads • grains and cereals	• dermatitis or eczema • photophobia • cracked lips • split nails
Niacin	• vegetables • fish • dairy • unrefined cereals • lean meat • legumes and nuts • eggs • poultry • whole wheat breads and grains	• pellagra (skin and gastrointestinal lesions, nervous mental disorders) • lack of energy • diarrhea or gastrointestinal disturbances • headaches • anxiety, tension, depression
Pantothenic acid (B_5)	• eggs • lentils • unrefined grains • vegetables	• energy production • synthesis of hormones and blood cells • used to make neurotransmitter acetylcholine (ACh)
B_6 (water-soluble)	• meats • vegetables • whole grain cereals	• abnormal brain wave patterns and convulsions • dermatitis • cracks at corners of mouth • irritation of sweat glands
Folic acid (Folacin) (water-soluble)	• leafy green vegetables that have not been overcooked • citrus fruits • eggs • organ meats • whole grains • seeds, nuts, legumes	• neural tube birth defects • anemia • gastrointestinal difficulties • glossitis (inflammation of the tongue) • anxiety, tension, or depression • poor memory • fatigue

Table 12–5. Vitamins

Vitamin	Nutritional Sources	Results of Deficiency
B_{12} (water-soluble)	• fish • eggs • meat • dairy produce	• pernicious anemia • neurological disorders
Biotin (water- soluble)	• vegetables • nuts and seeds • fish • eggs	• dermatitis and eczema • premature gray hair • fatigue • depression • muscle discomfort, including cramps
C (Ascorbic acid) (water-soluble)	• citrus fruits • tomatoes • green peppers • cabbage family	• frequent colds • lack of energy • bleeding or tender gums • degeneration of muscles • failure of wounds to heal • anemia • scurvy
D (fat-soluble)	• cod-liver oil • fish • dairy • eggs • sunlight	• rickets in children • osteoporosis in adults • joint pain or stiffness • backache • tooth decay • muscle cramps • hair loss
E (fat-soluble)	• wheat germs • unrefined vegetable oils • seeds, nuts, beans • fish • whole grains	• anemia • easy bruising • slow wound healing
K (fat-soluble)	• green-leafy vegetables • cabbage family • milk	• unable to clot blood

Sources: Adapted from *Mayo Clinic Family Health Book* (2nd ed.), [CD–ROM], by Mayo Clinic, 1994, Available: IVI Publishing, 7500 Flying Cloud Drive, Minneapolis, MN 55344-3739; *Exercise Physiology: Energy, Nutrition and Human Performance* (4th ed.), by W. D. McArdle, F. I. Katch, & V. L. Katch, 1991, Philadelphia: Lea & Febiger; *Nutrition: Medicine of the Future* [Online] by P. Shepherd, 1997, available: *http://www.trans4mind.unet.com/nutri.htm*; and *Understanding Normal and Clinical Nutrition* by E. N. Whitney, & C. B. Cataldo, 1983, St. Paul, MN: West.

Minerals

Minerals are inorganic elements or compounds that are essential constituents of all cells (*Taber's Cyclopedic Medical Dictionary*, 1997). The three main functions include (a) providing structure in the formation of bones and teeth; (b) maintaining function of normal heart rhythm, muscle contraction, nerve conduction, and acid-base balance of the body; and (c) regulating the cellular metabolism (McArdle et al., 1991). Major minerals are found in large quantities in the body; trace minerals are found in minute quantities (e.g., <.01%). Major minerals are listed in Table 12–6.

Table 12–6. Major Minerals (listed in order of importance)

Minerals	Sources	Major Function
Calcium (Ca)	• dairy products • sardines • salmon • kidney beans • dark green leafy vegetables	• building bones and teeth • protects against osteoporosis • transmission of neural impulses and muscular contractions
Phosphorus (P)	• animal protein • nuts and legumes • dairy products • oatmeal • eggs • barley and lentils	• combines with calcium to build bones and teeth • combines with B vitamins to stimulate energy metabolism
Potassium (K)	• cereal • dried peas • fruits and vegetables • meats	• transmission of neural impulses and muscular contractions • critical to maintaining heartbeat
Sulfur (S)	• any protein	• produces skin and growth of nails
Sodium (Na)	• salt (NaCl) • abundant in food supply	• transmission of neural impulses and muscular contractions
Chlorine (Cl)	• salt (NaCl)	• transmission of neural impulses and muscular contractions • modulates fluid exchange in body cells • aids in digestion when present in hydrochloric acid (HCl)
Magnesium (Mg)	• whole grains • fruits and vegetables	• glucose metabolism enabling release of energy • transmission of neural impulses and muscular contractions
Iron (Fe)	• abundant in many vegetables, fruits, and poultry • nuts • legumes • lettuce • whole wheat grains	• part of hemoglobin and essential to the transportation of oxygen in the blood • part of enzymes needed for cell respiration

Sources: Adapted from *Exercise Physiology: Energy, Nutrition and Human Performance* (4th ed.), by W. D. McArdle, F. I. Katch, & V. L. Katch, 1991, Philadelphia: Lea & Febiger; *Taber's Cyclopedic Medical Dictionary*, 1997, Philadelphia; F. A. Davis; and *Understanding Normal and Clinical Nutrition* by E. N. Whitney, & C. B. Cataldo, 1983, St. Paul, MN: West.

Water

Water, although not important as a food nutrient, is essential in converting bodily processes, such as when protein is converted to amino acids. Water is involved in all metabolic activities within the cells, and it acts as a transporting agent of the body. It is the principal component of blood, lymph, and tissue fluid and secretions of the body. Forty to 60 percent of a person's weight is water. Water comes from liquids, fruits, and vegetables and is produced during the process of metabolism. The recommended daily intake of water for adults is about five 8-ounce cups (McArdle et al., 1991).

What Is a Healthy Diet?

In planning a healthy diet, the therapist should work with the client to consider the following issues (U.S. Department of Health and Human Services, Public Health Services, 1988):

▶ reducing consumption of saturated fats and cholesterol

▶ increasing consumption of vegetables, fruits, whole-grain foods, fish, poultry, lean meats, and low-fat dairy products

▶ increasing consumption of complex carbohydrates and fibers through whole-grain foods, cereal products, vegetables, and fruits

▶ limiting intake of sodium by reducing the number of packaged foods or not adding salt to foods at the table

▶ reducing or eliminating alcohol in the diet

▶ reducing sugar, especially processed sugar

▶ increasing calcium in the diet by including nonfat or low-fat dairy products

▶ increasing the amount of iron, especially for children, adolescents, or women of child-bearing age through the use of lean meat, beans, cereal, and whole-grain products

▶ balancing the number of calories consumed with the energy expended through activities. For example, the average adult age 23 to 50 expends about 2,200 calories a day. If one is to lose weight, then the caloric intake should be below 2,200 calories. A client who is either more active or less active will need more or less calories, respectively, to maintain his or her present weight. For example, a male who weighs 170 pounds will use approximately 1.5 calories per minute lying at ease, but 11 calories per minute playing basketball, 9 calories per minute mowing the lawn, 7 calories per minute playing golf, 11 calories per minute running, and 6 calories per minute when engaged in moderate walking on asphalt.

Incorporating Nutrition into an Occupational Therapy Program

Individuals with psychosocial dysfunction who have been hospitalized or institutionalized should have their nutrition assessed after returning to independent living to ensure (a) that their needs are being met and (b) that they can develop an adequate diet. Cooking groups are an important part of psychosocial occupational therapy and are used frequently in therapy. These groups allow the client to practice independent skills (ADL), develop social interactions, increase self-esteem, and develop good nutritional habits. During these cooking groups, there should be opportunities for the therapist to discuss the benefits of good nutrition and exercise and for clients to raise questions or concerns. Psychoeducational approaches, where the therapist can present nutrition in a more formal setting, should be considered.

HERBAL MEDICINE

The use of herbs in the treatment of disease has been traced back to the Neanderthal man, some 60,000 years ago (Solecki, 1975). What are herbs? How are they used as medicine? And what is the evidence for their effectiveness? Herbs are plants, not ordinarily used as food, but are claimed to have medicinal qualities. "All cultures have long folk medicine histories that include the use of plants. Even in ancient cultures, people methodically and scientifically collected information on herbs and developed well-defined herbal pharmacopoeias" (Workshop on Alternative Medicine, 1994, p. 183). The origin of many prescription drugs comes from plants. So the use of plants as medicine is not unusual. Throughout the world herbs are being self-prescribed, used by Oriental doctors, homeopaths, naturopaths, holistic physicians, and also traditional practitioners. Health care professionals, including occupational therapists, should be aware of how herbs are marketed to the public and the growing literature, examining the effects of herbs on preventing and treating diseases. Herbal products currently are not regulated as drugs by the U.S. Food and Drug Administration (FDA). Herbs are considered food supplements like vitamins, and manufacturers and distributors of herbs cannot claim in selling herbs that they have a medicinal value. Otherwise the FDA would have to approve their distribution. Many scientists and physicians believe that herbs as well as vitamin supplements are worthless or even potentially dangerous and do not recommend that clients explore their use (Herbert, 1986; Snider, 1991). In spite of this, millions of people throughout the world take supplements of vitamins and herbs daily. Vitamin supplements and herbs are advertised in health magazines and sold over the counter in supermarkets, discount stores, pharmacies, and health food stores. The consumer also has easy access to herbs.

What are some of the most common herbs? Mark Mayell (1997), in *Natural Health Magazine*, described the medicinal qualities of 25 herbs. For example, *cayenne pepper* reduces pain; *chamomile tea* can induce sleep; *gingko* improves energy, mood, and brain function; *ginseng* can increase your energy and sex drive; *kava* can reduce anxiety from stress; *St. John's wort* can reduce depression; *valerian* relieves anxiety, insomnia, headaches, and menstrual cramps. Are these medicinal claims valid and have they been verified or confirmed through research? A panel on herbal medicine comprised mostly of physicians and researchers recommended that the Office of Alternative Medicine, established in 1991 by the U.S. Congress, "should hold a research organizational conference to facilitate planning in herbal research" (Workshop on Alternative Medicine, 1994, p. 202). However, there has been research on the medicinal value of herbs. For example, Nordfors and Hartvig (1997), in a study of 25 clinical trials comparing St. John's wort with a placebo and established antidepressants, found that St. John's wort was effective in decreasing the depressed symptoms in 61 to 75 percent of the patients. They found the side effects of the herb were mild and much less than the antidepressant drug. Other studies in Germany have confirmed the medicinal effects of St. John's wort in decreasing depression in individuals with mild, moderate, and severe depression (Linde et al., 1996). Other studies of herbs have confirmed the effectiveness of *ginseng* on patients with non-insulin-dependent diabetes (Sotaniemi, Haapakoski, & Rautio, 1995); *garlic* as an inhibitor of cancer (Cheng, Meng, Tzeng, & Lin, 1995; Lea, 1996); *valerian* in reducing anxiety (Bourin, Bougerol, Guitton, & Broutin, 1997); *chamomile* as an anxiolytic and mild sedative (Viola et al., 1995); *gingko* as effective in mountain sickness (Roncin, Schwartz, & D'Arbigny, 1996); and *green tea* as effective in preventing cancer (Jankun, Selman, Swiercz, & Skrzypczak-Jankun, 1997).

ALTERNATIVE TREATMENT

Focusing Questions

▶ What is alternative medicine?

▶ How do we evaluate an alternative treatment technique?

▶ How do we evaluate the effectiveness of an alternative treatment technique?

Definition and Prevalence

Alternative medicines are approaches that are not taught in medical school and are not considered to be in the mainstream of medical practice. Novey (2000) lists six principles of alternative medicine:

▶ healing power of nature, meaning that the body has the inherent ability to restore health

▶ treatment of the whole person by taking into consideration the interaction of the physical, spiritual, mental, emotional, genetic, environmental, and social factors

▶ "do no harm" in the application of the alternative treatment, although it is important for the clinician to be aware of the interactions, especially between herbs and medication, that can cause adverse effects

▶ identify and treat the cause of the illness because symptoms are usually expressions of the bodies attempt to heal itself

▶ prevention, the ultimate goal of alternative medicine, is accomplished by change of lifestyle

▶ physician or therapist as a teacher encourages the client to engage in healthy practices

Eisenberg et al. (1998), in a follow-up survey on the use of alternative medicines among the general population, found the following:

> Use of at least 1 of 16 alternative therapies during the previous year increased from 33.8% in 1990 to 42.1% in 1997 (*P* < or = .001). The therapies increasing the most included herbal medicine, massage, megavitamins, self-help groups, folk remedies, energy healing, and homeopathy. The probability of users visiting an alternative medicine practitioner increased from 36.3% to 46.3% (*P* = .002). In both surveys alternative therapies were used most frequently for chronic conditions, including back

problems, anxiety, depression, and headaches. There was no significant change in disclosure rates between the two survey years; 39.8% of alternating therapies were disclosed to physicians in 1990 vs. 38.5% in 1997. The percentage of users paying entirely out-of-pocket for services provided by alternative medicine practitioners did not change significantly between 1990 (64.0%) and 1997 (58.3%; *P* = .36). Extrapolations to the US population suggest a 47.3% increase in total visits to alternative medicine practitioners, from 427 million in 1990 to 629 million in 1997, thereby exceeding total visits to all US primary care physicians. An estimated 15 million adults in 1997 took prescription medications concurrently with herbal remedies and/or high dose vitamins (18.4% of all prescription users). Estimated expenditures for alternative medicine professional services increased 45.2% between 1990 and 1997 were conservatively estimated as $21.2 billion in 1997, with at least $12.2 billion paid out-of-pocket. This exceeds the 1997 out-of-pocket expenditures related to alternative therapies were conservatively estimated at $27.9 billion, which is comparable with the projected 1997 out-of-pocket expenditures for all US physician services. (p. 1569)

Recent Research in Alternative Medicine

Novey (2000), in his book entitled *Clinician's Complete Reference to Complementary & Alternative Medicine*, lists alternative systems of medical practice and cites evidence for their efficacy. These are described in the following paragraphs.

▶ *Acupuncture.* More than 2,300 studies were carried out between 1970 and 1997 using individuals from various diagnostic categories, including addictions and psychiatric disorders (Klein & Trachtenberg, 1997). Additional detail regarding the efficacy of acupuncture can be found in a compendium written by Birch and Hammerschlag (1996).

▶ *Aroma therapy.*

> Aromatherapy works very well on insomnia, stress and emotional problems, particularly if touch is involved. The author would put the success rate in this area as high as 75% based on published research, case studies, and personal clinical experience. . . Aromatherapy can be a useful ingredient of a multiple-disciplinary pain management team. (Buckle, 2000, 659)

▶ *Light therapy.* This procedure is the application of shining light on a person's body into acupuncture points or the eyes to balance or restore health (Wallace, 2000). Light therapy has been effective with patients with seasonal affective disorders (Avery, 1998; Eastman, Young, Fogg, Liu, & Meaden, 1998; Lewy et al., 1998; Terman, Terman, & Ross, 1998).

▶ *Magnetic field therapy.* This method uses magnets in treating patients. The FDA has approved it for use in bone fractures (Pawluk, 2000). Magnetic therapies have been used in the treatment of venous ulcers (Ieran et al., 1990; Stiller et al., 1992), diabetic neuropathy (Weintraub, 1998), and reducing the pain in post-polio syndrome (Vallbona, Haywood, & Jurida, 1997).

▶ *Massage therapy.*

> Massage may enhance the immune system. A study suggests an increase in cytotoxic capacity associated with massage (Ironson et al., 1996). A study of chronic fatigue syndrome subjects found that a group receiving massage therapy had lower depression, emotional distress, and somatic symptom scores, more hours of sleep, and lower epinephrine and cortisol levels than a control group (Field et al., 1997). (Greene, 2000, p. 344)

▶ *Qi gong.* This method of alternative medicine incorporates "meditation, movement exercises, self-massage, and special healing techniques to regulate internal functions of the human body" (Londorf & Winn, 2000, p. 231).

▶ *Relaxation therapy.* Relaxation therapy includes physiological and psychological changes that are achieved through refocusing techniques, conscious breathing and meditation, and body awareness. Refocusing techniques includes redirecting thoughts by defusing the negative feeling attached to an everyday event. Conscious breathing and meditation are techniques of abdominal breathing while seated in a relaxed position. In body awareness, the client becomes aware of muscle tension, increased heart rate, body temperature, and pain. The goal is to help integrate body and mind to achieve a relaxation response (Sultanoff & Zalaquett, 2000). In recent studies, relaxation therapy has been effective in reducing (a) anxiety (Rasid & Parish, 1998), (b) migraine headaches in pediatric clients (Sartory, Muller, Metsch, & Pothmann, 1998), and (c) the damaging effects in coronary diseases (Dath, Mishra, Kumaraiah, & Yavagal,1997; van Dixhoorn, 1998).

▶ *Rolfing.* Rolfing has been shown to be effective in the treatment of individuals with chronic low back pain (Cottingham & Maitland, 1997).

▶ *Spiritual healing and prayer.*

> In a more recent study (Koenig, George, & Peterson, 1998), predictors of depression outcome were examined in a sample of 87 hospitalized older adult patients at Duke Hospital. . . .Significant predictors

of outcome included family history of depression, low quality of life, declining physical functioning, and low social support. We also measured religious attendance, frequency of private religious activities, and intrinsic religiosity. All religious measures were associated with a faster remission of depression, although only intrinsic religiosity achieved statistical significance. We discovered that religion appears to be particularly beneficial for persons with chronic disability that is unresponsive to medical treatments. (Koenig, 2000, pp. 135–136)

▶ *Therapeutic guided imagery.* "Therapeutic guided imagery allows patients to enter a relaxed state of mind and then focus their attention on images associated with the the issues they are confronting" (Rossman & Bresler, 2000, p. 65). Currently it is being used for relaxation, to reduce anxiety in depression, and to help patients prepare for surgery (Tusek, Church, Strong, Grass, & Fazio, 1997).

▶ *Therapeutic touch.* "Therapeutic touch can be defined as the exchange of life force energies between two or more people with the expressed purpose of health, changing, communicating, and growing in a health spiritual and physical manner" (Ledwith, 2000, p. 462). This method of healing has been demonstrated to be effective in reducing pain and anxiety in patients with burns (Turner, Clark, Gauthier, & Williams, 1998).

▶ *Tai Ch'i.*
Evidence shows that Tai Ch'i is an effective treatment for many cardiovascular ailments, including heart disease, arteriosclerosis, skeletal deterioration, and fractures due to falls (Kessenich, 1998). Tai Ch'i is also effective in improving intellectual functions in children. In addition to its physiologic effectiveness, individuals that practice Tai Ch'i report an increased sense of well-being and a willingness to continue with an exercise program (Kutner, Barnhart, Wolf, McNeely, & Xu, 1997; Lai, Lan, Wong, & Teng, 1995). (Liu & Morgan, 2000, p. 224)

Additional evidence for the effectiveness of Tai Ch'i comes from Lai, Lan, Wong, & Teng, 1995.

▶ *Trager® approach.* In this approach, the therapist trains the client to develop awareness of relaxation and tension through the use of touch and repetitive rhythmic and pleasant motions. The purposes are to decrease pain, increase neuromuscular control, reduce anxiety, hypertension, and hyperactivity (Liskin, 2000). One study reported in the occupational therapy literature showed improvement with patients with hand disorders using the Trager® method (Cooper, Liskin, Moorehead, 1999).

Evaluation of an Alternative Treatment Technique

How can an alternative treatment technique be evaluated by an occupational therapist when clients raise issues about these techniques with the therapist? The criteria that follow can be used to guide the therapist in judging whether there is scientific or objective evidence to support the use of the technique.

▶ The alternative treatment technique does no harm psychologically or biologically in the short term and there are no harmful cumulative effects.

▶ The effectiveness of the treatment technique can be validated, through self-evaluation, a standardized test, or a physical measure.

► A standardized methodology for administering the alternative treatment can be replicated, such as the prescribed dosage of a vitamin, herb, or drug; exercise protocol; relaxation technique; or applying a device or object to the body (e.g., TENS unit or biofeedback device).

► The alternative treatment can be feasibly and easily implemented or self-administered or demonstrated by a teacher, therapist, or other professional.

► The treatment method (e.g., teaching biofeedback, Rolfing, or Feldenkrais) can be taught in a sequential, hierarchical order without a costly or unrealistic fee.

► There is a scientific explanation for how the treatment method works (e.g., exercise may be effective in preventing heart disease because it has been shown that aerobic exercise over time can create collateral circulation that increases blood flow).

► The treatment technique fits into a theory that explains the phenomena (e.g., the relationship between germ theory and antibiotics).

► There are clinical studies (case studies, quasi-experimental studies with no control group, or retrospective studies) demonstrating that treatment is effective.

► There are highly controlled double-blind experimental studies demonstrating treatment effectiveness.

Assumptions

► Scientific method is the most effective way to evaluate the effectiveness of treatment method.

► Effectiveness of treatment is based on patient report of reduced symptoms, increased functioning, or physiological evidence.

Assessment

Alternative treatment methods are already being used in occupational therapy. The reader can use the questionnaire that follows as a guideline in exploring the use of alternative treatment methods in practice. The therapist should apply the objective criteria as listed in evaluating the effectiveness and clinical usefulness of the alternative treatment method.

Survey of Alternative Treatment Methods Used in Occupational Therapy[1]

ALTERNATIVE HEALING QUESTIONNAIRE

1. Age _____ 2. Male/Female _____ 3. Full/Part time _____ 4. Years of Practice _____

5. Education: (circle one)

   a. C.O.T.A.   b. BS/BA in OT   c. Masters in OT   d. Ph.D.   e. other

6. List your specialty area(s) of practice:

   _____

7. List your cultural background influence on attitude toward alternative healing:

   _____

8. From the attached chart, identify all the alternative healing methods you use in *practice* (Y/N) and rank the methods you use most ("1" being most frequently used).

9. From the chart, identify the alternative healing methods you use in your *personal life* (Y/N) and rank the methods you use most ("1" being most frequently used).

10. From the list of alternative healing methods, what areas would you be interested in learning more about? ("1" being the most interested in)

11. From the methods used in practice please identify *how you learned* about these healing techniques. Place a check mark in the appropriate column.

12. How are you **reimbursed** for alternative healing in your clinical practice of OT? (Please check YES or NO)

	YES	NO
A. Insurance	_____	_____
B. Patient payment	_____	_____
C. Medicare/Medicaid	_____	_____
D. Hospital daily rate	_____	_____
E. Other_____		

[1] This survey was designed by F. Stein, V. J. Knotts, L. Baldwin, J. Jurkowski, & P. Reynolds (1997).

Survey of Alternative Treatment Methods Used in Occupational Therapy
ALTERNATIVE HEALING QUESTIONNAIRE

Alternative Healing Methods:	In Practice? Y/N Rank	In Personal Life? Y/N Rank	How did you learn about the method(s)?						
			University Course	Cont Educ. Class	Private Study	Home Study Course	Trained on Job	Literature Review	TV Media
I. Active Body Work									
1. Aerobic Exercise									
2. Alexander Technique									
3. Aqua Therapy									
4. Controlled Breathing									
5. Feldenkrais									
6. Progressive Relaxation									
7. Rolfing									
8. ROM Dance									
9. Tai Ch'i									
10. Yoga									
II. Passive Body Work									
1. Acupressure									
2. Massage									
3. Myofacial Release									
4. Reflexology									
5. Therapeutic Touch									
III. Cognitive Control									
1. Aroma Therapy									
2. Autogenics									
3. Ayurveda									
4. Biofeedback									

Survey of Alternative Treatment Methods Used in Occupational Therapy ALTERNATIVE HEALING QUESTIONNAIRE									
	In Practice?	In Personal Life?	How did you learn about the method(s)?						
Alternative Healing Methods:	Y/N Rank	Y/N Rank	Uni-versity Course	Cont Educ. Class	Private Study	Home Study Course	Trained on Job	Liter-ature Review	TV Media
5. Dream Therapy									
6. Humor									
7. Hypnotherapy									
8. Meditation									
9. Relaxation Response									
10. Spirituality									
11. Visualization									
IV. Physical Agent Modalities									
1. Electrical Stimulation									
2. Fluidotherapy									
3. TENS									
4. Ultrasound									
V. Diet									
1. Herbal or Botanical									
2. Homeopathy									
3. Naturopathy									
4. Nutritional or Vitamins									
VI. IADL Functionals									
1. Hippotherapy									
2. Horticulture									
3. Pet Therapy									

Survey of Alternative Treatment Methods Used in Occupational Therapy ALTERNATIVE HEALING QUESTIONNAIRE									
	In Practice?	In Personal Life?	How did you learn about the method(s)?						
Alternative Healing Methods:	Y/N Rank	Y/N Rank	Uni- versity Course	Cont Educ. Class	Private Study	Home Study Course	Trained on Job	Liter- ature Review	TV Media
VII. Creative Arts									
1. Art Therapy									
2. Bibliotherapy									
3. Dance									
4. Music									
5. Poetry									
6. Psychodrama									
7. Storytelling									
OTHER									

Definitions to be used when filling out the questionnaire:

I. Active Body Work

1. *Aerobic exercise*: Use of exercise that impacts on cardiovascular system to improve, correct, or alternate a variety of physical problems or conditions.

2. *Alexander technique*: It is a method of bringing the way we move under our conscious control and avoiding a buildup of muscular tension. It involves balance and movement therapy and it is used to improve postural habits that are currently causing fatigue.

3. *Aqua therapy*: Therapeutic use of water, hot or cold, fresh or mineral.

4. *Controlled breathing*: Learning to exhale, let go, and breathe slowly through abdominal control, with the aim of reducing stress.

5. *Feldenkrais*: Learning new patterns of movement to enhance the communication between the brain and body by improving a person's awareness of physical and mental performance.

6. *Progressive Relaxation*: Procedure that involves identifying a local state of tension, and relaxing it away by learning to control all of the skeletal musculature through systematic muscle tension and relaxation.

7. *Rolfing*: Deep massage of the tissues around muscles. The purpose is to increase the range of motion of the joints and to enhance suppleness.

8. *ROM dance*: It is movement therapy comprised of expressive dance and relaxation techniques. It incorporates joint motion in all ranges to help individuals with joint and muscle limitations. It is an educational process that assists an individual in improving one's movement functioning through hands-on repatterning and verbal instruction.

9. *Tai Ch'i*: An old Chinese system designed to develop ch'i within the body. It can be used to rejuvenate, to heal and prevent illness and injuries, and also to lead to spiritual enlightenment. It is based on principles of rhythmic movements, equilibrium of body, effective breathing and development of life forces in the body through a series of slow-moving, circular movements.

10. *Yoga*: The term yoga, as used in the Western world, has been associated almost exclusively with physical postures and regulation of breathing. The aim in a spiritual sense is to achieve harmony of self and universe.

II. Passive Body Work

1. *Acupressure*: Compression of blood vessels by means of needles and pressure points in surrounding tissues.

2. *Massage*: Manipulation, methodical pressure, friction, and kneading of the body.

3. *Myofacial release*: Treatment for myofacial pain may follow a three-pronged approach that focuses on treating both the pain and the dysfunction. The three aspects of this approach are manual therapy, movement and exercise, and education. Whole body "hands-on" approach to release soft tissue (muscle) from abnormal grip of tight fascial (connective tissue).

4. *Reflexology*: Massage of reflex points on feet and hands to encourage health and well-being.

5. *Therapeutic touch*: A treatment seeking to relieve symptoms by use of touch. Healing of imbalanced energy (vital life force) through the use of laying on of hands.

III. Cognitive Control

1. *Aroma therapy*: The use of essential oils from plants to enhance general health and appearance.

2. *Autogenics:* Focusing attention on formerly unconscious events occurring during relaxed states is part of effective autogenic training. Self-regulation is involved in reaching a desired relaxed state.

3. *Ayurveda*: An ancient Hindu medical practice that strives to improve health by harmonizing mind, body, and spirit. It utilizes herbal remedies, massage therapy, yoga, and pulse diagnosis.

4. *Biofeedback*: A training program designed to develop one's ability to control the autonomic (involuntary) nervous system. After learning the technique, the patient may be able to control heart rate, blood pressure, and skin temperature or to relax certain muscles. The patient learns by using monitoring devices that sound a tone or show a visual display when changes in pulse, blood pressure, brain waves, and muscle contractions occur. Relaxation therapy such as meditation is often used to mediate the change.

5. *Dream therapy*: Using dreams to gain access to unconscious mind by means of examining content of dreams. Using a dream diary is helpful in this procedure. The use of dreams and the dream state to accomplish physical and emotional healing involving both interpretation and active participation in the dream process.

6. *Humor*: Any communication that is perceived by any of the interacting parties as humorous and leads to laughing, smiling, or a feeling of amusement.

7. *Hypnotherapy*: Treatment by inducing an alternative state of consciousness so the

individual feels relaxed and has little pain.

8. *Meditation*: It involves taking a comfortable position in a quiet environment, regulating breathing, having a physically relaxed and mentally calm attitude while focusing on a mental image or word.

9. *Relaxation response*: The physiological reaction that is sought and produced by sitting serenely and alone in a quiet place with eyes closed and arms and hands relaxed, paying careful attention to breathing, and repeating a brief word or phrase at each respiratory cycle. The aim is to reach a tranquil mental state that refreshes the mind and body.

10. *Spirituality*: It is an individual's focus on meaning in life and connection to the universe. It is the higher purposes that give meaning to life and it is evident through faith and beliefs.

11. *Visualization*: Imagining the working's of one's own body or inner experiences or visualizing natural scenes to encourage relaxation, healing, and well-being.

IV. Physical Agent Modalities

1. *Electrical stimulation*: Using tools that give off an electrical stimulus to help with facilitation of muscular control.

2. *Fluidotherapy*: A dry heat modality consisting of cellulose particles held in a container and moved in air. The turbulence of the mixture generates a thermal effect when objects are immersed in the medium.

3. *TENS*: Application of mild electrical stimulation to skin electrodes placed over a painful area. It causes interference with transmission of painful stimuli, providing noninvasive pain relief that works by stimulating the endorphins.

4. *Ultrasound*: Inaudible sound in the frequency range of approximately 20,000- to 10-billion cycles per second. Ultrasound has different velocities in tissues that differ in density and elasticity. This property permits the use of ultrasound in outlining the shape of various tissues and organs in the body. Use of ultrasound from diagnostic and therapeutic purposes requires special equipment.

V. Diet

1. *Herbal/Botanical*: Using forms of plants such as herbs for prevention and treatment of illnesses.

2. *Homeopathy*: School of medicine, founded by Dr. S. C. F. Hahnemann in the late 18th century, based on the theory that large doses of drugs that produce symptoms of a disease in healthy people will cure the same symptoms when administered in very small amounts. This is loosely based on the theory that "like cures like." Using natural remedies of specially prepared plants and minerals to boost the body's own defense mechanisms and healing processes.

3. *Naturopathy*: A therapeutic system that does not use drugs but employs natural forces such as light, heat, air, water, massage, herbs, healthy food, and vitamins.

4. *Nutritional/Vitamins*: The application of special foods and vitamins to maintain health and to prevent illness.

VI. IADL/Functional

1. *Hippotherapy*: "Treatment with the help of the horse." It aims to strengthen, stretch, and relax the muscles, enhance the motor coordination of the rider, and to attain psychological goals such as increase in self-esteem.

2. *Horticulture*: The science or art of cultivating fruits, vegetables, flowers, and plants.

3. *Pet therapy*: The therapeutic use of pets, to create an animal-human bond, which may improve a patient's physical and emotional health.

VII. Creative Arts

1. *Art therapy*: Use of art as a therapeutic tool.

2. *Bibliotherapy*: Nonphysical, psychotherapeutic technique in which the patient is encouraged to read books that are inspir-

ing and related to the patient's illness or experiences. Used in treating mental illness.

3. *Dance*: To move using series of rhythmical motions and steps. Dance is a good form of exercise and expression.
4. *Music*: The use of music for relaxation by creating an emotional climate.
5. *Poetry*: A composition designed to convey a vivid and imaginative sense of experience. Can be insightful in discovering what a person is feeling and thinking.
6. *Psychodrama*: A form of group psychotherapy in which patients act out assigned roles. The therapeutic goals are to reduce emotional symptoms and to encourage personal growth.
7. *Storytelling*: Reminiscing about events in a person's life and recapturing visual scenes. It can also be a life review of an individual.

BIBLIOGRAPHY FOR ADDITIONAL INFORMATION IN ALTERNATIVE TREATMENTS

The following annotated bibliography can be useful for students exploring alternative treatment methods in occupational therapy. Most of these references come from the occupational therapy literature. The bibliography was prepared with the help of Jacie Jurkowski, OTR.

PAM (Physical Agent Modalities)

Carroll, S. G., & Meeny, C. F. (1993). Electrical stimulation for restoring independent feeding in a man with quadriplegia. *American Journal of Occupational Therapy, 47*, 739–742.
The investigators applied NMES (neuromuscular electrical stimulation) to an individual with quadriplegia (C4–C5) to improve his strength and endurance of the anterior and middle fibers of the deltoid muscle. The exercises were used to prepare him to feed himself independently. After a 3-week period of NMES and a 12-session exercise program 5 days a week the client was able to feed himself. In a 6-month follow-up, the client was still feeding himself.

Humphry, R., & Taylor, E. (1991). Survey of physical agent modality use. *American Journal of Occupational Therapy, 45*, 924–931.
Nine hundred and 97 surveys were sent to occupational therapists who worked in the area of Physical Disabilities. Six hundred twenty-nine of the surveys were completed and the results showed that the most commonly used physical agent modality (PAM) was hot and cold packs and that most of the therapists learned about PAM on the job.

King, T. I. (1996). The effect of neuromuscular electrical stimulation in reducing tone. *American Journal of Occupational Therapy, 50*, 62–64.
Dr. King compared neuromuscular electrical stimulation (NMES) and passive stretch in reducing chronic wrist spasticity in an individual who had experienced a CVA. He found that both methods were effective in reducing spasticity.

King, T. I. (1992). The use of electromyographic biofeedback in treating a client with tension headaches. *American Journal of Occupational Therapy, 46*, 839–842.
EMG biofeedback was used to treat a client with tension headaches. The treatment included nine outpatient visits, applying EMG, resistive exercises, and relaxation therapy. After 4 weeks, the patient was pain free from headaches and was more functional in home activities.

Pet Therapy

Ferrie, P., Rovner, B., Shmuely, Y., & Zisselman, B. (1996). A pet therapy intervention with geriatric psychiatry inpatient. *American Journal of Occupational Therapy, 50*, 47–57.
A pilot study of individuals in a geriatric psychiatry unit who received pet therapy or exer-

cise for a 1-week period. Those in the pet therapy group showed improvement in feelings on an outcome measure scale. The need for more research in the area of pet therapy was recommended.

Fick, K. M. (1993). The influence of an animal on social interactions of nursing home residents in a group setting. *American Journal of Occupational Therapy, 47*, 529–534.

The results of the study showed increased social interactions after a dog was introduced to residents in the nursing home.

Humor

MacRae, A., & Vergeer, G. (1993). Therapeutic use of humor in occupational therapy. *American Journal of Occupational Therapy, 47*, 678–683.

The results of the survey indicated that humor was effective in (a) building rapport between occupational therapists and physical therapists, (b) increasing productivity, (c) relieving stress, and (d) building personal relationships between coworkers.

Exercise

Casby, J. A., & Holm, M. B. (1994a). Occupationally embedded exercise versus rote exercise: A choice between occupational forms by elderly nursing home residents. *American Journal of Occupational Therapy, 49*, 397–404.

The investigators found that patients would rather play basketball than do rote exercises. The clients also showed more functional improvement with basketball than with rote exercises.

Music

Casby, J. A., & Holm, M. B. (1994b). The effect of music on repetitive disruptive vocalizations of persons with dementia. *American Journal of Occupational Therapy, 48*, 883–889.

Classical music, favorite music, and no music were compared with three elderly patients diagnosed with dementia of the Alzheimer type who had repetitive disruptive vocalizations. The authors found that the use of music was effective for two of the three patients.

Recreational Activities/Leisure

McGruder, J. E., & Taylor-Siegel, L. P. (1996). The meaning of sea kayaking for persons with spinal cord injuries. *American Journal of Occupational Therapy, 50*, 39–46.

The investigator interviewed three clients with spinal cord injury (SCI) about their sea kayaking experience. The participants concurred that the novelty, challenge, safety, and sociability helped them in building self-confidence.

Pasek, P. B., & Schkade, J. K. (1996). Effects of a skiing experience of adolescents with limb deficiencies: An occupational adaptation perspective. *American Journal of Occupational Therapy, 50*, 24–31.

The authors found that after a 6-day ski trip, which resulted in increased mastery of the skill of skiing, the adolescents felt that their self-esteem was increased.

Relaxation Techniques

Courtney, C., & Escobedo, B. (1990). A stress management program: Inpatient to outpatient continuity. *American Journal of Occupational Therapy, 44*, 306–310.

The author applied exercise, assertiveness training, arts and crafts, relaxation training, and stress management techniques in a psychoeducational program. Follow-up results showed that the treatment was effective in increasing relaxation and decreasing anxiety.

Engel, J. M. (1992). Relaxation training: A self-help approach for children with headaches. *American Journal of Occupational Therapy, 46*, 591–596.

The results showed a decrease of severity, frequency, and intensity of headaches for 10 children practicing relaxation techniques daily for 6 weeks.

Lysaght, R., & Bodenhamer, E. (1990). The use of relaxation training to enhance functional outcomes in adults with traumatic head injuries. *American Journal of Occupational Therapy, 44,* 797–802.

Relaxation training with EMG biofeedback was effective in increasing functional skills in four adults with traumatic brain injuries.

Tse, S., & Barley, D. M. (1992). Tai Ch'i and postural control in the well elderly. *American Journal of Occupational Therapy, 46,* 295–300.

The study showed that Tai Ch'i increased the participants' postural control on three of five balance tests.

REFERENCES

American College of Sports Medicine. (1978). The recommended quantity and quality of exercise for developing and maintaining fitness in health adults. *Medicine and Science in Sports, 10,* vii–ix.

American Occupational Therapy Association. (1993). Purposeful activity. [Position paper]. *American Journal of Occupational Therapy, 47,* 1081–1082.

American Occupational Therapy Association. (1994). *Uniform terminology for occupational therapy* (3rd ed.). Rockville, MD: Author.

Åsberg, M., Perris, C., Schalling, D., & Sedvall, G. (1987). The CPRS—development and applications of a psychiatric rating scale. *Acta Psychiatrica Scandinavia, 271*(Suppl.), 1–27.

Avery, D. H. (1998). A turning point for seasonal affective disorder and light therapy research? *Archives of General Psychiatry, 55,* 863–864.

Beck, A. T., Ward, C. H., Mendelson, M., Mock, J., & Erbaugh, J. (1961). An inventory for measuring depression. *Archives of General Psychiatry, 4,* 561–571.

Birch, S., & Hammerschlag, R. (1996). *Acupuncture efficacy: A compendium of controlled clinical studies.* Tarrytown, NY: National Academy of Acupuncture and Oriental Medicine.

Björntorp, P., & Krotkiewski, M. (1985). Exercise treatment in diabetes mellitus. *Acta Medica Scandinavica, 217,* 3–7.

Blair, S. N., Kohl, H. W., Paffenbarger, R. S., Clark, D. G., Cooper, K. H., & Gibbons, L. W. (1989). Physical fitness and all–cause mortality: A prospective study of healthy men and women. *Journal of the American Medical Association, 273,* 2093–2098.

Blue, F. R. (1979). Aerobic running as a treatment for moderate depression. *Perceptual and Motor Skills, 48,* 228.

Blumenthal, J. A., Fredrikson, M., Kuhn, C. M., Ulmer, R. A., Walsh-Riddle, M., & Appelbaum, M. (1990). Aerobic exercise reduces levels of cardiovascular and sympathoadrenal responses to mental stress in subjects without prior evidence of myocardial ischemia. *American Journal of Cardiology, 65,* 93–98.

Blumenthal, J. A., Fredrikson, M., Matthews, K. A., German, D., Steege, J., Walsh–Riddle, M. A., Kuhn, C., Rifai, N., & Rodin, J. (1991). Stress reactivity and exercise training in pre- and postmenopausal women. *Health Psychology, 10,* 384–391.

Bosscher, R. J. (1993). Running and mixed physical exercises with depressed psychiatric patients. *International Journal of Sport Psychology, 24,* 170–184.

Bouchard, C., Deprés, J–P., Tremblay, A. (1993). Exercise and obesity. *Obesity Research, 1,* 133–147.

Bourin, M., Bougerol, T., Guitton, B., Broutin, E. (1997). A combination of plan extracts in the treatment of outpatients with adjustment disorder with anxious mood: Controlled study versus placebo. *Fundamental Clinical Pharmacology, 11,* 127–132.

Brollier, C., Hamrick, N., & Jacobson, B. (1994). Aerobic exercise: A potential occupational therapy modality for adolescents with depression. *Occupational Therapy in Mental Health, 12,* 19–29.

Brown, D. R., Wang, Y., Ward, A., Ebbeling, C. B., Fortlage, L., Puleo, E. et al. (1995). Chronic psychological effects of exercise and exercise plus cognitive strategies. *Medicine and Science in Sports and Exercise, 27,* 756–775.

Buckle, J. (2000). Aromatherapy. In D. W. Novey, *Clinician's complete reference to complementary &*

alternative medicine (pp. 651–666). St. Louis: Mosby.

Callen, K. E. (1983). Mental and emotional aspects of running. *Psychosomatics, 24*(2), 133–151.

Carroll, S. G., & Meeny, C. F. (1993). Electrical stimulation for restoring independent feeding in a man with quadriplegia. *American Journal of Occupational Therapy, 47,* 739–742.

Casby, J. A., & Holm, M. B. (1994a). Occupationally embedded exercise versus rote exercise: A choice between occupational forms by elderly nursing home residents. *American Journal of Occupational Therapy, 48,* 397–404.

Casby, J. A., & Holm, M. B. (1994b). The effect of music on repetitive disruptive vocalizations of persons with dementia. *American Journal of Occupational Therapy, 48,* 883–889.

Cheng, J. Y., Meng, C. L., Tzeng, C. C., & Lin, J. C. (1995). Optimal dose of garlic to inhibit dimethylhydrazine-induced colon cancer. *World Journal of Surgery, 19,* 621–626.

Cooper, C., Liskin, J., & Moorhead, J. F. (1999). Dyscoordinate co-contraction: Impaired quality of movement in patients with hand disorders. *Occupational Therapy Practice, 4*(3), 40–45.

Cottingham, J., & Maitland, J. (1997). A three-paradigm treatment model using soft tissue mobilization and guided movement-awareness techniques for patients with chronic back pain: A case study. *Journal of Orthopedic Sports Physical Therapy, 26,* 155–167.

Cotton, D. H. G. (1990). *Stress management: An integrated approach to therapy.* New York: Brunner/Mazel.

Courtney, C., & Escobedo, B. (1990). A stress management program: Inpatient to outpatient continuity. *American Journal of Occupational Therapy, 44,* 306–310.

Cox, J. P., Evans, J. F., & Jamieson, J. L. (1979). Aerobic power and tonic heart rate responses to psychological stressors. *Personality and Social Psychology Bulletin, 5,* 160–163.

Crews, D. J., & Landers, D. M. (1987). A meta-analytical review of aerobic fitness and reactivity to psychosocial stressors. *Medicine and Science in Sports and Exercise, 19*(Suppl.), S114–S120.

Dath, N. N. S., Mishra, H., Kumaraiah, V., & Yavagal, S. T. (1997). Behavioural approach to coronary heart disease. *Journal of Personality Clinical Studies, 13,* 29–33.

Davis, G. M. (1993). Exercise capacity of individuals with paraplegia. *Medicine and Science in Sports and Exercise, 25,* 423–432.

de Coverley Veale, D. M. W. (1987). Exercise and mental health. *Acta Psychiatrica Scandinavica, 76,* 113–120.

Dey, S. (1994). Physical exercise as a novel antidepressant agent: Possible role of serotonin receptor subtypes. *Physiology and Behavior, 55,* 323–329.

Dey, S., Singh, R. I., & Dey, P. K. (1992). Exercise training: Significance of regional alterations in serotonin metabolism of rat brain in relation to antidepressant effect of exercise. *Physiology and Behavior, 52,* 1095–1099.

DiPietro, L. (1995). Physical activity, body weight, and adiposity: An epidemiologic perspective. *Exercise and Sports Sciences Review, 23,* 275–303.

Dishman, R. K. (1988). Overview. In R. K. Dishman (Ed.), *Exercise adherence: Its impact on public health* (pp. 1–9). Champaign, IL: Human Kinetics.

Dishman, R. K., & Gettman, L. R. (1980). Psychobiological influences on exercise adherence. *Journal of Sport Psychology, 2,* 295–310.

Doyne, E. J., Chambless, D. L., & Beutler, L. E. (1983). Aerobic exercise as a treatment for depression in women. *Behavior Therapy, 14,* 434–440.

Doyne, E. J., Ossip–Klein, D. J., Bowman, E. D., Osborn, D. M., McDougall-Wilson, I. B., & Neimeyer, R. A. (1987). Running versus weight lifting in the treatment of depression. *Journal of Consulting and Clinical Psychology, 55,* 748–754.

Drinkwater, B. L. (1993). Exercise in the prevention of osteoporosis. *Osteoporosis International, 1,* S169–S171.

Dubos, R. (1979). Medicine evolving. In D. S. Sobel (Ed.), *Ways of health: Holistic approaches to ancient and contemporary medicine* (pp. 21–44). New York: Harcourt Brace Jovanovich.

Eastman, C. I., Young, M. A., Fogg, L. F., Liu, L., & Meaden, P. M. (1998). Bright light treatment of winter depression: A placebo-controlled trial. *Archives of General Psychiatry, 55,* 883–889.

Eisenberg, D. M., Davis, R. B., Ettner, S. L., Appel, S., Wilkey, S., Van Rompay, M., Kessler, R. C. (1998). Trends in alternative medicine use in the United States, 1990–1997: Results of a follow-up national survey. *Journal of American Medical Association, 280*, 1569–1575.

Engel, J. M. (1992). Relaxation training: A self-help approach for children with headaches. *American Journal of Occupational Therapy, 46*, 591–596.

Etnyre, B. R., & Abraham, L. D. (1986). Gains in range of ankle dorsiflexion using three popular stretching techniques. *American Journal of Physical Medicine, 65*, 189–196.

Ewart, C. K. (1989). Psychological effects of resistive weight training: Implications for cardiac patients. *Medicine and Science in Sports and Exercise, 21*, 683–688.

Ewbank, P. P., Darga, L. L., & Lucas, C. P. (1995). Physical activity as a predictor of weight maintenance in previously obese subjects. *Obesity Research, 3*, 257–263.

Fagard, R., Bielen, E., Hespel, P., Lijnen, P., Staessen, J., Vanhees, L., et al. (1990). Physical exercise in hypertension. In J. H. Laragh & B. M. Brenner (Eds.), *Hypertension: Pathophysiology, diagnosis, and management* (Vol. 2, pp. 1985–1998). New York: Raven.

Fagard, R. H., & Tipton, C. M. (1994). Physical activity, fitness and hypertension. In C. Bouchard, R. J. Shepard, & T. Stephens (Eds.), *Physical activity, fitness, and health: International proceedings and consensus statement* (pp. 633–655). Champaign, IL: Human Kinetics.

Ferrie, P., Rovner, B., Shmuely, Y., & Zisselman, B. (1996). A pet therapy intervention with geriatric psychiatry inpatient. *American Journal of Occupational Therapy, 50*, 47–57.

Fick, K. M. (1993). The influence of an animal on social interactions of nursing home residents in a group setting. *American Journal of Occupational Therapy, 47*, 529–534.

Field, T., Hernandez-Reif, M., Seligman, S., Krasnegor, J., Sunshine, W., Rivas-Chacon, R., Schanberg, S., Kuhn, C. (1997). Chronic fatigue syndrome: Massage therapy effects on depression and somatic symptoms in chronic fatigue syndrome. *Journal of Chronic Fatigue Syndrome, 3*, 43–51.

Fillingim, R. B., & Blumenthal, J. A. (1993). The use of aerobic exercise as a method of stress management. In P. M. Lehrer & R. L. Woolfolk (Eds.), *Principles and practice of stress management* (2nd ed., pp. 443–462). New York: Guilford.

Fisher, N. M., Gresham, G. E., Abrams, M., Hicks, J., Horrign, D., & Pendergast, D. R. (1933). Quantitative effects of physical therapy on muscular and functional performance in subjects with osteoarthritis of the knees. *Archives of Physical Medicine and Rehabilitation, 74*, 840–847.

Fransen, M., Margiotta, E., Crosbie, J., & Edmonds, J. (1997). A revised group exercise program for osteoarthritis of the knee. *Physiotherapy Research International, 2*, 30–41.

Green, H. J., Jones, L. L., & Painter, D. C. (1990). Effects of short-term training on cardiac function during prolonged exercise. *Medicine and Science in Sports and Exercise, 22*, 488–493.

Greene, E. (2000). Massage therapy. In D. W. Novey, *Clinician's complete reference to complementary & alternative medicine* (pp. 338–348). St. Louis: Mosby.

Greist, J. H., Klein, M. H., Eischens, R. R., Faris, J., Gurman, A. S., & Morgan, W. P. (1979). Running as treatment for depression. *Comprehensive Psychiatry, 20*, 41–54.

Hambrecht, R., Niebauer, J., Marburger, C., Grunze, M., Kälberer, B., Hauer, K, Schlierf, G., Kubler, W., & Schuler, G. (1993). Various intensities of leisure-time physical activity in patients with coronary artery disease: Effects on cardiorespiratory fitness and progression of coronary atherosclerotic lesions. *Journal of the American College of Cardiology, 22*, 468–477.

Hamilton, M. (1960). A rating scale for depression. *Journal of Neurology, Neurosurgery, and Psychiatry, 23*, 56–61.

Haskell, W. L., Alderman, E. L., Fair, J. M., Maron, D. J., Mackey S. F., Superko, H. R., Williams, P. T., Johnston, I. M., Champagne, M. A., Krauss, R. M., et al. (1994). Effects of intensive multiple risk factor reduction on coronary atherosclerosis and clinical cardiac events in men and women with coronary artery disease: The Stanford Coronary Risk Intervention Project (SCRIP). *Circulation, 89*, 975–990.

Herbert, V. (1986). Unproven (questionable) dietary and nutritional methods in cancer prevention and treatment. *Cancer, 58*(Suppl.), 1930–1941.

Humphry, R., & Taylor, E. (1991). Survey of physical agent modality use. *American Journal of Occupational Therapy, 45*, 924–931.

Ieran, M., Zaffuto, S., Bagnacani, M., Annovi, M., Moratti, A., & Cadossi, R. (1990). Effect of low frequency pulsing electromagnetic fields on skin ulcers of venous origin in humans: A double blind study. *Journal of Orthopedic Research, 8*, 276–282.

Ironson, G., Field, T., Scafidi, F., Hashimoto, M., Kumar, M., Kumar, A., Price, A., Goncalves, A., Burman, I., Tenteman, C., Patarca, R., & Fletcher, M. A. (1996). Massage therapy is associated with enhancement of the immune system's cytotoxic capacity. *International Journal of Neuroscience, 84*, 205–217.

Jacobs, B. L. (1994). Serotonin, motor activity, and depression-related disorders. *American Scientist, 82*, 456–463.

Jacobson, E. (1929). *Progressive relaxation.* Chicago: University of Chicago.

Jankun, J., Selman, S. W., Swiercz, R., Skrzypczak-Jankun, E. (1997, June 5). Why drinking green tea could prevent cancer. *Nature, 387*(6633), 561.

Jeffery, R. W. (1995). Community programs for obesity prevention: The Minnesota Heart Health Program. *Obesity Research, 3*(Suppl.), 283S–288S.

Kaplan, K., Mendelson, L. B., & Dubroff, M. P. (1983). The effect of a jogging program on psychiatric inpatients with symptoms of depression. *The Occupational Therapy Journal of Research, 3*, 173–175.

Kessenich, C. R. (1998). Tai ch'i as a method of fall prevention in the elderly. *Orthopedic Nursing, 17*, 27–29.

Kielhofner, G. (Ed.). (1985). *A model of human occupation: Theory and application.* Baltimore: Williams & Wilkins.

King, T. I. (1992). The use of electromyographic biofeedback in treating a client with tension headaches. *American Journal of Occupational Therapy, 46*, 839–842.

King, T. I. (1996). The effect of neuromuscular electrical stimulation in reducing tone. *American Journal of Occupational Therapy, 50*, 62–64.

Klein, L. J., & Trachenberg, A. I. (comp.). (1997). *Acupuncture: January 1970 through October 1997.* Bethesda, MD: National Library of Medicine. Retrieved February 14, 2001, from the World Wide Web: *http://www.nlm.nih.gov/pubs/cbm/ acupuncture.html.*

Koenig, H. G. (2000). Spiritual healing and prayer. In D. W. Novey, *Clinician's complete reference to complementary & alternative medicine* (pp. 130–140). St. Louis: Mosby.

Koenig, H. G., George, L. K, & Peterson, B. L. (1998). Religiosity and remission from depression in medically ill older patients. *American Journal of Psychiatry, 155*, 536–542.

Kutner, N. G., Barnhart, H., Wolf, S. L., McNeely, E., & Xu, T. (1997). Self-report benefits of Tai Ch'i practice by older adults. *Journals of Gerontology. Series B: Psychological Sciences and Social Sciences, 52B*, 242–246.

Lai, J. S., Lan, C., Wong, M. K., & Teng, S. H. (1995). Two-year trends in cardiorespiratory function among older Tai Ch'i Chuan practitioners and sedentary subjects. *Journal of American Geriatric Society, 45*, 1222–1227.

Lea, M. A. (1996). Organosulfur compounds and cancer. *Advances in Experimental Medical Biology, 401*, 147–154.

Lechin, F., van de Dijs, B., Orozco, B., Lechin, A. E., Baez, S., Lechin, M. E., Rada, I., Acosta, E., Arocha, L., Jimenez, V., et al. (1995). Plasma neurotransmitters, blood pressure, and heart rate during supine resting, orthostasis, and moderate exercise in dysthymic depressed patients. *Biological Psychiatry, 37*, 884–891.

Ledwith, S. (2000). Therapeutic touch. In D. W. Novey, *Clinician's complete reference to complementary & alternative medicine* (pp. 462–471). St. Louis: Mosby.

Lewy, A. J., Bauer, V. K., Cutler, N. L., Sack, R. L., Ahmed, S., Thomas, K. H., Blood, M. L., & Jackson, J. M. (1998). Morning vs. evening light treatment of patients with winter depression. *Archives of General Psychiatry, 55*, 890–896.

Linde, K., Ramirez, G., Mulrow, C. D., Pauls, A., Weidenhammer, W., & Melchart, D. (1996, August 3). St. John's wort for depression—An overview and meta-analysis of randomized clinical trials. *British Medical Journal, 313*(7052), 253–258.

Liskin, J. (2000). Trager® approach. In D. W. Novey, *Clinician's complete reference to complementary & alternative medicine* (pp. 472–482). St. Louis: Mosby.

Liu, Y., & Morgan, T. M. (2000). Tai Ch'i. In D. W. Novey, *Clinician's complete reference to complementary & alternative medicine* (pp. 219–230). St. Louis: Mosby.

Londorf, D., & Winn, M. (2000). Qi gong. In D. W. Novey, *Clinician's complete reference to complementary & alternative medicine* (pp. 231–244). St. Louis: Mosby.

Lubin, B. (1981). Additional data on the reliability and validity of the brief lists of the depression adjective check lists. *Journal of Clinical Psychology, 37*, 809–811.

Lysaght, R., & Bodenhamer, E. (1990). The use of relaxation training to enhance functional outcomes in adults with traumatic head injuries. *American Journal of Occupational Therapy, 44*, 797–802.

MacRae, A., & Vergeer, G. (1993). Therapeutic use of humor in occupational therapy. *American Journal of Occupational Therapy, 47*, 678–683.

Martin, M. J., Hulley, S. B., Browner, W. S., Kuller, L. H., & Wentworth, D. (1986). Serum cholesterol blood pressure, and mortality: Implications from a cohort of 361,662 men. *Lancet, 2*, 933–936.

Martinez, M. E., Giovannucci, E., Spiegelman, D., Hunter, D. J., Willett, W. C., & Colditz, G. A. (1997, July 2). Leisure-time physical activity, body size, and colon cancer in women: Nurses' Health Study Research Group. *Journal of National Cancer Institute, 89*, 948–955.

Martinsen, E. W. (1994). Physical activity and depression: Clinical experience. *Acta Psychiatrica Scandinavica, 377*, 23–27.

Martinsen, E. W., Hoffart, A., & Solberg, O. (1989). Comparing aerobic with nonaerobic forms of exercise in the treatment of clinical depression: A randomized trial. *Comprehensive Psychiatry, 30*, 324–331.

Martinsen, E. W., Medhus, A., & Sandvik, L. (1985). Effects of aerobic exercise on depression: A controlled study. *British Medical Journal, 291*, 109.

Mayell, M. (1997, September/October). 23 power herbs. *Natural Health, 27*(5), 115–120, 122, 124, 126, 128, 130, 132, 164–175.

Mayo Clinic. (1994). *Mayo clinic family health book* (2nd ed.). [CD–ROM]. (Available: IVI Publishing, 7500 Flying Cloud Drive, Minneapolis, MN 55344–3739)

McArdle, W. D., Katch, F. I., & Katch, V. L. (1991). *Exercise physiology: Energy, nutrition and human performance* (3rd ed.). Philadelphia: Lea & Febiger.

McArdle, W. D., Katch, F. I., & Katch, V. L. (1996). *Exercise physiology: Energy, nutrition and human performance* (4th ed.). Philadelphia: Lea & Febiger.

McAuley, E., Mihalko, S. L., & Bane, S. M. (1997). Exercise and self-esteem in middle-aged adults: Multidimensional relationships and physical fitness and self-efficacy influences. *Journal of Behavioral Medicine, 20*, 67–83.

McGruder, J. E., & Taylor-Siegel, L. P. (1996). The meaning of sea kayaking for persons with spinal cord injuries. *American Journal of Occupational Therapy, 50*, 39–46.

Meeusen, R., & De Meirleir, K. (1995). Exercise and brain neurotransmission. *Sports Medicine, 20*, 160–188.

Mittleman, M. A., Maclure, M., Tofler, G. H., Sherwood, J. B., Goldberg, R. J., & Muller, J. E. (1993). Triggering of acute myocardial infarction by heavy physical exertion: Protection against triggering by regular exertion. *New England Journal of Medicine, 329*, 1677–1683.

Mongeau, R., Blier, P., & de Montigny, C. (1997). The serotonergic and noradrenergic systems of the hippocampus: Their interactions and the effects of antidepressant treatment. *Brain Research— Brain Research Reviews, 23*(3), 145–195.

Montgomery, S. A., & Åsberg, M. (1979). A new depression scale designed to be sensitive to change. *British Journal of Psychiatry, 134*, 382–389.

National Sporting Goods Association. (1997). *Snowboarding leads 1996 sport growth while exercise walking remains America's favorite activity.* Retrieved August 29, 1997, from the World Wide Web: *http://www.fitnesslink.com/feature/stats.htm.*

Nelson, B. W., O'Reilly, E., Miller, M., Hogan, M., Wegner, J. A., & Kelly, C. (1995). The clinical effects of intensive, specific exercise on chronic low back pain: A controlled study of 895 consecutive patients with 1-year follow up. *Orthopedics, 18*, 971–981.

Nelson, M. E., Fischer, E. C., Dilmanian, F. A., Dallal, G. E., & Evans, W. J. (1991). A one–year walking program and increased dietary calcium in postmenopausal women: Effects on bone. *American Journal of Clinical Nutrition, 53*, 1304–1311.

Niebauer, J., Manbrecht, R., Schlierf, G., Marburger, C., Kalberer, B., Kubler, W., & Schuler, G. (1995). Five years of physical exercise and low fat diet: Effects on progression of coronary artery disease. *Journal of Cardiopulmonary Rehabilitation, 15*, 47–64.

Nordfors, M., & Hartvig, P. (1997). St. John's wort against depression in favour again. *Lakartidningen, 94*, 2365–2367.

North, T. C., McCullagh, P., & Tran, Z. V. (1990). Effects of exercise on depression. *Exercise and Sport Sciences Reviews, 18*, 379–415.

Novey, D. W. (2000). *Clinician's complete reference to complementary & alternative medicine.* St. Louis: Mosby.

Ornish, D., Brown, S. E., Scherwitz, L. W., Billings, J. H., Armstrong, W. T., Ports, T. A., et al. (1990). Can lifestyle changes reverse coronary heart disease? The Lifestyle Heart Trial. *Lancet, 336*, 129–133.

Paffenbarger, R. S., Hyde, R. T., Wing, A. L., & Hsieh, C. C. (1986). Physical activity, all-cause mortality, and longevity of college alumni. *New England Journal of Medicine, 314*, 605–613.

Pasek, P. B., & Schkade, J. K. (1996). Effects of a skiing experience of adolescents with limb deficiencies: An occupational adaptation perspective. *American Journal of Occupational Therapy, 50*, 24–31.

Pawluk, W. (2000). Magnetic field therapy. In D. W. Novey, *Clinician's complete reference to complementary & alternative medicine* (pp. 164–175). St. Louis: Mosby.

Powell, K. E., Spain, K. G., Christenson, G. M., & Mollenkamp, M. P. (1986). The status of the 1990 objectives for physical fitness and exercise. *Public Health Reports, 100*, 147–158.

President's Council on Physical Fitness and Sports. (1996). *Physical activity and health: A report of the surgeon general.* Pittsburgh, PA: U.S. Department of Health and Human Services, Centers for Disease Control and Prevention, National Center for Chronic Disease Prevention and Health Promotion.

President's Council on Physical Fitness and Sports. (1997). *Manual.* [Online]. Available: *http://www.virtual–fitness.com/exrguide.htm* [1997, Aug 29].

Rape, R. N. (1987). Running and depression. *Perceptual and Motor Skills, 64*, 1303–1310.

Rasid, Z. M., & Parish, T. S. (1998). The effects of two types of relaxation training on students' levels of anxiety. *Adolescence, 33*, 99–101.

Roncin, J. P., Schwartz, F., & D'Arbigny, P. (1996). EGb 761 in control of acute mountain sickness and vascular reactivity to cold exposure. *Aviation Space and Environmental Medicine, 67*, 445–452.

Rosenfeld, I. (1996). *Dr. Rosenfeld's guide to alternative medicine: What works, what doesn't—and what's right for you.* New York: Random House.

Ross, C. E., & Hayes, D. (1988). Exercise and psychologic well-being in the community. *American Journal of Epidemiology, 127*, 762–771.

Rossman, M. L., & Bresler, D. E. (2000). In D. W. Novey, *Clinician's complete reference to complementary & alternative medicine* (pp. 65–72), St. Louis: Mosby.

Roth, D. L., & Holmes, D. S. (1985). Influence of physical fitness in determining the impact of stressful life events on physical and psychologic health. *Psychosomatic Medicine, 47*, 164–173.

Sartory, G., Muller, B., Metsch, J., & Pothmann, R. (1998). A comparison of psychological and pharmacological treatment of pediatric migraine. *Behavioral Research Therapies, 36*, 1155–1170.

Shepherd, P. (1997). *Nutrition: Medicine of the future.* [Online]. Retrieved February 11, 2001, from the World Wide Web: *http://www.trans4mind.unet.com/nutri.htm.*

Smith, C. W. (1991). Exercise: Practical treatment for the patient with depression and chronic fatigue. *Primary Care, 18*, 271–281.

Snider, S. (1991, May). Beware the unknown brew: Herbal teas and toxicity. *FDA Consumer, 25*, 13–33.

Soares, J., Naffah-Mazzacoratti, M. G., Cavalheiro, E. A. (1994). Increased serotonin levels in physically trained men. *Brazilian Journal of Medical and Biological Research, 27*, 1635–1638.

Solecki, R. S. (1975). Shanidar IV: A Neanderthal flower burial of northern Iraq. *Science, 190*, 880.

Sotaniemi, E. A., Haapakoski, E., & Rautio, A. (1995). Ginseng therapy in non-insulin-dependent diabetic patients. *Diabetes Care, 18*, 1373–1375.

Stefanic, M. L., & Wood, P. D. (1994). Physical activity, lipid and lipoprotein metabolism, and lipid transport. In C. Bouchard, R. J. Shaphard, & T. Stephens (Eds.), *Physical activity, fitness, and health: International proceedings and consensus statement* (pp. 417–431). Champaign, IL: Human Kinetics.

Stein, F., Knotts, V. J., Baldwin, L., Jurkowski, J., & Reynolds, P. (1997). *Survey of alternative treatment methods used in occupational therapy.* Unpublished paper. (Available from F. Stein, University of South Dakota, Department of Occupational Therapy, 414 E. Clark St., Vermillion, SD 57069)

Stephens, T., & Craig, C. L. (1990). *The well-being of Canadians: Highlights of the 1988 Campbell's Survey.* Ottawa: Canadian Fitness and Lifestyle Research Institute.

Stephens, T., Jacobs, D. R., & White, C. C. (1985). A descriptive epidemiology of leisure-time physical activity. *Public Health Reports, 100*, 147–158.

Stiller, M. J., Pak, G. H., Shupack, J. L., Thaler, S., Kenny, C., & Jondreau, L. (1992). A portable pulsed electromagnetic field (PEMF) device to enhance healing of recalcitrant venous ulcers: A double-blind placebo-controlled clinical trial. *British Journal of Dermatology, 127*, 147–154.

Sultanoff, B. A., & Zalaquett, C. P. (2000). Relaxation therapies. In D. W. Novey, *Clinician's complete reference to complementary & alternative medicine* (pp. 114–129), St. Louis: Mosby.

Taber's cyclopedic medical dictionary. (1997). Philadelphia: F. A. Davis.

Terman, M., Terman, T. S., & Ross, D. C. (1998). A controlled trial of timed bright light and negative air ionization for treatment of winter depression. *Archives of General Psychiatry, 55*, 875–882.

Towner, E. A., & Blumenthal, J. A. (1993). The efficacy of exercise in the management of hypertension. *Homeostasis, 34*, 338–345.

Tse, S., & Barley, D. M. (1992). Tai chi and postural control in the well elderly. *American Journal of Occupational Therapy, 46*, 295–300.

Turner, J. G., Clark, A. J., Gauthier, D. K., & Williams, M. (1998). The effect of therapeutic touch on pain and anxiety in burn patients. *Journal of Advance Nursing 28*, 10–20.

Tusek, D. L., Church, J. M., Strong, S. A., Grass, J. A., & Fazio, V. W. (1997). Guided imagery: A significant advance in the care of patients undergoing elective colorectal surgery. *Diseases of the Colon Rectum, 40*, 172–178.

U.S. Department of Health and Human Services, Public Health Services. (1988). *The surgeon general's report on nutrition and health.* [Online]. Retrieved February 11, 2001, from the World Wide Web: *http://www.mcspotlight.org/media/reports/surgen_rep.html#1.*

Vallbona, C., Haywood, C. F., & Jurida, G. (1997). Response of pain to static magnetic fields in postpolio patients: A double blind pilot study. *Archives of Physical Medicine Rehabilitation, 78*, 1200–1203.

Van Deusen, J., & Harlowe, D. (1987). The efficacy of the ROM dance program for adults with rheumatoid arthritis. *American Journal of Occupational Therapy, 41*, 90–95.

van Dixhoorn, J. (1998). Cardiorespiratory effects of breathing and relaxation instruction in myocardial infarction patients. *Biological Psychology, 49*, 123–135.

Viola, H., Wasowski, C., Levi de Stein, M., Wolfman, C., Silveira, R., Dajas, F., Medina, J. H., & Paladine, A. C. (1995). Apigenin, a component of Matricaria recutita flowers, is a central benzodiazephine receptor-ligand with anxiolytic effects. *Planta Medica, 61*, 213–216.

Wallace, L. B. (2000). Light therapy. In D. W. Novey, *Clinician's complete reference to complementary & alternative medicine* (pp. 154–163, 701). St. Louis: Mosby.

Weintraub, M. I. (1998). Chronic submaximal magnetic stimulation in peripheral neuropathy: Is there a beneficial therapeutic relationship? *American Journal of Pain Management, 8,* 12–16.

Weyerer, S. (1992). Physical inactivity and depression in the community: Evidence from the Upper Bavarian Field Study. *International Journal of Sports Medicine, 13,* 492–496.

Whitney, E. N., & Cataldo, C. B. (1983). *Understanding normal and clinical nutrition.* St. Paul, MN: West.

Workshop on Alternative Medicine. (1994). *Alternative medicine: Expanding medical horizons.* (NIH Publication No. 94–066). Washington, DC: Government Printing Office.

Zung, W. K. (1965). A self–rating depression scale. *Archives of General Psychiatry, 12,* 63–74.

13

Creative and Expressive Arts and Their Application to Psychosocial Treatment

> *Briefly, these principles hold that arts, crafts, skill, drama, intellectual pursuits in classes and study groups, involvement in a nursery-school or greenhouse program, are productive, creative, recreative activities in their own right, with implications for personal growth and development, in any individual. These activities can be highly "therapeutic" for anyone, since they promote changes in a positive direction, offer a structure for daily life, support competence, and enhance the dignity and identity of the person involved.*
>
> — J. M. Erikson, with D. Loveless & J. Loveless, 1976, *Activity, Recovery, Growth: The Communal Role of Planned Activities*, p. 59.

Operational Learning Objectives

By the end of this chapter, the learner will:

1. Define creativity.

2. Discriminate between teaching expressive arts and using expressive arts in therapy.

3. Understand the dimensions in creative expressive arts, such as art, music, dance, poetry, puppetry.

4. Discuss the dynamics of the creative artists who were mentally ill.

5. Apply art as a creative modality in therapy.

Focusing Questions for the Chapter

▶ What is creativity?

▶ How can creativity be used in treatment?

▶ What are the different creative therapies which can be incorporated?

▶ What is the difference between pure creativity and expressive therapies?

▶ What is the relationship between a creative artist and the symptoms of mental illness?

▶ How can we incorporate art and music therapy into a comprehensive or holistic treatment program?

▶ What is the difference between art or music education and art or music therapy?

One of the major themes of this book is the application of creative problem solving by the occupational therapist in treating individuals with mental illness by empowering them to solve everyday life situations. The occupational therapist working with individuals with mental illness attempts to release the creative and expressive processes of the client so that the individual can develop a sense of self and insight into understanding his or her feelings. This does not mean that the client will become a painter like Picasso or a musician like Beethoven, but rather that he or she can use more effectively the creative potential every human being possesses. There are numerous examples of creative artists such as the painter Van Gogh, the novelist Dostoevski, the dramatist Strindberg, the dancer Nijinsky, and others who suffered the anguish and sufferings of emotional illness, yet in spite of it were able to create masterpieces.

Crutchfield (1961), in discussing the creative process, proposed that it is universally found in every individual, not only the notable. In every individual are all of the relevant cognitive and motivational processes that account for creative behaviors. The premise of this argument is that occupational therapists should attempt to help individuals with mental illness discover and develop their inherent human potential. In this way, the occupational therapist works in concert with the individual with mental illness to discover new insights into the self, experiment with new ways of approaching problems of living and coping with stress, and express feelings to facilitate growth and recovery.

The application of crafts is an important consideration in releasing creative potential within the individual client. Kleinman and Stalcup (1991) reported that "[c]rafts, as one type of purposeful activity, have been a traditional therapeutic modality in occupational therapy (Levine, 1987; Reed, 1986) and are commonplace in child psychiatry programs . . . [however] it may be that the therapeutic efficacy of craft activities has not yet been adequately demonstrated by research" (p. 325).

Drake (1999), in her textbook *Crafts and Rehabilitation*, analyzes major crafts used clinically by therapists. Using such crafts as woodworking, leatherwork, needlework, copper tooling and metal craft, mosaics, ceramics, weaving, latchhook, macramé, and other fiber crafts, she analyzes each according to its application in physical dysfunction, pediatrics, and geriatrics. In her analysis, she states

> Many clients improve, while others deteriorate. A craft that the client may have accomplished or been proficient in at an earlier period may still be simplified.
>
> This is central to occupational therapy—to match or adapt the activity to the client. By approaching each craft with the sure knowledge that it can be made simpler or more complex according to the needs of the clients, the therapist can be confident that a client is allowed to choose a craft that fits his or her self-concept. (p. 33)

Teaching the Arts Versus Creative Expression in Therapy

The goal of traditional art education is to instruct the individual in technical skills so that the student is able to imitate the "Masters" in art movements such as impressionism, expressionistic, abstraction, minimalism, and pop art. "In effect, this aim is to induce him to produce pictorially on a level that may be beyond his comprehension and that has no relationship to his personality" (Schaefer-Simmern, 1948, p. 5).

> Instruction in art—sometimes a part of occupational therapy, sometimes labeled art therapy—began appearing in mental hospitals in the 1940s and 1950s. The early art therapist was often a person with training in art media whose function was to provide rudimentary instruction in techniques to patients. This was to keep the patient soothed by encouraging him to copy landscapes, religious figures and so on; to fill time; or to allow him to express emotions in a presumably nonthreatening way. If the patient did produce something meaningful or personal, it would be sent to his therapist or ward physician, who would probably note it; with rare exceptions, that would be that. (Fagan, J., 1973, p. xii)

John Dewey's influence in art education led to the emphasis on creative expression: "Normally and naturally, artistic activity is the way in which one may 'gain in the strength and stature, the belief in his own powers, and the self-respect, which make artistic activity constructive in the growth of personality'" (Dewey, 1948, p. x). Art therapy is an extension of creative expression, and is used in the treatment process. Initially, art therapy was influenced by psychoanalytic theory.

> Psychoanalytic treatment holds as postulate that in order to leave the past we must relive and resolve it in all its complexity of pain, confusion, hate, and love. The creative task of expressive therapy, as with all therapies, is to help patients separate and leave old conflicts so that their world can be met with fresh eyes and new perceptions. (Robbins, 1980, p. 38)

Assumptions

The assumptions underlying this chapter are:

▶ Spontaneity in the expressive arts is a legitimate adjunct to psychotherapy for individuals with a psychosocial dysfunction.

▶ Artists and individuals with mental illness or psychosocial dysfunction share certain unique experiences such as withdrawal, alienation, extreme anxiety, depression, euphoria, and an active fantasy life.

▶ Artists often respond to these experiences by producing art that reflects these experiences.

▶ Therapists can elicit feeling and meanings from their clients' paintings and drawings, which might reflect their (the clients') inner lives.

THE RELATIONSHIP BETWEEN CREATIVITY AND MENTAL ILLNESS

The act of creation is a humanizing experience that brings to the forefront the greatest gifts of man. Leonardo da Vinci devising methods of flying, Frank Lloyd Wright designing a building for a museum, Jonas Salk discovering a vaccine to protect against polio, and the NASA scientist designing a land rover to explore the surface of Mars are diverse examples of the commonality in art, architecture, scientific medicine, and engineering of man's greatest accomplishments. Creativity in the service of the ego, to paraphrase Ernest Kris (1952), is a guiding force in man. Rollo May (1975) in his work, *The Courage to Create*, stated that modern man living at a time of ambiguity, stress, and lack of direction must discover "new forms, new symbols, new patterns on which a new society can be built" (p. 21).

M. C. Richards (1964), the potter and poet, stated in her work, *Centering*, "The artist and craftsman . . . is continually willing his work. He devotes his life to acts which are a personal commitment to value. He [or she] is, to varying degrees, an example of a practicing initiative. A creative person . . . using his lifetime to find his original face, to awaken his own voice, beyond all learning, habit, thought: to tap life at its source" (p. 43). The act of creation to Richards is a personal expression of one's innermost thoughts and feelings. For the creative artist the commitment to produce something original is an intrinsic motivator. Many times, creative artists have made a commitment to devote their lives to very arduous work.

What is the relationship between creativity and the process of mental illness as it relates to art as a therapeutic media? It is not unusual for many creative artists to have shared some of the same intense or distorted experiences as the client with mental illness. However, it is not assumed that to be a creative artist you must be schizophrenic or mentally ill, nor is the converse true. If we look upon the process of mental illness as one aspect of the range of human potential and as a certain unique experience as Laing (1967) implies, then the creative expression of the individual with mental illness becomes a vehicle to be encouraged. More specifically, the expressive arts can be used as therapeutic media.

In understanding the concept of creativity, we have used the definition by George Domino (1969) who, in a study entitled "Maternal Personality Correlates of Son's Creativity," proposed that

Creativity is a process characterized by:
- Originality, novelty or freshness of approach;
- adaptiveness to reality in that it must solve a problem, achieve a goal, in general be a reality oriented response;
- the original insight or approach must be developed or elaborated. (pp. 180–181)

Three factors should be considered when applying this concept of creativity to the treatment process in occupational therapy: (a) the role of the occupational therapist as a creative treatment agent in facilitating growth and recovery in the client; (b) the exploration of creative activities in expanding the behavior repertoire and life experiences of the client; and (c) the creation of an environment that fosters growth and recovery.

Rationale for the Use of the Expressive Arts in Occupational Therapy

Thompson and Blair (1998), in a thoughtful discussion of the use of creative arts in occupational therapy, provided an eclectic framework for promoting arts and crafts in mental health practice. In order for the expressive arts to be therapeutic, the occupational therapist must be able to discover in the patient or client the most appropriate activity to release the individual's creative forces (Brienes, 1995; Rhyne, 1973). The selection of the activity, whether suggested by the therapist, self-selected by the client, or jointly discovered by the occupational therapist and client should be related to the innate creative potential of the individual. The selection of the activity must meet the psychological needs of the client if it is to have any curative value. The occupational therapist, knowing the client's personal history and working in alliance with the client, utilizes the creative process in stimulating within the client growth experiences that enable the client to recover.

Another way to analyze the occupational therapists' goals with individuals with mental illness is to identify the potential inherent qualities of activities to change an individual's behavior. Spontaneous art is an example of a therapeutic modality that can be used creatively with clients with psychosocial disorders (Blair, 1990). It is an example of how creativity can be used as a positive force in helping the individual to express powerful feelings through an activity. The relationships among creativity, mental illness, and spontaneous art are explored in the following sections.

> This suggests that occupational therapists need to make an effort to present material in a way that is as attractive and as stimulating as possible. As a result, their clients will hopefully engage with it and maximize their opportunities for achieving optimal experiences through it. Carefully thought out and presented creative art activities could therefore be an important addition to groups that aim to teach clients more adaptive interpersonal skills, though purely verbal interaction. It is hoped that, with a more eclectic framework to support the use of creative activities, occupational therapists will feel that creative arts are a useful medium, even where therapy has clear cognitive-behavioural, human-occupational or other underlying paradigms, other than a psychodynamic one. (Thompson & Blair, 1998, p. 60).

The Creative Artist

The life of a creative artist can be very introspective and lonely. It is also, by its very nature, divergent and nonconforming. The creative artist may, for example, consciously decide to forego a conventional life and live a precarious, insecure existence such as a bohemian. The story of Paul Gauguin, the French Impressionist painter who rejected a middle-class life of a banker to become an artist is a symbolic, recurrent theme in lives of many artists. Success during the lifetime of a creative artist is rare. For every Picasso there are thousands of creative

artists who are not recognized during their lifetime. This is understandable because the creative artist is in the forefront of expressing new concepts. For example, abstract art was initially rejected by art critics and the public at large. Generally, new ideas in architecture, music, dance, and poetry take a generation before being universally accepted.

There are similarities between the introspective, lonely, nonconforming life of the creative artist and the withdrawn, inner existence of the individual with mental illness. There are also similarities in the everyday struggles that exist in both lives. However, there are vast differences in directions and life goals between the creative artist and the individual with schizophrenia. The creative artist struggles to express his or her ideals and talents in a poem, painting, piece of music, sculpture, dance, or invention. On the other hand, the individual with mental illness often is blocked in expression, unable to communicate, and imprisoned in his or her own psychological world. Perhaps one factor in the effective treatment of these individuals is to encourage spontaneous expressions and develop individual talents that can release creative energy. As occupational therapists we need to examine the creative world of our clients. In doing so we expand our understanding of their problems and enhance our ability to help them.

Similarly, the creative artist shows characteristics that parallel those of the withdrawn, alienated, fantasy-ridden individual who has fled from the existence of life in the presence of extreme anxiety. If we examine the lifestyles of the creative artist and the individual with chronic mental illness, we often find a commonality that sometimes results in the creative artist becoming mentally ill or the individual with mental illness producing artistic creations. Examples of artists who have produced creative masterpieces during extreme periods of depression, isolation, euphoria, and states of mysticism are numerous in the literature (Lange-Eichbaum, 1932). For example, Goya painted vivid frescoes of scenes depicting his inner conflicts while actively hallucinating (Guidol, 1966). Van Gogh, during periods of severe depression, was able to paint expressive landscapes of the land he loved (Meier-Graete, 1933). Coleridge wrote *Kubla Khan* while in a fantasy-like state produced by opium (Hyslop, 1925). Kafka during deep depressions was able to write stories revealing feelings of paranoid oppression (Brod, 1960). The artist is thus able to create while in periods of emotional turbulence or to utilize childlike feelings in expression such as those by Paul Klee identified by Ernest Kris (1952) as using regression in the service of the ego. In other words, the creative artist is able to utilize aspects of his life experiences that for the individual with mental illness may be immobilizing or disabling in daily tasks.

Lawrence Kubie (1961) in his book, *Neurotic Distortion of the Creative Process*, pointed out that many psychologically ailing artists, writers, musicians, and scientists refuse therapy out of a fear that in losing their illness they will lose not only their much prized "individuality" but also their creative zeal and spark. However, as a psychoanalyst, Kubie felt that the creative artist would become more productive if he lost his illness. This point is controversial. Freud (1948), on the other hand, felt that creativity may serve as a vehicle for solving personal conflicts experienced by the individual artist. Perhaps without a feeling of dissonance or disturbance the individual lacks the motivation to create. Wordsworth (Ghiselin, 1952) in defining what a poet is in a preface to the second edition of his lyrical ballads, stated:

> To these qualities he had added a disposition to be affected more than other men by absent things as if they were present, an ability of conjuring up himself passions, which are indeed

far from being the same as those produced by real events. (p. 83)

Wordsworth's feelings seem very similar to the description of hallucinations in clients with schizophrenia who generate visual and auditory experiences based on intrapsychic conflicts. Erik Erikson (1950) described the schizophrenic process in a young girl, Jean, who retreated into a centrifugal world where she was the center of her own reality. Jean developed bizarre behavior patterns during her childhood and adolescence. These included being terrified by a large, soft ball or a paper crackling. She was unable to communicate verbally to another person. She remained in essence a separate entity closed off from the world. However, Jean had musical ability. Quoting Erikson (1950):

> At my next visit, I heard someone practicing some phrases of Beethoven's first sonata, and innocently remarked on the strong and sensitive touch. I thought a gifted adult was playing. To find Jean at the piano was one of the surprises which are so gripping in working with these cases. (p. 180)

This example serves to reinforce the thesis that individuals with schizophrenia are able to create in spite of their illness if they are provided an environment that encourages expression.

The Goertzels (1962) in their study, *Cradles of Eminence*, found that many of the giants of literature, art, music, science, and invention came from broken homes marked by family upheaval and discontinuity. The unhappiness created by the disharmony from the environment is not unlike the family disturbances of those with mental illness. However, in response to these problems the creative artist mobilizes his or her energies in activities that release these feelings, for example, Eugene O'Neil's creation of the harsh reality of the play "Long Day's Journey into Night," Thomas Wolfe's recreating insecure fantasies in "You Can't go Home Again," Schuman composing a symphonic masterpiece in a period of bereavement, or Van Gogh, who in spite of an emotional breakdown completing 150 paintings during a year he spent in a mental hospital (Elgar, 1958). Kris (1952) in his book, *Psychoanalytic Explorations in Art*, suggests that the creative individual is distinguished from the individual with psychosis in whom flexibility of regression is also found by his (the person with psychosis) inability to channel the expression. These examples strongly support the thesis that the creative artist is able to produce significant works of art in spite of periods of emotional illness.

ART THERAPY

Art of Individuals with Schizophrenia

"A Survey of the Literature on Artistic Behavior in the Abnormal" by Anastasi and Foley (1940) reveals that the spontaneous productions of clients in mental hospitals during the 1800s were first put on public display as a sort of curiosity. Dr. Cesare Lombroso, an Italian psychiatrist, and Dr. Hans Prinzhorn, a German psychiatrist, were foremost in presenting collections of "psychotic art" gathered from insane asylums throughout Europe. Their purpose was to show the similarity between the art forms created by individuals with psychosis, children's art, and the artistic productions of primitive natives. Dr. Prinzhorn presented this "esthetic" approach to "psychotic art" and he interpreted the client's art productions in view of universal "creative forms." However, the interest in the sheer aestheticism of "psychotic art" has little significance today.

According to Anastasi and Foley (1940), the most important work done in the field before 1900 was by Dr. Max Simon, a French psychiatrist, who noted that some clients paint imagined agonies, misfortunes, and persecutions. With the advent of Freud and psychoanalysis, "psychotic art" began to be interpreted as a very significant expression of inner motives and conflicts in the client. Freud's theory of determinism, stated, in substance, that certain acts of man, be it a slip of the tongue, the forgetting of a name, or even the painting of an incoherent scene, may at first appear to be meaningless. However, when subjected to psychoanalytic investigation, these productions represent levels of unconscious feelings and ideations. "Psychotic art," as an accessory to Freudian analysis, had a new dimension with the interpretation of symbols in the art productions by individuals. The interpretations of "psychotic art" through psychoanalysis opened the way for clinical representations of its use (Gianascol, 1954).

Art has long been used with individuals with schizophrenia as an adjunct to psychotherapy (Naumburg, 1950). Art has served as a communication link between the client and therapist. Generally, we find in schizophrenia that the individual has difficulty maintaining interpersonal relationships. However, the individual with schizophrenia "telegraphs" his inner conflict through bizarre speech, inappropriate action, and withdrawal. Psychoanalysts have pointed out that the speech of individuals with schizophrenia has a definite meaning and content even though it may be quite distorted and incomprehensible to the observer. Art can be utilized to record the individual's desire to communicate and to reflect his or her inner world. Harry Stack Sullivan (Kasanin, 1954) noted that individuals with schizophrenia use personal symbols in their language to maintain their feelings of self-security. The personal symbols of individuals with schizophrenia can be seen in their art productions where hallucinations or delusions are represented.

Contrary to the common belief that individuals with schizophrenia live in a continual state of fantasy, Goldstein and Scherrer (1941) presented evidence that there is a similarity between the concrete reality thought processes in the individual with organic brain damage and in the individual with schizophrenia. Thinking is reduced to primitive, elemental, "concrete" performance that corresponds to the simplicity and superficiality of their behavior. The implication of Goldstein's work is that the individual with schizophrenia communicates in his or her personal language, which represents "concrete" reality on his or her own terms. In other words, the individual with schizophrenia desires to communicate on a simple level but has difficulty communicating his or her inner world to the "other" person. The individual with schizophrenia uses personal symbols and refuses to understand symbols outside of himself. He or she tends to be literal in his or her thinking without the use of abstracts and generalizations. In "schizophrenic art" we can see the personal symbols that reflect concrete problems to the client. Some artists portray dreams and uninhibited thought in the manner of "schizophrenic patients." The artist usually presents recognizable objects in a disassociated manner through a process of unrepressed creative activity. The result of this process is a highly personalized painting that has symbolic meaning to the artist. In the same way as the surrealist artist, the individual with schizophrenia should be able to express his inner life without repression (Matthews, 1965). The relation between the artist and the individual with schizophrenia is described by Robbins (1994):

> The world of Picasso's Guernica is upon you as you encounter the reality of schizophrenia. Ravaged and pained forms, distorted phantoms and ghosts, confusion and panic float in and obscure your vision. The art therapist's very being is rocked as the power of unconscious symbols of the patient's faraway past are reactivated. The gloom and ache of lost battles and the piercing deadness of something empty and gone become present. Schizophrenia takes on many shapes and forms. However, all schizophrenics have in common a sense of defeat and retreat from external reality. For some, this loss virtually began at birth so that not even a glimmer of a self to be rediscovered or reborn is provided. There are chronic and acute patients, non-differentiated patients, as well as more encapsulated patients with crystallized versions of pain and terror; their diagnoses read catatonic, paranoid, and hebephrenic. Each patient hopefully has a distillation of a self to be rediscovered, an ego to be regenerated, and a reality that needs reintroduction. The self within awaits contact. Perhaps art may be a way to find courage and hope by putting the various pieces of a fragmented self into a new whole. (p. 108)

Spontaneous art can be an excellent mode of expression for the individual with schizophrenia (Wilson, 1987). "Many art therapists could produce examples in which a schizophrenic child or adult has regained the capacity to symbolize and increase his sense of reality through the regular production of artwork" (Wilson, 1987, p. 50).

Art as a Creative Modality for the Occupational Therapist

The use of art as a therapeutic technique is most effective in a clinical setting where the client can participate in an art group. The paintings can be either discussed in the group as a group therapy session directed by a therapist or the artwork can be analyzed as an adjunct to individual therapy (Wadeson, 1980). Usually , the client with schizophrenia preserves his artistic style rigidly so that the group will not influence his productions. The client can be acclimated to the group situation by establishing rapport. The therapist can guide the individual to his own style of painting in a permissive atmosphere. After the individual becomes comfortable in the group, every effort of the therapist is directed toward encouraging the individual to paint spontaneously.

The interpretation of the client's art production is in relation to the individual factors in his or her life. The characteristics of the productions that are most valuable are the graphic evidence of the individual's intrapsychic world and communication messages (Heine & Steiner, 1986; Pickford, 1967). The art production is interpreted in view of the manifest content (what is actually painted) and the latent content (personal symbolization). The derivative meaning is based on the dynamics of the latent content. Interpreting the client's art productions is done in conjunction with overall treatment. In treatment facilities where individual therapy is not practiced, the patient's productions can be discussed in a group under the therapist's direction. In the group setting, the patient's personal problems and conflicts can be worked out by an externalization of subjective thoughts and emotion.

A study of psychiatric art (Anastasi & Foley, 1940) found that the subject matters most frequently painted by patients with schizophrenia were the following:

► representation of delusional ideas

► reproduction of hallucinations and illusions

► predominance of religious themes

► allegories

► supernatural and fabulous creations

► ambitious projects—maps, plans

► portrayal of gory, gruesome objects, as well as scenes of ruin and catastrophe

► sexual themes

This list shows precisely how art can reflect the problems of the individual.

Art can also be used to document the client's progress or mood states (Heine & Steiner, 1986). At first, for example, the client's work may reflect extreme incoherence or peculiarity; later it may show signs of his or her interests and a new awareness of reality. Repressed desires and fears can be represented in the artwork in the form of personal symbols. Interpretation of spontaneous art productions usually comprises four areas: (a) the client's technique, (b) the client's use of the media, (c) color symbolism, and (d) the form and organization of the subject matter depicted.

The client's techniques can reveal many aspects of his or her personality. For instance, the very precise and mechanical artist who is interested in detail and clarity usually presents an obsessive, compulsive personality. The client who works very slowly and is consequently unproductive can reflect depression. The indecisive client who must work first on scrap paper before using canvas can represent an insecure person, one who has feelings of inadequacy. A guarded thinking individual with paranoia will be secretive about his or her work and fearful of the therapist's interpretation. Some clients will work rapidly and in an agitated manner, revealing unresolved tensions. The prolific client, who produces art on a large scale, may be working out delusions of grandeur. Sometimes the art productions are destroyed, thereby informing the therapist that the client feels worthless and self-destructive. The rigid, negativistic client may refuse to discuss the paintings or drawings.

Art Interpretation (Psychodynamic Approach)

Observing the client's use of the media will allow the therapist to gain insight about a client's problems. When only part of the media is used, the client may perceive the environment as hostile. Large forms on the paper or canvas may express expansiveness and grandiosity. Hostility and aggression toward the environment may show themselves in heavy thick lines that almost tear through the media. On the other hand, light thin strokes may represent a fear of the environment.

The client's use of color may provide additional insight. Color often is used to reflect emotional tone. For example, red may denote strong passion while the use of blacks and browns may show depression. Purple is sometimes used by individuals with paranoia to represent delusions of grandeur. Blue may tell of a desire to control the environment. The use of yellow alone can denote hostility. Orange is significant as being a "warm" color. Green can mean feelings of well-being and security.

Individuals with schizophrenia typically use color without integrating it with form, disassociating between their feelings and ideas. Their art productions may seem bizarre when they attempt to juxtapose color and tone. A client can attempt to control impulsive color combinations and by doing so indicate the desire to restrain emotionality. Drawings of people can reveal perception of body image. Is the painting an integrated whole or is it a disorganized mass? Are colors in harmony with each other? Is the painting a representation of a scene from the past? The answers to these questions can provide a guide to the extent of the individual's inner conflicts.

It should be possible for a therapist to allow the individual with mental illness to use art to nonverbally communicate his or her inner feelings. The methods used in art therapy should allow a client an opportunity to express creativity and simultaneously enhance therapy. Spontaneous art therapy is a creative medium that can provide the individual with schizophrenia a nonverbal channel of communication.

In a current application of the psychodynamic approach to art therapy, Benetton (1995), an occupational therapist, described a case study treating a patient with psychosis where the therapist used art interpretation in helping the client work out his conflicts. In this approach, the therapist combined transference (a psychoanalytic technique) with traditional art therapy.

Frye (1990) has applied the use of art as an expressive framework to clients with multiple personalities. Her rationalization of the use of art is noted in the following statement:

> Because of its holistic and activity-oriented approach, occupational therapy has much to offer in the treatment of patients with multiple personality disorder. Purposeful activity has been examined under many frames of reference for both its intrinsic and therapeutic value. This paper draws support for the use of expressive modalities with patients with multiple personality disorder largely from the object-relations framework, which grew from early psychoanalytic approaches in occupational therapy developed by Azima in 1959, Fidler and Fidler in 1963, and later expanded by Mosey in 1970. (p. 1015)

Her perspective in the use of the expressive arts can be expanded to clients with various psychosocial disorders:

> Expressive art is used in a variety of settings by many therapies, most frequently by art therapy, as a highly specialized psychoanalytic vehicle of self-discovery. Occupational therapy uses art to promote mastery over those life experiences that prevent independence. . . . Occupational therapists can use art activity as an expressive framework for creating a therapeutic alliance with the patient. (p. 1013)

Art Therapy and Behavioral Therapy

Art therapy can also be approached from a behavioral model (DeFrancisco, 1983; Roth, 1987; van Sickle & Acker, 1975). In this approach, operant conditioning, modeling, and reinforcement are used to help the client participate in self-expression through art. Marks and Gelder (1966, as cited in Roth, 1987) suggested that there are similarities between the psychodynamic and behavioral approaches when used in art therapy:

> They include (1) giving of advice and encouragement by the therapist; (2) conveying to the patient an expectation of improvement; (3) encouraging the patient to recognize current sources of stress and repetitive patterns of behavior; (4) manipulating the environment; (5) decreasing anxiety gradually: Psychotherapists emphasize correct timing of graduated interpretations to prevent patients experiencing excessive anxiety; this is very similar to behavior therapists gradually presenting anxiety-laden stimuli during desensitization (Roth, 1987, p. 217)

DANCE THERAPY

Dance therapy is the use of dance "as a carefully guided tool to produce desirable physiological, emotional, and/or behavioral changes in emotionally or physically handicapped persons" (Hood, 1959, p. 18). As with art therapy, dance therapy can provide the occupational therapist a media for empowering clients to overcome the debilitating experiences of mental illness.

The assumptions underlying dance therapy as expressed by Levy (1988) include:

► "Dance therapy is a form of psychotherapy differentiated from traditional psychotherapy in that it utilizes psychomotor expression as its major mode of intervention" (p. xi).

► The body and mind are inseparable; dance is an activity that unifies body, mind, and spirit.

► Movement therapy can promote health and growth in the individual.

► A dance can be used as a cathartic experience in an individual.

► Dance therapy traces its earliest experience to modern dance.

► Dance therapy originated from the work of Freud in psychoanalysis.

► The history of dance therapy began in the 1940s where most dance therapists worked with clients with psychiatric disorders in state mental hospitals.

► The theories of the neo-psychologists Reich, Adler, Sullivan, Jung, and Schilder were used by dance therapists in explaining the relationship between nonverbal communication and psychotherapy.

► The work of Rogers and Maslow introduced to dance therapy the humanistic theory, which proposes the uniqueness of individuals and the release of creative and expressive potential.

► Dance therapy, like music therapy, art therapy, and psychodrama, uses nonverbal expression for communicating feelings and unconscious thoughts.

► Dance can be used to express symbolism using imagery, fantasy, recollections, and enactment.

Marion Chase Technique

One technique developed by Marion Chase (Chaiklin, 1975) involved warm-up, theme development, and closure. In warm-up, individuals do exercises such as mirroring movements, forming a circle of dancers, and physical stretching. In theme development, the dance therapist uses verbal interpretation of the individual's movements to clarify for the individual what is being expressed nonverbally. The dance therapist also observes tension and rigidity in the muscles of the dancer. A group process is used to discuss individual's movements and posture. In closure, the individuals have an opportunity to express their feelings toward the experience (Chaiklin, 1975).

Range of Motion (ROM) Dance

Occupational therapists have incorporated the principles of Tai Ch'i relaxation, biofeedback, and occupational therapy theories in treating clients in a holistic approach to maintaining physical function (Van Deusen & Harlowe, 1987). The ROM dance has been shown to be effective in increasing range of motion in clients diagnosed with arthritis. According to Van Deusen and Harlowe, developers of this program, the goals and values in this technique are as follows:

- To assist participants in following any medical recommendations provided by their personal physicians and therapists for involvement in daily exercise and rest routines
- To increase the frequency, enjoyment, and perceived benefit of involvement in daily exercise and rest
- To enhance the ability to cope with stress and pain through the use of relaxation techniques
- To provide a forum for group interaction concerning personal health care management
- To provide selected health education experiences
- To improve body awareness
- To promote an experience of well-being

The program's use of an expressive dance form for maintaining range of motion reflects occupational therapy principles more fully than does routine exercise. It emphasizes the creative use of relaxation and pain management techniques during prescribed rest periods to increase the benefits and perceived value of rest as a daily activity. (p. 91)

The use of ROM Dance therapy may be efficacious for clients with psychosocial dysfunction, as the aims and purpose are holistic in nature and conducive to relieving stress.

MUSIC THERAPY

Music therapy is the skillful use of music and musical elements by an accredited music therapist to promote, maintain, and restore mental, physical, emotional, and spiritual health. Music has nonverbal, creative, structural, and emotional qualities. These are used in the therapeutic relationship to facilitate contact, interaction, self-awareness, learning, self-expression, communication, and personal development. (Canadian Association for Music Therapy, 1994, p. 3)

The use of music therapy assumes that:

► Music can be used to change emotions.

► Music can be used to stimulate emotions and arouse physiological systems.

► Music can be used for relaxation purposes.

► Music can be used as a purposeful activity in occupational therapy in helping an individual to perform. "Considering the holistic philosophy of occupational therapy, its broad client base, and its traditional use of creative and purposeful activity, music would seem to be an ideal modality" (MacRae, 1992, p. 275).

► Music can facilitate mood changes, alter states of awareness, modify one's consciousness, and increase affective response (MacRae, 1992, p. 275).

► Music is nonverbal and may be perceived as nonthreatening (Friedman, 1960).

► "Physicians whose sole task is caring for the mentally ill have long realized that music is one of the best medicines for the mind" (Podolsky, 1954, p. 11).

In his book, *Music Therapy*, Podolsky describes a number of case studies in which music has been used successfully with clients with mental illness who were hospitalized. He reports on the use of the "iso" principle, developed by Dr. Altshuler. This principle is based on the use of music that is identical to the mood of the client by matching mood to a musical selection. For example, clients who were depressed were aroused using a music selection with andante tempo, reflecting slow, steady music, while individuals with mania were relaxed with allegro music, a tempo that is very fast and lively. Clinicians have reported that listening to selected pieces of music has been effective in reducing anxiety and moderating anger (Girard, 1954a, 1954b), reducing depression and fatigue (Herman, 1954a, 1954b), reducing hostility (Hilliard, 1954), working out grief (Brown, 1954), and reducing hypertension (Sugarman, 1954).

A number of studies have shown the efficacy of using music to treat individuals with physical and psychosocial illness. Casby and Holm (1994), occupational therapists, examined the effect of classical music on reducing the repetitive and disruptive vocalization of three individuals with Alzheimer's disease who were residents of a long-term care facility. Using a single-subject research design, they found that use of relaxing classical music and favorite music significantly decreased the number of vocalizations in two of the three subjects. Marley (1984) examined the use of music with hospitalized infants and toddlers (ages 5 weeks to 36 months) who demonstrated stress behaviors, such as frequent crying, throwing of objects, body tension, lethargy, and lack of vocalization. Use of relaxation, didactic games, movement, and songs seemed to be effective in reducing these behaviors. In a review of the literature on the use of music with children with autism,

Nelson, Anderson, and Gonzales (1984) found music to be an effective therapeutic media. Staum and Flowers (1984) used music training with a child with autism as a reinforcement when teaching ADL skills. The therapist capitalized on the child's enjoyment and response to music.

MacRae (1992) has argued eloquently for the use of music in occupational therapy:

> I believe that music is not only a legitimate healing tool, but also an appropriate expression of the philosophy of occupational therapy. Music is a vocational activity for some and an active or passive leisure pursuit for others. It is a pleasurable, intrinsically motivating activity that can be easily graded and used to promote overall health through relaxation and movement. Music is both versatile and powerful in that it has the potential to involve all of the components of occupational performance—motor, sensory, cognitive, social, and emotional. In this paper, I describe the healing effects of music and discuss its present and potential uses in occupational therapy. (p. 275)

In support of her argument, MacRae cited several studies (Farber, 1982; Miller, 1979; Silberzahn, 1988). Music (a) increases reality orientation to persons, places, and things (Miller, 1979); (b) is useful with comatose clients for auditory input (Farber, 1982); and (c) appears to be related to learning and memory (Silberzahn, 1988).

Music has been used with a psychodynamic approach, using psychoanalytic theory (Pavlicevic, 1997). "Within a psychoanalytic framework, it offers a structure to demonstrate the use of energy with its harmony and disharmony as well as counterpoint, to describe the temporal nature of our most primitive experience" (Shields & Robbins, 1980, p. 256).

In an extensive review of the literature, Maranto (1993) concluded that

> Music is a method of treatment that humankind has relied on for many centuries.

Although music is a complex stimulus, and responses to music are equally complex, research has supported its effectiveness as a treatment modality with many clinical problems. Because music is a personal and unique experience to each individual, research methodology has yet to reveal an operational paradigm for its many applications. In spite of this, clinical uses of music are fairly widespread and successful. Recent research, particularly that concerning the immune system's responsiveness to music and the entrainment possibilities of music, will certainly open many new frontiers to music therapy practitioners. Among the reasons for the existence of music in virtually every culture, its ability to elicit and maintain human health and well-being stands out. (pp. 432–433)

OTHER CREATIVE ARTS THERAPIES

The creative arts therapies include art therapy, dance/movement therapy, drama therapy, music therapy, psychodrama, and poetry therapy. These therapies use arts modalities and creative processes during intentional interventions in therapeutic, rehabilitative, community, or educational settings to foster health, communication, and expression; promote the integration of physical, emotional, cognitive, and social functioning; enhance self-awareness; and facilitate change. (National Coalition of Arts Therapies Association, n.d., p. 1)

The National Coalition of Arts Therapist Associations (NCATA) was established in 1979 to promote the use of creative or expressive arts as therapeutic modalities. Besides the use of art, music, and dance therapy as therapeutic media for individuals with mental illness, play therapy (Axline, 1947), bibliotherapy (McFarland, 1952), psychodrama (Moreno, 1947), puppetry (Phillips, 1996), and poetry (Leedy, 1960) have also been used by occupational therapists. Each of these therapeutic modalities is useful in help-

ing the client deal with his or her unconscious feelings or anxieties in a symbolic manner.

Play Therapy

Play therapy is used with children as a means of enabling them to express their feelings (e.g., fears, anger, disappointments) within the context of a safe environment (Jeffrey, 1990). (See Chapter 4 under occupational behavior frame of reference for a discussion of the use of play in development.) In the occupational therapy setting, play has many purposes.

> It is used to establish a therapeutic relationship with a child by providing a neutral shared experience. The inanimate play object provides a link between therapist and child without, at this stage, feelings being revealed. The play assists the assessment processes, that is, diagnostic, behavioral, developmental and continuous assessment. The child through different play activities, can regress and use play symbolically to release tension and aggression. His unconscious and conscious needs and conflicts can be enacted with the play materials, as well as expressing fears, fantasies, etc. By interpreting all these activities the therapist helps the child to gain insight and he can alter his attitudes, improve his way to relating to adults and peers, and practice these new skills in the social setting of play-group therapy. The child develops new skills, and uses his creativity, which can sublimate basic needs in a socially acceptable way and he receives praise and recognition so that his confidence and self-image are improved. (Jeffrey, 1990, pp. 248–249)

Psychodrama and Other Creative Therapies

Psychodrama (Moreno, 1947), sometimes called sociodrama, explores individual psychodynamics through dramatic methods by enacting or reenacting situations that are of emotional significance to the client. It was developed by Jacob Moreno, a psychiatrist, who used psychoanalytical concepts such as projection, introjection, identification, and role reversal. There are five variables within psychodrama:

▶ *Stage*, which is the living space or simulated environment

▶ *Protagonist*, who portrays the client's involvement in his or her own life by free and spontaneous acting

▶ *Director*, who is the therapist and controls the psychodrama by selecting the protagonist situation, the auxiliary egos, and asking the audience for their feedback. The director maintains the flow of the psychodrama by eliciting responses from the protagonist, providing reality therapy through consensual validation, and restraining negative acting out on the part of the protagonists or the auxiliary egos

▶ *Auxiliary egos*, who are the significant individuals in the protagonist's life, such as a parent, siblings, friends, and spouse and who are actors within the psychodrama. The auxiliary egos are sometimes portrayed as an extension of the client's alter egos

▶ *Audience*, who are other clients in the psychodrama group whose role is to be supportive to the protagonist and to help the protagonist resolve some of the interpersonal or emotional issues with the help of the therapist. The members of the audience may also identify with the protagonist and gain insight into their own interpersonal relationship and issues

Psychodrama and related techniques have been used by occupational therapists since the 1930s (Beagan, 1990; Guile, 1983; Nobel, 1933; Phillips, 1996; Ruscombe-King, 1983; Schuman, Marcus, & Nesse, 1973).

▶ *Puppetry*, a related drama, is used frequently with children to explore feelings and to enact conflictual situations. The child speaks through the puppet, thus making it a less fearful or threatening situation.

▶ *Bibliotherapy* is a therapeutic technique in which the therapist recommends books to the client based on content and specific relevance. This technique uses books to help people solve problems by enabling them to identify with characters who have overcome severe hardship or mental illness. When used in group therapy, bibliotherapy provides a method for structuring interactions between the therapist and clients based on mutual sharing of literature (Pardeck & Pardeck, 1989; Riordan & Wilson, 1989). Bibliotherapy has been used by occupational therapists since the 1940s (Hart, 1943; McFarland, 1952; Schneck, 1944).

▶ Another form of bibliotherapy is *poetry therapy*. "Poetry Therapy is a specific and powerful form of bibliotherapy, unique in its use of metaphor, imagery, rhythm, and other poetic devices" (National Association of Poetry Therapy [NAPT], n.d., p. 1). Poetry therapy employs poetry and other forms of literature to promote one's understanding of the self and the individual in society, to accept or change one's feelings and behavior, and to heighten both mental and social wellness (National Association of Poetry Therapy). As with other therapies, poetry therapy has been used by occupational therapists (Walsh, 1988).

SUMMARY

In summary, creative and expressive arts have been an integral part in the history of occupational therapy. Occupational therapists have explored the use of various creative media in treating individuals with mental illness. Psychodynamic, cognitive-behavioral, and human occupation frames of references have been used in guiding practice and interpreting the creative product, whether it is a painting, poem, interpretative dance, musical piece, or dramatization. The potential for using the creative arts in therapy is still evolving.

REFERENCES

Anastasi, A., & Foley, J. P. (1940). A survey of the literature on artistic behavior in the abnormal. *Psychological Monographs, 52*(6), 1–71.

Axline, V. M. (1947). *Play therapy.* New York: Ballantine.

Beagan, D. (1990). Spontaneity and creativity in the NHS: Starting a new group. T*he British Journal of Occupational Therapy, 48,* 370–374.

Benetton, M. J. (1995). A case study applying a psychodynamic approach to occupational therapy. *Occupational Therapy International, 2,* 220–228.

Blair, S. C. (1990). Occupational therapy and group psychotherapy. In J. Creek (Ed.), *Occupational therapy and mental health principles, skills and practice* (pp. 193–210). Edinburgh: Churchill Livingstone.

Brienes, E. (1995). *From clay to computers.* Philadelphia: F.A. Davis.

Brod, M. (1960). *Franz Kafka: A biography.* New York: Schocken.

Brown, L. W. (1954). Music therapy for acute grief. In E. Podolsky (Ed.), *Music therapy* (pp. 130–135). New York: Philosophical Library.

Canadian Association for Music Therapy. (1994). *What music therapy is.* Canadian Association for Music Therapy/ Association de Musicothérapie du Canada Annual General Meeting, Vancouver, British Columbia, May 6, 1994. Retrieved February 14, 2001, from the World Wide Web: *http://www.musictherapy.ca/*

Casby, A., & Holm, M. (1994). The effect of music on repetitive disruptive vocalizations of persons with dementia. *American Journal of Occupational Therapy, 48,* 883–889.

Chaiklin, S. (1975). Dance therapy. In S. Arieti (Ed.), *American handbook of psychiatry.* New York: Basic Books.

Crutchfield, R. (1961). *The creative process.* In Proceedings of the conference on "The Creative Person" (pp. VI-1–VI-16). Berkeley: University of California, Institute of Personality Assessment and Research and Liberal Arts Department.

DeFrancisco, J. (1983). Implosive art therapy: A learning-theory-based, psychodynamic approach. In L. Gantt & S. Whitman (Eds.), *The fine art of therapy* (pp. 74–79). Alexandria, VA: American Art Therapy Association.

Dewey, J. (1948). Foreword. In H. Schaefer-Simmern, *The unfolding of artistic activity: Its basis, processes, and implications* (pp. ix–x). Berkeley: University of California.

Domino, G. (1969). Maternal personality correlates of sons' creativity. *Journal of Consulting and Clinical Psychology, 33*(2), 180–183.

Drake, M. (1999). *Crafts in therapy and rehabilitation* (2nd ed.). Thorofare, NJ: SLACK.

Elgar, F. (1958). *Van Gogh: A study of his life and work.* New York: Frederick A. Praeger.

Erikson, E. (1950). *Childhood and society.* New York: W. W. Norton.

Erikson, J. M. (1976). *Activity, recovery, growth: The communal role of planned activities.* New York: W. W. Norton.

Fagan, J. (1973). Foreword. In J. Rhyne, *The gestalt art experience* (pp. xi–xiii). Monterey, CA: Brooks/Cole.

Farber, S. D. (1982). *Neurorehabilitation: A multisensory approach.* Philadelphia: W. B. Saunders.

Freud, S. (1948). *Leonardo da Vinci.* (A. A. Brill, Trans.). London: Routledge and Kegan Paul.

Friedman, S. M. (1960). One aspect of the structure of music. *Journal of the American Psychoanalytic Association, 8,* 427–449.

Frye, B. (1990). Art and multiple personality disorder: An expressive framework for occupational therapy. *American Journal of Occupational Therapy, 44,* 1013–1022.

Ghiselin, B. (1952). *The creative process: A symposium.* New York: New American Library.

Gianascol, A. J. (1954). Psychiatric potentialities of art. *Journal of Nervous and Mental Disease, 120,* 238–244.

Girard, J. (1954a). Moderating anger with music. In E. Podolsky (Ed.), *Music therapy* (pp. 107–111). New York: Philosophical Library.

Girard, J. (1954b). Music therapy in the anxiety states. In E. Podolsky (Ed.), *Music therapy* (pp. 101–106). New York: Philosophical Library.

Goertzel, V., & Goertzel, M. G. (1962). *Cradles of eminence.* Boston: Little, Brown.

Goldstein, K., & Scherrer, M. (1941). Abstract and concrete behavior: An experimental study. *Psychological Monographs, 53*(2), 1–151.

Guidol, J. (1966). *Francisco DeGoya Y. Lucientes.* New York: Harry N. Abrams.

Guile, L. A. (1983). Psychodrama—As part of an integrated therapeutic programme. *The Australian Occupational Therapy Journal, 30,* 65–69.

Hart, R. E. (1943). Paving the road to health with books. *Occupational Therapy and Rehabilitation, 22,* 228–233.

Heine, D., & Steiner, M. (1986). Standardized paintings as a proposed adjunct instrument for longitudinal monitoring of mood states: A preliminary note. *Occupational Therapy in Mental Health, 6*(3), 31–37.

Herman, E. P. (1954a). Music therapy in depression. In E. Podolsky (Ed.), *Music therapy* (pp. 112–115). New York: Philosophical Library.

Herman, E. P. (1954b). Relaxing music for emotional fatigue. In E. Podolsky (Ed.), *Music therapy* (pp. 116–120). New York: Philosophical Library.

Hilliard, B. (1954). Music therapy for emotional disturbances. In E. Podolsky (Ed.), *Music therapy* (pp. 121–129). New York: Philosophical Library.

Hood, C. (1959, February). The challenge of dance therapy. *Journal of Health–Physical Education–Recreation, 30,* 17–18.

Hyslop, T. B. (1925). *The great abnormals.* London: Phillip Alan.

Jeffrey, L. I. H. (1990). Play therapy. In J. Creek (Ed.), *Occupational therapy and mental health: Principles, skills and practice.* Edinburgh: Churchill Livingstone.

Kasanin, J. S. (1954). *Language and thought in schizophrenia.* Los Angeles: University of California.

Kleinman, B. I., & Stalcup, A. (1991). The effect of graded craft activities on visuomotor integration in an inpatient child psychiatry population. *American Journal of Occupational Therapy 45,* 324–330.

Kris, E. (1952). *Psychoanalytic exploration in art.* New York: International Universities Press.

Kubie, L. S. (1961). *Neurotic distortions of the creative process.* New York: The Noonday Press.

Laing, R. D. (1967). *The politics of experience.* New York: Ballantine.

Lange-Eichbaum, W. (1932). *The problem of genius.* (E. E. Paul & C. Paul, Trans.). New York: Macmillan.

Leedy, J. J. (1960). *Poetry therapy.* Philadelphia: Lippincott.

Levy, F. J. (1988). *Dance movement therapy: A healing art.* Reston, VA: American Alliance for Health, Physical Education, Recreation, and Dance.

MacRae, A. (1992). Should music be used therapeutically in occupational therapy? *American Journal of Occupational Therapy, 46,* 275–277.

Maranto, C. D. (1993). Music therapy and stress management. In P. M. Lehrer & R. L. Woolfolk (Eds.), *Principles and practice of stress management* (2nd ed., pp. 407–442). New York: Guilford.

Marks, I. M., & Gelder, M. G. (1966). Common ground between behaviour therapy and psychodynamic methods. *British Journal of Medical Psychology, 39,* 11–23.

Marley, L. S. (1984). The use of music with hospitalized infants and toddlers: Descriptive case study. *Journal of Music Therapy, 21,* 128–132.

Matthews, J. H. (1965). *An introduction to surrealism.* University Park: Pennsylvania State University Press.

May, R. (1975). *The courage to create.* New York: Bantam.

McFarland, J. H. (1952). A method of bibliotherapy. *American Journal of Occupational Therapy, 6,* 66–73, 95.

Meier-Graete, J. (1933). *Vincent Van Gogh.* New York: The Literary Guild of America.

Miller, K. J. (1979). *Treatment with music: A manual for allied health professionals.* Kalamazoo, MI: Western Michigan University.

Moreno, J. L. (1947). *Psychodrama.* Beacon, NY: Beacon House.

National Association of Poetry Therapy (NAPD). (n.d.). *Poetry Therapy—A Form of Bibliotherapy.* Retrieved February 14, 2001, from the World Wide Web: *http://www.poetrytherapy.org/articles/pt.htm#back-to-top*

National Coalition of Arts Therapies Association (NCATA). (n.d.). *NCATA.* Retrieved February 14, 2001, from the World Wide Web: *http://www.ncata.com/*

Naumburg, M. (1950). *Schizophrenic art: Its meaning in psychotherapy.* New York: Grune and Stratton.

Nelson, D. L., Anderson, V. G., & Gonzales, A. D. (1984). Music activities as therapy for children with autism and other pervasive developmental disorders. *Journal of Music Therapy, 21,* 101–116.

Nobel, T. D. (1933). The use of dramatics and stage craft in the occupational treatment of mentally ill patients. *Occupational Therapy and Rehabilitation, 12*(2), 73–81.

Pardeck, J. T., & Pardeck, J. A. (1989). Bibliotherapy: A tool for helping preschool children deal with developmental change related to family relationships. *Early Child Development and Care, 47,* 107–129.

Pavlicevic, M. (1997). *Music therapy in context: Music, meaning and relationship.* London: Jessica Kingsley Publishers.

Phillips, M. E. (1996). Looking back: The use of drama and puppetry therapy during the 1920s and 1930s. *American Journal of Occupational Therapy, 50,* 229–233.

Pickford, R. W. (1967). *Studies in psychiatric art: Its psychodynamics, therapeutic value, and relationship to modern art.* Springfield, IL: Charles C. Thomas.

Podolsky, E. (1954). Music and mental health. In E. Podolsky (Ed.), *Music therapy* (pp. 11–23). New York: Philosophical Library.

Rhyne, J. (1973). *The gestalt art experience.* Monterey, CA: Brooks/Cole.

Richards, M. C. (1964). *Centering in pottery, poetry, and the person.* Middletown, CT: Wesleyan University Press.

Riordan, R. J., & Wilson, L. S. (1989). Bibliotherapy: Does it work? *Journal of Counseling and Development, 69,* 506–508.

Robbins, A. (1980). *Expressive therapy: A creative arts approach to depth-oriented treatment.* New York: Human Sciences Press.

Robbins, A. (1994). Clinical considerations. In A. Robbins (Ed.), *A multi-modal approach to creative art therapy* (pp. 103–115). London: Jessica Kingsley Publishers.

Roth, E. A. (1987). A behavioral approach to art therapy. In J. A. Rubin (Ed.), *Approaches to art therapy: Theory and technique* (pp. 213–232). New York: Bruner/Mazel.

Ruscombe-King, G. (1983). Psychodrama: A treatment approach to alcoholism. *The British Journal of Occupational Therapy, 46*(7), 185–187.

Schaefer-Simmern, H. (1948). *The unfolding of artistic activity: Its basis, processes, and implications.* Berkeley: University of California.

Schneck, J. M. (1944). Studies in bibliotherapy. *Occupational Therapy and Rehabilitation, 23,* 316–323.

Schuman, S. H., Marcus, D., & Nesse, D. (1973). Puppetry and the mentally ill. *American Journal of Occupational Therapy, 27,* 484–486.

Shields, A., & Robbins, A. (1980). Music in expressive therapy. In A. Robbins (Ed.), *Expressive therapy: A creative arts approach to depth-oriented treatment.* New York: Human Sciences.

Silberzahn, M. (1988). Integration in sensorimotor therapy. In H. L. Hopkins & H. D. Smith (Eds.), *Willard and Spackman's occupational therapy* (7th ed., pp. 127–141). Philadelphia: Lippincott.

Staum, M. J., & Flowers, P. J. (1984). The use of stimulated training and music lessons in teaching appropriate shopping skills to an autistic child. *Music Therapy Perspectives, 1*(3), 14–17.

Sugarman, P. (1954). A musical program for emotional high blood pressure. In E. Podolsky (Ed.), *Music therapy* (pp. 151–154). New York: Philosophical Library.

Thompson, M., & Blair, S. E. E. (1998). Creative arts in occupational therapy: Ancient history or contemporary practice? *Occupational Therapy International, 5,* 49–65.

Van Deusen, J., & Harlowe, D. (1987). The efficacy of the ROM dance program for adults with rheumatoid arthritis. *American Journal of Occupational Therapy, 41,* 90–95.

van Sickle, K. G., & Acker, L. E. (1975). Modification of an adult's problem behavior in an art therapy setting. *American Journal of Art Therapy, 14,* 117–120.

Wadeson, H. (1980). *Art psychotherapy.* New York: John Wiley.

Walsh, A. C. (1988, May 26). Writing poetry helps O.T. cope with tragedy. *OT Week, 2*(20), 6, 30.

Wilson, L. (1987). Symbolism and art therapy: Theory and clinical practice. In J. A. Rubin (Ed.), *Approaches to art therapy: Theory and technique* (pp. 44–62). New York: Bruner/ Mazel.

CHAPTER

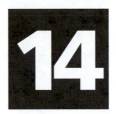

Quality Assurance, Continuous Quality Improvement, Reimbursment, and Documentation

Rita Chang, M.S., OTR

> *One cannot be in the practice of any of the health professions today without being keenly aware of the many forces shaping one's future roles and responsibilities.*
>
> — W. L. West (1967), *The 1967 Eleanor Clark Slagle Lecture: Professional Responsibility: In Times of Change*, p. 10.

Operational Learning Objectives

By the end of this chapter, the learner will:

1. Discuss the evolution of quality assurance in mental health care.

2. Identify important events in the development of quality assurance.

3. Distinguish among credentialing, licensure, privileging, and practice standards as they relate to quality assurance.

4. Distinguish among the different roles of the American Occupational Therapy Association, the National Board for Certification in Occupational Therapy, and State Licensing Boards.

5. Discuss the concept of Quality Assurance.

6. Identify the three-part process in evaluating quality.

7. Describe the role of measurement in assessing quality.

8. Identify two methods occupational therapists can employ to ensure quality services.

9. Discuss the evolution of Continuous Quality Improvement.

10. Distinguish between Quality Assurance and Continuous Quality Improvement.

11. Discuss the basic tenets of Continuous Quality Improvement.

12. Discuss the roles of documentation in occupational therapy.

13. Identify the fundamental elements of documentation.

14. Define problems to be addressed in a client's treatment plan.

15. Write a clear, concise SOAP note

16. Understand federal entitlements, such as Medicare and Medicaid, and other programs for reimbursing mental health services.

QUALITY ASSURANCE

When an individual seeks the professional services of an occupational therapist, how does the client know that the services provided are beneficial? How does this individual know that the occupational therapist is qualified and skilled in the various assessments and modalities being utilized? Health care quality has evolved from a time of unquestioned belief in the health care professional to a new era of "checks and balances," which hold the professional accountable for a commitment to "quality" with regard to ethics, education, lifelong learning, and care provided. Quality assurance is a means of regulating and enhancing the quality of health care. According to Joe (1992):

Quality assurance asks and answers questions such as the following: Is the care being provided to a given group of patients/clients having the expected or desired effects? If so, to what extent? If not, what changes are likely to produce the intended outcomes? Are these changes feasible? Is this an area in which expenditures of health care efforts and resources are apt to produce considerable improvement, or might these be better directed to some other, more fruitful area? If a plan for improvement has been implemented, has it actually been successful? (p. 251)

These questions are being asked by third-party payers, health care providers, health care facilities, accrediting bodies, and health care consumers. The answers come in the form of continuous outcomes measurements. Quality assurance and outcomes measurements are very closely related. The data from standardized outcomes measurements are being collected by compatible computer systems, which allow health care facilities, third-party payers, accrediting bodies, government, and health care consumers to compare outcomes and costs and to gauge the quality of services being provided within a facility and among similar health care providers. As Joe (1992) predicted, quality assurance is tied to cost control, reimbursement, and health care service promotion.

HISTORICAL NOTES ON QUALITY ASSURANCE

Standards regarding the practice of health care date as far back as the Hippocratic oath, written in the 4th century B.C., which was the embodiment of medical ethics. Concerns regarding quality assurance in mental health care evolved outside of the medical field. Care for the "insane," prior to the 16th century, resided primarily with religious orders, benefactors, and penal institutions (Wells & Brooks, 1988). According to Ellenberger (1974), the beginnings of quality assurance in mental health care can possibly be traced to Juan Cuidad Duarte, a 16th century Spanish merchant who suffered a transient psychotic episode. After his "treatment" through flogging, Duarte recovered and founded a hospital dedicated to the humane treatment of those with mental illness. After his death, he was canonized as Saint John of God, and the Order of Charity for the Service of the Sick was established to implement his practices throughout Europe

(Wells & Brooks, 1988). This order is believed to have influenced Phillippe Pinel and Jean-Etienne Esquirol, who were pioneers in reforming psychiatric care (Wells & Brooks, 1988). With the establishment of psychiatric hospitals and development of training in psychiatry at the university level in the 19th century, the study of mental disorders eventually achieved the status of a legitimate academic discipline (Wells & Brooks, 1988). The credentialing of graduates in psychiatry from medical schools was also a means of regulating standards in mental health care.

A rising concern regarding the overall quality of medical education in the United States arose in the late 19th century. As a result of this concern, the American Medical Association created the Council on Education. In 1908, this council co-sponsored with the Carnegie Foundation, a review of North American medical schools. This resulted in a report from Abraham Flexner (1910), which criticized the poor quality of medical education with regard to the curricula and the school laboratory facilities. The Flexner report was instrumental in the closing of 60 of the existing 155 North American medical schools (Joe, 1992). Flexner suggested that uniform standards, based on a systematic approach, should be used to regulate the quality of medical school education.

In 1912, the Third Clinical Congress of Surgeons of North America proffered a resolution that revolutionized the concept of quality assurance:

> Some system of standardization of hospital equipment and hospital work should be developed, to the end that those institutions having the highest ideals may have proper recognition before the profession, and that those of inferior equipment and standards should be stimulated to raise the quality of their work. (Davis, 1960, p. 476)

The American College of Surgeons (ACS) was founded in 1913 and the members developed several standards for quality assurance programs. The Hospital Standardization Program, developed in 1917, required medical staff to review their performance through clinical record review (Affeldt, Roberts, & Walczak, 1983). According to Langsley (1980), ACS also initiated an evaluation of surgical competence based on an assessment of outcomes. By assessing compliance with its standards, ACS introduced the process of hospital accreditation. According to Graham (1982), only 90 of the 692 hospitals covered in the first accreditation survey were approved.

The Joint Commission on Accreditation of Healthcare Organizations (JCAHO, formerly known as the Joint Commission on Accreditation of Hospitals) was established in 1951 by the American College of Physicians, the American College of Surgeons, the American Hospital Association, and the American Medical Association (Wells & Brooks, 1988). Most states now mandate JCAHO accreditation for licensure, and most third-party payers require it for reimbursement (Joe, 1992). Until 1980, the JCAHO accreditation councils developed standards for mental health services for long-term facilities, institutions for individuals with mental retardation, impatient facilities for individuals with mental illness, and long-term public facilities for children and adolescent (Affeldt, Roberts, &Walczak, 1983).

Professional Standard Review Organizations (PSRO)

The Medicare and Medicaid programs (developed in 1965 under Public Law 89–94) affected not only the development of JCAHO, but also other quality assurance programs. This law mandated quality assurance programs for facilities seeking reimbursement for Medicare (Title XVIII) and Medicaid (Title XIX). A committee at each facility, composed of physicians, was required to carry out retrospective utilization reviews. For each review, the committee determined whether hospitalization was medically necessary and whether appropriate care was given. The requirement of mandatory review was controversial and did little to contain rapidly rising costs of Medicare and Medicaid. As a result, Congress passed legislation to establish Professional Standard Review Organizations (PSROs) in 1972. The individual PSROs consisted of physicians and other health care professionals in a PSRO region designated by the Secretary of Health, Education and Welfare. The primary purpose of PSROs was to perform required quality assurance reviews for reimbursing facilities and individual providers for services delivered under Medicare, Medicaid, or Maternal and Child Health program benefits. The four major goals of PSROs were:

1. Assure that health care services are of acceptable professional quality.
2. Assure appropriate utilization of health care facilities at the most economical level consistent with professional standards.
3. Identify quality and utilization problems in health care practices and work toward their improvement.
4. Obtain voluntary correction of inappropriate or unnecessary practitioner and facility practices and recommend appropriate sanctions against practitioner and facilities. (Stein, 1985, p. 23)

The utilization of PSROs initially raised very strong reactions. Physicians were concerned about restrictions on their autonomy, and health care providers were concerned about confidentiality of the patient. Despite objections to mandated review, peer review programs were developed in the late 1960s and early 1970s by the American Psychiatric Association and the American Psychological Association to evaluate psychiatric care provided under the Civilian Health and Medical Program of the Uniformed Services (CHAMPUS).

The Peer Review Improvement Act was incorporated in 1982 secondary to costs associated with PSROs. PSROs were replaced by peer review organizations (PROs). According to federal regulations, each state was required before the end of 1984 to designate a single PRO to act on its behalf in monitoring the quality of care for Medicare beneficiaries. The PROs were under a 2-year contract with the Federal Health Care Financing Administration (HCFA) (Joe, 1992). Reviews conducted by PROs are required to be objective and include the monitoring of inappropriate admissions, patient/client deaths, and inappropriate use of restraints.

DEFINITION OF QUALITY ASSURANCE

What constitutes "quality" mental health care? What is quality assurance and why is it necessary? Quality is a subjective term that depends upon how it is assessed, the standards and criteria used in evaluation, and the values of those who seek to define it. The definition of quality is always subject to change and is open to various interpretations.

According to Rodriguez (1988), an ideal system of quality assurance would ensure optimal care for all patients. Thus care for everyone would be available, appropriate, and efficacious and would be provided without consideration of costs. According to Ostrow, Williamson, and Joe (1983), a system like this is preferred by both the patient and the provider; however, the driving forces of quality of care include not only the provider and the patient but economic considerations as well.

Rapidly rising costs in health care have all but obliterated the days of extended inpatient mental health hospitalizations. In the early 1970s, the cost of mental health care would not have been a major factor in defining quality or quality assurance. In the 1980s, concern regarding the availability of Medicare spurred third-party payers to limit and cap rather than expand benefits. This trend posed a threat to the future of mental health services, frequently the first health services sacrificed during economic recession (Rodriguez, 1988). According to Rodriguez (1988), concerns about the consequences of federal budget restraints and rising program costs might result in impediments to quality of care, containment of quality assurance activities, limited access to services, and inadequate provision of care. Inpatient mental health hospitalizations now average 3 to 5 days and there is a greater trend toward outpatient services or partial hospitalization. Mental health hospitalizations are often closely monitored by utilization review boards (URBs). The primary function of URBs is to document medical necessity and to ensure appropriate utilization of services.

Health care payers (e.g., insurance companies, Medicare, and Medicaid) are increasingly influencing the course of mental health care. With managed care, patients are often restricted to a specific number of days or dollar allowances for inpatient or outpatient services. This is an ethical dilemma for mental health professionals, who feel that therapy is compromised by the limits placed by the payers. Individual differences among clients occur in recovery from a mental illness. For example, recovery from depression varies, not only from patient to patient but from hospitalization to hospitalization as well. Treatment of mental illnesses also varies. This poses a challenge for payers who may have difficulty comprehending the variations in treatment for patients in mental health. In psychosocial practice, a thorough and appropriate documentation is vital to being reimbursed. According to Rodriguez (1988), the tendency of mental health professionals to limit

clinical information placed in medical records, attributing it to "privileged communications," makes it difficult for payers and their agents to understand the value of the mental health care. Tension between providers and payers is common as providers become frustrated with the constraints of coverage and payers struggle to stabilize the costs of mental health care.

A consensus among patients, mental health care providers, and payers determines what constitutes quality. Once standards of quality are established, objective measures of quality assurance can be determined. According to the Institute of Medicine, quality assurance is a system "to make health care more effective in improving the health status and satisfaction of a population within the resources which society and the individual have chosen to spend for that care" (as cited in Joe, 1992, p. 255). Donabedian (1982) reinforced that sentiment by stating that "Quality consists in a precise matching of services to needs, without excess or deficit" (p. 116). According to Williamson et al. (1982), "quality assurance encompasses both the traditional concept of quality (that is, a high degree of effectiveness in providing care) and cost containment (that is, an efficient use of resources)" (p. xvii).

CREDENTIALING

Credentialing, licensure, privileging, and practice standards are also included under the rubric of quality assurance. These practices are used to ensure that only competent professionals are providing care. Credentialing for occupational therapists is currently carried out by the National Board for Certification in Occupational Therapy (NBCOT). In the 1930s, the American Occupational Therapy Association (AOTA) initiated and implemented registration for occupational therapists. In 1986,

AOTA created the American Occupational Therapy Certification Board (AOTCB) as a separate authority to conduct the entry-level certification program (NBCOT, 1996). AOTCB changed its name to NBCOT in 1996. In March 1999, NBCOT and AOTA signed an agreement that acknowledged NBCOT as the lawful owner of the federal certification mark registrations for the titles "Occupational Therapist Registered®" (OTR) and "Certified Occupational Therapy Assistant®" (COTA). Through ownership of the titles, NBCOT has the exclusive authority to determine certification standards. Eligibility requirements for certification are: (a) graduation from an approved occupational therapy education program accredited by the Accreditation Council for Occupational Therapy Education (ACOTE), (b) successful completion of supervised fieldwork, and (c) a passing score on the National Occupational Therapy Certification Examination. NBCOT established a new policy requiring the successful completion of an English language examinations that took effect in March, 1997 (NBCOT, 1996). Individuals whose first language is English are exempt from this policy.

> Licensure is the process by which an agency of government grants permission to an individual to engage in a given occupation upon finding that the applicant has attained the minimal degree of competence necessary to ensure that the public health, safety, and welfare will be reasonably well protected. (U.S. Department of Health Education and Welfare, 1977, p. 17)

Licensure requirements vary from state to state. They not only protect the title of occupational therapists and certified occupational therapists, but regulate practices under state licensure laws as well. Table 14–1 illustrates the different roles of AOTA, NBCOT, and State Licensing Boards in ethical and disciplinary actions. AOTA has developed standards of practice for its members

Table 14–1. Agencies for Ethical and Disciplinary Action[1]

Agency/Board	Responsibility	Jurisdiction	Sanctions
American Occupational Therapy Association (AOTA) (Standards & Ethics Commission and Judicial Board)	• Enforce/support AOTA Code of Ethics • SEC review allegations of unethical conduct, confidentiality • Send findings to Judicial Board of OTs appointed by President of AOTA • Council decides whether to discipline	AOTA members only	• Ranges from public censure to permanent loss of membership
National Board for Certification in Occupational Therapy (NBCOT) (Disciplinary Action Committee)	Protect public from persons whose behavior reflects incompetence, a breach of ethics, or impairment.	Certified OT practitioners and those eligible for certification	• Reprimand or • Suspend or revoke certification (depending on seriousness of the misconduct)
State Licensing Board (Not all states have licensure)	Varies state by state—all are responsible for monitoring scope of practice, supervision, role delineation.	Licensees or Certificate holders	• Reprimand • Temporarily suspend or permanently revoke license/certification

[1]Disciplinary Action Information Exchange Network maintains a listing of names and sanctions against people disciplined by AOTA or NBCOT.
Source: Reprinted with permission. Personal communication, K. Kniepman, (September, 1997).

as guidelines for the provision of occupational therapy services. The guidelines serve as minimum standards for occupational therapy practice (AOTA, 1992).

ASSESSMENT OF QUALITY IN HEALTH CARE

Donabedian (1980) proposed that the evaluation of quality care includes three parts: (a) structure or input, (b) process, and (c) outcome. *Structure* refers to the physical characteristics, materials, and financial resources of the institution. If the physical plant or financial resources are inadequate, the quality of care is compromised (Zusman, 1988). *Process* refers to the way the institution carries out its work. This includes procedures at two levels: (a) activities related to providing care including treatment and rehabilitation practices and (b) activities related to the organization of the services such as its policies and the operation of clinical teams (Lavendar, Leiper, Pilling, & Clifford, 1994). *Outcome measurement* refers to the effects of services provided to the patient. Outcome measurement becomes increasingly more important in the current climate of managed health care.

Sperry (1997) referred to a paradigm shift in the practice of psychiatry and behavioral health as the "outcomes revolution." According to Sperry (1997), the current era is characterized by an increasing emphasis on quality and accountability of psychiatric practice based on outcomes measurement. Changes in diagnostic evaluation, treatment emphasis, and measurement of therapeutic change describe this paradigm shift. This is a critical time for occupational therapists to validate treatment through research to ensure their role in psychosocial practice. The outcomes revolution focuses on function, the basic premise of occupational therapy. Diagnostic evaluation is emphasizing personality assessment less and focusing more on assessing functional life skills in self-care, work/productivity, and leisure. According to Sperry (1997), "focused functional assessment is rapidly replacing this kind (personality assessments) of diagnostic evaluation because clinicians and managed care organizations value evaluations that provide tangible and clinically relevant treatment targets and markers of therapeutic change" (p. 96). Treatment emphasis is shifting away from classical psychoanalytic treatment and moving toward cognitive behavioral treatment combined with medication to reduce symptoms and increase functional capacity. This change emphasizes that measurement occurs continuously, rather than only before and after treatment. This emphasis is not unlike the treatment plans and progress notes routinely written by occupational therapists.

Occupational therapists need to be responsible for monitoring the quality of their services. Although institutions are currently shifting from quality assurance to continuous quality improvement (CQI), there are methods occupational therapists can employ to ensure quality on both individual and organizational levels.

In 1972, Baum outlined the departmental audit as a tool to be used for assessing services of a department, determining priorities, and accomplishing objectives. According to Baum (1972), it is possible to (a) define problem areas through the systematic use of an internal audit, (b) establish procedures, (c) develop standards, and (d) assess staff performance as it relates to the department's objectives. Baum's Departmental Audit consists of 10 sections: departmental organization, departmental management, physical facilities, personnel, purchasing of supplies, departmental budget, patient treatment, volunteer services, and educational programs. Stein (1985) adapted Baum's criteria specifically for an Occupational Therapy Department in a psychosocial facility (Table 14–2).

THE NEED FOR DOCUMENTATION

Goal Attainment Scaling

Documentation is another important mechanism by which occupational therapists can chart quality care. Ottenbacher and Cusick (1989) introduced a method of evaluating the effectiveness of a therapeutic intervention called *goal attainment scaling*. Goal attainment scaling is an objective method of documentation that allows the therapist to document the effectiveness of occupational therapy interventions and demonstrate clinical accountability. Goal attainment scaling consists of the following steps:

1. *Identifying an overall objective*: The patient, family, therapist, and any other professionals or individuals involved identify an appropriate goal. Goals should relate to function and should be relevant to the patient's life.

2. *Identify specific problem areas that should be addressed*: Problem areas are prioritized and then reduced to observable, measurable components.

3. *Specifically identify what behaviors or events will indicate improvement in each of the areas selected in step 2*: The therapist identifies the behavior or event that will be measured.

4. *Determine the methodology that will be used to collect the desired information*: The therapist determines how the information will be collected, who will collect it, and in what environment the evaluation data will be collected.

5. *Select the expected level of performance*: The therapist and patient determine the long-term goal.

6. *Identify the most favorable outcome, the least favorable outcome, and intermediate levels of the client's performance*: Five realistic levels of performance are defined. Each level is then assigned a numeric value, with 0 indicating the expected level of performance and −2 and +2 indicating the least and most favorable outcomes, respectively (Ottenbacher & Cusick, 1989).

7. *Complete the Goal Attainment Scale*: Once the Goal Attainment Scale has been completed, ascertain whether there are overlapping levels, gaps between levels, or more than one indicator in a problem area. Only one descriptor can be used for each outcome.

8. *Assess patient's level of function*: Ascertain the client's current status on the Goal Attainment Scale and determine future assessments to evaluate progress.

Goals are then weighted and the scores are used in a formula that results in goal attainment score. The formula generates a standardized *T*-score that reflects the patient's performance with regard to the expected outcome level. Ottenbacher & Cusick (1993) caution against using Goal Attainment scaling as a means of assessing functional status. Rather, its strength is in the evaluation of individualized longitudinal change. According to Ottenbacher & Cusick (1993), "Goal attainment scaling is a flexible evaluation methodology that can address the documentation and accountability concerns facing health care providers" (p. 353). It provides therapists with a method of quantifying documentation. Goal attainment scaling is an example of an outcome measure and a quality assurance tool.

Smith, Cardillo, Smith, & Amezaga (1998) researched the use of Improvement Scaling as a measurement of patient's progress during treatment. Smith et al. (1998) described Improve-

Table 14–2. The Departmental Audit

Section I: Organization of the Department

▶ Is there an administrative organizational chart showing the relationship between the clinical director of the psychiatric facility and the Occupational Therapy Department?

▶ Does the Occupational Therapy Department have written objectives regarding:

- evaluation of patient's performance?
- short-term and long-term treatment goals?
- criteria for assessing improvement?
- criteria for recommending discharge?
- list others

▶ Are the occupational therapy objectives consistent with the overall philosophy and goals of the institution?

▶ Does the director of the Occupational Therapy Department communicate with clinical director and other professional staff through:

- team meetings?
- informal meetings?
- regular appointments?

▶ Are there written job descriptions for each position?

▶ Are staff being utilized consistent with their role delineations?

▶ Does the Occupational Therapy Department have written procedures that have been approved by the administration in relation to:

- referral of patient to OT?
- hours of treatment?
- emergency information?
- space utilization?
- list of therapeutic groups?
- reimbursement procedures?
- personnel policies?
- student restraining program?

Section II: Department Management

▶ Are staff required to write yearly goals?

▶ What criteria are used in evaluating staff performance?

▶ Are there regular staff meetings?

▶ Are the staff given opportunities to attend educational conferences and workshops?

▶ Does the department have an adequate filing system?

▶ Is there a logical formula to determine patient-staff ratio?

▶ Is there a plan to increase staff morale and job satisfaction?

Section III: Physical Facilities

▶ Is there adequate space for treatment groups, storage of supplies, and staff offices?

▶ Are equipment and supplies adequate for treatment needs?

▶ Are facilities and equipment properly maintained?

Section IV: Personnel

▶ Is there an orientation program for new employees?

▶ Are employee salaries and benefits competitive with comparable institutions?

▶ Are personnel files confidential and kept current?

Table 14–2. The Departmental Audit

Section V: Purchasing of Supplies

▶ Is there a written procedure for requesting supplies and equipment?

▶ Is there an inventory control for supplies?

Section VI: Departmental Budget

▶ Is there an adequate budget to meet the needs of the department?

▶ Are there monthly or periodic budget expenditure reports?

▶ Is the department able to generate enough income from patient treatment to maintain itself?

▶ Does the department head, in consultation with staff, plan an annual budget?

Section VII: Patient Treatment

▶ Do all therapists treat under a psychiatrist's referral?

▶ Is there an ethical statement guiding treatment?

▶ Are progress notes written regularly?

▶ Is there a current written treatment plan for each patient?

▶ Are medical records on each patient current?

▶ Are the following services utilized in occupational therapy?

- self-care evaluations
- vocational evaluations
- behavioral evaluations
- sensory-motor evaluations
- group treatment
- individual treatment

Section VIII: Volunteer Service

▶ Is there a volunteer program?

▶ Are volunteers involved in the following areas?

- patient aides
- clerical duties
- setting up and cleaning up
- inventory control

Section IX: Public Relations

▶ Does the department have an active program of informing the general public about occupational therapy?

▶ Does the department relate to consumer groups such a local Mental Health Association and Alliance for Mentally Ill?

▶ Does the department provide tours for the public?

Section X: Educational Programs

▶ Is the department affiliated with colleges and universities in providing clinical education experiences?

▶ Does the department provide Level I and Level II field work?

▶ Is the department active in joint research with colleges or universities?

▶ Does the department sponsor continuing education workshops?

ment Scaling (IMS) as a more efficient format of Goal Attainment Scaling "which has all of the essential elements of Goal Attainment Scaling and improves on it by including the advantages of standardization" (p. 337). According to Smith et al. (1998), IMS may be used in continuous quality activities to document patients' achievement of individual treatment goals and also provide third-party payers and managed care organizations proof of the effectiveness of treatment. Use of IMS continues to be researched. Although initially developed for use in rehabilitation, Smith et al. (1998) are developing a version of IMS that would be appropriate for mental health.

The JCAHO (1980) stated:

> Although complete and accurate patient records are important for continuity of care and for legal purposes, assessment of documentation in patient records by itself, does not constitute effective review. Each support service should examine care that is directly related to the health and well being of patients. (p. 3)

Joe (1992) reinforced this belief when she stated the following:

> In 1955, the organization (JCAHO) first began to stress the importance of medical audits. By 1974, hospitals were mandated to audit medical records and make quarterly reports. In 1981, judging that the audit system was producing good medical records, but not necessary better care, the Joint Commission began urging the introduction of additional monitors (measures of important outcomes of patient/client care) and a focus on problem resolution. (p. 253)

The challenge in applying documentation as a measure of quality assurance is to use documentation as a guide for treatment and a means of improving patient care rather than a simple recording mechanism. According to Bent (1988), "Quality enhancement procedures can be reasonably carried out if the documentation system provides the elements of information and organization required by quality assurance procedures" (p. 107). Without proper documentation and accountability, occupational therapists may compromise their role in mental health.

The Role of Documentation

Documentation plays a multifaceted role in psychosocial occupational therapy. It is a method of communication, a key reimbursement tool, a requirement for accreditation and licensure, and a therapist's major defense in legal liability cases. As a communication tool, documentation is a means for occupational therapists to convey a patient's plan of care to other professionals and to insurance carriers. When clearly written, documentation allows review agencies to determine that the course of occupational therapy provided is justified. A medical record is also the patient's "receipt" of services and reinforces the medical necessity for mental health care. In legal liability cases, documentation is the therapist's only defense in indicating that care was not only necessary but was also provided. Its importance is emphasized by Joint Commission on Accreditation of Healthcare Organizations (JCAHO, 1990) and Health Care Financing Administration (HCFA). Both agencies include documentation review as a component of accreditation and the licensing process. Good documentation reflects good treatment planning and implementation in psychosocial occupational therapy in mental health settings. Documentation that is poor or incomplete includes inappropriate, immeasurable, or unattainable goals. Good documentation affects occupational therapy's accountability in mental health services. According to Gillette (1982),

> the practice claims of the profession must be established in order to provide ample evidence

of the value of occupational therapy to consumers of the service and to other health care providers as well. In the absence of careful and thorough documentation, members of a profession such as occupational therapy will not receive appropriate recognition nor adequate reimbursement for their services. (p. 499)

When documentation is systematic, problem-focused, and objective and includes appropriate, measurable goals, it not only increases occupational therapy's accountability, but it can also be an effective means of quality assurance and outcome measurement. Effective documentation requires practice in writing clearly, attention to detail, and timeliness. Currently many psychosocial occupational therapists treat patients in groups more often than on an individual basis. Therapists may fall behind in writing progress notes due to time constraints. This can have detrimental effects on the implementation of patient care. McAninch (1984), in a review of psychiatric records, stated the following:

> The comprehensiveness of the assessment affected the adequacy or inadequacy of the treatment plan. If the treatment plan was ill-defined and vague, progress notes to indicate the implementation of treatment became increasingly anecdotal. Discharge summaries and aftercare planning were limited by the completeness of the records in the above mentioned areas. (p. 183)

Structure and Elements of Documentation

The problem oriented medical record (POMR), introduced by Lawrence Weed (1964), provides a structure for the elements of documentation. Using POMR, the occupational therapist organizes a patient's records into four sections: database, problem list, treatment planning, and progress notes. This structure provides an objective and systematic method for document-

ing a patient's background history and progress (Stein, 1985). POMR is not the only format used for documentation, but it appears to be the most common. Bent (1988) suggested an alternative method, Service by Objectives (SBO), to document psychosocial treatment. According to Bent (1982), SBO includes a client-information base, sufficient information to develop service goals, a strategy for treatment, and a systematic review of the service plan, with replanning, if indicated. The concepts of SBO can be incorporated into POMR when problems are well defined and appropriate goals and objectives are stated.

The elements provided in occupational therapy documentation need to reflect the perspective of the professional in a manner that validates occupational therapists' role in psychosocial practice. Recognizing the need for effective documentation, AOTA has provided guidelines (Thomson & Foto, 1995) that include a description of fundamental elements of documentation.

Types of Documentation include:

I. *Evaluation Report*: Used to document the initial contact with the consumer, the data collected, the interpretation of the data, and the intervention plan. When an abbreviated evaluation process is used, such as screening, it is documented using only limited content areas applicable to the consumer and situation. It includes the following areas.

  A. Identification and Background Information

    1. Name, age, sex, date of admission, treatment diagnosis, and date of onset of current diagnosis

    2. Referral source, services requested, and date of referral to occupational therapy

    3. Medical history and secondary problems or preexisting conditions, prior therapy

4. Precautions and contraindications
5. Pertinent history that indicates prior levels of function and support systems
6. Present levels of function in performance areas determined by examination
7. Performance contexts determined by examination
8. Consumer and family expectations

B. Assessment Results
1. Tests and assessments administered and the results
2. References to other pertinent reports and information
3. Summary and analysis of evaluation findings
4. Projected functional outcome(s)

C. Intervention or treatment plan
1. Long-term functional goals
2. Short-term goals
3. Intervention or treatment procedures
4. Type, amount, frequency, and duration of intervention or treatment
5. Recommendations

II. *Contact, Treatment, or Visit Note*: Used to document individual occupational therapy session or care coordination. May be very brief, such as in the use of a checklist, flow chart, or short narrative type notation.

A. Attendance and participation
B. Activities, techniques, and modalities
C. Assistive/adaptive equipment, prosthetics, and orthotics if issued or fabricated, and specific instructions for the application and/or use of the item
D. Consumer's response to therapy

III. *Progress Report*: Used periodically to document care coordination, interventions, progress toward functional goals, and to update goals and intervention or treatment plan.

A. Activities, techniques, and modalities
B. Consumer's response to therapy, and the progress toward short- and long-term goal attainment and comparison with previous functional status

C. Goal continuance
D. Goal modification when indicated by the response to therapy or by the establishment of new consumer needs
E. Change in anticipated time to achieve goals
F. Assistive/adaptive equipment, prosthetics, and orthotics if issued or fabricated, and specific instructions for the application and/or use of the item
G. Consumer-related conferences and communication
H. Home programs
I. Consumer/caretaker instruction
J. Plan

IV. *Reevaluation Report*: Used to document sessions in which portions of the evaluation process are repeated or readministered. Usually occurs monthly or quarterly, depending on the setting.

A. Tests and assessments readministered and the results
B. Comparative summary and analysis of previous evaluation findings
C. Reestablishment of projected functional outcome(s)
D. Update of intervention or treatment plan

V. *Discharge or Discontinuation Report*: Used to document a summary of the course of therapy and any recommendations.

A. Therapy process
B. Goal attainment
C. Functional outcome
D. Home programs
E. Follow-up plans
F. Recommendations
G. Referral(s) to other health care providers and community agencies

Thomson & Foto (1995) also state that each consumer of occupational therapy service must have a case record maintained as a permanent file.

Identification and Background Information

The occupational therapist is not the only professional who will be documenting the patient's progress. In addition to the occupational therapist, psychiatrists, psychologists, nurses, and social workers make up the multidisciplinary or interdisciplinary team. In order for occupational therapists to provide holistic care to the patient, it is important to share with the other professionals, the results of assessments, the problems identified by the therapist and patient, and the course of treatment.

Documentation is a strong communication tool—but only when it relays to other professionals what the occupational therapist objectively observes. The occupational therapist gathers the needed information through an evaluation of the patient. Assessments may be in the form of patient/family interview, chart review, observation, or standardized instruments. Questions to be considered in evaluating a patient include:

▶ Who is this person?

▶ Why is this person seeking treatment?

▶ Are there any precautions or contraindications of which others should be aware?

▶ What is the diagnosis?

▶ What is this person's medical history and any preexisting conditions?

▶ What were this person's prior levels of functioning?

▶ What are this person's present levels of functioning in performance areas?

▶ What are the performance contexts or environments in which the person engaged in occupation?

▶ What are the goals of this person? Of the family?

The answers to these questions can portray a complete and concise picture of the client seeking treatment. Insufficient information or extraneous information in the medical records will negate the importance of the review.

According to Lynch and Stein (1986), "How the patient assessment is documented is equally important as what is documented" (p. 7). Not only must an assessment be thorough, but it must also be clear and precise in conveying information.

For consistency and thoroughness, it is recommended that a standardized form, appropriate for the occupational therapist, be used. According to Siegel and Fischer (1981)

> Structured recording . . . standardizes both the collection and the recording of information. This makes it more likely, though not certain, that the information on the form will be complete and comparable from one patient to another, which becomes increasingly important as the care-review process relies more on patients' records. Moreover, completely structured data entry provides accessible and readable information very suitable for statistical analysis. (p. 46)

An example of a structured assessment form is illustrated in Table 14–3. It is important to remember to complete all parts of a structured form. If any section is deferred, referred, or inappropriate, a notation needs to be made so that other professionals will understand why it is not completed.

Assessment Results

If any assessment such as the *Kohlman Evaluation of Living Skills* (KELS; Thomson, 1992), *Allen Cognitive Level Test* (ACL; Allen, 1985), *Mini Mental State Evaluation* (MMSE; Folstein, Folstein, & McHugh, 1975) is used, a thorough write-up of each assessment is required. If a standardized procedure is not fol-

Table 14-3. Structured Data Collection Form

I.   Source of Data

Patient Interview	Patient Self-Assessment	Chart Audit
Task Observation	Other	

Precautions_____

II.   Level of Assistance

7   Complete Independence

6   Modified Independence: requires specialized equipment or more than a reasonable time

5   Stand by Cognitive Assistance

4   Minimal Cognitive Assistance (can complete 75%)

3   Moderate Cognitive Assistance (can complete 50%)

2   Maximal Cognitive Assistance (can complete 25%)

1   Total Cognitive Assistance (completes <25%)

Comments/Clarification_____

_____

III.   Functional Performance Area: for each functional performance area, the therapist should provide the level of assistance (from II) and make comments and clarifications relative to the task.

1.   Self-Care

  a. overall grooming
  b. overall hygiene

2.   Instrumental Activities of Daily Living

  a. safety
  b. home management
  c. money management
  d. parenting skills
  e. educational activities
  f. vocational activities
  g. socialization
  h. support systems

3.   Play/Leisure Activities

  a. use of community resources
  b. range of leisure activities

4.   Sensory-Motor

  a. mobility
  b. coordination
  c. proprioception
  d. hearing/vision
  e. body scheme

5.   Cognition

  a. concentration/attention
  b. orientation
  c. memory
  d. ability to follow directions
  e. problem solving

Table 14-3. Structured Data Collection Form

6. **Psychosocial**
a. self-esteem
b. coping skills
c. impulsivity
d. judgment
e. emotional identification
f. communication skills

lowed or if there are extraneous variables (such as unavoidable distractions) in the assessment, it is important to note this. *If an assessment or treatment is not documented, whether or not it was completed, it never happened.*

An occupational therapist uses the information collected in an assessment to develop a problem list that will be addressed during the course of the patient's treatment. A problem is any condition or situation that decreases the patient's ability to function in daily life and could be related to the cause of the patient's hospitalization. At a time when the average patient's length of stay in an acute inpatient mental health facility is approximately 3 to 5 days, it is important to address problems related to a patient's level of function. Questions that can assist the occupational therapist in identifying functional problems include (Dean & Zarn, 1996):

▶ What are the problems as stated by the patient?

▶ What are the patient's goals in treatment?

▶ What are the results of an assessment?

▶ What is the level of the patient's functioning in work, ADLs, IADLs, social skills, leisure, and cognition?

▶ What are the patient's expectations in treatment?

▶ Are the goals of the therapist congruent with the patient's goals? If not, how can the differences be resolved?

▶ What is the primary problem to be treated first?

▶ Can the patient's needs be met by the therapist, the family, or other health professionals?

Problems can be classified as active, inactive, deferred, referred, revised, and resolved. An *active* problem is present in the patient, identified in goals, addressed in treatment, and recorded in progress notes. *Inactive* problems have affected the patient in the past; however, they are not active presently. For example, a patient may have attempted suicide in the past, but is not suicidal now. These problems have the potential to become active or impact treatment; however, they will probably not be addressed in short-term treatment. *Deferred* problems either take little effort from staff to manage (e.g., high blood sugar levels or monitoring of blood sugar levels), or they will not be actively treated but may be considered later on. *Revised* problems are problems that are actively changed secondary to obtaining additional information and by clarifying a patient's current problem. *Resolved* problems have reached a state at which they no longer need to be addressed by treatment staff.

The occupational therapist should keep problem statements simple and concrete. They need to be individualized and defined in objective, functional, and measurable terms. A baseline for the comparison of progress should also be included. A template that can be used to define problems is as follows:

▶ The patient is experiencing (*identify the problem*) as evidenced by (*an observable measure*) leading to (*the problem's impact on function*).

An example of a problem statement is:

▶ The patient is experiencing decreased ability to complete bathing as evidenced by patient not bathing even when urged by family members. This leads to patient's decreased ability for independent self-care.

▶ *Baseline*: Patient has not bathed for the past week per family report.

In the scenario below (Lynch & Stein, 1986), a problem is identified and used to formulate a patient care plan.

Intervention or Treatment Plan

A well-written treatment plan provides direction for treatment and focus for the occupational therapist and the patient. It directly addresses the identified problems and should be given to or discussed with the patient to increase his or her investment and motivation in the treatment plan. A treatment plan is an occupational therapist's means of communicating the patient's plan of care to the other professionals and also as a means of emphasizing the patient's need for occupational therapy services. Thus the treatment plan needs to be clear, complete, and accurate (Stein, 1985).

The elements of the treatment plan include the problem, long-term functional goals, short-term goals, interventions directly related to the goals, and any recommendations. Problems should be identified in the assessment stage. A treatment goal is a general statement of what is expected to occur at the end of a sequence of therapy sessions. The treatment goal needs to be accompanied by measurable treatment objectives. Treatment objectives are more specific than the goal and relate exactly *what* intervention or treatment procedure will be used, *how* the behavior will be measured, the *frequency* of addressing the behavior, and the *duration* of the intervention. Goals need to be achievable, easily understood, and appropriate to the patient's individualized treatment plan. An example of goal and objective identification related to the

---

Scenario: This is a twenty-five-year-old white male admitted from a group home. Patient has been extremely fearful since a fight with another resident. Patient cannot sleep, stays awake for fear of reprisal. Patient wears soiled, wrinkled clothing and his hair is unkempt. Patient paces the floor throughout interview.

Problem Statement	*Preferred Terminology*
1. Cannot sleep	1. Insomnia
2. Worried about resident retaliation	2. Excessive anxiety due to fear of another resident
3. Unkempt appearance	3. Inadequate self-care

Source: From "Evaluating Occupational Therapy Psychiatric Care Through Medical Documentation," by J. J. Lynch & F. Stein, 1986, p. 62. *Occupational Therapy in Mental Health*, 6(3).

preceding scenario is is portrayed in Table 14-4 (Lynch & Stein, 1986, p. 63).

Throughout a patient's hospitalization, individual treatment plans need to be reviewed and modified to reflect the patient's progress. When objectives are achieved, new objectives will need to be established to guide treatment toward resolution of the problems. As new problems surface, goals and objectives related to these problems will need to be identified. If objectives are not met, they need to be reviewed and the following questions should be asked (Dean & Zarn, 1996):

- Was the right method used for treatment?
- Was the objective set too high?
- Is it the right objective?

- Is the objective clear?
- Is the right problem addressed?
- Is more information needed?
- Are other factors entering in the picture of which you were not aware?
- Might it take longer than expected? (p. 18)

Objectives should then be either rewritten or terminated with an explanation on the treatment plan as to why they were not achieved. Each facility will have its own policy regarding establishment and review of treatment plans. It is recommended that an individual treatment plan be established within 72 hours of admission and reviewed at least once a week.

It is important to remember that the treatment plan is the primary source of communica-

Table 14–4. Patient Care Plan

PROBLEM NUMBER	PROBLEM	GOAL	OBJECTIVE	APPROACH
1.	Insomnia	Return to patient's normal sleeping pattern	After 2 weeks of daily relaxation therapy, patient will sleep through 3 of the next 5 nights	• Schedule one 60-min relaxation session a day, 5 times a week for the next 2 weeks • Encourage patient to use techniques daily
2.	Excessive anxiety due to fear of fellow resident	Reconcile difference between patient and fellow resident	By discharge, patient will have met with resident and resolved differences to the satisfaction of both parties and as deemed appropriate by therapist	• Meet with patient daily on individual basis to discuss circumstances of conflict • Schedule at least two conferences with other resident to discuss conflict • Research the histories of both parties • Schedule a meeting of both parties and therapist
3.	Inadequate self-care	Exercise personal hygiene care	By discharge patient will select and prepare wardrobe without assistance and complete proactive hygienic care to satisfaction of therapist	• Assess functional abilities in self-care • Based on assessment, assign responsibilities for self-care

tion with the other professionals, insurance carriers, and quality assurance reviewers. It provides others with an understanding of the patient's ability to function and eliminates any ambiguity regarding the effect of the patient's mental illness. It is a systematic approach to treatment and identifies the need for occupational therapy.

Progress Report

The progress report or note should document the patient's ongoing treatment and also include any reevaluations. (See the outline previously provided by Thomson and Foto, 1995.) The style of progress notes may vary from facility to facility. The problem-oriented medical record (POMR; Weed, 1964) is most commonly used in occupational therapy. When using POMR, a SOAP-style progress note is used. Only one problem should be addressed in each SOAP note. According to Stein (1985), in this manner the note will clearly state the problem and how the patient feels about the problem; what the clinician observes, performs, or measures; and finally, what the clinician intends to do—in clear, measurable terms. When documenting a SOAP-style note, the following guidelines should be used:

S = Subjective information. This is any information the client or other person tells you. This information may be "directly quoted" or paraphrased.

O = Objective information. This is information that you directly test or observe. This section does not include judgment—just the facts and nothing but the facts.

A = Assessment. Not to be confused with the results of an assessment (which belong in O). This is the section which calls for professional judgments. It includes clinical reasoning and predictions based on your professional opinion.

P = Plan. This is the section which outlines your treatment strategies and recommendations and states goals. (Neufeld, personal memorandum, 1997)

Additional guidelines and helpful hints for writing SOAP notes are provided in Table 14–5.

Progress Note Guidelines

Some practical suggestions for writing SOAP notes follow.

▶ *Be timely.* Complete all assessments, plans, and documentation on time. Document as soon as possible (ASAP) after therapy sessions or occurrences.

▶ *Be objective.* Include the facts: Patient appears to be hallucinating vs. Patient pacing in room and talking to self. Upon staff inquiry, patient states Julius Caesar is walking with patient in room.

▶ *Be specific.* Patient had difficulty sleeping vs. Patient slept a total of 2 hours.

▶ *Be complete, not verbose.* Note what is significant to the treatment plan and the patient's condition, such as changes in affect, change in physical condition, changes in cognition, changes in thoughts of self-harm.

▶ *Write legibly in black ink.* If you or no one else can read what is written, it was never recorded.

▶ *Use only approved correct abbreviations* and use them sparingly. These may vary from facility to facility.

▶ *Do not include irrelevant comments* or jokes! For example, patient is just a spoiled

Table 14–5. SOAP Note

	Initial Note	Progress Note	Discharge Note
S	Significant information reported by the patient, family, or staff on the illness; a person's roles, attitudes, goals; living situation, family or teacher contributions.	Patient report of response to treatment	A summary of report from patient, family, and/or staff on overall treatment issues, benefits, feelings, and perceptions
O	Patient's Medical History: • "Chart reviewed. . . ." • Results of assessments • Clinical observations • "Not tested because. . ."	List problem and report observed responses to treatment under each problem. (Problem #1. Decreased ADL Performance, etc.)	State each problem # and summarize progress made for each.
A	Therapist's judgment and analysis of the situation. Identify deficits that cause functional limitations. Identify rehabilitation potential. Identify and state problems (can list incomplete database as problem).	• Therapist's judgment on the response to treatment. • Status of goals; if achieved. • Provide reasoning for new problems identified and state with problem #.	• Therapist's judgment of patient progress of overall treatment, current functional performance, and interpretation of why or why not successful. • Reasoning for discharge recommendations which will be stated in P. • Status of all goals stated. • Date when goal achieved. If not achieved, state unresolved or chronic.
P	Treatment strategies. • Treatment (Tx) frequency and duration. Goals: LTG and STG. • Who, what, what assist, time frame, conditions. • STG: performance component • LTG: functional outcome • RUMBA	• Modify treatment plan/strategies or continue treatment plan. • State new goals. • Make recommendation.	• Recommendations (for additional OT, home health, need for other services, etc.). • Home Program or instructions if given to patient or family. Follow-up or precautions given.

Source: Reprinted with permission. Personal communication from P. Neufeld (September, 1997).

brat; patient is just being difficult, let him suffer! (This has actually been noted in documentation.)

▶ *Do not use white-out or scratch out errors.* Check with facility regarding errors on documentation. Usually, a line should be drawn through the error and initials and date should be written by error.

▶ *Complete all sections of a note.* Explain any sections not completed on preprinted formats.

▶ *Be consistent with the treatment plan and other documentation* included on the chart.

Thomson & Foto (1995) stated that the following elements should also be present in a client's case record:

▶ Consumer's full name and case number on each page of documentation

▶ Date stated as month, day, and year for each entry; time of intervention; and length of session

▶ Identification of type of documentation and department name

▶ Practitioner's signature with a minimum of initial of first name, last name, and professional title

▶ Signature of the recorder directly at the end of the note without space left between the body of the note and the signature

▶ Countersignature by a Registered Occupational Therapist (OTR) on documentation written by students and Certified Occupational Therapy Assistants (COTA) when required by law or the facility

▶ Compliance with confidentiality standards

▶ Acceptable terminology as defined by the facility (p.1035)

Discharge or Discontinuation Report

This report is the final communication regarding a patient's course through therapy and can be written in a SOAP format as well. It emphasizes the gains made through occupational therapy. It can increase the occupational therapist's accountability if the initial problems, goals, and objectives were identified correctly and written well. It is important for the clinician to compare the patient's goal attainment and functional outcome to the goals and functional levels in the evaluation report. The results of this comparison can be used for quality assurance and outcome measurement purposes.

Summary of the Process of Documentation

Proper documentation is extremely critical for the reimbursement of occupational therapy services in mental health. At present, there is a high rate of denials of reimbursement from Medicare for occupational therapy in skilled nursing facilities (SNF) and partial hospital settings. Fiscal intermediaries (FIs), insurance companies that administer Medicare claims, many times do not understand the occupational therapists' role in mental health care. Quite often, occupational therapy is confused with activity or recreational therapy, which is not covered by Medicare. FIs have also stated that they do not understand why a patient with mental illness, and no evidence of a physical disability would require the *physical rehabilitation* services of an occupational therapist. This implies that their knowledge of occupational therapy is limited to physical rehabilitation rather than functional rehabilitation or habilitation. Documentation is the primary method that occupational therapists have for justifying the need for occupational therapy and emphasizing its unique services in mental health. In this new era of treatment outcomes, it is imperative that clinicians provide documentation that supports the efficacy and cost effectiveness of occupational therapy. Occupational therapists need to take a proactive role in increasing their accountability. Through proper documentation, not only can occupational therapists assure the quality of their services, but they can also validate the necessity for their services in a mental health setting as well.

CONTINUOUS QUALITY IMPROVEMENT

Continuous Quality Improvement (CQI) is founded on management principles developed by a statistician, W. Edwards Deming (1982). Deming formed many of his theories during World War II when he applied statistical methods in industry to improve the quality of military production. After the war Japanese industrialists invited Deming to share his theories regarding industrial production. At that time, the label "made in Japan" was synonymous with inferior products and the Japanese wanted to change that perception. Deming encouraged them to base their product design on what their consumers wanted and then to continuously study and improve their products and production systems. Deming's basic premise was that constant research and improvement of product design and production systems would allow an industry to prepare for the future and efficiently meet (and often surpass) consumer demands. Within 4 years of applying Deming's theories, the reputation of Japanese products improved as well as the quality of the finished products. Although U.S. industry dominated supplying consumer goods during the time of Japanese industrial reconstruction, it began to lose markets in the 1970s and 1980s. Ironically, U.S. companies started to examine what had made the Japanese companies successful. Through systematic adoption of Deming's techniques, U.S. organizations redesigned their work procedures leading to significant increases in efficiency, effectiveness, and market success (Chowanec, 1994). Deming's principles emphasizing the process of quality production and a team-oriented approach to change processes are used to improve the quality of services. These theories are the basis of continuous quality improvement in health care (Gillem, 1988).

As the costs of health care have continued to rise, so has the demand for cost-effective, high-quality health care. Continuous quality improvement theories were introduced to health care after it became evident that quality assurance methodology alone was not able to improve health care. In 1987, the JCAHO, under its Agenda for Change, began the process of changing its quality assurance standards to the continuous quality framework (JCAHO, 1991). According to Schyve, JCAHO's vice president for research and standards in 1991, CQI was seen as an evolutionary process that would build on the strengths of traditional quality assurance, while discarding its more ineffective approaches (Koska, 1991). Since 1997, the JCAHO Hospital Accreditation Standards have emphasized the improvement of organization performance rather than quality assurance standards. According to the Accreditation Standards, the goal of improving organization performance is to ensure that the organization designs processes well and systematically monitors, analyzes, and improves its performance to upgrade patient outcomes (JCAHO, 1999). JCAHO proposes that an organizations approach to improving its performance includes: (a) designing processes, (b) monitoring performance through data collection, (c) analyzing current performance, and (d) improving and sustaining improved performance (p.1).

What is Continuous Quality Improvement?

Although CQI and QA are regarded as two separate entities, CQI can be seen as an extension of quality assurance. Whereas QA identifies problems within a system, CQI addresses continuous improvement of the system via inspection of system processes. Rather than addressing only short-term goals, CQI looks at future functioning and encourages organizations to broaden their perspective. The following is an explanation of CQI, based on basic CQI tenets of O'Leary and O'Leary (1992).

▶ *CQI is, first and foremost, internally driven, not an external mandate.* As occupational therapists we learn that we need to involve our clients when assisting them with goal development. Unless treatment goals are client-centered, there is little impetus for the client to achieve them. Quality assurance methods are driven mostly by external requirements, which often gives recipients the feeling that their goals and standards are being developed for them without consideration for their interests. It is not surprising that quality assurance has fostered a "you versus us" mentality and has often led to feelings of resentment. CQI theory emphasizes that an organization needs to have its own investment in improving its ability in providing care. This is demonstrated by JCAHO providing standards for improving performance rather than mandating specific CQI procedures. JCAHO (1997) emphasizes that hospitals have "a planned, systematic, hospital wide approach to process design and performance measurement, assessment, and improvement" (p. 137). By following JCAHO's standards, an organization utilizes CQI concepts in a manner that is beneficial to its own unique system. According to O'Leary and O'Leary (1992), the intent of JCAHO's standards is to stimulate organization creativity in solving problems and capitalizing on opportunities for improvements.

▶ *CQI recognizes that error-free care cannot be guaranteed but rather emphasizes that the quality of care can always be continuously improved.* It is not realistic for occupational therapists to expect that all of our clients with the same diagnosis will reach the same level of accomplishment at the end of treatment. Nor do we expect that a client will not have some days when learning skills are difficult. When clients are having a difficult day in treatment, we encourage them and assist them with problem-solving to simplify their tasks. We try to provide an

environment that allows for mistakes and fosters achievement. The title "quality assurance" often leads some to believe that quality in health care can be guaranteed and that mistakes can be eliminated. In this type of environment, we would expect frustration and denial of difficulty from our clients. It should be no surprise that the quality assurance mentality may encourage defensiveness and an inclination toward "covering up" mistakes. The CQI model emphasizes learning from mistakes and leads the involved parties to assemble appropriate clinical, management, and support services staff to address the underlying issues (O'Leary & O'Leary, 1992). CQI does not tolerate mistakes more than quality assurance; however, it focuses less on penalties and more on correction and prevention.

▶ *CQI focuses on systems first and individuals second.* When working with our clients on new techniques, skills, and use of adaptive equipment, occupational therapists must always take into consideration the environments to which their clients are returning rather than focusing only on their clients' disabilities. It is not very useful to devote limited therapy time to work on budgeting skills when the client is not responsible for budgeting at home. CQI focuses on considering possible problems in the system (environment) rather than concentrating on problems within the individual. Drs. Juran and Deming have maintained since the early 1950s that at least 85 pecent of an organization's failures are the fault of management-controlled systems whereas workers control fewer than 15 percent of the problems (Scholtes, 1988). If this is the case, it would be more effective and efficient to concentrate on difficulties within the system than to blame the individual worker. In mental health care, clients very rarely work with occupational therapists alone. Teamwork is essential in mental health care, especially in an acute, inpatient setting. Other than direct client care, there are many processes involved from the time the client is admitted to the program to the time the client is discharged. When something adverse occurs, the quality assurance mentality may focus on the fault of an individual; however, rarely is just one individual involved when there is a problem in a system. Through concentration on fixing blame, employee satisfaction drops and job burnout may increase. The feelings of frustration and helplessness in the staff are not unlike what a client would experience while working on an inappropriate goal.

▶ *CQI is an organization-wide set of activities.* CQI is not something to be undertaken by one profession alone. When an occupational therapist works with a client on communication skills, she or he communicates this goal to the other members of the team. By relating this goal, the therapist ensures that the other team members are aware of what the client is attempting to accomplish. CQI is a mind set that requires everyone in the organization to work with each other in accomplishing improved performance. A health care organization is a complex system of interdependencies; few issues of any consequence can be addressed effectively solely within an individual department (O'Leary & O'Leary, 1992). According to JCAHO (1999), "performance-improvement activities are most effective when they are planned, systematic, and organization-wide and when all appropriate individuals and professions work collaboratively to plan and implement them" (p. 6). An

occupational therapy department cannot stand alone and will not be able to carry out the CQI philosophy without support of the entire organization. Each person in a health care organization provides some contribution in a client's care and needs to be invested in improving performance for CQI to work.

▶ *CQI requires leadership commitment.* The decision to incorporate CQI concepts affects an entire organization and needs to begin at the senior leadership positions. According to Scholtes (1988), the most frequent cause of failure in any quality improvement effort is uninvolved or indifferent top and middle management. Managers must lead the transformation effort to ensure long-lasting success. An occupational therapist should not teach a client a social skill without being able to demonstrate its use and effectiveness. Why would hospital staff take stock in a new philosophy that is not supported and used by top managers in the organization? CQI calls for managers to be educators and leaders rather than bosses. According to Berwick, Godfrey, and Roessner (1990), it takes several years for the "new" quality culture to take root. It is important for organization leaders to educate themselves, become proficient in CQI design, and adopt CQI principles in their own practice before attempting to engage the entire organization in the new philosophy.

▶ *CQI requires performance measurement.* Before working with a client, an occupational therapist assesses his or her level of functioning. The client and the therapist then work together to establish relevant, understandable, measurable, behavioral, and achievable goals. By doing this, a client's progress can be measured throughout treatment. CQI encourages decision making based on data rather than hunches, looking for root causes of problems rather than reacting to superficial symptoms, and seeking permanent solutions rather than relying on quick fixes (Scholtes, 1988). Through the use of flowcharts, Pareto charts[1], cause and effect diagrams, opera-

tional definitions, and various other charting mechanisms, the CQI process focuses on systematic monitoring, evaluation, and improvement of the effectiveness and efficiency of work procedures rather than on inspection of the finished product (Chowanec, 1994). Constant assessment, through reliable and valid feedback mechanisms, allows processes to be analyzed and improved. Both outcomes and processes need to be measured in order for perform-

---

[1]A Pareto chart is a series of bars whose heights reflect the frequency or impact of problems (Scholtes, 1988).

Table 14-6. Dimensions of Performance

1. DOING THE RIGHT THING	
The *efficacy* of the procedure or treatment in relation to the patient's condition	• The degree to which the patient's care and services have been shown to accomplish the desired or projected outcome(s)
The *appropriateness* of a specific test, procedure, or service to meet the patient's needs	• The degree to which the care and services provided are relevant to the patient's clinical needs, given the current state of knowledge
2. DOING THE RIGHT THING WELL	
The *availability* of a needed test, procedure, treatment, or service to the patient who needs it	• The degree to which appropriate care and services are available to meet the patient's needs
The *timeliness* with which a needed test, procedure, treatment, or service is provided to the patient	• The degree to which the care and services are provided to the patient at the most beneficial or necessary time
The *effectiveness* with which tests, procedures, treatment, and services are provided	• The degree to which the care and services are provided in the correct manner, given the current state of knowledge, to achieve the desired or projected outcome for the patient
The *continuity* of the services provided to the patient with respect to the other services, practitioners, and providers and over time	• The degree to which the patient's care is coordinated among disciplines, among organizations, and over time
The *safety* of the patient and others to whom the services are provided	• The degree to which the risk of an intervention and risk in the care environment are reduced for the patient and others, including the health care provider
The *efficiency* with which care and services are provided	• The relationship between the outcomes (results of care) and the resources used to deliver patient care and services
The *respect and caring* with which care and services are provided	• The degree to which those providing care and services do so with sensitivity and respect for the patient's needs, expectations, and individual differences • The degree to which the patient or a designee is involved in his or her own care and service decisions

Source: From *Comprehensive Accreditation Manual for Long Term Care 1998–1999* by Joint Commission on Accreditation of Healthcare Organizations [JCAHO], 1998. Retrieved February, 14, 2001, from the World Wide Web: *http://www.jcaho.org/ standard/ltc-pi.html*

ance improvement. A list of the dimensions of performance is provided in Table 14–6.

▶ *CQI is organized around patient care, not organization structure.* With health care professionals losing their autonomy to managed care and the influence of rising health care costs, it is easy for them to lose sight of the basic principal of health care: care for the patient. As mentioned earlier, very rarely is only one department involved in patient care. It should only make sense that evaluation of care be conducted by a multidisciplinary team. Quality assurance encourages an individual department to monitor the quality of care provided by that department. CQI proposes that those involved in the care of the patient should also together be involved in the review of that care (O'Leary, 1993). This approach also lessens the practice of finger-pointing and blaming certain departments. Each team member involved in a client's care needs to consider herself or himself a vital link in the provision of quality care. In fact, Berwick, Godfrey, and Roessner (1990) noted that each employee in an organization has a "triple role" of customer, processor, and supplier. When assessing a patient through a chart review, an occupational therapist is a "customer" of the professional who has recorded information in the chart. While using this information in developing a treatment activity, the occupational therapist is considered a "processor." When working with the client on the treatment activity, the occupational therapist takes on the role of "supplier." With all of these processes occurring in the varying roles of professionals, time and resources are wasted in looking for faults in the individual practitioners rather than processes.

▶ *Is QA still needed?* Although QA has all but disappeared from JCAHO literature, its role in health care should not be eliminated. Credentialing, licensure, and practice standards continue to ensure that professionals have achieved a certain level of education and the abilities necessary for practice. QA continues to identify the outliers of performance (Booth, 1993), and coupled with CQI activities, can assist with evaluation and resolution of individual performance. Schyve and Prevost (1990), stated that

> As we are learning to master the methods of quality assurance, a new conceptual approach focused on quality improvement is being advocated. But this new approach is not a derailment for health care practitioners committed to improve patient care quality. Rather, it is a progressive step that builds upon the concepts and methods of quality assurance. Whereas quality assurance tends to focus on correcting problems in patient care quality—especially individual practitioners' problems—quality improvement focuses on finding opportunities to improve quality by changing systems as well as individual practitioner behavior. (p. 61)

According to Booth (1993), a sound appreciation and consistent application of the principles of QA remain the technical bedrock on which the more "spiritual" aspects of quality improvement can flourish. Adoption of QI methods should not diminish the use of QA activities. Evaluation of structure, process, and outcome will continue to be necessary, and the results from these evaluations can be used in CQI activities.

▶ *CQI, OT, and mental health.* According to Sluyter (1996), the principles and techniques of CQI have only recently been applied to the field of mental health. Despite the few reports regarding CQI in mental health settings, Sluyter (1996) analyzed CQI along cultural, technical, strategic, and structural dimensions in 10 mental health centers and found that the philosophy and techniques of CQI are as applicable to the mental health sector as they are to health care in general. The Texas Department of Mental Health and Mental Retardation was one of the first major state agencies using a system-wide effort to implement CQI as a resolution to a major lawsuit (Rago & Gilbert, 1996). According to Rago and Gilbert (1996), the CQI program (a) enhanced understanding of treatment and service delivery as a system, (b) provided the basis for using data to support decision-making at all levels within the hospital and across hospitals, (c) formally defined the care staff's role in the organizational structure with regard to the quality of services and associated decision-making, and (d) provided a basis for the administrator to use numeric goals.

McFarland, Harmann, Lhotak, and Wieselthier (1996) recommend asking the following questions prior to assessing need for a CQI program:

> Does your organization embrace CQI philosophically? Is customer-focused quality and value viewed as a strategic concept? Is there a strong future orientation and willingness to make long term commitments to stakeholders? Are people (especially the leadership) open to intensive critique? (p. 42)

Rago and Gilbert (1996) introduced the Quality System Oversight (QSO) CQI program for system-wide mental health hospitals. McFarland, Harmann, Lhotak, and Wieselthier (1996) provide a CQI program for a community mental health center based on Malcolm Baldrige National Quality Award Criteria. Elliot (1996) recommended using a double loop learning process to continuously evaluate the CQI process once it is in place.

Examination of CQI and its basic tenets indicates that its philosophies are not too estranged from some of the philosophies incorporated into occupational therapist's daily practice. With the increasing focus on the quality of care provided and CQI and performance measures, it is important to remember why all of this is taking place: People are in need of good mental health care and employees are in need of a healthy work environment. Only through the complete teamwork of a mental health care organization and investment in improving quality can employees, clients, and the entire organization benefit. The CQI philosophy, when followed appropriately, can provide a means of achieving this goal of excellence in performance.

REIMBURSEMENTS, FEDERAL ENTITLEMENTS, AND OCCUPATIONAL THERAPY COVERAGE[2]

Medicare

Medicare was established under Title XVII of the Social Security Act in 1965.

Beneficiaries: People who are 65 years of age or older, some people under age 65 who have disabilities, and people with end-stage renal disease (permanent kidney failure that is treated with dialysis or a transplant). Mental health beneficiaries are required to have a specific psychiatric diagnosis.

Settings: Hospital inpatient and outpatient settings, skilled nursing facilities, physician's

---

[2]Much of this material has been obtained from Scott and Somers (1992) and Goldman and Megra (1997).

offices, private practice, outpatient rehabilitation facilities, hospices, rehabilitation agencies, and home health agencies

Part A: The Hospital Insurance Program pays for hospital inpatient, skilled nursing facility, home health care, and hospice care. Medicare payments to hospitals for inpatient treatment are made via diagnostic related group (DRG) payments. The DRG system disburses a predetermined fixed sum to hospitals for each discharged patient based on the DRG into which the patient is coded. Mental health coverage provided by free standing psychiatric hospitals is exempt from the DRG system. In lieu of DRG, mental health hospitals and mental health units in acute care general hospitals, are reimbursed on a retrospective basis based on reasonable costs incurred under the Congressional Tax Equity and Fiscal Responsibility Act (TEFRA) methodology. Payment for psychiatric hospitalization only occurs when treatment is "active." Active treatments are those which can be expected to improve a patient's condition. Mental health occupational therapy is covered under the provision that requires hospitals to have a sufficient number of qualified therapists to provide comprehensive therapeutic activities for psychiatric inpatients. Coverage is limited to 190 days over the life of the beneficiary.

Part B: The Supplementary Medical Insurance Program pays for medical and other services (e.g., durable medical equipment & surgical supplies), hospital outpatient, physician, and other professional services, clinical laboratory services, and home health care. Mental health occupational therapy is covered for patients with a psychiatric diagnosis meeting specific conditions from the American Psychiatric Association's *Diagnostic and Statistical Manual of Mental Disorders* (DSM–IV, APA, 1994). Reimbursement for services is limited to 62.5 percent of actual expenses incurred in a calendar year.

Reimbursement for services provided by a Medicare-certified occupational therapist in independent practice is determined by a fee schedule measuring "resource-based relative value scale . . . [which] . . . assigns relative values for work, office expense, and malpractice, adjusted for geographic variations in cost, and converted to a dollar amount by a conversion factor" (American Psychiatric Association, 1995). Medicare Part B also covers partial hospitalizations that are intensive and comprehensive outpatient mental health programs. The intent of partial hospitalization is to prevent relapse or inpatient hospitalization for individuals who do not require 24-hour care, have adequate support systems outside the hospital setting, have a psychiatric diagnosis, and are not judged to be dangerous to self or others. Occupational therapy services, requiring the skills of a qualified occupational therapist, are covered if the services provided are reasonable and necessary for treatment of the patient's conditions and are reasonably expected to improve or maintain the patient's condition and functional level. Fiscal intermediaries who have differing policies regarding reimbursement for mental health occupational therapy vary from state to state. A physician is required to prescribe, supervise, and review a patient's individual treatment plan, which is developed by the entire treatment team with input from the patient.

Civilian Health and Medical Program of the Uniformed Services (CHAMPUS)

CHAMPUS is the U.S. Department of Defense program of health care.

Beneficiaries: Dependents of active duty armed forces members and retired armed forces members

Settings: Inpatient and outpatient hospitals

CHAMPUS shares costs of health care with civilian providers. Civilian coverage for dependents precedes CHAMPUS. CHAMPUS also pays for services through fiscal intermediaries. Inpatient and outpatient mental heath care is provided under the basic program of CHAMPUS. Mental health occupational therapy services are obtained through civilian providers and are covered if deemed medically necessary by a supervising physician and intended to help the patient overcome or compensate for a disability resulting from an illness, injury, or the effects of a CHAMPUS-covered condition. Occupational therapists are required to be employees of providers authorized by CHAMPUS and must render services in connection with CHAMPUS organized care.

Federal Employees Health Benefit Program

Beneficiaries: Federal government employees and retirees

Settings: Varying

This program is implemented by various private plans and is subject to only general federal laws and regulations regarding services provided (surgical, medical, hospital, etc.). Mental health occupational therapy varies from plan to plan.

Medicaid

This program was established under Title XIX of the Social Security Act.

Beneficiaries: Certain groups of low-income persons. Some mandatory Medicaid eligibility groups are: low-income families with children who meet certain of the eligibility requirements in the State's AFDC plan in effect on July 16, 1996; Supplemental Security Income (SSI)

recipients (or in states using more restrictive criteria—persons who are aged, blind, disabled); infants born to Medicaid-eligible pregnant women; children under age 6 and pregnant women whose family income is at or below 133 percent of the federal poverty level; recipients of adoption assistance and foster care under Title IV-E of the Social Security Act; Medicare beneficiaries who have low income and limited resources; special protected groups who may keep Medicaid for a period of time (HCFA, 1999). This is administered by states within federal guidelines pertaining to eligibility, types and range of services, payment levels for services, and administrative operating procedures.

Settings (can vary in different states): Inpatient hospital services, nursing homes, rural health clinics, outpatient hospitals, home health services, medical day treatment settings, hospice, and school medical services

Psychosocial occupational therapy is covered under optional Medicaid services. Federal regulations define the types of services states are required to provide to categorically and medically needy Medicaid beneficiaries and selected optional services states may include in their Medicaid programs (Goldman & Megna, 1997). Coverage varies from state to state.

Private Payment Insurance Systems

Beneficiaries: Employees and consumers of such systems

Settings: Varying

There are thousands of private health insurance systems in the United States. Coverage varies from provider to provider. State insurance codes guide coverage requirements for both non-profit and profit private health plans. Federal standards established in the Employee Retirement Income Security Act (ERISA) govern the self-funded plans that are provided by employers. There are also many plans under Blue Cross/Blue Shield that are quasi-independent. Standards are not set by a sole governing body, which causes coverage to vary from state to state.

Prepaid Health Plans, Health Maintenance Organizations (HMOs), or Preferred Provider Organizations (PPOs)

Beneficiaries: Enrolled members
Settings: Varying

Services are limited to a geographical area and with PPOs, certain health providers. HMOs are governed by federal regulations and often enroll Medicare beneficiaries. Mental health care services provided to Medicare beneficiaries by HMOs are subject to regulations of Medicare. Services covered by HMOs and PPOs will vary from program to program.

REFERENCES

Affeldt, J. E., Roberts, J. S., & Walczak, R. M. (1983). Quality assurance—Its origin, status, and future direction: A JCAH perspective. *Evaluation and Health Professions, 7,* 45–255.

Allen, C. (1985). *Occupational therapy for psychiatric diseases: Measurement and management of cognitive disabilities.* Boston: Little, Brown.

American Occupational Therapy Association (AOTA). (1992). Standards of practice for occupational therapy. *American Journal of Occupational Therapy, 46,* 1082–1085.

American Psychiatric Association. (APA). (1994). *The diagnostic and statistical manual of mental disorders.* Washington, DC: Author.

American Psychiatric Association. (1995). *Medicare and mental health care: Problems and prospects for change.* Washington, DC: Author.

"Answering Service." (1980). *Quality Review Bulletin, 6*(4).

Baum, C. (1972). A management tool: The departmental audit. *The American Journal of Occupational Therapy, 26*(6), 299–301.

Bent, R. J. (1982). The quality assurance process as a management method for psychology training programs. *Professional Psychology, 13,* 98–104.

Bent, R. J. (1988). Education for quality assurance. In G. Stricker & A. R. Rodriguez (Eds.), *Handbook of quality assurance in mental health.* New York: Plenum.

Berwick, D. M., Godfrey, A.B., & Roessner, J. (1990). *Curing health care: New strategies for quality improvement.* San Francisco, CA: Jossey-Bass.

Booth, F. V. (1993). ABC's of quality assurance. *Critical Care Management, 9*(3), 477–489.

Chowanec, G. D. (1994). Continuous quality improvement: Conceptual foundations and application to mental health care. *Hospital and Community Psychiatry, 45*(8), 789–793.

Davis, L. (1960). *Fellowship of surgeons: A history of the American college of surgeons.* Springfield, IL: Charles C. Thomas.

Dean, J., & Zarn, A. (1996, August). *Treatment planning process for partial hospitalization programs.* Paper presented at the annual conference of the Association for Ambulatory Behavioral Healthcare, Minneapolis, MN.

Deming, W. E. (1982). *Quality, productivity, and competitive position.* Cambridge: Massachusetts Institute of Technology, Center for Advanced Engineering Study.

Donabedian, A. (1980). *Explorations in quality assessment and monitoring* (Vol. 1). Ann Arbor, MI: Health Administration Press.

Donabedian, A. (1982). *Explorations in quality assessment and monitoring* (Vol. 2). Ann Arbor, MI: Health Administration Press.

Ellenberger, H. F. (1974). Psychiatry from ancient to modern times. In S. Arieti (Ed.), *American handbook of psychiatry. Vol 1: The foundation of psychiatry* (2nd ed., pp. 3–27). New York: Basic Books.

Elliot, R .L. (1996). Double loop learning and the quality of quality improvement. *Journal on Quality Improvement, 22*(1), 59–66.

Flexner, A. (1910). *Medical education in the United States and Canada: A report to the Carnegie Foundation for the Advancement of Teaching* (Bulletin No. 4). New York: Carnegie Foundation.

Folstein, M. F., Folstein, S. E., & McHugh, P. R. (1975). Mini–mental state: A practical method for grading the cognitive state of patients for the clinician. *Journal of Psychiatric Research, 12,* 189–198.

Gillem, T. R. (1988). Deming's 14 points and hospital quality: Responding to the consumer's demand for the best value health care. *Journal of Nursing Quality Assurance, 2,* 70–78.

Gillette, N. P. (1982). Nationally speaking—A data base for occupational therapy: Documentation through research. *American Journal of Occupational Therapy, 36,* 499–501.

Goldman, A., & Megna, R. (1997). *Medical assistance program.* Madison: Wisconsin Legislative Bureau.

Graham, N. (1982). Historical perspective and regulations. In N. Graham (Ed.), *Quality assurance in hospitals* (pp. 3–13). Rockville, MD: Aspen.

Joe, B. E. (1992). Quality assurance. In J. Bair & M. Gray (Eds.), *The occupational therapy manager* (pp. 251–258). Rockville, MD: American Occupational Therapy Association.

Joint Commission on Accreditation of Healthcare Organizations (JCAHO). (1980). *The QA guide.* Chicago: Author.

Joint Commission on Accreditation of Healthcare Organizations. (1990). *Primer on indicator development and application.* Oakbrook Terrance, IL: Author.

Joint Commission on Accreditation of Healthcare Organizations (JCAHO). (1991). *An introduction to quality improvement in health care.* Oakbrook Terrace, IL: Author.

Joint Commission on Accreditation of Healthcare Organizations. (1997). *Hospital accreditation standards.* Oakbrook Terrace, IL: Author.

Joint Commission on Accreditation of Healthcare Organizations. (1998). *Comprehensive Accreditation Manual for Long Term Care 1998–1999.* Oakbrook Terrace, IL: Author. Retrieved February 14, 2001, from the World Wide Web: *http://www.jcaho.org/standard/ltc-pi.html*

Joint Commission on Accreditation of Healthcare Organizations. (1999). *Automated comprehensive accreditation manual for hospitals. The official handbook.* Oakbrook Terrace, IL: Author.

Koska, M. T. (1991). New JCAHO standards emphasize continuous quality improvement. *Hospitals, 65*(15), 41–42.

Langsley, D. G. (1980). Quality assurance in psychiatric treatment. *National Association of Private Psychiatric Hospitals Journal, 11,* 13–17.

Lavendar, A., Leiper, R., Pilling, S., & Clifford, P. (1994). Quality assurance in mental health: The QUARTZ system. *British Journal of Clinical Psychology, 33,* 451–467.

Lynch, J. J., & Stein, F. (1986). Evaluating occupational therapy psychiatric care through medical documentation. *Occupational Therapy in Mental Health, 6*(3), 53–66.

McAninch, M. (1984). Quality assurance in the residential and outpatient mental health setting. *Quality Review Bulletin, 10*(6), 181–185.

McFarland, D., Harmann, L., Lhotak, C., & Wieselthier, V. F. (1996). The quest for TQM in a community mental health center: Using the Baldrige criteria as a framework. *Journal on Quality Improvement, 22*(1), 37–47.

National Board for Certification in Occupational Therapy (NBCOT). (1996). *National Board for Certification in Occupational Therapy: What it is. What it does.* Gaithersburg, MD: Author.

O'Leary, D. S. (1993). The measurement mandate: Report card day is coming . . . Almost every reform proposal includes a requirement for measuring performance outcomes and report performance information. *Joint Commission Journal on Quality Improvement, 19,* 487–491.

O'Leary, D. S., & O'Leary, M. R. (1992). *From quality assurance to quality improvement.* Oakbrook Terrace, IL: Joint Commission on Accreditation of Healthcare Organizations.

Ostrow, P. C., Williamson, J. W., & Joe, B . E. (1983). *Quality assurance primer.* Rockville, MD: American Occupational Therapy Association.

Ottenbacher, K. J., & Cusick, A. (1989). Goal attainment scaling as a method of clinical service evaluation. *The American Journal of Occupational Therapy, 44*(6), 519–525.

Ottenbacher, K. J., & Cusick, A. (1993). Diminutive versus evaluative assessment; some observations on goal attainment scaling. *The American Journal of Occupational Therapy, 47*(4), 349–354.

Rago, B., & Gilbert, D. A. (1996). QI as a resolution to a major lawsuit. *Journal on Quality Improvement, 22*(1), 48–57.

Rodriguez, A. R. (1988). An introduction to quality assurance in mental health. In G. Stricker & A. R. Rodriguez (Eds.), *Handbook of quality assurance in mental health.* New York: Plenum.

Scholtes, P. R. (1988). *The team handbook: How to use teams to improve quality.* Madison, WI: Joiner.

Schyve, P. M., & Prevost, J. A. (1990). From quality assurance to quality improvement. *Psychiatric Clinics of North America, 13*, 61–71.

Scott, S. J., & Somers, F. P. (1992). Payment for occupational therapy services. In J. Bair & M. Gray (Eds.), *The occupational therapy manager* (pp. 317–332). Rockville, MD: American Association of Occupational Therapy.

Siegel, C., & Fischer, S. K. (1981). *Psychiatric records in mental health care.* New York: Brunner/Mazel.

Sluyter, G. V. (1996). Application of TQM to mental health: Lessons from ten mental health centers. *Journal on Quality Improvement, 22*(1), 67–75.

Smith, A., Cardillo, J. E., Smith, S. C., & Amezaga, A. M. (1998). Improvement scaling (rehabilitation version). A new approach to measuring progress of patients in achieving their individual rehabilitation goals. *Medical Care, 36*(3), 333–347.

Sperry, L. (1997). Treatment outcomes: An overview. *Psychiatric Annals, 27*(2), 95–99.

Stein, F. (1985). *Documentation and quality assurance in psychiatric occupational therapy.* Unpublished manuscript. (Available through F. Stein, University of South Dakota, Department of Occupational Therapy, 414 E. Clark St., Vermillion, SD 57069)

Thomson, L. K. (1992). T*he Kohlman Evaluation of Living Skills* (KELS; 3rd ed.). Rockville, MD: American Occupational Therapy Association.

Thomson, L. K., & Foto, M. (1995). Elements of clinical documentation (revision). *The American Journal of Occupational Therapy, 49*, 1032–1035.

U.S. Department of Health, Education, and Welfare. (1977). *Credentialing health manpower.* (Publication No. (05)77-50057). Washington, DC: Government Printing Office.

Weed, L. L. (1964). Medical records, patient care and medical education. *Irish Journal of Medical Science, 6*, 271–282.

Wells, K. B., & Brooks, R. H. (1988). Historical trends in quality assurance for mental health services. In G. Stricker & A. R. Rodriguez (Eds.), *Handbook of quality assurance in mental health* (pp. 39–63). New York: Plenum.

West, W. L. (1967). The 1967 Eleanor Clark Slagle Lecture: Professional Responsibility in times of change. *The American Journal of Occupational Therapy, 22*(1), 9–15.

Williamson, J. W., Bard, D. M., Fee, E., Garg, M. L., Hudson, J. I., Ingbar, M. L., Jesse, W. F., Karst, D. R., Nevins, M. M., Noren, J., Stritter, S. T., & Wilson, R. (1982). *Teaching quality assurance and cost containment in health care.* San Francisco: Jossey-Bass.

Zusman, J. (1988). Quality assurance in mental health care. *Hospital and Community Psychiatry, 29*, 1286–1290.

CHAPTER

15

Evaluating and Designing Clinical Research Studies[1]

> *One should not be too ready to embrace a conjecture that comes into the mind; it must be submitted to most careful scrutiny before being accepted even as a tentative hypothesis, for once an opinion has been formed, it is more difficult to think of alternatives.*
>
> — William Ian Beardmore Beveridge (1950), *The Art of Scientific Investigation*, p. 69.

Operational Learning Objectives

By the end of this chapter, the learner will:

1. Differentiate research as a scientific task from clinical practice.

2. Distinguish between applied and basic research.

3. Generate a research question related to the learner's area of interest in clinical practice.

4. Critically evaluate the published literature in psychosocial occupational therapy.

5. Identify the factors in treatment that potentially can affect outcome.

6. Identify external variables that need to be controlled in clinical research.

7. Outline a protocol for clinical research using single-subject or group design.

---

[1]Portions of this chapter are based on "Evaluating Psychiatric Treatment Methods through Clinical Trials Research" by F. Stein (1980) and *Clinical Research in Occupational Therapy* (4th ed.) by F. Stein and S. K. Cutler (2000).

8. Design a subject informed consent form that is consistent with the ethics of human research.

RESEARCH IN PSYCHOSOCIAL OCCUPATIONAL THERAPY

Applied Versus Basic Research

As an applied profession occupational therapy traditionally has relied on knowledge generated from research findings in the natural and social sciences. In a way occupational therapy has rested on the foundation of knowledge built through centuries of laboratory and clinical investigations. The practice of psychosocial occupational therapy has direct links with the fields of psychology, sociology, and psychiatry. Research findings in the social sciences often directly impact on the practice of occupational therapy. For example, if a psychological researcher finds that a behavior modification program is effective in teaching social skills in students with behavior disorders, this information can be further tested by occupational therapists in teaching social skills activities to a group of clients. Research provides the knowledge base for clinical practice.

▶ What is research?

▶ What is the difference between applied and basic research?

▶ How does research relate to clinical practice?

▶ What is the relationship between research and the practice of psychosocial occupational therapy?

▶ What topics are appropriate for occupational therapists to investigate?

▶ How can published research be critically evaluated and incorporated into clinical practice?

Research is the systematic and objective investigation into a topic, by stating a hypothesis or guiding question and collecting primary data (Stein, 1976). It includes quantitative and qualitative designs. As a generalization we can state with a fair amount of confidence that effective clinical practice rests on the findings of valid clinical research. Research can be equated with the scientific method that is directed at the discovery of knowledge. The scientific method, the essential ingredient of research, contains seven steps that the researcher performs: (a) asking a feasible question, (b) examining previous literature, (c) stating an hypothesis or guiding question, (d) designing an objective methodology, (e) collecting data, (f) analyzing the results, and (g) stating the conclusions. Both applied and basic research use the scientific method in discovering new knowledge. The difference lies in the focus of the investigation.

In applied research the investigator chooses research topics that are related to human problems with the results being directly aimed at solving these problems. For example, the occupational therapist as an applied researcher, can be concerned with the problems that clients with psychosocial disorders may have in self-regulating their feelings, taking responsibility for their own self-care, being able to work, engaging in leisure-time activities, interacting with others, and actualizing their potentialities. These are applied problems, which are research topics of direct interest to the clinical practitioner.

The applied researcher can attack these problems from a number of directions, depending on the research objectives. The researcher may be interested in developing a new evaluation instrument for measuring stress management or assessing the client's degree of involvement in leisure activities. Another research approach may involve designing a survey of families of children with autism with the research objective of evaluating the interactions between the family members and the child with autism. Still another example may involve determining the efficacy of using biofeedback therapy in reducing anxiety with individuals who are depressed.

In basic or pure research, the investigator raises questions that are not necessarily directly related to clinical application. For example, the basic researcher may be interested in the neurophysiology of the limbic system, the mechanisms of neurotransmitters, the reactions of the immune system to stress in animal models, or the critical stages of play in typical children. The focus of basic research in the natural or social sciences is the acquisition of knowledge that underlies human or animal functions. These research questions usually relate to structure, mechanisms, and typical developmental landmarks. Although the results of basic research may not have direct application, they do lay the foundation for applied research and, in the long run, may affect practice.

Both applied and basic research efforts are appropriate for the researcher in occupational therapy. Often the distinction between applied and basic research is blurred. Some studies have both an applied and a basic research focus. This is probably a positive characteristic. For example, a researcher interested in the development of play behavior in typical children may also be interested in the use of play with children with behavior disorders as a means of facilitating the acquisition of social skills. In this example, the researcher would investigate the developmental landmarks related to the acquisition of play behavior in typical children as the basis of devising a hierarchical treatment program that facilitates social skills through play behavior.

GENERATING RESEARCH IN PSYCHOSOCIAL OCCUPATIONAL THERAPY

How does the clinician generate a research problem? The first stage in research is to ask a question. Research questions in psychosocial occupational therapy, for example, can relate to the design of a new test to evaluate independent living skills or to determine whether a treatment method is effective. Generating a research question comes about from identifying a gap in knowledge. For example, psychiatric researchers continually evaluate new treatment approaches to determine their effectiveness. Throughout the history of psychiatry, somatic techniques, psychotherapeutic approaches, and sociological interventions have been tried, evaluated, and many times discarded. In the past, psychiatric researchers have raised the following questions:

▶ Is electroconvulsive therapy effective in reducing the symptoms of depression?

▶ Is psychoanalytic psychotherapy effective in increasing the self-esteem of clients with schizophrenia?

▶ Is lithium effective with individuals with manic depression?

▶ Is aversive therapy effective in increasing the communication skills of children with autism?

▶ Is the humanist approach the most effective model to use when working with children with conduct disorders?

▶ Are Ritalin® or other stimulants effective in reducing symptoms of hyperactivity or inattention in individuals with ADHD?

Characteristics of a Research Study

A good research study has the following characteristics:

▶ The research question is understandable. The terms used in the research question conform to accepted terminology of the discipline (e.g., DSM–IV [APA, 1994], Uniform Terminology Application to Practice [AOTA, 1994], or contemporary usage in clinical practice). This is especially important in accurately identifying diagnostic groups, psychological tests, treatment techniques, and outcome criteria.

▶ The research question is relevant to clinical practice. A preliminary search of the research literature should be undertaken to locate related studies. The result of the preliminary research should establish the relevancy of the research question.

▶ The outcome variables or therapeutic goals in the research study are measurable. For example, standardized tests are used to measure a desired outcome such as increased self-esteem, decreased anxiety, or increased communication skills.

▶ Clinical observations provide supportive evidence for the research questions that are generated. For example, the psychosocial occupational therapist may observe that clients with schizophrenia have difficulty initiating and establishing friendships. This observation can generate the following research questions: Do adults with schizophrenia have fewer friendships than typical adults? How can the occupational therapist increase the social skills of individuals with schizophrenia?

▶ The research question leads into a feasible methodology. From the research question, the investigator will be able to select participants, identify a test to measure outcome, and design a procedure that will control for systematic extraneous variables (e.g., gender, intelligence, and education).

The next step in generating a research topic is to become familiar with the background literature. The researcher strives to become an expert in the area by examining primary research sources related to the topic. A literature search is carried out to identify relevant journal articles. It is critical, in this process, that the researcher evaluate the internal and external validity of the study. This is done by evaluating the

▶ objectivity of the researcher

▶ manner in which the variables were controlled

▶ methodology for selecting participants

▶ use of a control group

▶ statistical analyses performed on the results.

Clinical Research

Evaluation of psychosocial treatment is a fertile area for clinical researchers in occupational therapy. Few comprehensive studies have analyzed treatment techniques in depth. As a result, there are controversies in the selection of treatment techniques for individuals with psychosocial dysfunction. For example, controversy still exists on the efficacy of psychotherapeutic techniques (e.g., psychoanalysis, choice or use of medications, application of electroconvulsive therapies, use of behavior modification techniques, and sensory-integration therapy). Why do these controversies continue?

First, there have been disagreements on a conceptual level in identifying, diagnosing, and treating mental illness. On one extreme, individuals believe that mental illness is not a disease, but a social and cultural discrepancy (Laing, 1967; Szasz, 1974). On the other hand, others believe that mental illness is either (a) a disease that can be caused by an organic brain dysfunction, such as viral infection (Torrey,

1991) or structural anomaly (Hedaya, 1996). A third group considers mental illness to be a diathesis-stress disorder, which posits that individuals have a genetic predisposition and vulnerability and stress precipitates episodes of the disorder (Neuchterlein & Dawson, 1984; Norman & Malla, 1993; Sapolsky, 1998). Theorists have differed in their approaches to psychiatry when advocating specific treatment techniques for the broad area of mental illness. Many times, researchers have failed to acknowledge the individual needs of the client and the differential effects of treatment. For example, researchers apply knowledge to a diagnostic group, such as personality disorders, without recognizing the individual differences among subjects.

The second reason for the controversies in psychiatric rehabilitation is the lack of comprehensive studies to validate practice. Much of the research in psychosocial practice is fixed at a two-variable research stage model in which researchers are still looking for the single cause of mental illness and the "magic bullet cure" (e.g., the overuse of Prozac® in treating individuals with depression). If progress is to occur in psychiatric rehabilitation, in-depth studies using multifactorial designs to measure treatment effectiveness must be initiated.

A holistic view in investigating psychiatric treatment methods is necessary to avoid the trap of two-variable research that lacks an analysis of interactional effects. For example, suppose depression is the result of an interaction between genetics, family dynamics, biological structure and ineffective methods to regulate stress. An investigator studying exclusively the relationship between genetics and depression produces mixed results because he or she has not taken the other major factors into account. He or she will not be able to generalize results for clients with depression. The following dia-

gram hypothetically illustrates the interactions among the three independent variables (genetics, family dynamics, stress management) and the dependent variable (diagnosis of depression). Individuals who have positive family dynamics and self-regulation are least likely to develop episodic depression even if they have a genetic vulnerability factor. Depression would have a high probability of occurring if there is an interaction among the three variables, genetic predisposition for depression, negative family dysfunction, and ineffective stress management.

	Ability to Self-regulate Stress	Inability to Self-regulate Stress
Positive Family Dynamics	Lowest depressive risk	
Negative Family Dynamics		Highest depressive risk

This hypothetical example shows the complex factors involved in analyzing the etiology of a mental illness. It is highly probable that many psychiatric illnesses result from this type of interactional pattern. However, only through painstaking research will it be possible to identify interactional effects.

Models of Clinical Research

In carrying out research in psychosocial occupational therapy, a number of research models can be implemented (Stein & Cutler, 1996; 2000). Stein and Cutler described eight models for clinical research:

I. *Experimental (Prospective Design)*: In this design, the researcher manipulates the causes and examines the effects in a highly controlled setting. Interactional effects of variables can be observed empirically. For example, the researcher compares the effectiveness of social skills training versus arts and crafts in reducing psychotic symptoms.

II. *Methodological*: Measuring instruments, curriculum, or therapeutic procedures and approaches are constructed. Innovated technology in allied health, rehabilitation, or special education become important in this model. For example, a clinician develops an instrument to identify leisure interests to use with individuals with psychosocial disorders.

III. *Evaluation*: The research performs a critical analysis of health care, delivery systems, or educational programs. Thus, the effectiveness of systems and treatment programs are objectively assessed. For example, the researcher evaluates the effectiveness of a forensic psychiatry unit that includes occupational therapy.

IV. *Heuristic*: In this model, the researcher is interested in discovering possible causative factors in chronic disabilities, and analysis of time, space, and cost factors in treatment. Further research can be generated by identifying significant variables. For example, the investigator seeks to identify environmental factors in a nursing home that encourage clients' involvement in activities.

V. *Correlational (Retrospective Design)*: This model is used to test relationships between nonmanipulated variables in order to gain knowledge of factors that are assumed to have an associational relationship. For example, the researcher identifies factors that are related to the onset of symptoms associated with ADHD.

VI. *Clinical or Qualitative*: In-depth study of individuals, groups, or systems to understand the underlying dynamics that affect them. For example, the clinician examines how individuals with schizophrenia adjust to changes in work environments.

VII. *Survey*: Researchers using this model describe general characteristics of homogenous populations. For example, the clinician surveys individuals with depression to determine how they deal with stress.

VIII. *Historical*: Past events are reconstructed and investigated using primary sources to understand contemporary problems. The researcher examines the history of occupational therapy in psychosocial practice by identifying individuals and events that impacted present-day practice.

In this chapter, the emphasis is on retrospective and prospective single-subject design.

CRITIQUE OF CLINICAL RESEARCH STUDIES

When evaluating the validity of research studies, the following questions are proposed.

I. Title

   A. Was the target population identified (e.g., individuals with borderline personality)?

   B. What treatment methods (independent variables) were compared (e.g., stress management training, social skills training, prescriptive exercise)?

   C. What was the outcome (dependent variables) or desired improvement (e.g., decrease in anxiety or hyperactivity, increase in social skills or working ability)?

II. Need for the Study

   A. What was the significance of the problem related to clinical practice (e.g., provides a treatment protocol for individuals in forensic units)?

B. What was the implied intention of the researcher in evaluating the effectiveness of a specific treatment method (e.g., document effectiveness for reimbursement)?

C. What was the justification for the study (e.g., to determine if a program should be continued or eliminated)?

III. Literature Review

A. Were the landmark studies cited?

B. Were the references current (e.g., within last 5 years)?

C. Did the literature review support the need for the study?

D. What was the incidence and prevalence of the psychosocial disorder being studied?

E. Was the literature review exhaustive (e.g., use of research studies from a variety of journals, objective by using studies from different perspectives)?

F. What retrieval methods were used in identifying literature (e.g., MEDLINE, CINAHL, OT databases, PsychLit)?

IV. Methodology

A. Were the participants a representative sample of a target population?

B. Was there a comparative control group?

C. Were reliable and valid tests used in the study?

D. Can the research procedure be replicated?

E. Was the hypothesis clearly stated or was there a guiding question?

F. Was an informed consent procedure used before collecting data?

V. Results

A. How were data collected?

B. What statistical techniques were used to analyze data?

C. How were data displayed (e.g., charts, figures, tables)?

VI. Conclusion

A. Were the conclusions consistent with statistical results?

B. Were the results of the study consistent with previous literature?

C. Were limitations of methodology identified?

D. Can results be applied to clinical practice?

E. Did the investigators suggest further research studies?

SINGLE-SUBJECT DESIGN

Single-subject research can provide an objective strategy for clinicians to compare and validate the effectiveness of treatment methods. In single-subject research, the therapist carefully documents the effects of treatment in a client over a period of time. Comparable treatment methods can be alternated in blocks of time. For example, a treatment is used for a 3-week period and the outcome of the treatment method is evaluated. Then a different treatment is used with the same client for another 3-week period, and the outcome is evaluated. The client's improvement for both treatments are correlated.

One method for carrying out single-subject designs without setting up experimental and control groups beforehand is to alternate treatment methods randomly for clients as they are admitted to a clinical service. Another method is for the therapist to alternate treatment methods for a specific client with the client serving as his or her own control. When a therapist alternates treatment techniques, the treatment techniques selected should be appropriate and based on the occupational therapist's sound judgment.

In single-subject research, the therapist's major concern is with evaluating the effectiveness of a specific treatment method for a specific client. The therapist evaluates the client, defines behavioral objectives for treatment, applies the best treatment method, and then reevaluates the improvement the client has made at the time of discharge. The conclusion is that, if the client improved, then the treatment intervention was successful. If the treatment method is successful, the therapist assumes that the treatment method can be applied to similar clients. However, before one can generalize in this way, the research study should be replicated with clients with similar diagnoses to validate results.

It is also frequently suggested that one treatment method is better than other comparable methods in treating clients with similar diagnoses. Some therapists assume that the method can be applied to a wide range of clients, for example, applying sensory integration therapy with all children who are diagnosed with ADHD. Again, this must be confirmed by comparing the effectiveness of sensory integration with other methods. Another assumption that therapists hold is that the treatment method is the only factor in accounting for a client's improvement. Other factors that clinicians must examine if their results are to be considered valid are the client's motivation, therapist's relationships, environmental factors, and sensitivity of outcome measure. In addition, without a control group, there is also a question of whether improvement occurred because of the therapist's attention to the client (i.e., the Hawthorne effect).

Evaluation of Treatment and Treatment Outcome

Researchers and clinicians have various definitions of what improvement in a patient means. For the researcher, the dependent variable "improvement" is operationally defined and measurable, and the independent variables or treatment methods that caused the improvement are clearly identified. However, the therapist, working with clients every day, uses behavioral criteria for evaluating a client's progress. For example, these criteria may be ability to work, to be independent in self-care, to have less symptoms of a psychosocial disability, and to have more positive social skills. The clinician applies the results from individual case studies from his or her clinical practice to support or negate a method of treatment, whereas the researcher presents a controlled study relating the treatment methods to measurable variables. The discrepancy between the researcher and the therapist in their understanding of what constitutes treatment, what variables affect outcome, and what represents improvement, is critical in any discussion comparing a researcher with a clinician. Table 15–1 summarizes the differences between researchers and clinicians in evaluating treatment outcome.

The effects of interaction between the therapist and client, treatment method and client, and environmental context and client make it difficult for researchers to isolate the specific variables causing specific results. These relationships are schematically shown in Figure 15–1. Before the researcher can determine if one treatment method is more effective than another method, he or she must identify and control the possible extraneous variables that could influence the results. These four areas of influence include the client, the therapist, and the environmental context as well as the treatment method.

Table 15-1. Researcher–Clinician Comparison for Evaluating Treatment Outcome

Variables Affecting Outcome	Researcher	Clinician
Treatment technique	*Independent variables* (treatment method): experimental variable that is manipulated, operationally defined, and can be replicated in other studies.	Clinical method that can be modified, and adapted to the needs of the patient and the experiences of the therapist.
Other potential factors	*Systematic extraneous variables*, such as age, gender, and SES, which must be controlled by matching participants, making random assignments to treatment groups, or narrowing the scope of the treatment.	Individual factors in the client that account for the improvement in some and the regression or no improvement in others.
Assessment procedures	*Operational definition and measurement of improvement* (pre/post) after establishing criteria and controlling for the Hawthorne effect.	Clinical impression of client's progress based on the therapist's initial evaluation and subsequently observed changes.

Source: Adapted from *Clinical Research in Occupational Therapy* (4th ed.), by F. Stein and S. K. Cutler, 2000, p. 74, San Diego, Singular Publishing Group.

The researcher also must account for the interactional effects among variables. For example, a therapist with a penchant for order may be more effective using a cognitive behavioral treatment method than a therapist who, with a strong need to nurture, uses a client-centered method. A treatment method that is effective with one therapist may not be as effective with another therapist. The importance of therapist characteristics is recognized by clinicians. That is, a supervisor will assign clients to therapists based on the clinician's preferences. A therapist may, for example, prefer working with children, adults, males, females, or clients with certain diagnoses. Therapists' preferences for working with specific clients are usually indicative of personality variables. However, the self-selecting process of the therapists for a specific treatment method, a specific setting, or a designated diagnostic group may be limited by the therapist's education and experience. As therapists gain insight into their own skills and perceived effectiveness in working with clients, they develop specific preferences. For the clinical researcher who is evaluating the effectiveness of a treatment procedure, sensitivity to and awareness of the interactional effects of variables on treatment outcome are necessary.

All of these factors, (client, treatment method, therapist, and environment) potentially can affect outcome. For example: What specific treatment method by what specific therapist for what specific client in what specific environment is effective as measured by what specific test instrument?

CONTROL OF FACTORS AFFECTING CLIENT IMPROVEMENT IN PERFORMANCE AREAS AND PERFORMANCE COMPONENT

When controlling the factors that may account for client improvement, the researcher must consider the following questions within each of the variables listed below:

Treatment Methods (examples)

- Biofeedback
- Cognitive-behavioral
- Exercise
- Medication
- Psychoeducational
- Relaxation therapy
- Sensory integration
- Stress management

Client Characteristics

- Diagnosis (DSM-IV)
- Cognitive style
- Cultural background
- Education
- Demographics
- Gender
- Intelligence
- Occupation
- Personality

Changes in Performance Areas and Performance Components

Environmental Context

- Changes in life situations
- Copers
- Housing (halfway house, hospital)
- Interpersonal relationships
- Stressors
- Treatment setting

Therapist Variables

- Cognitive style
- Competence
- Cultural background
- Education
- Experience
- Interests
- Personality
- Values

Therapist Variables

▶ Is age or gender of the therapist significant in affecting outcome?

▶ Is cognitive style, that is, the characteristic way that the individual perceives the world (e.g., field independence or field dependence) a factor?

▶ How does the therapist's personality affect change?

▶ Are the levels of education, experience, and competence factors in improvement?

▶ Are there cultural or ethnic factors that facilitate or hinder client progress?

▶ What other qualities of the therapist can potentially affect client improvement?

▶ What are the effects of interactions of co-therapists who are simultaneously treating the same client?

Client Variables

▶ Do specific demographic factors such as age, gender, marital status, or socioeconomic status (SES) affect treatment outcome?

▶ How does the diagnosis and severity of illness affect treatment?

▶ How does the client's intelligence, education, and occupation affect the treatment process?

▶ Does the congruence between the personality of the client and therapist affect outcome?

Treatment Method Variables

▶ Is special training needed in applying the treatment method?

▶ Is there a treatment protocol (i.e., standard procedure) to apply to clients?

▶ How does medication, if applicable, affect treatment?

▶ How does the frequency, duration, and intensity of individual treatment sessions affect the outcome?

▶ Does group treatment affect outcome?

▶ Is there an underlying theoretical explanation for the effect of the treatment on client improvement?

Environmental Variables

▶ Does the setting where treatment takes place (e.g., hospital, CMHC, client's home, RTC, or supported employment) affect outcome?

▶ Does the client attend a support group?

▶ Do physical variables in the treatment setting (e.g., lighting, background sound, color, temperature, atmospheric pressure, visual distractions) affect the treatment outcome?

Figure 15–2 describes graphically the interaction between the therapist and treatment outcome variables.

External Variables Affecting Change in Performance Areas and Performance Components

The *placebo effect* is defined as the client's ability to produce a psychological or physiological change through variables such as self-suggestion and therapist expectation. For example, a therapist may implant in the client's mind the idea that a specific treatment method, such as

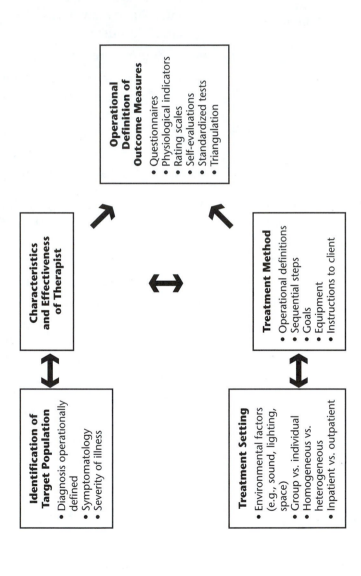

Figure 15-2. Interactional effects of treatment method, therapist, client, and environmental context. (Adapted from *Clinical Research in Occupational Therapy* (4th ed.), by F. Stein and S.K. Cutler. 2000, p.76, San Diego: Singular Publishing Group.)

biofeedback, relaxation therapy, meditation, or exercise, will produce beneficial results in the client's psychosocial functioning. Historically, placebos were used in drug studies in order to isolate the effects or actions of specific drugs. However, it was found that some clients reported improvements in their conditions from placebos. The powerful effect of psychological attitudes and emotions on the autonomic nervous system, which, in turn, regulates the internal physiological environment is probably the underlying reason for the placebo effect. If acute depression and the accompanying symptoms of insomnia, fatigue, and lack of appetite can be produced by verbal cues, for example, talking about the death of a loved one, then perhaps psychological cues such as the therapist's expectancy of improvement can produce beneficial changes in the client. In single-subject research, it is important to use the placebo effect as a motivating force to increase the probability of improvement. On the other hand, the researcher must control the placebo effect by combining it with the specific treatment methods that are being compared.

The *Hawthorne effect* is similar to the placebo effect inasmuch as it is self-produced by the client. The effect was initially observed in an experiment carried out by the Western Electric Corporation in Hawthorne, New York in 1939 (Homans, 1965; Roethlisburger & Dickson, 1939). The purpose of that study was to investigate the effects of varying physical conditions (independent variables) on increased output rate (dependent variables). "The increased in the output rate . . . could . . . be related to . . . the development of an organized social group in a peculiar and effective relation with its supervisors" (Homans, 1965, p. 596). They found that production increased as a result of the attention that was given to the workers, rather than the specific variables intended to produce a favorable working condition. The workers continued to increase their production even after the favorable working conditions were removed. On analyzing the results and from interviews with the workers, they found that the major factor in improved production was the workers' attitude that the management gave the worker deferential treatment. The Hawthorne effect was a common occurrence in psychiatric treatment when clients were segregated into intensive care units, afforded special care, or involved in programs such as sensory integration treatment, behavior therapy, or reality orientation. In every innovative program the Hawthorne effect is present. In single-subject research the Hawthorne effect is minimized by controlling the amount of time and attention given to the client in each treatment method being compared. For example, in a study comparing biofeedback to relaxation therapy in reducing anxiety, the researcher would program time and researcher attention equally to clients in both treatment conditions.

Experimenter bias is the conscious or unconscious influence of the researcher in producing results that are desired. This can be blatant in the case of a researcher who has received advanced training in a specific treatment method such as biofeedback, sensory integration, cognitive therapy, and relaxation therapy and wants to reassure himself or herself that the treatment method is effective. The biased researcher has accepted the efficacy of the treatment method and will not accept contrary evidence. This preset view produces bias and reduces objectivity. Research bias is controlled by a double-blind study where the investigator and subjects are unaware of which subjects are in the experimental or control group. In single-subject designs it is important to control researcher bias by having an objective clinician or research assistant implement the treatment design and collect data.

Protection of Subjects in Research

Institutions receiving federal support for the conduct of research involving human subjects are required to establish a committee that examines the possible risks and benefits of the research (Institutional Review Board [IRB.]). The composition of the IRB. based in universities, CMHC, and hospitals includes individuals responsible in the institution for reviewing and approving research proposal. The researcher meets with the IRB. to discuss the possible risks and the controls used to minimize their effects. The purpose of the IRB. is not to pass on the validity of the research, except in instances where children or other vulnerable populations are involved or where the risks are excessive as in research that involves adverse physical, psychological, or chemical reactions. The researcher should also provide a method that protects the subject's identity. The following outline of a proposal for a single-subject research study includes a section on the informed consent procedure that guarantees the subject's anonymity and states the potential risks involved in the research.

Proposal for Single-Subject Research

Title of Study. Include in the title: (a) the independent variable, which is usually the treatment method in experimental designs; (b) the dependent variable, which is the behavior to be changed; (c) participant, such as a representative sample of the target population; and (d) the setting where the research is to take place.

Example of single-subject research title:

The Effect of Biofeedback Training (*independent variable*) on the Development of Communication Skills (*dependent variable*) in a Child (*participant*) with Autism Attending a Residential Treatment Program (*treatment setting*).

The Research Problem. In this section of the research proposal, the investigator justifies the need for the study by relating epidemiological data in terms of prevalence and incidence of the disorder to support the significance of the problem and need for study. If the participant of the study is an individual with severe depression, the rationale for using a specific treatment method would be discussed as well as the potential implications of the results in the field of occupational therapy.

The Literature Review. The investigator reports previously published studies related to present investigation. The use of a database search (e.g., MEDLINE, CINAHL, PsychLit, OT databases) is a necessary part of the research process. It is essential to document previous research in planning the methodology.

A number of Web sites, listed below, describe the most current research studies and give information about the various psychosocial disorders and disabilities. These sites will be helpful when planning a research study. (See also Appendix D.)

▶ *http://www.mentalhealth.com/p.html*

▶ *http://www.medweb.emory.edu/MedWeb/*

▶ *http://netpsych.com/*

▶ *http://www.human-nature.com/odmh/index.html*

▶ *http://www.nimh.nih.gov/*

▶ *http://www.informatik.fh-luebeck.de/icd/welcome.html*

▶ *http://www.nami.org/*

▶ *http://www.healthgate.com/HealthGate/MEDLINE/search.shtml*

▶ *http://www.ncbi.nlm.nih.gov/PubMed/*

▶ *http://www.nida.nih.gov/NIDAHome1.html*

Operational Definitions. The exact procedure used to select a participant for the study, treatment method (independent variable), outcome measure (dependent variable), and setting for treatment are delineated.

The participant is defined by screening criteria that includes variables such as diagnosis (from DSM–IV [APA, 1994]), age, intelligence, SES, gender, and other factors that could potentially effect the results of the study. For example, in a study of autism the screening criteria for subject inclusion could be further defined as male, aged 5 to 8 years old, with an intelligent quotient of at least 85 and coming from a middle-class family.

Treatment method should be described in enough detail so that the experiment can be replicated by other researchers. Factors to be considered in defining a treatment method include a manual of directions, time in carrying out treatment, training requirements of therapist, and standardized equipment, if used. It is not sufficient to say that behavior management, SI, or exercise was used with the subject. The exact method in operationalizing the treatment must be described precisely.

Outcome measure is defined as the specific standardized test or procedure that is used to measure the effects of the treatment method. Desired outcomes, such as increased self-esteem, social skills, increased self-care skills, job satisfaction, and assertiveness or reduced anxiety, depression, hostility, somatic complaints, delusions, and hallucinations, are defined by specific psychological tests, scales, inventories, or other standardized procedures. Reliability and validity data are reported when describing the outcome measure.

Treatment setting is defined as the environment in which the research takes place. The treatment setting in psychosocial research can include a psychiatric hospital, CMHC, school, Veterans' Administration Hospital, day treatment facility, outpatient clinic, vocational setting, residential treatment school, and client's home.

Measurement of Dependent Variables. There are four scales of measurement in science: nominal, ordinal, interval, and ratio. These four scales of measurement are hierarchical in complexity. The nominal scale is the most basic and is applied when categorizing variables. In psychosocial research the nominal scale measurement is used when diagnosing clients (e.g., schizophrenia or depression). In analyzing outcome, nominal scale measurement can be used when the researcher sets up two categories designating either improvement or no improvement. Ordinal scale measurement is used when analyzing the degree of improvement such as, "minimally improved," "moderately improved," and "much improved." It is a step up from nominal scale measurement; however, it still has a large degree of subjectivity. Interval scale measurement is continuous and represents a quantitative measurement. Examples of interval scale measurement are blood pressure recordings from a blood pressure cuff or heart rate. There are few pure interval scale measurements in psychosocial research. Ratio scale measurement implies a continuous interval scale with an absolute zero such as measuring weight with a scale or grip strength on a dynamometer.

Validity of Research Study. External validity represents the general reliability of results to an target population. External validity is an estimate of the confidence in applying the results from a case study to a target population. External validity is increased as a study is replicated and consistent results are reported. For example, if a study is carried out in different geographic areas by several investigators with similar findings, the confidence in the validity of the results is enhanced. Single-subject research should be replicated to increase external validity and to generalize results to a target population.

Internal validity represents the degree of experimental rigor in controlling for extraneous variables that potentially could affect the outcome of the study. The researcher should try to control for the affect of outside factors by initially listing all extraneous variables and then describing how they are controlled. For example, in a study of sensory integration techniques with individuals with schizophrenia to increase socialization, the researcher would select a subject based on a priori screening criteria.

Treatment Methodology. The basic design in evaluating treatment effectiveness with one subject has been described by various researchers such as Barlow and Hersen (1984), Yin (1993), Stake (1995), Krishef (1991), Tripodi (1994),

Ottenbacher and Bonder (1986), Kazdin (1982), and Alberto and Troutman (1998). The research design is based on dividing treatment intervention into baseline, intervention and return to baseline (ABA design). Figure 15–3 gives an example of an ABA design. In this example, the time for each intervention is 2 weeks. The dependent variable, increased relaxation, is measured before and after the intervention (e.g., biofeedback). The data are analyzed by noting the changes in relaxation measures following treatment.

Informed Consent Procedure. In all research involving human subjects, the researcher must develop a written informed consent form that the participant or legal guardian, in cases of

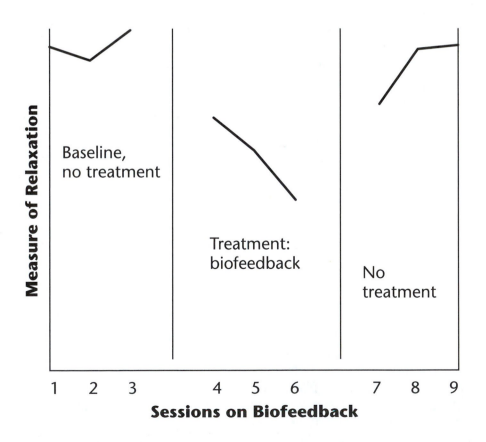

Figure 15-3. Example of an ABA design.

minors, must sign and agree to before becoming a participant in a research investigation.

The informed consent document should include the following information:

1. The participant's name should not be used in reporting results.

2. The results of the study will only be used for advancing scientific knowledge.

3. The subject has been informed of the purposes and details of the experimental procedures involving time commitments, place where data collection will be done, and any compensation for the subject's time.

4. The potential risks, both psychological and physical, stated in clear and easily understood language.

5. The participant will be informed that he or she can refuse to participate in the study or withdraw at any time without any penalty or prejudice to the participant.

Figure 15–4 is an example of an informed consent form

In summary, single-subject research enables the investigator in psychosocial occupational therapy to identify the specific factors that interact and affect change in the subject. It is no longer productive to continue to use reductionistic two-variable research in identifying effective treatment techniques. Reductionistic means simplifying complex concepts into simpler concepts. An example is treating a complex illness that has multifactorial causes with a simple rem-

---

Dear Participant:

The purpose of this study is to find out if a new treatment method helps people to cope better with their stress.

If you agree to participate in the study, you will spend three hours a week in a biofeedback laboratory learning how to relax your forehead muscles. The procedure is painless and there are no psychological or physical risks. The results of the study will be used only for advancing scientific knowledge, and your name will not appear in any written or oral account of the research. You may withdraw from the study at any time without any penalty or prejudice.

The study will take place in the occupational therapy department and will involve your participation for five weeks for a total of 15 hours.

Any questions regarding this study should be referred to _____ at the following telephone number.

Sincerely,

Researcher's signature

I have received a complete explanation of the study and procedures and agree to volunteer/participate as a subject.

_____   _____

Name of participant   Date

Figure 15-4. Example of an Informed Consent Form.

edy, such as taking medication. In this book, we have emphasized a holistic comprehensive approach to understand the causes and treatment of psychosocial illness. This is in direct contrast to a reductionistic approach.

SUMMARY

Clinical research is, by its very nature, dependent on repeated replication over time. Research in heart disease is an example of how cumulative data compiled over a period of 25 years led to the identification of risk factors in myocardial infarction. The same process can be applied to psychosocial research if clinicians and researchers will combine efforts by documenting the multiple causes, interactional effects, and results that are observed in treatment of individuals with psychosocial dysfunction. One of the potential benefits of clinical research is increasing the specificity in identifying treatment methods in occupational therapy that can be used effectively with individuals who are mentally ill.

REFERENCES

Alberto, P. A., & Troutman, A. C. (1998). *Applied behavioral analysis*. Columbus, OH: Prentice Hall/Merrill.

American Occupational Therapy Association. (1994). *Uniform terminology for occupational therapy: Application to practice* (3rd ed.). Rockville, MD: Author.

American Psychiatric Association. (1994). *Diagnostic and statistical manual of mental disorders* (4th ed.). Washington, DC: Author.

Barlow, D. H., & Hersen, M. (1984). *Single-case experimental designs*. New York: Pergamon.

Beveridge, W. I. B. (1950). *The art of scientific investigation*. New York: W. W. Norton.

Hedaya, R. (1996). *Understanding biological psychiatry*. New York: W. W. Norton.

Homans, G. (1965). Group factors in worker productivity. In H. Proshansky & B. Seidenberg (Eds.), *Basic studies in social psychology* (pp. 592–604). New York: Holt, Rinehart, & Winston.

Kazdin, A. E. (1982). *Single-case research designs: Methods for clinical and applied settings*. New York: Oxford University Press.

Krishef, C. H. (1991). *Fundamental approaches to single subject design and analysis*. Malabar, FL: Krieger.

Laing, R. D. (1967). *The politics of experience and the bird of paradise*. Middlesex, UK: Penguin.

Neuchterlein, K. H., & Dawson, M. E. (1984). A heuristic vulnerability/stress model of schizophrenic episodes. *Schizophrenia Bulletin, 10*, 300–312.

Norman, R. M. G., & Malla, A. K. (1993). Stressful life events and schizophrenia. I: A review of the research. *British Journal of Psychiatry, 162*, 161–166.

Ottenbacher, K. J., & Bonder, B. (Eds.). (1986). *Scientific inquiry: Design and analysis issues in occupational therapy*. Rockville, MD: American Occupational Therapy Foundation.

Roethlisburger, F. J., & Dickson, W. J. (1939). *Management and the worker*. Cambridge, MA: Harvard University Press.

Sapolsky, R. M. (1998). *Why zebras don't get ulcers: An updated guide to stress, stress-related diseases, and coping*. New York: Freeman.

Stake, R. E. (1995). *The art of case study research*. Thousand Oaks, CA: Sage.

Stein, F. (1976). *Anatomy of research in allied health*. Cambridge, MA: Schenkman.

Stein, F. (1980). Evaluating psychiatric treatment methods through clinical trials research. *Occupational Therapy in Mental Health, 1*(2), 1–14.

Stein, F., & Cutler, S. K. (1996). *Clinical research in allied health and special education* (3rd ed.). San Diego: Singular Publishing Group.

Stein, F., & Cutler, S. K. (2000). *Clinical research in occupational therapy* (4th ed.). San Diego: Singular Publishing Group.

Szasz, T. S. (1974). *The myth of mental illness: Foundations of a theory of personal conduct* (Rev. ed.). New York: Harper & Row.

Torrey, E. F. (1991). A viral-anatomical explanation of schizophrenia. *Schizophrenia Bulletin, 17,* 15–18.

Tripodi, T. (1994). *A primer on single-subject design for clinical social workers.* Washington, DC: National Association of Social Workers.

Yin, R. K. (1993). *Applications of case study research.* Newbury Park, CA: Sage.

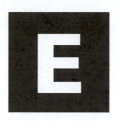

Epilogue

To me, writing this book with Sue Cutler was like a journey through time. We explored the corpus of literature written about the methods used in treating individuals with mental illness. Occupational therapy has a strong link with naturalistic healing, moral treatment, the arts and crafts movement, creative expression, psychodynamic interpretations, behavioral medicine, holistic treatment, and the wellness model. To practice as a psychosocial occupational therapist is in the best traditions of community and social service. What we do has a tremendous impact on the individual we treat and his or her family and friends. Clinical practice in mental health is primarily in the community where it belongs. We no longer have to isolate individuals in human warehouses away from their communities and families. Occupational therapists have a tradition of doing what is best for the client. In our work we focus on the daily roles and occupations that define the individual.

What is the future for psychosocial occupational therapists? In an article in OT Week (1997), "Taking the Pulse of Mental Health OTs," the authors discussed a survey completed by 285 mental health practitioners. "Decreased client length of stay, followed by consolidation or merging of services were identified most often as the key challenges facing today's mental health OT practitioner" (p. 9). Other observations centered around (a) the interventions that "will need to address functional outcomes that interface with managed care" (p. 9), (b) the most common diagnoses treated (i.e., schizophrenia, mood disorders, and anxiety disorders), (c) the most common interventions used (i.e., coping skills, social skills, crafts, and leisure activities), and (d) the frame of reference most often employed in "evaluation and treatment" (p. 9) (i.e., Model of Human Occupation and Cognitive Behavioral).

Although the trend in the last 10 years has been a decreasing number of occupational therapists entering psychosocial practice, the theories and practices in occupational therapy have continued to be used by other mental health professionals. The importance of occupational therapy in treating individuals with mental illness is an important aspect of the holistic approach to treatment and will continue to be used in treating patients with physical as well as mental disabilities.

REFERENCE

American Occupational Therapy Association. (1997, May 22). Taking the pulse of mental health OTs. *OT Week, 11,* 9.

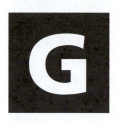

Glossary

Activity analysis is a detailed examination of a task into performance components such as perceptual, cognitive, psychological, and cultural factors. The significance and meaning of a task to an individual is considered as well as the sequential steps necessary in completing task.

Activity group therapy was originally developed by Slavson (1943) for treating children with behavior disorders. Slavson advocated a permissive environment where children act out their impulses through play and behavioral infractions. The goal of therapy is to help the child develop inner controls.

Acupuncture is an ancient Chinese treatment technique that is based on the concept of a vital energy flow or life force (ch'i), which is thought to circulate through the body along meridians similar to the blood vessels or neural circuits. Practitioners of acupuncture insert needles into identified meridians of the body to relieve pain. Some scientists explain that the effectiveness of acupuncture is that endorphins (opiates) are released when a needle is placed in the meridian point. Acupuncture is also being used in a number of illnesses such as drug addiction and asthma. Research results have been encouraging.

Adaptation is an adjustment of a person to his or her environment; a reaction to a stressor or environmental demand by an individual. Adaptation can also refer to the modification of an environment (e.g., addition of more structure to the daily schedule) or equipment, or materials (e.g., providing cues in the work environment to enable the individual to function independently in work, leisure, or self-care).

Adaptive skills refer to a newly learned behavior that helps the individual to be independent in performance areas.

Adult day care provides supervised social, recreational, and health related services for clients who have cognitive, emotional, and physical impairments. Individuals with Alzheimer's disease can benefit from day care. Caregivers can also benefit from the respite that allows them to continue their activities and to work.

Aerobic exercise is repetitive movements of major muscle groups while the body utilizes large amounts of oxygen that is transported through the arteries, as in walking, running, dancing, biking, and swimming. It has been shown to be an effective activity in treating depression and anxiety (Wykoff, 1993).

Affect refers to the mood of an individual such as depressed, angry, happy, manic, anxious, relaxed, guilty, envious, or hostile.

After-care clinic is usually a state- or locally funded agency that is an extension of the state or county hospital designed to provide a transition to the community. Services provided can include supervision of medication, counseling and psychotherapy, vocational placement, and occupational therapy.

Alexander technique is a body technique to correct the posture of the head, neck, and spine by bringing the way we move under our conscious direction and avoiding a buildup of muscular tension. It involves balance and movement therapy used to improve postural habits currently causing fatigue. Anecdotal evidence claims that it is effective in relieving tension headaches, neck and back pain, and muscle spasms.

Alternative medicines are approaches that are not taught in medical school and are not considered to be in the mainstream of medical practice.

Alzheimer's disease is a chronic, progressive disorder that most often occurs in people over 65 years old. It is characterized by memory loss, personality deterioration, confusion, disorganization, language distortions, sleep and eating disturbances, and a complete breakdown in self-care functions.

Anorexia nervosa is an eating disorder most common in females 12 to 21 years old characterized by a fear of being obese and refusal to maintain normal body weight. The disorder results in emaciation, amenorrhea, body image disturbances, anxiety, and other emotional reactions.

Antisocial personality disorder is characterized by behaviors such as lying, stealing, aggressiveness, substance abuse, criminal activity, and disregard for authority and discipline. The individual lacks moral and ethical standards, empathy toward others, and is unable to feel guilt.

Synonymous terms are sociopathic and psychopathic personality.

Anxiety is a feeling of apprehension, worry, uneasiness, fear of the future, or dread. Physiological symptoms such as disturbed breathing, increased heart rate, increased sweating, hand tremors, and dizziness frequently accompany anxiety.

Anxiety disorders are exaggerated fears that prevent or limit an individual from performing normal activities or behavior. They include panic disorders, phobias, stress disorders, and obsessive-compulsive behaviors. Many times physical symptoms occur with anxiety disorders such as heart palpitations, sweating, hand tremors, chest pain, shortness of breath, dizziness, and nausea.

Aphasia is a language impairment where the client is unable to communicate or comprehend speech and/or written words.

Apraxia is a motor dysfunction with difficulty in coordination of voluntary movement.

Aqua therapy is the therapeutic use of water, hot or cold, fresh or mineral.

Aroma therapy is the use of essential oils from plants to enhance general health and appearance. There is evidence that oil of lavender and sandalwood are effective in producing a calming effect.

Arousal is the physiological state of readiness or stimulation of an individual to act, as in Selye's (1974) theory of stress, or in the ability to attend to a task.

Art therapy is the use of art as a therapeutic tool that provides the opportunity for nonverbal expression, communication, and growth.

Asperger's syndrome characterized by obsessive thinking, solitary activity, difficulty with emotional bonding, egocentricity, poor social skills, and lack of eye contact. They have sometimes been referred to as "high-functioning autism." Rote memory is highly developed.

Assertiveness training is a technique used in behavior therapy to assist individuals with social skills to become more assertive in their interpersonal relationships. Role-playing and behavior rehearsal are used in the technique.

Assessment is the critical appraisal of a client's interests, personality, aptitude, physical capacity, intelligence, and functional abilities. Methods of assessment include standardized psychometric tests, clinical observations, performance scales, facility generated procedures, and client interviews.

Attention-Deficit Hyperactivity Disorder (ADHD) refers to the symptoms of inattention, hyperactivity, and impulsiveness that interfere with a child's, adolescent's or adult's ability to learn, work continuously, and engage in leisure activities. The disorder also impacts on interpersonal relationships. Ritalin®, which is the trade name for methylphenidate hydrochloride, is frequently prescribed for ADHD. Cognitive-behavioral therapy and relaxation therapy are appropriate and effective treatment methods.

Autism is a pervasive developmental disorder characterized by extreme withdrawal; difficulty establishing relationships with parents or peers, communicating with others or using language, or completing self-care activities; an inward turning toward self; and highly repetitive or stereotypical actions.

Autogenic training is a system of self-regulation of the autonomic nervous system in which the client uses visualization, deep diaphragmatic breathing, and "mind-quieting phrases," such as "my hands are heavy and warm." Biofeedback can be combined with autogenic training (Norris & Fahrion, 1993).

Autogenics involves focusing attention on formerly unconscious events occurring during relaxed states. Self-regulation is involved in reaching a desired relaxed state.

Aversion therapy is a form of behavior therapy in which punishment or unpleasant stimuli are used to extinguish maladaptive behavior such as alcoholism, drug abuse, sexual deviance, and self-mutilation.

Avoidant personality disorder is characterized by social avoidance, lack of friends, inhibition of feelings, feeling of inadequacy, and hypersensitivity to criticism. An individual tends to be a loner and does not seek out social groups or friendships.

Ayurveda is an ancient Hindu medical practice that strives to improve health by harmonizing mind, body, and spirit. It utilizes herbal remedies, massage therapy, yoga, and pulse diagnosis.

Behavior therapy is the application of treatment techniques based on the principles of learning theories that include aversion therapy, contingency management, and systematic desensitization. The purpose is to change maladaptive behavior through positive reinforcement, modeling behavior, and conditioning.

Bibliotherapy is a therapeutic technique in which the therapist recommends books to the patient based on the content of the book and its specific relevance to the patient in working out problems. Reading groups can be incorporated with group therapy.

Biofeedback is a method in which the client becomes aware of internal processes such as heart rate, blood pressure, finger temperature, or muscle tension as a means to control function. The client learns by using monitoring devices that sound a tone or show a visual display when changes in pulse, blood pressure, brain waves, and muscle contractions occur. Biofeedback is usually combined with a relaxation technique so that the client can produce beneficial changes in one's physiology. The client can apply the information learned from biofeedback to reduce one's stress. A training program is designed to develop the ability to control the autonomic (involuntary) nervous system. After learning the technique, the client may be able to control heart rate, blood pressure, and skin temperature or to relax certain muscles.

Biopsychosocial approach implies that an etiology of a disease has biological, psychological, and sociological determinants such as genetic, developmental, and environmental factors. In treatment biopsychosocial implies a holistic multimodal treatment approach encompassing medication, psychological counseling, exercise, nutrition, stress management, and cultural considerations.

Bipolar disorder is an affective illness characterized by episodes of mania and depression. Symptoms of the disorder fluctuate from extreme euphoria, delusions of grandeur, and frantic activity to profound sadness, guilt, lowered self-esteem, fatigue, and suicidal ideation.

Body image is the individual's subjective concept of his or her physical appearance based on conscious or unconscious feelings toward self.

Borderline personality disorder is marked by an inability to discover meaning in one's life, a feeling of emptiness, and difficulty in maintaining long-term relationships. Emotional outbursts, sadness, fear, and suicidal ideation are frequently experienced.

Bulimia is an eating disorder marked by recurrent or continuous episodes of binge eating followed by self-induced vomiting, fasting, and diarrhea. Individual may engage in excessive exercise. Depression and an overly concern about body shape frequently accompany bulimia.

Case management is a comprehensive system of treating individuals with mental illness that includes evaluating client's needs, developing feasible goals, arranging for services in the community, and monitoring the client's progress and follow-up (Baker & Intagliata, 1992).

Catatonia is a clinical symptom of motor dysfunction manifested by marked rigidity, waxy flexibility, stupor, and frantic overactivity.

Catecholamine is derived from the amino acid tyrosine. It has a vital function in the brain of stimulating the nervous system, cardiovascular function, metabolic rate, temperature, and smooth muscles. It plays a key role in arousing the autonomic nervous system (sympathetic response). Dopamine and norepinephrine are catecholamines.

Catharsis is a term used by Freud to describe how repressed ideas or traumatic experiences are brought to the consciousness during psychotherapy. In general terms it refers to the free expression of negative feelings, such as fear and anxiety, which are released through expressive media such as art, music, poetry, or dance.

Chaining is a behavioral therapy technique in which an activity is broken down into task intervals for the client to learn in a sequential manner. Forward chaining is carrying the task from the first step until completion. On the other hand, backward chaining starts with the last step in the task and works backward in sequence to the first step.

Chiropractic care is a discipline of health practice that examines the relationship between the structure and position of the spinal column to the onset of diseases, pain syndromes, and neurophysiological effects. Chiropractors emphasize prevention and health maintenance, as well as treatment. The major treatment method is spinal manipulation in which the chiropractor uses his or her hands to mobilize, adjust, manipulate, massage, or stimulate the client's spine.

Circadian rhythm is the awake, sleep, and activity cycle in animals during a 24-hour period. Individuals can track their circadian rhythm by recording the average hours of sleep needed during a 24-hour period and their activity level during the day.

Client-centered therapy is a type of psychotherapy developed by Rogers (1951), which emphasizes the relationship between the client and therapist, and empowers the client to facilitate psychological growth. Also known as nondirective therapy.

Clinical observation is a method of observing client's verbal and nonverbal behavior in a treatment setting.

Codependency refers to an individual's addiction that is shared with a significant other such as a spouse. Addictions such as alcohol, drugs, gambling, or smoking may be reinforced by the codependent individual.

Cognition is the mental activity of perceiving, thinking, reasoning, evaluating, remembering, planning, and making decisions. The act of cognition includes memory (perception, encoding, storage, and retrieval of information), attention, language, and executive functioning.

Cognitive impairments are dysfunctions in memory (perception, encoding, storage, and retrieval of information), attention, language, and executive functioning (Spaulding, 1994).

Cognitive therapy as conceptualized by Beck (1976) is defined as a verbal therapy that helps the client to examine his or her thoughts, impulses, and feelings that are contributing to a disorder. The first principle of cognitive therapy is that the way people structure a situation determines how they feel and behave. For example, if they interpret a situation as dangerous, they feel anxious and prepare to protect themselves. Behavioral techniques are used by cognitive therapists to help clients develop new approaches in dealing with everyday activities by helping them to monitor their behavior and to try out new behaviors.

Community Mental Health Center (CMHC) is an outgrowth of the Community Mental Health Center Act of 1963. The CMHC was conceptualized as an alternative to long-term institutionalization for individuals with mental illness. CMHCs provide five basic mental health services: inpatient hospitalization when needed, outpatient care, partial hospitalization, emergency mental health services, and consultation and education to community groups and agencies.

Community support program (CSP) was an initiative of the National Institute of Mental Health in response to the deinstitutionalization of individuals with chronic mental illness. CSP supplied funds to public hospitals, community mental health centers, and county and social service agencies to provide comprehensive services, including psychosocial rehabilitation to those with chronic mental illness. Community support system (CSS) was a major thrust of CSP.

Community support system (CSS) is a model that tries to meet the needs of individuals with mental illness, such as health and dental, housing, income support, entitlement (Medicare, Medicaid), and employment, through a case management approach.

Complementary medicine is another term for alternative medicine. It refers to the innovations or alternative approaches to traditional medicine. Relaxation therapies, body work, humor, and therapeutic use of vitamins and herbs are examples of complementary medicine.

Concurrent validity is the degree of correlation with another standardized instrument. For example, a new test of stress management is correlated with an established test of stress management that has high reliability and validity.

Construct validity is the extent to which the test measures a theoretical construct. For example, generating test items based on a theoretical construct such as Selye's Theory of Stress (Selye, 1974) to develop a test on stress management.

Content or face validity is the extent to which the test matches the content of the task or material. For example, a test on self-concept has content validity if the questions on the test deal with issues of self-concept.

Contingency management is a group of techniques used in behavior therapy in which the client establishes a contract with the therapist to modify a behavioral response by shaping the consequences of that response. For example, the client will receive a token for positive interpersonal communications.

Continuous Quality Improvement (CQI) is a systems approach to improving the quality of care of an organization, hospital, or agency. In this approach, creativity, trial and error, individual leadership, and achievable and measurable goals are emphasized.

Controlled breathing involves learning to use abdominal muscles in breathing slowly with the aim of reducing stress and anxiety.

Course of an illness is the predicted stages of an illness based on clinical observations of the illness and epidemiological studies of stages in an illness. For example, 90 percent of individuals who have a single manic episode experience future episodes. Another example is the progressive nature of Alzheimer's disease where the individual deteriorates in stages.

Crisis intervention is a 24-hour service that is made available to clients with mental illness to reduce the stress on the client or family members. Problems such as a loss of job, broken friendships, drug-related problems, or criminal offenses can many times put the individual into a crisis. A case manager or mental health professional can provide support by linking the individual to resources in the community. Telephone hot lines open and accessible to the individual can be extremely important in alleviating a crisis.

Dance is movement by using a series of rhythmical motions and steps. It is a good form of exercise and expression of emotions.

Dance therapy is the use of dance or movement as a carefully guided tool to release tension, develop awareness, acceptance of self, and effective social interactions (Hood, 1959; Levy, 1988).

Day treatment centers (DTCs), previously referred to as day hospitals, were established in the United States in the 1950s for individuals who were discharged from mental hospitals and needed a period of transitional services. The services provided are comprehensive and include medication management, counseling, group therapy, and occupational therapy. The occupational therapist plays an important role in the DTCs in helping individuals in the performance areas of work, self-care, and leisure. A guiding philosophy of the DTC is to treat the individual as a member of the community where he or she lives.

Deinstitutionalization is the process of discharging individuals from large state or county hospitals into community facilities such as day treatment centers, or supportive housing such as halfway houses, group homes, and residential treatment centers.

Delusion is a false belief without substance such as believing that people are reading one's mind, or food is being poisoned, or people are plotting against the individual.

Dementia is a broad term that refers to progressive chronic disorders of the brain characterized by memory loss, confusion, disorientation, personality deterioration, depression, and a complete breakdown in self-care functions. Alzheimer's disease, Pick's disease, Huntington's chorea, and organic brain syndrome associated with alcoholism can lead to dementia.

Dependent personality disorder describes an individual with an extreme need to be taken care of by another individual. The disorder usually begins in childhood and is characterized by passivity, submissiveness, indecisiveness, poor self-confidence, and a need to be nurtured and supported.

Depression is a mood disorder that can be characterized as mild, moderate, or severe. Symptoms of depression include eating dysfunction, sleeping disturbance, fatigue, low self-esteem, inability to concentrate, difficulty in making decisions, feelings of hopelessness, and sadness. *See Dysthymic disorder.*

Diathesis is a predisposition or vulnerability to a specific disease, disorder, or condition. A diathesis-stress refers to the precipitating of an episode of symptoms leading to a disease through a stressful event or stressors in the environment.

Disability is any restriction or lack (resulting from an impairment) of ability to perform an activity in the manner or within the range considered normal for a human being. These human activities include walking, running, speaking, writing, dressing, feeding oneself, or listening. A psychiatric disability results from the symptoms of an illness such as delusions or hallucinations that can prevent an individual from engaging in everyday human interactions. The symptoms of depression can cause an individual to become disabled in working (World Health Organization [WHO], 1980).

Dopamine is a catecholamine neurotransmitter that occurs naturally in the brain and effects arousal in the autonomic nervous system. An overabundance of dopamine has been implicated as a factor in the etiology of schizophrenia. A paucity of dopamine is associated with Parkinson's disease and tardive dyskinesia. L-dopa, the precursor of dopamine, is used in the treatment of Parkinson's disease.

Down syndrome is a type of mental retardation that is caused by a genetic defect where an extra chromosome (21 or 22) is present at birth. The individual's intellectual potential can range from educable to profound mental retardation. Early sensory stimulation programs, gross motor activities, special education, and vocational preparation are critical aspects of habilitation programs for individuals with Down syndrome.

Dream therapy is a method of using dreams, as in psychoanalysis, to gain access to the unconscious by examining the content of dreams. Using a dream diary is helpful in this process. The use of dreams and the dream state to accomplish physical and emotional healing involves both interpretation and the active participation of the client in the dream process.

Dysthymic disorder represents a chronically depressed mood occurring over a period of at least 2 years in which the individual experiences the symptoms of depression for most of the day.

Dystonia is a motor disorder that is characterized by stiffening in muscles and sudden contractions or "jerky" movements of the arms, neck, or face. It is sometimes a side effect of long-term usage of antipsychotic drugs.

Electrical stimulation involves applying an electrical stimulus to help facilitate muscular control.

Electroencephalograph (EEG) is an instrument for detecting and recording the electrical potential produced by the brain cells. Brain-wave activity is recorded indicating alpha, beta, delta, and theta rhythms, which describe the range of cycles per second of the amplitude of the signal. An individual producing alpha waves (8 $\frac{1}{2}$ to 12-second waves) is usually in a very relaxed state, while beta waves (15 to 30 seconds) are indicative of normal consciousness. EEG is used in biofeedback training.

Electromyograph (EMG) is an instrument to record the electrical activity of muscles by applying surface electrodes (transducers) or needle electrodes into the muscle. Along with the EMG, an oscilloscope and amplifier are used in biofeedback to record muscle activity, for example, the frontalis muscles in relaxation therapy.

Endorphin is a polypeptide component found naturally in the brain that acts as a natural analgesic by binding to opiate receptor sites. Some researchers have found that endorphins are produced by aerobic exercise, such as jogging and fast walking.

Epidemiology is the statistical study of incidence, prevalence, and distribution of diseases in a population and health-related events. The results are applied to the control of diseases and used in analyzing health problems among specific populations.

Ergonomic job analysis is an open-ended process that includes a detailed inspection, description, and evaluation of the workplace, equipment, tools, work methods, and the human factors that impact on performing a job (Keyserling, Armstrong, & Punnett, 1991).

Ergonomics risk factors are variables related to performing a job that can potentially lead to injuries, illnesses, or diseases. These factors can include the environment, for example, extreme temperature, poorly designed tools, an uncomfortable chair, work methods such as using poor lifting techniques, undue or continual stress, and repetitive motions.

Etiology is the examination of the cause or causes of an illness or disease. There are predisposing and precipitating factors that lead to the onset of a disease. Most mental illnesses have multiple risk factors such as genetic, physiological, developmental, psychological and sociological factors that can predispose a vulnerable individual to mental illness. Stress and sudden losses can precipitate an episode of mental illness in an individual who is vulnerable.

Evaluation is the overall judgment of an individual's behavior, characteristics, aptitudes, and present functioning that is gained through specific tests, clinical observations, and procedures that can be used for treatment planning or discharge recommendations.

Executive functions of the brain are higher level cognitive tasks such as abstraction, sequential organization, motor planning, and decision-making.

Expressed emotion (EE) is a concept related to a family's psychological interactions with a family member who is mentally ill (e.g., has a diagnosis of schizophrenia). The criteria for high expressed emotion is based on factors such as negative comments about family member, personal criticism, dissatisfaction with individual's behavior, lack of warmth expressed toward individual, and constant worry about individual. An indication of high expressed emotion toward a family member with mental illness has been linked to a higher relapse rate in individuals with schizophrenia living in the community than those individuals living in household with low expressed emotion (Brown, Birley, & Wing, 1972).

Extinction refers to the elimination or inhibition of behavior by not reinforcing behavior.

Feldenkrais method is a motor therapy that involves learning new patterns of movement to enhance the communication between the brain and body. The method includes lying on one's back, sitting, or standing while becoming aware of each movement. The therapist or instructor may use massage to reduce one's stress or muscular tension. The purposes of this method are to reduce joint pain, improve joint mobility, increase muscle coordination, and improve posture.

Fetal Alcohol Syndrome (FAS) refers to a child with a disability exhibiting intellectual and learning deficits, ADHD, and deficient growth patterns. It is caused by intake of alcohol by the mother during pregnancy. Facial characteristics include small head, eyes, and jaws; a wide, flat nose bridge; and lack of a groove between the lip and the nose.

Flashback is a recurrence of a traumatic event, memory trace, emotion, or perceptual experience. It is present in individuals with posttraumatic stress disorders.

Flat affect refers to dull, unresponsive emotions where the client has difficulty expressing feelings.

Fluidotherapy is the application of a dry heat modality consisting of cellulose particles held in a container and moved in air. The turbulence of the mixture generates a thermal effect when objects are immersed in the medium.

Frame of reference is based on a theoretical model or theory that generates a specific evaluation and treatment techniques in clinical practice. Psychodynamic, model of human occupation, cognitive-behavioral, and sensory integration are frames of reference in psychosocial occupational therapy.

Framework for support (Trainor & Church, 1984) is a model based on self-help; family, friends, and neighbors; community resources; and the formal mental health system. An important premise of this approach is that individuals with mental health problems should be empowered to control their own lives (Carling, 1995).

Functional refers to the degree of a client's independence in the performance areas of work/productivity, self-care, and leisure.

Functional Capacity Assessment (FCA) is a comprehensive and systematic approach that measures the client's overall physical ability such as muscle strength, endurance, joint range of motion, ambulation, sitting, standing, and lifting that are related to work activities. Examples of FCAs are *Isernhagen Work System Functional Capacity Evaluation Procedures, Baltimore Therapeutic Equipment, Key Functional Capacity Assessment, and Blankenship System.*

Galvanic Skin Response (GSR) is the change in the electrical resistance of the skin reflecting the individual's emotional state. What is being measured is the conductive pathway of a sweat gland which is associated with an individual's sympathetic response. The GSR is traditionally used in "lie detector" tests.

General systems theory is a model of understanding the relationships between people and organizations, and between parts and wholes (von Bertalanffy, 1950).

Gestalt therapy is a form of humanistic psychotherapy developed by Perls (1969) that emphasizes the client's awareness of the perceptual environment and the "here and now." It utilizes self-awareness exercises to teach the client to be sensitive to the sensory stimuli in the environment.

Global Assessment of Function (GAF) Scale considers the client's functioning on a graded scale of 1 to 100 with 1 indicating that the client is a persistent danger to self or others and 100 indicating that an individual is functioning at a superior level in a wide range of activities, has many positive qualities, and no symptoms. The scale is based on a mental health-mental illness continuum (APA, 1994).

Goal Attainment Scaling (GAS) is a tool used to describe the personal goals of clients on five possible levels of outcome for each goal. For example, a client can identify lack of assertiveness as a personal problem. A therapeutic strategy is implemented to help the client to improve (Ottenbacher & Cusick, 1989).

Group dynamics is the study of the factors and conditions that affect the actions in a group, for example, the building of group cohesion and leadership functions.

Habilitation is the development of function in the performances of work, leisure, and self-care in an individual with a developmental disability such as autism or childhood schizophrenia. In some cases adults with chronic mental illness who have not developed functional abilities are taught these competencies for the first time and are considered to be habilitated rather than rehabilitated.

Habituation refers to the daily adaptive behavior or routines of an individual as described in the Model of Human Occupation.

Halfway house is a supportive housing environment where clients are provided a structured and supportive setting. Frequently clients are given communal responsibilities for maintenance and kitchen tasks. Its purpose is to provide a transition from a hospital to independent living in the community.

Hallucination is a false perception such as seeing, hearing, or smelling a sensation that does not exist in reality. The individual with a hallucination is unable to distinguish between the real and the imagined sensation.

Handicap is a disadvantage for a given individual, resulting from an impairment or a disability that limits or prevents the fulfillment of a normal role depending on age, sex, and social and cultural factors. A psychiatric handicap is the inability to perform normal role functions as a student, worker, husband, wife, father, or mother or to engage in work, leisure activities, or be independent in self-care or social functioning. The handicap can also be aggravated by environmental factors such as stigma which produces a negative attitude toward individuals with mental illness and thereby prevents the individual from obtaining employment (World Health Organization [WHO], 1980).

Health Maintenance Organization (HMO) is a prepaid group health care program that provides diagnostic treatment services, ambulatory care, hospitalization, and surgery with an emphasis on prevention.

Herbal/botanical is a method of using forms of plants for prevention and treatment of illnesses.

Hippo therapy is treatment with the help of the horse. It aims to strengthen, stretch, and relax the muscles, enhance the motor coordination of the rider and to attain psychological goals such increased self-esteem.

Histrionic personality disorder is characteristic of individuals who are prone to exaggerate, act out or demonstrate feelings, and show explosive personality reactions. In this disorder the individual strives for excitement and surprise in relationships with others. Others characterize individuals as vain, self-centered, demanding, and shallow.

Holistic medicine is a comprehensive approach to treatment considering the physical, social, psychological, spiritual, and economic needs of the client. Holistic methods include diet therapy, exercise, stress management, and relaxation therapy as well as traditional treatments.

Homeopathy is a school of medicine, founded by Dr. S. C. F. Hahnemann in the late 18th century, based on the theory that large doses of drugs that produce symptoms of a disease in healthy people will cure the same symptoms when administered in very small amounts. This is loosely based on the theory that "like cures like." Homeopathic physicians use natural remedies of specially prepared plants and minerals to boost the body's own defense mechanisms and healing processes.

Homeostasis refers to the state of dynamic equilibrium that the internal body organisms strive to maintain through feedback mechanisms and regulatory functions. Cannon (1932) described the processes in the body in maintaining normal values such as heart rate, blood pressure, salt, water, blood sugar, and hemoglobin. Homeostasis also refers to the body's reaction to disease such as T-cell production to fight infection.

Horticulture is the science and art of gardening and cultivating fruits, vegetables, flowers, and plants. Horticulture is used as a therapeutic modality.

Humanism refers to a system of beliefs and a theory of knowledge that emphasizes the acceptance of diverse cultural values, capacities, and achievements of human beings. In treatment, it represents the unconditional acceptance of the individual, even when a behavior is unacceptable. It is also related to the humane treatment of individuals with mental illness during the 19th century termed Moral Treatment.

Humanitarianism refers to the promotion of social betterment through social action groups that provide aid, welfare, and opportunities to those in poverty or survivors of wars and natural disasters.

Humor is any communication that is perceived by any of the interacting parties as humorous and leads to laughing, smiling, or a feeling of amusement. Humor can be used as a stress reducing method in treatment. There is some evidence that humor stimulates neuropeptides and endorphins that can relieve pain.

Hypnotherapy is treatment by inducing an alternate state of consciousness in which the individual feels relaxed and with little pain.

Hypothalamic-pituitary-adrenocortical axis refers to the complex interactions that occur in the autonomic nervous system that involve neurotransmitters and hormonal secretions. It plays an important role in the stress reaction and in maintaining the health of the individual in homeostatic reactions.

Imagery is a relaxation technique that involves visualizing relaxing scenes with one's eyes closed. Many practitioners recommend that the client rotate his or her eyes inward and upward as a warm-up technique before visualizing colors, objects, abstract ideas, and significant people in one's life.

Impairment is any loss or abnormality of physiological, psychological, or anatomical structure or function such as blindness, deafness, astereognosis, mental retardation, or lack of pain sensation. A psychiatric impairment is for example a delusion, hallucination, severe anxiety, phobia, depression or any other symptom that interferes with carrying out normal human activities (World Health Organization [WHO], 1980).

Incoherence is incomprehensible speech or thinking.

Innate intelligence is the inherited biological aptitudes and abilities of an individual.

Institutionalization is an insidious process where, over many years, an individual living in an institution, for example, a state mental hospital, develops apathy, flattened affect, hopelessness, dilapidated appearance, and dependency on others for carrying out activities of daily living.

Interdisciplinary team comprises individuals from different disciplines who work cooperatively in generating treatment goals in collaboration with the client.

Intervention refers to the application of treatments, techniques, methods, drugs, or surgery to improve the patient's condition.

Intrinsic motivation refers to the internal motivation to achieve or perform an activity without external rewards. For example, an artist will continue painting without expecting any reward or praise. Individuals with intrinsic motivation have an internal locus of control.

JCAHO is an acronym for the Joint Commission on the Accreditation of Hospitals.

Job burnout is a debilitating condition caused by chronic occupational stress which results in depleted energy, lowered resistance to illness, job dissatisfaction, pessimism, increased inefficiency, and absenteeism.

Job coach is a counselor or therapist who provides support to the employed client.

Kinesthesia is perception of position, weight, and movements for example such as throwing a ball at a target.

Leisure is a major occupation and performance area that relates to the individual's use of free time. It is related to intrinsic motivation, quality of life, personal freedom, life satisfaction, relaxation, health, lifestyle, amusement, self-actualization, and pleasure. Leisure occupations include a wide range of activities such as gardening, sports, hobbies, social clubs, music, and traveling, that are related to the specific interests of an individual. Cultural, psychological, social, developmental, family, and educational, factors may influence leisure choices.

Locus of control relates to an individual's view that events can either be influenced by self (internal locus of control) or are predetermined or influenced by others (external locus of control).

Massage is the manipulation, methodical pressure, friction, and kneading of the body to reduce stress, increase relaxation, and reduce muscle tension.

Measurement scale is a system of assigning scores to a trait or characteristic.

Measures of central tendency include the mean (average score), mode (the most frequent score), and the median (the 50th percentile or middle score).

Measures of variability include the standard deviation (the degree of dispersion in the scores), and the range (the difference between the high and low scores).

Medicaid is a federally mandated entitlement program that provides medical care for individuals who are indigent.

Medical model is the traditional approach to diagnosing, preventing, and treating diseases. It is based on the scientific method of hypothesis, testing, and experimental design. In the medical model the physician focuses on detecting disease and treating it primarily through drugs and surgery. The physician is seen as the expert in treating the patient. A client-centered approach, behavioral medicine, or alternative medicine, and holistic medicine are contrasted with the traditional medical model which has been attacked as being reductionistic.

Medicare is a federally mandated entitlement program that reimburses hospitals, physicians, and health care workers in providing services to individuals 65 years and older.

Meditation involves taking a comfortable position in a quiet environment, regulating breathing, and having a physically relaxed and mentally calm attitude while focusing on a mental image or word.

Mental retardation (MR) is characterized by subnormal intellectual aptitude or potential which affects an individual's functional abilities to work, engage in leisure activities, be independent in self-care, and establish and maintain interpersonal relationships. MR can range from mild, moderate, or severe to profound disability.

Model of Human Occupation (MOHO) is an occupational therapy frame of reference that is based on the theory of general systems. Role acquisition, environmental and temporal adaptation, and skills development are emphasized in treatment. Volition, habituation, and performance are key concepts (Kielhofner, 1997).

Modeling behavior is a technique used in behavior therapy to help the client acquire social skills by observing and then imitating behavior.

Mood disorders include disturbances of affect such as depression, mania, and bipolar disorders.

Moral treatment was a movement during the 19th century that developed as a reaction to the inhumane care of the mentally ill who up until that time were abused and poorly treated. Arts and crafts, farming, and creative activities were emphasized in moral treatment.

Multidisciplinary team is comprised of professionals from various disciplines who assess and treat clients autonomously and meet regularly to coordinate treatment.

Multiple personality disorder refers to the presence in individuals of two or more personalities that are distinct and can alternate in certain situations. Each personality is usually not aware of the other personalities.

Music therapy is the use of music for relaxation by creating an emotional climate or the instruction on how to play a musical instrument with the goals, for example, of increasing self-esteem or a feeling of accomplishment.

Myofacial release is a method for treating myofacial pain that considers both the origin of the pain and the resulting dysfunction. The three aspects of this approach include manual therapy, movement and exercise, and patient education. A whole body "hands-on" approach is used to release soft tissue (muscle) from abnormal grip of tight fascial (connective tissue).

Narcissistic personality disorder describes an individual who shows signs of grandiosity toward self, fantasies of power over others, omniscience, self-importance, vanity, and a strong need for admiration by others and opportunities for exhibiting self. Sometimes the individual shows a lack of empathy and understanding toward others.

National Board for Certification in Occupational Therapy (NBCOT) was created by AOTA in 1986 as a separate authority to conduct entry level certification programs and to monitor professional standards of practice for occupational therapists.

Naturopathy is based on a therapeutic system that does not advocate the use of drugs. The naturopath employs natural forces such as light, heat, air, water, massage, herbs, healthy food, and vitamins in treating individuals with a dysfunction.

Negative symptoms are losses or lessening of human functions such as the loss of motivation, withdrawal from social interactions, apathy, flattening of affect, loss of words to say, and loss of critical thinking or problem solving ability such as in making decisions. Negative symptoms are associated with schizophrenia.

Neurosis is a term that was first defined in the DSM–I (1952) as psychoneurotic and referred to behaviors in individuals marked by anxiety, avoidance, feelings of inadequacy, phobias, unhappiness, excessive guilt, and obsessive behavior. Currently in the DSM–IV (1994) these behaviors are indicative of personality disorders.

Object relations is a concept derived from psychoanalytic theory. It operates on a conscious or unconscious level. The concept is based on the initial bonding relationship between the mother and the infant. This interpersonal and intrapsychic experience is the basis for all dyadic relationships (e.g., sibling, friend, spouse, employee-employer, colleague, or acquaintance) and becomes the basis for the individual's sense of self. Life experiences can modify one's intrapsychic perception of engagement in object relations.

Obsessive-compulsive personality disorder is present in an individual who has a morbid concern with neatness, orderliness, perfection, and ritualistic or repetitive behavior. Symptoms include extreme preoccupation with details that interferes with task completion, excessive time at work at the expense of leisure, overconscientiousness regarding ethical or legal standards, lack of flexibility in decision making, a miserly spending attitude, and the hoarding of objects.

Occupational stress is the sum of the factors in the work environment that negatively affect the individual's psycho-physiological adjustment or homeostasis.

Occupational therapy is the application of purposeful activities to prevent disability and injury in individuals who are at risk and to develop and restore functions in individuals who are disabled. Functional activities include the ability to work, to be independent in self-care, to engage in leisure activities and to be effective in social interactions. The effectiveness of occupational therapy will depend on the therapist's ability to establish a therapeutic relationship and to select a purposeful activity that is meaningful to the client in producing a desired outcome.

Occupations are the culturally and personally meaningful and purposeful activities that humans engage in during their everyday lives. These occupations include the major functions of life such as work, leisure, play, self-care, rest, sleep, and social interactions.

On-the-job evaluations are situations in which the client is evaluated while employed.

Operant conditioning is a type of behavior therapy in which an individual's positive behavior is reinforced and negative behavior is not reinforced. Behavior is shaped by reinforcing sequential steps in a hierarchical manner.

Orthomolecular medicine is the study of the relationship between vitamins in the body and the onset of diseases such as the relationship between B complex vitamins and psychiatric disorders. Orthomolecular practitioners recommend megadoses of vitamins in treating specific psychiatric disorders.

Outcome is the result of a treatment intervention. Outcomes research is the investigation of treatment methods in producing desired outcomes such as the decrease of negative symptoms in individuals with schizophrenia.

Outcome measure is a specific test, procedure, or tool that is used to measure the results of a treatment intervention.

Panic disorder is an anxiety disorder characterized by panic attacks and is accompanied by acute anxiety, terror or fright, hyperventilation, sweating, chest pain, dizziness, and a feeling of losing control of self. Panic attacks can occur suddenly lasting for minutes with a sense of imminent danger or impending disaster. A panic disorder can lead to agoraphobia (fear of being in public and being alone).

Paradigm is a conceptual model that becomes universally accepted. For example during the age of institutionalization (1920–1950) in the United States the paradigm for treating mental illness was through hospitalization. In the 1960s a shift in the paradigm occurred by the Community Mental Health Movement.

Paradoxical intention (Frankl, 1967) is a behavior therapy technique that is based on the theory that individuals develop fears and tensions because of anticipatory anxiety. In using this technique, the individual is told to think of something he fears most or to create a negative emotion such as anxiety. By creating a negative feeling, the individual begins to cognitively control the symptom. It has been used as a successful technique with those who stutter who consciously produce stuttering and by doing so, control the speech.

Paranoid personality disorder is marked by extreme suspiciousness and distrust of others. An individual with this disorder attributes hidden motives and agendas of hostility directed by others toward self. The individual is easily offended, tends to misread and distort verbal and nonverbal communications, and is hypervigilant.

Paranoid schizophrenia is a subcategory of schizophrenia characterized by delusions, irrational beliefs, excessive suspicion, and feeling of persecutions by others.

Parataxic distortion refers to the "uncommunicative, unintelligible, and misleading statements in allegedly communicative interpersonal contexts" (Sullivan, 1963, p. 23).

Parkinson's disease is a chronic progressive nervous disorder occurring in later life, characterized by masklike facial expressions, intention tremor, slowing of voluntary movements, rigidity and weakness of muscles, and a peculiar gait.

Partial hospitalization includes day, evening, night, and weekend day treatment programs for individuals who need a supportive environment during a period of crisis but are able to avoid hospitalization and to stay in the community.

Participating action research (PAR) is a qualitative research model in which the researcher and participants in the research are both actively involved in the conceptualization, design, implementation, and interpreting of results.

Passive-aggressive personality disorder is characterized by stubbornness, procrastination, indecisiveness, envy, and resistance to requests and demands from others. The individual with this disorder tends not to be overtly hostile but through indecision and defiance creates negative confrontations with others.

Percentage (%) is the number of cases per hundred.

Percentile is a point in a distribution that defines where a given percentage of the cases fall. For example, the 89th percentile is the point where 89 percent of the cases are at or below this point.

Perception is the capacity to recognize sensory stimuli such as visual, tactile, auditory and proprioceptive stimuli in a meaningful way.

Performance areas are derived from the uniform terminology in occupational therapy (AOTA, 1994) and refer to the areas of work/productivity, self-care, and leisure.

Performance components include cognitive, sensory, perceptual, and psychosocial aspects of performance.

Personal resources to cope with stress are the individual assets and environmental supports an individual can use in alleviating stressors.

Personality is the complex of characteristics, behavioral traits, and attitudes that distinguish an individual from others.

Personality disorders comprise a number of disorders including anti-social, histrionic, paranoid, passive-aggressive, obsessive-compulsive, schizoid, narcissistic, borderline, and avoidant types. The disorder usually begins during childhood or adolescence and continues into adulthood. Many times the disorder leads to self-defeating behaviors that interfere with the individual's ability to adapt to changes in the environment and to meet societal expectations.

Pet therapy is the therapeutic use of pets, to create an animal-human bond, which may improve a patient's physical and emotional health.

Phenomenological refers to the subjective experiences and feelings of an individual. Depressed feelings and delusions in an individual with mental illness can be considered phenomenological symptoms.

Phobia is an abnormal fear or irrational dread of a specific object (e.g., spiders), activity (e.g., flying), or situation (e.g., being in an open plain).

Physical agent modalities (PAMs) are modalities applied by a therapist to a client such as transcutaneous electrical nerve stimulation (TENS), ultrasound, diathermy, and hydrotherapy that use electricity, water, heat, cold, light, or sound for therapeutic purposes.

Poetry therapy is the use of poetry to help clients to express their feelings and innermost thoughts. The poetry is designed to convey a vivid and imaginative sense of experience. It can be insightful in discovering a person's fantasies, desires, and fears.

Positive symptoms in a psychiatric illness such as schizophrenia represent an excess or distortion of normal functions, for example, normal suspicion becomes delusional thinking or illusions become hallucinations. Other examples of positive symptoms include disorganized speech and thinking, bizarre dressing, and exaggerated postures or hand movements.

Posttraumatic stress disorder is an anxiety disorder that occurs in response to a traumatic event such as a war time experience, natural disaster, airplane crash, parental abuse, or physical/mental torture. The symptoms include recurring vivid memories of the past experience causing insomnia, recurrent nightmares, hypervigilance, and other symptoms related to anxiety. The disorder can last for many years.

Postrotary nystagmus (PRN) is a normal reaction of the eyes in reaction to the body being rotated in a swing. The eyeballs respond by constantly moving in a cyclical direction. PRN is assessed by therapists using sensory integrative therapy.

Predictive validity is the extent to which a test can predict success or accuracy over a period of time, for example, predicting a client's ability to live in the community after discharge from the hospital.

Prevocational evaluation is a program to assess a client's ability to work, for example, in a sheltered workshop, competitive employment, or as homemaker.

Problem-oriented medical record (POMR) is a systematic method of recording progress notes in the patient's chart that prioritizes the symptoms and problems and a plan to treat these problems. The initial notes are periodically evaluated and progress notes are recorded. SOAP notes are part of a problem-oriented record.

Prodromal refers to coming before the initial stage of a disease such as severe anxiety precipitating an episode of depression in a vulnerable individual.

Professional Standard Review Organization (PSROs) were founded by the U.S. Congress in 1972 to ensure that health care services provided under Medicare, Medicaid, or Maternal and Child Health programs were of acceptable professional quality.

Prognosis is a clinical forecast of the probable course of the illness and the eventual outcome of the disease or condition. For example, the prognosis of an individual diagnosed with schizophrenia will depend on the age of the initial onset, the severity of symptoms, intelligence level, and environmental factors.

Progressive relaxation is a treatment method developed by Edmund Jacobson (1929, 1978). The method is based on tensing and relaxing muscle groups in the body systematically. The procedure involves identifying a local state of tension and relaxing it away by learning to control all of the skeletal musculature through systematic muscle tension and relaxation.

Proprioception is the perception by muscles, tendons, and the labyrinth in the ear, of movements and positions of bodily parts (e.g., the awareness of position of shoulder with eyes closed).

Psyche is a term derived from the Greek that means soul or mind.

Psychedelic is a term popularized in the 1960s during the "hippie era" that referred to an altered state of consciousness and visual hallucinations produced by drugs such as mescaline, psilocybin, or lysergic acid diethylamide (LSD).

Psychiatric diagnostic interview is an exploration of the patient's symptoms and problems; past psychiatric treatments, hospitalizations, and medications; medical history of past diseases, allergies, and bodily injuries; family history of mental illness; psychosocial development, education, occupation, family relationship, friendships, and sexual experiences; mental status examination: assessment of appearance, behavior, current mood, cognition, suicidal or homicidal thoughts, and reality testing.

Psychiatric rehabilitation is a multidisciplinary approach with the goal of restoring function in social skills, self-care, leisure, and work (Anthony, 1979). Psychiatric rehabilitation refers to restoring function in an individual with a psychiatric disability.

Psychoanalysis is a systematic method of psychotherapy founded by Sigmund Freud that employs free association, dream analysis, analyses of transference, and other psychodynamic techniques to help an individual understand the unconscious feelings and desires that shape his or her personality and behavior.

Psychodrama is a form of group psychotherapy in which patients act out assigned roles. The therapeutic goals are to reduce emotional symptoms and encourage personal growth. The psychodrama includes a protagonist who is the center of the drama, alter egos who help the protagonist to think through identified issues, a director who sets the stage and scenes, and an audience who comment on the actions and give insight to the protagonist.

Psychodynamic refers to the understanding of the conscious and unconscious forces that motivate behavior, cause symptoms, and shape one's personality. Psychotherapists such as psychoanalysts use a psychodynamic approach in treating individuals with mental disorders.

Psychomotor agitation describes the state of a client who is in constant motion with severe restlessness, pacing, wringing of hands, and purposeless activity accompanied by a high level of anxiety.

Psychoneuroimmunology is the study of the relationships and interactions between the mind, central nervous system, autonomic nervous system, and endocrine system. It represents the effects of psychological states on the immune system. It has been found in some studies that extreme stress reactions can dampen the immune system and leave the individual vulnerable to disease.

Psychopathic pertains to antisocial behavior such as violence, criminal activity, physical or sexual abuse, or related behaviors that reflect a lack of moral and ethical standards. Synonymous terms are sociopathic and antisocial reaction.

Psychosis is a severe mental disorder characterized by delusions, hallucinations, thinking disturbances, and inability to perform activities of daily living such as in schizophrenia, extreme depression, dementia, and chronic alcoholism .

Psychosomatic medicine refers to the study of the relationship of psychological factors and the etiology of physical and psychiatric disorders. Current investigators in psychosomatic medicine examine both the physical and psychological factors as causes and effects and treat mind and body as one.

Psychotherapy is a treatment technique that relies primarily on the verbal interactions between the therapist and client. The methods used in psychotherapy vary considerably depending on the theoretical model espoused by the therapist. In general the phases in psychotherapy include (a) establishing a therapeutic alliance with the client, (b) understanding the client's problems and making a tentative diagnosis, (c) helping the client to understand and gain insight into the causes of his or her problems, (d) setting goals for treatment that are mutually acceptable by therapist and client, (e) implementing treatment where the client learns and tests out new behaviors, and (f) closure and discharge of the client.

Quality assurance is a system to measure the effectiveness of a hospital or treatment facility to meet standards of care established by governmental agencies or hospital associations. A quality assurance program in a hospital includes an evaluation component to identify problems and an action component to improve patient care.

Quality of life is a concept that implies that individuals have the capacity to determine what brings them most happiness in their lives. Factors such as being with one's family, being in one's home, ability to travel independently, food choices, expressing oneself through music and art, socializing with friends, and working at an interesting job are components of quality of life.

Qi Gong is part of traditional Chinese medicine, along with accupuncture, application of herbs, and massage. This method of alternative medicine incorporates "meditation , movement exercises, self-massage, and special healing techniques to regulate internal functions of the human body" (Londorf & Winn, 2000, p. 231).

Range of motion dance (ROM dance) is a movement therapy comprised of expressive dance and relaxation techniques. It incorporates joint motion in all ranges to help individuals with joint and muscle limitations. It is also an educational process that assists individuals in improving their movement functioning through hands-on repatterning and verbal instruction.

Rational-emotive therapy (RET) is a direct psychotherapy technique originated by Albert Ellis (Ellis & Whiteley, 1979) that helps the client to problem solve by working through solutions and stating the options. The therapist frequently confronts the client with the consequences of his or her behavior and assigns homework problems for the client to try out new behaviors.

Raw score is the score obtained directly on the test before transforming it into a more meaningful comparison (e.g., z-score, percentile, or standard score).

Reality therapy is a psychotherapy technique introduced by Glasser (1965) that focuses on helping the client take responsibility for his or her behavior and to confront problems directly.

Reductionism refers to reducing complex situations, data, phenomena, and experiences to simple terms. An example is to treat major depression, a complex illness that affects an individual's ability to work, socialize with others, engage in leisure activities, and regulate one's self-care, by taking a drug to relieve symptoms. A holistic approach is in contrast to reductionistic treatment.

Reflexology is the application of massage of reflex points on feet and hands to encourage health and well-being.

Regression is a relapse or exacerbation of symptoms in which an individual's illness gets worse. For example, an individual who is making improvement from an episode of depression suddenly regresses with exaggerated feelings of suicide.

Rehabilitation is the restoration of function in an individual with an acquired disability.

Function relates to competence in an individual's ability to work, to be independent in self-care and leisure activities and to be able to have the social skills for effective personal interactions.

Reinforcement schedule is the time interval of rewarding a client in reinforcing behavior such as every time a client responds positively in an interpersonal encounter.

Relaxation response is a treatment method developed by Herbert Benson (1975) based originally on Transcendental Meditation. In this method the client is taught to have a passive attitude and to recite a verbal phrase to himself or herself while in a comfortable position. The physiological reaction that is sought is produced by sitting serenely and alone in a quiet place with eyes closed and arms and hands relaxed; paying careful attention to breathing; and repeating a brief word or phrase at each respiratory cycle. The aim is to reach a tranquil mental state that refreshes the mind and body.

Reliability is the extent to which a test gives consistent results when administered by different testers on different occasions. The major method used to measure reliability is test-retest. Other methods include split half and equivalency forms.

Remission is the lessening of symptoms or complete recovery from an illness. For example in an individual diagnosed with schizophrenia, the symptoms of hallucinations and delusions may disappear and the individual is able to work and engage in normal activities. Individuals may be in remission for weeks, months, or years.

Rolfing is the application of deep massage to the connective tissue, which is the wrapping that binds and connects muscles and bones (Rolf, 1977). The purpose of rolfing is to increase the range of motion of the joints and to enhance suppleness by stretching and unwinding the fas-

cia, which become thickened and stuck together causing pain and immobility in the client. The massage involves deep sliding movements to the neck, shoulder, torso, and lower extremities.

RUMBA is an acronym for *r*elevant, *u*nderstandable, *m*easurable, *b*ehavioral and *a*chievable. It is used as a guide in writing operational treatment objectives for clients.

Schizoid personality disorder is symptomatic of individuals who are withdrawn, introspective, oversensitive, seclusive, and detached from initiating and maintaining close relationships. The individual with a schizoid personality disorder tends toward working alone and has difficulty in expressing feelings.

Schizophrenia is a severe psychotic mental disorder that can be classified into subtypes such as paranoid, catatonic, disorganized, undifferentiated, and residual. A diagnosis of schizophrenia is made if symptoms such as delusions, hallucinations, thinking disorders, and disorganized behavior are present for at least 6 months. The symptoms of schizophrenia interfere with the individual's ability to carry out the normal role functions in work, leisure, self-care, and social interactions.

Schizoaffective disorders includes affective disorders such as depression and bipolar, which develop concurrently with psychotic symptoms such as delusions and hallucinations. It is a form of schizophrenia. Treatment includes a holistic plan with medication to decrease the symptoms of psychosis and depression or bipolar symptoms and psychosocial rehabilitation to help the individual integrate into the community.

Seasonal affective disorder (SAD) is a mood disorder accompanied by symptoms of depression such as fatigue, diminished concentration, sadness, sleep and eating disturbances, and a general malaise. It is thought to be caused by the diminishing of daytime sun in late fall and winter. Treatment includes light therapy, medication, stress management, and exercise.

Self is the individual's typical characteristics or personality that constitutes his or her identity. It is comprised of the affective, cognitive, and spiritual qualities that are distinctive.

Self-concept or self-image is the individual's perceptions, feelings, and attitudes about his or her own identity, values, capabilities, and weaknesses.

Self-efficacy is the individual's perception of being able to perform a functional task or occupation.

Self-esteem is the individual's appraisal of his or her competencies and abilities to succeed or master tasks that he or she is confronted with on a daily basis. An individual's self-esteem can be assessed as low or high depending on his or her self-confidence in performing a task.

Sensory Integration (SI) Therapy is an occupational therapy frame of reference that is based on developmental, neurological, and perceptual concepts. Vestibular stimulation, balance exercises, visual spatial awareness, motor planning, tactile exercises, and bilateral motor coordination activities are specific techniques used in treatment (Ayres, 1972).

Serotonin is a neurotransmitter in the central nervous system that occurs naturally in the brain. It plays an important role in mood behavior and sleep-wake cycle. The regulation of serotonin is important in treating depression.

Sheltered workshop is a supportive employment environment where individuals with disabilities produce a saleable product such as in assembly work or provide a service such as lawn maintenance. Individuals are usually paid on the basis of their productivity, which can be below or at comparable wages for the job performed. The work can be transitional to competitive employment or long term. Work adjustment

training is usually incorporated into the program.

Side-effects of medications are adverse effects in the individual that accompany the actions of a drug such as nausea, headaches, dizziness, hypertension, dryness of mouth, blurred vision, insomnia, and tardive dyskinesia.

Signs are objective findings of a disease or disorder that are observed by the clinician or measured objectively through a test. Psychiatric signs can be gathered through laboratory findings indicating brain lesions, through electroencephalograms indicating epilepsy, or through objective tests such as *Minnesota Multiphasic Personality Inventory*.

SOAP note is an organized method of recording a patient's progress. SOAP stands for *S*ubjective findings which are the reported symptoms of the patient; *O*bjective findings of the therapist; *A*ssessment, which is the documented analysis and summary of the findings; and *P*lan, which are the recommended treatments, therapeutic interventions, and further diagnostic tests, if necessary.

Social skills are comprised of skills in (a) attending/listening, (b) conversational, (c) supportive, (d) problem-solving, and (e) self-control. These skills include both verbal and nonverbal behaviors.

Sources of error in measurement are derived from the unreliability of the instrument, bias of the test administrator, unreliability of the client, or undesirable test environment.

Spirituality is an individual's focus on meaning in life and connectiveness to the universe. It is the higher purposes that give meaning to life and are evident through faith and beliefs.

Stigma implies a devaluation of an individual because of a disability. For example, the stigma attached to having a psychiatric disability is marked by a prejudiced attitude by a person who devalues an individual with mental illness.

Storytelling is reminiscing about events in a person's life and recapturing visual scenes. It can also be a life review of an individual.

Stress is a term that can mean the amount of pressure on an individual (stressor) or the end result such as (stress reactions).

Stress management is a general term that includes systematic treatment interventions to reduce the hyperarousal of the sympathetic nervous system. Biofeedback, progressive relaxation, relaxation response, meditation, yoga, Tai Ch'i, music therapy, exercise, and cognitive-behavioral therapies are examples of techniques used in a comprehensive stress management program.

Stress reactions are the psycho-physiological reactions in the individual that are the end results of stressors minus personal resources.

Stressors are the specific factors that precipitate a stress reaction.

Substance abuse is a psychiatric disorder in which the individual becomes dependent on a chemical substance such as alcohol, sedatives, hypnotics, anxiolytics, amphetamines, cocaine, opium, or heroin. Effects of substance abuse include delirium, psychosis, and cognitive mood disorders, sleep and eating disturbances, anxiety, and a general interference with functional activities of living.

Support groups are community groups like Alliance for the Mentally Ill (AMI), Recovery Incorporated, and Alcoholics Anonymous (AA) that meet regularly and provide opportunities for individuals with mental illness and their families and friends to discuss openly the problems associated with mental illness. Lectures, educational films, and literature are also available at support group meetings.

Supported employment is a concept first used with individuals with developmental disabilities. It includes job placement, work adjustment, advocacy, job coaching, and follow-up. The concept has been expanded to individuals with mental illness to include transitional employment and access to career development and training.

Supported housing refers to enabling individuals to live in affordable housing by improving access to existing housing through federal subsidies or cooperative ventures. Rental units, single-family homes, or public housing can be supported housing.

Symptoms are reported changes in an individual that are subjective sensations such as pain, hearing voices, anxiety, or seeing double images.

Syndrome refers to a group of symptoms or signs of an impairment or dysfunction. For example, Korsakoff's syndrome is characterized by delirium, hallucinations, memory disturbances, disorientation for time and space, confusion, and personality deterioration. Persian Gulf syndrome is characterized by respiratory and gastrointestinal disturbances, fatigue, muscle and joint pain, and memory impairment.

Systematic desensitization is a technique developed by Wolpe (1990) and used in behavior therapy for eliminating phobias in which the client is exposed to anxiety-producing stimuli in gradual increments until the phobia is eliminated.

Tactile defensiveness, conceptualized by Jean Ayres (1972), is a syndrome identified in the sensory integration literature in which an individual has an aversive reaction to being handled or touched.

Tai Ch'i is an old Chinese system designed to develop ch'i within the body. It can be used to rejuvenate, to heal and prevent illness and injuries, and also to lead to spiritual enlightenment. It is based on principles of rhythmic movements, equilibrium of body, effective breathing, and development of life forces in the body through a series of slow-moving, circular movements.

Tardive dyskinesia is a motor disorder that is similar to symptoms occurring in Parkinson's disease such as slow, rhythmic involuntary movements, tremors, and muscular weakness. It can occur as a side effect of long-term dosage of phenothiazines, which are tranquilizers used in the treatment of schizophrenia.

Task Analysis: *see* **Activity analysis**.

Terminal behavior refers to the target goal in behavior therapy such as the cessation of smoking, the reduction of temper tantrums, or elimination of phobias.

Test is essentially an objective and standardized measure of a sample of behavior (Anastasi, 1988). The main purpose of a test is to predict future performance.

Therapeutic community is a term first coined by Maxwell Jones (1953) to describe a treatment environment created in psychiatric hospitals or community mental health centers where community meetings of staff, patients, and family are held, patient government is encouraged, and each individual takes responsibility for housekeeping tasks.

Therapeutic milieu is an environment of support where clients feel comfortable in learning and developing social, cognitive, employment, leisure, and self-care skills while feeling empowered to change behavior.

Therapeutic social clubs are client-centered groups where individuals can socialize, and engage in recreational activities. They can be incorporated in hospitals or in the community as drop-in centers. Beard at Fountain House in New York City was an innovator in developing therapeutic social clubs.

Therapeutic touch is an alternative treatment technique where the therapist uses touch for

"the expressed purpose of health, changing, communicating, and growing in a health spiritual and physical manner" (Ledwith, 2000, p. 462).

Therapeutic use of self is a term conceptualized by Jerome Frank (1958), a psychotherapist. It refers to the therapist-client relationship.

Token economy is a technique of behavior therapy in which clients earn tokens for specific positive behaviors or mastery of skills. Token economies have been used in psychiatric hospitals and residential schools. Tokens can be exchanged for desired foods or privileges.

Transactional analysis (TA) is a psychotherapy technique developed by Berne (1961) that analyzes the roles that individuals take in interpersonal relationships such as parent (superego), child (id), or adult (ego).

Transcutaneous electrical nerve stimulation (TENS) is the application of mild electrical stimulation to skin electrodes placed over a painful area. It causes interference with transmission of painful stimuli. It is presumed to work by producing noninvasive pain relief by stimulating the release of endorphins or polypeptides.

Transdisciplinary team is comprised of professionals from various disciplines who share their roles with one another. For example, an occupational therapist may use family therapy or behavior management techniques in treatment sessions after consulting with the social worker or behavioral psychologist about the procedures.

Undifferentiated schizophrenia is diagnosed when an individual displays the major symptoms of schizophrenia such as hallucinations, delusions, and thinking disorders, but there is no single prominent feature.

Validity is the extent to which a test measures what it is designed to measure. Types of validity include face, content, concurrent, predictive, and construct.

Values clarification "is an intervention approach that utilizes a form of questioning and a set of activities or strategies to help individuals learn the valuing process" (Franklin, 1986, p. 41). This process helps an individual to choose, affirm, and act on his or her beliefs.

Vestibular stimulation refers to the stimulation of the vestibular system that controls equilibrium and reactions to gravity. Sensory integrative therapists use vestibular stimulation in treatment by using swings, hassocks, therapy balls, and scooter boards.

Visualization is imagining the working's of one's own body or inner experiences to encourage healing and well-being.

Vocational rehabilitation is the restoration of work functions in individuals with mental or physical disabilities.

Work is defined as paid or unpaid activity that contributes to subsistence, produces a service or product, and is culturally meaningful to the worker. Work can be driven by internal motivation if the individual engages in work purely for the inherent job satisfaction, pleasure, or self-accomplishment that results. For example, the creative artist or composer may be working to express a feeling or create a new composition without concern for material reward. The creative individual may spend many hours on work without pay as intrinsic motivation. On the other extreme is the individual who dislikes his or her job, such as a factory worker who works for subsistence only. This is an example of extrinsic motivation. Probably the highest level of job satisfaction is to work at a job that one enjoys and to be paid a high salary. This may be true for some professional athletes or successful artists. Most individuals work to support their standard of living while selecting a job that they

enjoy. Some individuals engage in full-time volunteer work in activities that they find rewarding. Housewives or house husbands work at home for no monetary compensation while performing full-time work in child care, household tasks, and cooking. All of these activities are work. For the occupational therapist, evaluating the client's work and the worker role are important aspects of treatment.

Work hardening is a multidisciplinary approach of applying a structured environment and supervised activities for injured workers. Activities include simulated work tasks, functional activities, cardiovascular reconditioning, body mechanics, and stress management (Demers, 1992).

Work samples are well-defined activities that are similar to an actual job. They can be used to assess an individual's vocational aptitude, worker characteristics, and vocational interests (Nadolsky, 1974). Examples of work samples include Valpar, Micro-Tower, and McCarron-Dial.

Yoga, as used in the Western world, has been associated almost exclusively with exercises, physical postures, and regulation of breathing. The aim is to achieve the harmony of body, mind, and spirit.

REFERENCES

American Occupational Therapy Association. (AOTA). (1994). *Uniform terminology for occupational therapy*: Application to practice. (3rd ed.). Rockville, MD: Author.

American Psychiatric Association. (1952). *Diagnostics and statistical manual: Mental disorders* (1st ed). Washington, DC: Author.

American Psychiatric Association. (1994). *Diagnostic and statistical manual of psychiatric disorders* (4th ed.). Washington, DC: Author.

Anastasi, A. (1988). *Psychological testing* (6th ed.). New York: Macmillan.

Anthony, W. A. (1979). *The principles of psychiatric rehabilitation.* Amherst, MA: Human Resources Press.

Ayres, A. J. (1972). *Sensory integration and learning disorders.* Los Angeles: Western Psychological Services.

Baker, F., & Intagliata, J. (1992). Case management. In R. P. Liberman (Ed.), *Handbook of psychiatric rehabilitation* (pp. 213–243). Boston: Allyn & Bacon.

Beck, A. T. (1976). *Cognitive therapy and emotional disorders.* New York: International Universities Press.

Benson, H. (1975). *Relaxation response.* New York: William Morrow.

Berne, E. (1961). *Transactional analysis in psychotherapy.* New York: Grove.

Brown, G. W., Birley, J. L. T., & Wing, J. K. (1972). Influence of family life on the course of schizophrenia disorder: A replication. *British Journal of Psychiatry, 121,* 241–258.

Cannon, W. (1932). *The wisdom of the body.* New York: Norton.

Carling, P. J. (1995). *Return to community building support systems for people with psychiatric disabilities.* New York: Guilford.

Demers, L. (1992). *Work hardening: A practical guide.* Stoneham, MA: Andover.

Ellis, A., & Whiteley, J. M. (Eds.). (1979). *Theoretical and empirical foundations of rational-–emotive therapy.* Pacific Grove: CA: Brooks/Cole.

Frank, J. (1958). The therapeutic use of self. *American Journal of Occupational Therapy, 12,* 215–225.

Frankl, V. (1967). *Man's search for meaning.* Boston: Beacon.

Franklin, D. (1986). A comparison of the effectiveness of Values Clarification presented as a personal computer program versus a traditional therapy group: A pilot study. *Occupational Therapy in Mental Health, 6*(3), 39–52.

Glasser, W. (1965). *Reality therapy; A new approach to psychiatry.* New York: Harper & Row.

Hood, C. (1959). The challenge of dance therapy. *Journal of Health, Physical Education, and Recreation, 30,* 17–18.

Jacobson, E. (1929). *Progressive relaxation.* Chicago: University of Chicago.

Jacobson, E. (1978). *You must relax* (4th ed.). New York: McGraw-Hill.

Jones, M. (1953). *The therapeutic community.* New York: Basic.

Keyserling, W. M., Armstrong, T. J., & Punnett, C. (1991). Ergonomic job analysis: A structured approach for identifying risk factors associated with overexertion injuries and disorders. *Applied Occupational Environmental Hygiene, 6,* 353–363.

Kielhofner, G. (1997). *Conceptual foundations of occupational therapy* (2nd ed.). Philadelphia: F. A. Davis.

Ledwith, S. (2000). Therapeutic touch. In D. W. Novey, *Clinician's complete reference to complementary & alternative medicine* (pp. 462–471). St. Louis: Mosby.

Levy, F. J. (1988). *Dance/movement therapy a healing art.* Reston, VA: The American Alliance for Health, Physical Education, Recreation, and Dance.

Londorf, D., & Winn, M. (2000). Qi gong. In D. W. Novey, *Clinician's complete reference to complementary & alternative medicine* (pp. 231–244). St. Louis: Mosby.

Nadolsky, J. M. (1974). The work sample in vocational evaluation: A consistent rationale. *Vocational Evaluation and Work Adjustment Bulletin, 7,* 2–5.

Norris, P. A., & Fahrion, S. L. (1993). Autogenic biofeedback in pyschophysiological therapy and stress management. In P. M. Lehrer & R. L. Woolfolk, P. (Eds.), *Principles and practices of stress management* (2nd ed., pp. 231–262). New York: Guilford.

Ottenbacher, K. J., & Cusick, A. (1989). Goal attainment scaling as a method of clinical service evaluation. *The American Journal of Occupational Therapy, 44*(6), 519–525.

Perls, F. (1969). *Gestalt therapy verbatim.* Moab, UT: Real People Press.

Rogers, C. (1951). *Client-centered therapy.* Boston: Houghton Mifflin.

Rolf, I. (1977). *Rolfing: The integration of human structures.* Santa Monica, CA: Dennis–Landman.

Selye, H. (1974). *Stress without distress.* Philadelphia: Lippincott.

Slavson, S. R. (1943). *An introduction to group therapy.* New York: The Commonwealth Fund.

Spaulding, W. D. (Ed). (1994). *Cognitive technology in psychiatric rehabilitation.* Lincoln: University of Nebraska Press.

Sullivan, H. S. (1963). *The fusion of psychiatry and social science.* New York: W. W. Norton.

Trainor, J., & Church, K. (1984). *A framework for support for people with severe mental disabilities.* Toronto: Canadian Mental Health Association.

von Bertalanffy, L. (1950). The theory of open systems in physics and biology. *Science, 111*, 23–29.

Wolpe, J. (1990). *The practice of behavior therapy* (4th ed.). Elmsford, NY: Pergamon.

World Health Organization (WHO). (1980). *International classification of impairments, disabilities, and handicaps* (ICIDH). Geneva, Switzerland: Author.

Wykoff, W. (1993). The psychological effects of exercise on non-clinical and clinical populations of adult women: A critical review of the literature. *Occupational Therapy in Mental Health, 12*(3), 69–106.

APPENDIX

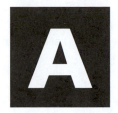

Diagnosis of Mental Disorders

Axis I. Clinical Syndromes and Other Conditions That May Be a Focus of Clinical Attention

---

Disorders Usually First Diagnosed in Infancy, Childhood, or Adolescence
- Learning Disorders
- Motor Skills Disorder
- Communication Disorders
- Pervasive Developmental Disorders (e.g., Autism, Asperger's, PDD)
- Attention-Deficit and Disruptive Behavior Disorders (e.g., ADHD, Conduct Disorder, Oppositional Defiant Disorder)
- Feeding and Eating Disorders of Infancy of Early Childhood (e.g., Pica)
- Tic Disorders (e.g., Tourette's Syndrome)
- Elimination Disorders (e.g., Encopresis, Enuresis)
- Other Disorders of Infancy, Childhood, or Adolescence (e.g., Separation Anxiety Disorder, Selective Mutism)

Delirium, Dementia, and Amnestic and Other Cognitive Disorders
- Delirium
- Dementia
- Amnesic Disorders
- Other Cognitive Disorders

Mental Disorders Due to a General Medical Condition Not Elsewhere Classified
- Catatonic Disorder Due to (*state general medical condition*)
- Personality Change Due to (*state general medical condition*)
- Mental Disorder Not Otherwise Stated (NOS) Due to (*state general medical condition*)

Substance-Related Disorders
- Alcohol-related Disorders (alcohol use or alcohol-induced)
- Amphetamine (or Amphetamine-like)-Related Disorders (amphetamine use or amphetamine-induced)
- Caffeine-Related Disorders (caffeine induced)

(continued)

- Cannabis-Related Disorders (cannabis use or cannabis induced)
- Cocaine-Related Disorders (cocaine use or cocaine induced)
- Hallucinogen-Related Disorders (hallucinogen use or hallucinogen induced)
- Inhalant-Related Disorders (inhalant use or inhalant induced)
- Nicotine-Related Disorders (nicotine use or nicotine induced)
- Opioid-Related Disorders (opioid use or opioid induced)
- Phencyclidine (or Phencyclidine-like)-Related Disorders (phencyclidine use or phencyclidine induced)
- Sedative-, Hypnotic-, or Anxiolytic-Related Disorders (use or induced)
- Polysubstance-Related Disorder
- Other (Or Unknown) Substance-Related Disorders

Schizophrenia and Other Psychotic Disorders

Mood Disorders
- Depressive Disorders
- Bipolar Disorders

Anxiety Disorders (e.g., panic attacks, phobias, Obsessive-Compulsive Disorder, Posttraumatic Stress Disorder)

Somatoform Disorders (e.g., Conversion Disorder, Pain Disorder)

Factitious Disorders (e.g., production or feigning symptoms to deceive clinician, malingering)

Dissociative Disorders (e.g., disorders that disrupt the ability to integrate consciousness, memory, identity, and perception)

Sexual and Gender Identity Disorders
- Sexual Dysfunctions
- Paraphilias
- Gender Identity Disorders

Eating Disorders (e.g., Bulimia, Anorexia)

Sleep Disorders
- Primary Sleep Disorders
- Sleep Disorders Related to Another Mental Disorder
- Other Sleep Disorders

Impulse-control Disorders Not Elsewhere Classified (e.g., Kleptomania, Pyromania, Pathological Gambling)

Adjustment Disorders (e.g., chronic maladaption to a psychosocial stressor not significant enough to be classified elsewhere)

Other Conditions That May Be a Focus of Clinical Attention
- Psychological Factors Affecting Medical Condition
- Medication Induced Movement Disorders
- Other Medication-induced Disorders
- Relational Problems
- Problems Related to Abuse or Neglect
- Attentional Conditions That May Be a Focus of Clinical Attention

---

Axis II. Personality Disorders and Mental Retardation.

Mental Retardation (mild, moderate, severe, profound)

Personality Disorders
- Paranoid Personality Disorder (overly suspicious)
- Schizoid Personality Disorder (difficulty in forming relationships)
- Schizotypal Personality Disorder (peculiarities in speech and behavior)
- Antisocial Personality Disorder (acting out toward others)
- Borderline Personality Disorder (instability and uncertainty related to behavior and identity)
- Histrionic Personality Disorder (overly reactive behavior)
- Narcissistic Personality Disorder (preoccupation with self)
- Avoidant Personality Disorder (social withdrawal in spite of need for personal relationships)
- Dependent Personality Disorder
- Obsessive–Compulsive Personality Disorder (preoccupation with details)
- Personality Disorder Not Otherwise Stated (NOS)

Axis IV. Psychosocial and Environmental Problems.

Problems on this Axis are classified into the following problem areas:

- Problems with the primary support group (e.g., death of a family member, physical or sexual abuse)
- Problems with the social environment (e.g., discrimination, living alone, adjustment to retirement)
- Educational problems (e.g., illiteracy, learning difficulties)
- Occupational problems (e.g., unemployment, stressful work environment)
- Housing problems (e.g., homelessness, unsafe neighborhood)
- Economic problems (e.g., poverty, poor budgeting, underemployment)
- Problems with access to health care services (e.g., inadequate or no health insurance, lack of access to health care provider)
- Problems related to interaction with the legal system/crime (e.g., criminal behavior, adjudication, incarceration)
- Other psychosocial and environmental problems (e.g., disasters, such as floods or earthquake, isolation from community services)

Axis V. Global Assessment of Functioning.

On this Axis, the client rating is based on the following general areas:

- 91–100: superior functioning (e.g., adolescent coming from a single-parent family achieving at a high academic level)
- 81–90: absent or minimal symptoms (e.g., a widow who is slightly depressed and successfully returns to work)
- 71–80: transient and expectable reactions to psychosocial stressors (e.g., an individual whose house has flooded expresses anger toward authorities as an aftermath)
- 61–70: mild symptoms (e.g., during a divorce, the child shows some decrease in academic performance)
- 51–60: moderate symptoms (e.g., individual living alone without many friends who rejects social overtures from others)
- 41–50: serious symptoms (e.g., an individual showing such anxiety that he or she is inability to function at work, in daily living activities, and has few or no leisure activities)
- 31–40: some or major impairment in reality testing, communication, or several areas of psychosocial judgment (e.g., symptoms, such as illogical thinking and depressed mood, interfere with the individual's ability to attend school, work, or show independence in self-care)
- 21–30: delusional or hallucinatory, serious impairment in communication or judgment, or inability to function in almost all areas (e.g., individual is severely dysfunctional and needs continual supervision to perform activities of daily living)
- 11–20: some danger of hurting self or others, occasionally fails to maintain minimal personal hygiene, or gross impairment in communication (e.g., individual cannot self-regulate behavior and is a threat to self and others)
- 1–10: persistent danger of severely hurting self or others, inability to maintain minimal personal hygiene, or serious suicidal act with clear expectation of death (e.g., individual needs 24-hour supervision to prevent injury to self or others)
- 0: inadequate information (e.g., no information is known about the individual's social functioning)

Source: Adapted from the *Diagnostic and Statistical Manual, Fourth Edition* (DSM–IV, 1994) and the *Diagnostic and Statistical Manual, Fourth Edition, Text Revision* (DSM-IV-TR™, 2000) American Psychiatric Association, Washington, DC. Author.

APPENDIX

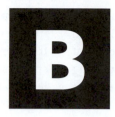

Severity of Psychosocial Stressors and Level of Functioning

The information presented here changed between the DSM–III-R (APA, 1987) and the DSM–IV (DSM, 1994) and is therefore presented here only for information. We feel that this scale helps to put the level of stressors into perspective.

In this part of the diagnostic evaluation, the clinician describes stressors in the individual's life that have had a significant effect on the onset of the disorder. The psychosocial stressor is interpreted as being a factor in precipitating the disorder within a year prior to the onset of the clinical syndrome of personality disorder.

Axis IV. Severity of Psychosocial Stressors

Code	Term	*Adult Examples*	*Child or Adolescent Examples*
1	None	No apparent psychosocial stressor	No apparent psychosocial stressor
2	Minimal	Minor violation of the law; small bank loan	Vacation with family
3	Mild	Argument with neighbor; change in work hours	Change in school teacher; new school year
4	Moderate	New career; death of close friend; pregnancy	Chronic parental fighting; change to new school; illness of close relative; birth of sibling
5	Severe	Serious illness in self or family; major financial loss; marital separation; birth of child	Death of peer, divorce of parents; arrest; hospitalization; persistent and harsh parental discipline
6	Extreme	Death of close relative; divorce	Death of parent or sibling; repeated physical or sexual abuse
7	Catastrophic	Concentration camp experience; devastating natural disaster	Multiple family deaths
8	Unspecified	No information or not applicable	No information or not applicable

Source: Adapted from the *Diagnostic and Statistical Manual–III-R (DSM–III-R)* by the American Psychiatric Association, 1987, Washington, DC: Author.

As with the previous table, this scale was changed between the DSM–III (APA, 1980) and the DSM–IV (APA, 1994); however, we feel that it helps put the level of adaptive functioning into perspective. We hope that it will help the new clinician.

Adaptive functioning includes social and interpersonal relationships with family and friends; occupational functioning as a worker, student, or homemaker; and involvement in leisure-time activities including recreation, sports, and hobbies.

Axis V. Highest Level of Adaptive Functioning in the Past Year

Levels	Adult Examples	Child or Adolescent Examples
1. SUPERIOR Usually effective functioning in social relationships, occupational functioning, and use of leisure time.	Single parent living in deteriorating neighborhood takes excellent care of children and home, has warm relations with friends, and finds time for pursuit of hobby.	A 12-year-old girl gets superior grades in school, is extremely popular among her peers, and excels in many sports. She does all of this with apparent ease and comfort.
2. VERY GOOD Better than average functioning in social relations, occupational functioning, and use of leisure time.	A 65-year-old retired widower does some volunteer work, often sees old friends, and pursues hobbies.	An adolescent boy gets excellent grades, works part-time, has several close friends, and plays banjo in a jazz band. He admits to some distress in "keeping up with everything."
3. GOOD No more than slight impairment in either social or occupational functioning.	A woman with many friends functions extremely well at a difficult job, but says "the strain is too much."	An 8-year-old boy does well in school, has several friends, but bullies younger children.
4. FAIR Moderate impairment in either social relations or occupational functioning or some impairment in both.	A lawyer has trouble carrying through assignments; has several acquaintances, but hardly any close friends.	A 10-year-old girl does poorly in school but has adequate peer and family relations.
5. POOR Marked impairment in either social relations or occupational functioning or moderate impairment in both.	A man with one or two friends has trouble keeping a job for more than a few weeks.	A 14-year-old boy almost fails in school and has trouble getting along with his peers.
6. VERY POOR Marked impairment in both social relations and occupational functioning.	A woman is unable to do any of her housework and has violent outburst toward family and neighbors.	A 6-year-old girl needs special help in all subjects and has virtually no peer relationships.
7. GROSSLY IMPAIRED Gross impairment in virtually all areas of functioning.	An elderly man needs supervision to maintain minimal personal hygiene and is usually incoherent.	A 4-year-old-boy needs constant restraint to avoid hurting himself and is almost totally lacking in skills.
8. UNSPECIFIED	No information available	No information available

Source: Adapted from the *Diagnostic and Statistical Manual–III (DSM–III)* by the American Psychiatric Association, 1980, Washington, DC: Author.

APPENDIX

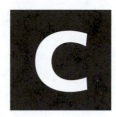

Role Delineation of the COTA

During the last twenty years, much effort has been directed toward the study of the first-year entry-level functions of the OTR and COTA. A document developed by the American Occupational Therapy Association entitled *Entry Level Role Delineation* was approved by the AOTA Representative Assembly in March 1981. The following principles and concepts were used initially in the development of this document:

▶ OTRs must be able to do all COTA roles and functions.

▶ The role delineation reflects present and future practice of occupational therapy.

▶ The role delineation reflects entry-level practice only, and may be used only for that level when used to develop educational *Essentials* or certification requirements.

▶ Entry level is defined as the first year of practice.

▶ Entry-level COTAs must receive direct supervision by an OTR professionally and legally during the first year of occupational therapy practice. COTAs are encouraged to participate in continuing educational programs provided by agencies and profes-

sional associations and to pursue other continuing education opportunities.

▶ Entry-level OTRs are certified for general practice and are able to independently provide services. Entry-level OTRs are encouraged to pursue continuing education, consultation, and other collaborative activities in their professional role.

▶ Employers should provide appropriate personnel for the supervision of new graduates.

▶ The role delineation addresses task and not "professional" behaviors that reflect ethical or value judgments.

Over the last 20 years, AOTA has updated the role delineation of COTAs and OTRs (AOTA, 1995; Margolis, Morgan, Dougherty, Halfon, & Petrone, 1997). These new roles include:

▶ The supervisor should consider current occupational standards and needs of therapy within the environment; complexity of evaluation and interventions employed; proficiencies of the supervisee; regulations, policies and procedures of the agency; state laws and regulations; and reimbursement requirements.

▶ The supervising therapist should spend a minimum of 3 to 5 direct contact hours per week with the full-time COTA. State regulations may require more stringent standards.

▶ Supervision may also include record reviews, observations of interventions and assessments, informal or formal meetings, functional supervision, or behavioral observations by other occupational therapy personnel.

▶ The OTR is ultimately responsible for the health and safety of each individual client receiving occupational therapy services under his or her supervision of the COTA.

▶ If an OTR delegates an assessment or intervention to the COTA, it is expected that results or findings will be consistent with the OTR by establishing service competencies.

▶ OTRs and COTAs must demonstrate actions that reflect nonjudgmental attitudes and values toward the client.

▶ The OTR evaluates clients to obtain or interpret the information necessary to plan an intervention. The COTAs role is to assist with data collection under the supervision of the OTR.

▶ The OTR initiates the evaluation process and delegates the appropriate assessments to be carried out by the COTA. The COTA may administer and score these assessments, but the OTR interprets the results with imput from the COTA to establish a treatment plan.

ADMINISTRATIVE ISSUES AND CONCERNS IN SUPERVISION OF COTAS

The American Occupational Therapy Association "Essentials and Guidelines for an Accredited Educational Program for the Occupational Therapy Assistant" (AOTA, 1991), the "Occupational Therapy Roles" (AOTA, 1993), and the "Guide for Supervision of Occupational Therapy Personnel" (AOTA, 1994) are only suggested guidelines. State licensure laws and the reimbursement codes for Medicare, Medicaid, and private insurance companies have had as much of an effect on actual practice and supervision issues as all three of these documents.

Some state occupational therapy associations have requested that on-site supervision be required for all billable COTA services and other states have been forced into that position through the political process of lobbying for licensure bills. In some states, COTAs receive a non-billable provider number after successful completion of the occupational therapy assistant National Board for Certification in Occupational Therapy (NBCOT) examination. This allows the OTR to bill for the COTAs services for a specific number of treatments with co-signature always required on all written evaluations and progress notes. OTRs taking vacations, attending workshops or conferences, or absent because of illness are required to have another OTR on the premises in order to fill in for any COTA supervision.

The on-site supervision requirement has prevented COTAs from functioning in any home service or community program without on-site supervision. As a result, other health workers such as home health aides, who receive a 6-week educational experience, have assumed these roles and jobs. There is nothing to prevent a COTA from accepting this job, but they can only be identified as a home health aide, not as a qualified person to do daily living skills and leisure time activities.

Emphasis in health care for the 21st century has been established in community and home health care programs coupled with the concern for reduction of cost of services. Development of these services will require lobbying for reimbursement coverage and utilization of all occupational therapy personnel for expansion of programs and cost effectiveness. It becomes apparent that if the community cannot afford occupational therapy services, they will be eliminated. Other health professionals are already being aggressive in their pursuit to assume the services that occupational therapy professionals provide.

The COTA, with OTR supervision, could provide particularly valuable services for clients with either a psychosocial or physical dysfunction . These services can include programs in the areas of physical restoration, daily living skills, work conditioning, leisure and play activities, therapeutic adaptations, wellness and prevention programs, and accessibility to home, work or community living. On-site supervision for the COTA would still be a necessity for the utilization of neurodevelopmental treatment techniques, sensory integration therapy, and the individual with acute physical disability or psychosocial dysfunction.

The intent of the original *Role Delineation* (AOTA, 1981) document was to make an honest effort at sorting out tasks, roles, and functions of the occupational therapy profession. The final format, however, relied on the catch-all phrase of "under direct supervision," which watered down the initial intent and left open the interpretation of current confusion. In addition, the role delineation only deals with the first year of practice and does not explore issues related to expertise gained through continuing education or amount of experience for either the OTR or COTA.

Clarifying and integrating a single role delineation philosophy for the COTA into practice, all of our standards, licensure, and reimbursement statements is an essential challenge that will be a positive additive for future growth and expansion of the occupational therapy profession. (See Appendix C: Table 1.)

Collaboration and Partnership

"The key to teamwork is collaboration. Meaningful collaboration results when each team member has mastered two requirements: (1) a clear understanding of each role; and (2) respect for the differences and similarities of each role" (Sands, 1998, p. 83). There is a trend in the profession to describe relationships between the OTR and the COTA as a partnership. Holmes (1993) stated "When the terms partner and collaboration are used to describe the relationship between the occupational therapist and the certified occupational therapy assistant, these words imply such elements as regard and respect for and knowledge of one's coworker" (p. 3). The OTR and COTA collaborate in the following ways (American Occupational Therapy Association, 1993):

▶ respond to requests for services

▶ develop treatment goals

▶ provide direct service

▶ adapt the enviroment using ergonomic principles

▶ communicate with other team members and caregivers

▶ document and record progress notes

▶ maintain treatment space and equipment

▶ monitor continuous quality improvement

▶ maintain and monitor standards of ethical behavior

Appendix C Table 1: Role Delineation for Entry-Level Occupational Therapists and Certified Occupational Therapy Assistants

	Entry-Level OTR	Entry-Level COTA
I. Referral	• Responds • Initiates • Supervises • Delegates	• Relays information • Initiates ADL referrals only
II. Occupational Therapy Evaluation		
1. Screening	• Collect • Formulate • Recommend • Document • Report	• Collect data as directed by OTR • Summarize • Record • Report own data to OTR
2. Assessment	• Interview client • Explain purpose of assessment and treatment • Select assessments • Administer standardized tests, clinical observations, and custom designed tests • Analyze and synthesize data • Report data • Make recommendations	• Contribute to the assessment • Assist in interviewing • Assist in observation to collect general data and report on selected skills • Administer standardized tests as directed by OTR • Report data as determined by OTR • Make recommendations to OTR
III. Program Planning	• Develop long- and short-term goals • Select occupational therapy interventions, including techniques, media, and purposeful occupation • Analyze task and activity components • Adapt techniques • Discuss OT goals with all involved • Coordinate program and treatment with other professionals	• Assist OTR in developing goals • Assist OTR in selecting techniques, media, and purposeful occupation • Analyze activities • Adapt techniques with OTR supervision • Discuss OT goals with all involved • Document and report initial goal setting as directed

Appendix C Table 1: Role Delineation for Entry-Level Occupational Therapists and Certified Occupational Therapy Assistants

	Entry-Level OTR	Entry-Level COTA
IV. Occupational Therapy Treatment	Engage client in purposeful and meaningful occupation in • physical living/daily living skills • psychological/emotional daily living skills • work skills • play/leisure • sensorimotor components • cognitive components • psychosocial components • therapeutic adaptations • prevention • Observe medical and safety precautions • Prepare and instruct a home program • Monitor client's program	• Under direction of OTR assist therapist in implementing purposeful and meaningfuloccupation • Observe medical and safety precautions • Assist in instruction of home program developed by OTR • Monitor client's program as directed by OTR
V. Program Continuation	• Formulate discharge and follow-up • Prepare home program • Instruct caregivers in continuity of treatment • Refer to other professionals • Recommend community resources • Summarize and document treatment progress	• Discuss need for discontinuation with OTR • Assist in preparation of home program • Assist in recommendation for environmental adaptations Recommend adaptations to environment • Assist in recommending community resources • Assist in summarizing and documenting treatment progress
VI. Service Management		
1. Administration	• Plan daily schedules • Prepare and order supplies • Determine space and equipment • Prepare and maintain records and budget • Prepare insurance forms for reimbursement • Compile and analyze group data • Conduct and participate in employee meetings • Follow departmental procedures • Seek and use consultation	• Plan daily schedules • Prepare and order supplies • Assist in analyzing group data • Participate in meetings • Follow procedures as mandates by the department
2. Personnel Supervision	• Recruit, select, orient, train, supervise, and evaluate COTAs • Orient, train, supervise, and evaluate Level I fieldwork students • Justify increasing personnel	• Supervise aides, volunteers, Level I OTA students • Assist in education of Level I students

Appendix C Table 1: Role Delineation for Entry-Level Occupational Therapists and Certified Occupational Therapy Assistants

	Entry-Level OTR	Entry-Level COTA
VII. Continued Education	• Plan and provide inservice education	• Assist in inservice education
	• Participate in continuing education and inservice programs	• Participate in continuing education and inservice programs
VIII. Public Relations	• Identify need and explain services to public	• Explain services to the public and professional groups

Sources: American Occupational Therapy Association. (1995). *COTA information packet (a guide for supervision).* Rockville, MD: Author; Margolis, D., Morgan, V., Dougherty, K., Halfon, K., & Petrone, P. (1997). *The OTR/COTA partnership: A blueprint for success.* Proceedings of the Annual Conference of the American Occupational Therapy Association, Orlando, FL, p. 27. Bethesda, MD: AOTA; American Occupational Therapy Association. (1994). Guide for supervision of occupational therapy personnel. *American Journal of Occupational Therapy, 48,* 1045–1046; American Occupational Therapy Association. (1991). Essentials and guidelines for an accredited educational program for the occupational therapy assistant. *American Journal of Occupational Therapy, 45,* 1085–1092; Schell, B. A. B. (1985). Guide to classification of occupational therapy personnel. *The American Journal of Occupational Therapy, 39,* 803–810.

REFERENCES

American Occupational Therapy Association. (1991). Essentials and guidelines for an accredited educational program for the occupational therapy assistant. *American Journal of Occupational Therapy, 45,* 1085–1092.

American Occupational Therapy Association. (1993). Occupational therapy roles. *American Journal of Occupational Therapy, 47,* 1087–1099.

American Occupational Therapy Association. (1994). Guide for supervision of occupational therapy personnel. *American Journal of Occupational Therapy, 48,* 1045–1046.

American Occupational Therapy Association. (1995). *COTA information packet (a guide for supervision).* Rockville, MD: Author.

Holmes, C. (1993, September). Challenging old paradigms. *Administration & Management Special Interest Section Newsletter, 9,* 3–4.

Margolis, D., Morgan, V., Doughterty, K., Halfon, K., & Petrone, P. (1997). *The OTR/COTA partnership: A blueprint for success.* Proceedings of the Annual Conference of the American Occupational Therapy Association, Orlando, FL, p. 27. Bethesda, MD: AOTA.

Sands, M. (1998). Practitioner's perspectives on the occupational therapist and occupational therapy assistant partnership. In M. E. Neistadt & E. B. Crepeau (Eds.), *Willard & Spackman's occupational therapy* (9th ed.; pp. 83–89). Philadelphia: Lippincott.

Schell, B. A. B. (1985). Guide to classification of occupational therapy personnel. *The American Journal of Occupational Therapy, 39,* 803–810.

APPENDIX

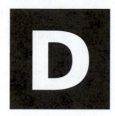

Useful Web Sites for Occupational Therapists, Students, and Researchers in Psychosocial Practice

Professional Organizations

American Occupational Therapy Association (AOTA)
http://www.aota.org/

Canadian Occupational Therapy Association (COTA)
http://www.caot.ca/

World Federation of Occupational Therapy (WFOT)
http://www.wfot.org.au/

British Association and College of Occupational Therapists
http://www.cot.co.uk/

World Psychiatric Association (WPA)
http://www.wpanet.org/

World Health Organization of the United Nations (WHO)
http://www.who.int/

World Federation for Mental Health (WFMH)
http://www.wfmh.org/

American Academy for Child and Adolescent Psychiatry (AACAP)
http://www.aacap.org/

American Psychiatric Association
http://www.psych.org/

American Psychological Association (APA)
http://www.apa.org/

Self-Help Groups

National Mental Health Association (NMHA)
http://www.nmha.org/

National Alliance for the Mentally Ill (NAMI)
http://www.nami.org/

The Alzheimer's Association
http://www.alz.org/

Bipolar and Depression
http://groups.yahoo.com/group/ros-esandthorns

Borderline Personality Disorder
http://groups.yahoo.com/group/welcometooz

Depression Support
http:// groups.yahoo.com/group/great-depression or
http:// groups.yahoo.com/group/melancholy

Schizophrenia
http:// groups.yahoo.com/group/schizophrenia

The Mental Health Net Self-Help Resources
http://mentalhelp.net/selfhelp.htm

Anxiety and Panic Disorders
http://www.soberrecovery.com/links/anxietyandpanicdisorde.html

Mental Health Information

Occupational Therapy Internet World
http://www.mother.com/~ktherapy/ot

About.com:The Human Internet
http://mentalhealth.about.com/health/mental-health/mbody.htm

ERIC
http://www.ericae.net
http://accesseric.org

Healthgate Medline
http://bewell.healthgate.com/

Internet Mental Health
http://www.mentalhealth.com/

Mental Health Net
http://mentalhelp.net/

National Association for Research in Schizophrenia and Depression (NARSAD)
http://www.mhsource.com/narsad/

Mental Health Source
http://www.mhsource.com/

Interpsych conferences
http://www.shef.ac.uk/~psysc/InterPsych/inter.html

Psychiatry and Mental Health
http://www.medscape.com/Home/Topics/psychiatry/psychiatry.html

DSM-IV Diagnoses and Codes

Numerical listing:
http://www.dr-bob.org/tips/dsm4n.html

Alphabetical listing:
http://www.dr-bob.org/tips/dsm4a.html

Governmental

National Institute of Mental Health (NIMH)
http://www.nimh.nih.gov/

Internet Grateful Med Medline Search, National Library of Medicine
http://igm.nlm.nih.gov/

APPENDIX

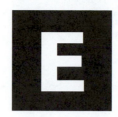

Calories Expended per Hour for Typical Activities

Activity	Weight		
	130 lbs	155 lbs	190 lbs.
Aerobics, general	354	422	518
Backpacking, general	413	493	604
Badminton	266	317	388
Basketball	354	422	518
Bicycling	236	281	345
Bicycling on stationary bike	295	352	431
Bowling	177	211	259
Calisthenics	266	317	388
Construction, outside, remodeling	325	387	474
Cooking or food preparation	145	176	216
Cross-country skiing	472	463	690
Dancing	266	317	388
Fishing	236	281	345
Gardening	295	352	431
General house cleaning	207	246	302
Golf	236	281	345
Hiking	354	422	518
Horseback riding	236	281	345
Jogging	413	493	604
Moving furniture	354	422	518
Mowing lawn	325	387	474
Raking lawn	236	281	345
Running	472	563	690
Shoveling snow	354	422	518
Sweeping garage or sidewalk	236	281	345
Swimming laps, freestyle	472	563	690
Tai ch'i	236	281	345
Throwing darts	148	176	216
Walking, slow pace	148	176	216
Walking a dog	207	246	302
Weight lifting	177	211	259
Yoga	236	281	345

Source: Adapted from *Calories Burned during Exercise and Activities*, developed from research of the *Medicine and Science in Sports and Exercise, The Official Journal of the American College of Sports Medicine*. Obtained June 27, 2001, from the World Wide Web: http://www.nutristrategy.com/activitylist.htm

INDEX

acquisitional frame of reference, 132

activity groups, 92

activity program
  and treatment methods, 77–78

acupuncture, 519–20

acute stress disorder, 216

additive effect, 314

aftercare clinic, 75

agoraphobia, 215

Alcoholics Anonymous
  Twelve Steps of, 223

alcoholism, 220–22

Allen Cognitive Levels, 257

alternative medicine
  definition, 519
  prevalence, 519
  recent research in, 519–21

alternative treatment, 521–22
  assessment, 522
  bibliography for additional information in, 529–31
  assumptions, 522

Alzheimer's disease, 15
  caregivers for individuals with, 226–27
  course of disease, 234–25
  definition, 224
  diagnosis, 225–26
  etiology and risk factors, 225
  incidence and prevalence, 225
  treatment, 226

analytic frame of reference, 132

anorexia nervosa, 15, 210

antianxiety or anxiolytic drugs, 317

antidepressants and mood stabilizers, 317–18, 323,

antipsychotic or neuroleptic drugs, 323

antisocial personality disorders, 209–10, 218

anxiety disorder(s), 14–16, 206, 214–16

acute stress disorder, 216

agoraphobia without history of panic disorder, 215
  due to a general medical condition, 216
  generalized anxiety disorder, 216
  panic disorder without agoraphobia (panic attack), 215
  panic disorder with agoraphobia, 215
  research evidence about, 217–18
  specific phobia, 215–16
  substance-induced anxiety disorder, 216
  social phobia, 216
  obsessive-compulsive disorder (OCD), 216
  posttraumatic stress disorder (PTSD), 216

aromatherapy, 520

art
  as a creative modality for the occupational therapist, 546–47

art therapy, 545–49
  and behavioral therapy, 548–49

asymmetrical tonic neck reflex, 154–55

attention deficit hyperactivity disorder (ADHD), 14
  characteristics of, 204

Attitudes Toward Mental Illness Scale, 2, 4

auditory-language dysfunction, 152–53

autism, 15, 205–6

autonomy, 231

aversive conditioning, 221

avoidant personality disorder, 218

Ayres, Jean, 152–55

Barth Time Construction, 258

Barton, W. E., 27

Bay Area Functional Performance Evaluation (BaFPE), 259

Beers, Clifford, 50–51

behavior assessment, 249

behavioral medicine, 138–39

behavioral theoretical model, 134–43

behaviorism, 134–37

    as related to cognitive behavioral theory, 137–38

behavior modification, 137

behavior therapy, 137–38

    as compared to traditional medicine, 140–41

Beveridge, William Ian Beardmore, 591

bibliotherapy, 553

bilateral integration, 152

bilateral motor coordination, 154

bioavailability, 310

biofeedback

    as a cybernetic model, 445–46

    as a process, 444–45

    autonomic nervous system and, 446–48

    definition, 444

    modalities, 447

        electroencephalogram, 449

        electromyographic (EMG), 447

        galvanic skin response (GSR), 449

        skin temperature feedback equipment, 449

    technology, 449–50

bipolar disorder, 14

blood-brain barrier, 310

Boys Town, 90–91

British empiricism, 135

bulimia, 210

Campbell, J. F., 391

Canadian Model of Occupational Performance (CMOP), 174–75, 260

career

    counseling programs, 402

    placement programs, 402

case management, 75

case study analysis, 201–2

case study (ies)

    in employment/vocational opportunities, 411–12

choreoathetoid movements, 155

classical conditioning, 135

clinical research, 594–95

    models of, 595–96

clinical research studies

    critique of, 596–97

    evaluating and designing, 591–608

cognitive-behavioral therapy (CBT) frame of reference

    assumptions, 145

    definition, 143–44

    principles of, 145

    research and methodology, 144–46

cognitive disability frame of reference, 146–49

cognitive treatment, 226

Cognitive Adaptive Skills Evaluation (CASE), 261

Comprehensive Occupational Therapy Evaluation (COTE), 262

comprehensive community mental health centers (CMHC), 66

certified occupational assistant (COTA), 56

    emergence of, 56–57

    in psychosocial practice, 194–96

Chapin, William, 18, 22–23

childhood depression, 206

Civilian Health and Medical Program of the Uniformed Services (CHAMPUS), 586–87

cognitive disability frame of reference, 146–49

communication aids, 472–73

community care model

    and the roles of the occupational therapist (1960–2000), 65–95

    applied to youth at risk, 86–88

    emergence of, 66–74

community living

    readjustment of patients to, 72–74

community mental health centers, 78–86

    occupational therapist's role in, 78–80

community mental health programs

    evaluating the effectiveness of, 92–95

    examples of, 90–91

    goals for, 70–72

    models for, 74–76

community residential treatment center (case study), 89

community support groups, 76

community treatment programs, 90–91

computerized assessment, 249

conditioned stimulus, 137

Continuous Quality Improvement (CQI)

    definition, 580–85

crafts, 540–41

creative arts therapies, 552–53
  see also art therapy; dance therapy; music therapy; and poetry therapy
creative process, 540
creativity
  relationship between mental illness and, 541–45
credentialing, 563–65
crisis response services, 75
cumulative effect, 314

daily life patterns
  continuity of, 34–35
dance
  and mental health, 37
dance therapy
  Marion Chase technique, 549–50
  range of motion (ROM) dance, 550
day treatment center
  activity program, 77–78
  goals and functions of, 76–78
  prototype of (The Support Network, Madison, WI), 81–83
  structure of, 77
dependent personality disorder, 218
depression, 210–14
  effects of exercise on, 504–7
  humor as a means to counteract, 439
design copying, 154
developmental frame of reference, 132
developmental theoretical model, 149–50
development of inner controls
  for youth at risk, 91
diagnoses
  coding, 199–200
Diagnostic and Statistical Manual (DSM-IV), 196–97
  assumptions in, 197–98
  classifications of, 199
  reliability and validity of, 200–1
diet
  healthy, 516–17
documentation
  and identification and background information, 572
  assessment results and, 572–75
  intervention and treatment plan in, 575–77
  need for, 566–69
  progress report in, 577–79

role of, 569–70
structure and elements of, 570–71
summary of process of , 579
drug(s)
  administration and absorption, 306–9
  antianxiety or anxiolytic, 317
  antidepressants and mood stabilizers, 317–18, 323
  antipsychotic, 323
  categorization of, 305
  classes of, 316–23
  definition, 302
  distribution, 309–10
  effects of, 311–12
  interactions of, 314
  mechanisms of actions and processes of, 312
  metabolism and elimination of, 310–11
  naming the, 304–5
  physiological barriers to absorption of, 310
  physiological dependency, 316
  physical dependency or addiction to, 316
  potency of, 314
  psychostimulants, 324, 326
  psychotherapeutic, 318–22
  response relationships, 312–14
  tolerance of, 315–16
DSM-IV (Diagnostic and Statistical Manual), 196–97
Dubos, R., 497
Dumazedier, J., 463
Dunton, Jr., William Rush, 51–52
dynamic treatment
  definition, 54
  development of, 54–56
dyspraxia, 152

eating disorders, 15–16, 210
education
  supported, 401–2
effective dosages, 313
ego, 116, 119–21
ego defense mechanisms
  introjection, 123
  isolation, 123
  projection, 123–25
  reaction formation, 125
  regression, 125–26
  repression, 126

sublimation, 126
turning against the self, 126
undoing, 127
ego psychology, 119–22
"Eight Stages of Man", 120–22
empathy, 232
employment
    casual, 399–400
    delivery of services for, 396–397
    for individuals with psychosocial disabilities,
        391–413
    full-time, 400
    in-home, 398–99
    part-time, 400
    principles of work for, 394–95
    self-, 400
    supported competitive, 85–86, 399
    support or follow along, 402
    theories of career development for, 393–94
    transitional, 399
    work as treatment and, 395–96
environmental mastery, 232
Erikson, Erik, 120–22, 544
Erikson, J. M., 539
exercise
    and mental health, 503–4
    as an alternative treatment, 530
    as part of therapy, 500–1
    beneficial effects of, 501–3
    definition, 498
    research on depression and, 504
    types or classifications of, 499–500
exercise program
    compliance and motivation to adhere to, 508–10
    components of, 507–8
exorcism, 38
experimenter bias, 603
extraocular muscle control, 155
eye-hand coordination, 153

families
    and mental illness, 18–23
Federal Employees Health Benefit Program, 587
Fidler, G. S., 129–32, 187
Fidler, J. W., 129–32, 187
figure-ground perception, 153
finger identification, 153

forensic psychiatry, 70
form and space perception, 152
frames of reference
    cognitive behavioral therapy (CBT), 143–44
    cognitive disability, 146–49
    occupational adaptation, 166–68
    occupational science, 168–70
    psychodynamic, 129–33
    Reilly's Work-Play, 170–73
    sensory integrative therapy, 151–62
Freud, Anna, 12
Freud, Sigmund, 112, 115–22
    and the tripartite mind (id, ego, superego),
        116–19
    and ego defense mechanisms, 123–25
Fromm, Erich, 123
Functional Assessment Scale (FAS), 263
functionalism, 135

Galen, 391
General Aptitude Test Battery (GATB), 400
generalized anxiety disorder, 216
Geriatric Depression Scale, 264
Geriatric Rating Scale (GRS), 265
Girls Town, 90–1
Gordon, Barbara, 18–19
graphesthesia, 153
group process, 359–84

halfway house, 74–75
Hamilton Depression Inventory (HDI), 266
Haas, Louis, 52–54
Hartmann, Heinz, 121
Hawthorne effect, 603
health maintenance organizations (HMOs), 588
health perspective, 35
Health Status Questionnaire (HSQ), 267
Hemphill, B. J., 241
herbal medicine, 517–18
hierarchical development, 91
Hippocrates, 32
histrionic personality disorder, 218
Hoch, P. H., 301
holistic approach
    in psychosocial practice, 1–23
    model for, 11–12
    steps in the, 191

and treatment for depression, 214–17
  role of nutrition in the, 511
holistic medicine, 15–18
homelessness, 69–70
humanism, 10–12
  definition, 10
humanistic caring, 12
humor
  as alternative treatment, 530
hypochondriasis
  of the remedies for, 44–45

id, 116, 120–21
incarceration, 70
Independent Living Skills Evaluation, (ILSE), 268
informed consent procedure, 606–7
initial interview
  assessment of client's symptoms during, 193–94
  purposes of, 190, 192
  structure of, 192–93
  therapeutic techniques during, 192
institutionalization
  negative effects of, 66–67
integration (of processes and attributes of an individual), 230
integration of function, 155
intimacy, 210

Jacobs Prevocational Skills Assessment (JPSA), 269
Jahoda, Marie, 227–33

Katz Adjustment Scale, 270
Kennedy, John F., 65
kinesthesia, 153
Kohlman Evaluation of Living Skills, 271

learning disabilities, 204
Leary, S., 359
leisure
  definition, 464–65
leisure activities/skills
  developing as alternative treatment, 530
  assumptions underlying, 465
  definition, 464–65
  identifying client interests in, 465–70
  purposes of, 470–71

life goals
  realistic, 35
Leisure Occupations Interest Inventory (LOII), 465–70
Leisure Occupations Sentence Completion, 466, 470
lethal dosage, 314
Life Satisfaction Index K (LSI-K), 272
light therapy, 520
localization of tactile stimuli, 153
Loewenstein Occupational Therapy Cognitive Assessment (LOTCA), 273
Loveless, D., 539
Loveless, J., 539

Magazine Picture Collage (MPC), 274
magnetic field therapy, 520
Maslow, A. H., 230
manic depressive illness (bipolar disorder), 14
manual form perception, 153
massage therapy, 520
Medicaid, 587
Medicare, 585–86
medications related to psychosocial issues, 301–55
meditation
  and progressive relaxation, 454–56
  and the relaxation response, 452
  definition, 450
  how does it work? 451–52
  recommendations to clients and therapists for using, 453–54
mental disorder
  definition of, 197
mental disorder, 9
mental health
  consultation, 75–76
  dance and, 37–78
  definition, 8–9
  exercise and, 35–36
  minimal, 10
  music and, 36–7
  naturalistic approach to, 32–38
  nutritional factors in, 33–34
  optimal, 10
mental health care
  equality of, 13
mental health problem, 9

mental health system
    reforms and shifts in the United States, 67–69
mental hygiene movement, 46–54
    Clifford Beers and, 50–51
mental illness
    attitudes toward, 2–8
    creativity and, 541–45
    definition, 8–9
    extended family and, 34
    homelessness and, 69–70
    incarceration and, 69–70
    families and, 18–23
    history of treatment of, 27–58
    incidence and prevalence of, 14–16
    inhumane era in the care of those with, 38–40
    moral treatment of those with, 40–42
    music and, 36
    nutritional factors in, 33–34
mental retardation, 204
Meyer, A., 1, 49–50
Milwaukee Evaluation of Daily Living Skills
        (MEDLS), 277
minimal dosage level, 313
Mini-Mental State (MMS), 278
Minnesota Multiphasic Personality Inventory
        (MMPI), 208
Model of Human Occupation (MOHO), 163–66
model for a therapeutic group, 373–81
modeling behavior, 91
mood disorders (affective disorders), 14, 16
    during young adulthood, 210–14
morning ritual, 440
Mosey, A. C., 109
    Three Frames of Reference, 132–33
motor accuracy, 154
muscle tone, 155
music
    and mental health, 36–37
    as alternative treatment, 530
music therapy, 550–52

narcissistic personality disorder, 218
National Institutes of Mental Health
    legislative chronology for, 68
Neary, John, 18–20
neuroleptic drugs, 323
NPI Interest Checklist, 279

nutrient, 511
nutrition, 509–16
    carbohydrates, 511–12
    in mental health, 33–34
    fats, 513
    incorporating into therapy, 517
    minerals, 515
    proteins, 512
    role of in a holistic program, 511
    vitamins, 513–15
    water, 516

obsessive-compulsive disorder (OCD), 216, 218
occupational adaptation, 166–68
occupational behavior
    frames of reference, 162–63
    theoretical model of, 162–75
occupational adaptation frame of reference, 166–68
Occupational Performance History Interview, 280
Occupational Questionnaire (OQ), 281
occupational science frame of reference, 168–70
occupational therapist
    art as a creative modality for the, 546–47
    community care model and the roles of the,
        65–95
    emphasis of, 53–54
    roles of the, 65, 78–80
occupational therapy
    and the mental hygiene movement, 46–54
    conceptual model of, 79–80
    emergence of, 27–57
    exercise as part of, 500–1
    facilities, 80–81
    implications for, 91–92
    incorporating nutrition into, 517
    in mental hospitals, 47–49
    insurance coverage for, 585
    process, 402–4
    profession of, 9–11
        emergence of the, 46–54
    psychotherapeutic nature of, 188–90
    survey of treatment methods used, 523–26
    treatment for alcohol abuse, 222
    treatment process, 139–42, 187–233
operant conditioning, 135
Outward Bound programs, 229

PAM (Physical Agent Modalities), 529
Parachek Geriatric Rating Scale, 282
panic disorder (panic attack), 215
paranoid personality disorder, 218
paranoid schizophrenia, 20
partial hospitalization, 74
perception of reality, 231–32
performance
    areas and component, 599–604
    component
Performance Assessment of Self-Care Skills (PASS),
    283
personal care
    skills necessary for independent living, 472
personality and conduct disorders, 206
    antisocial or psychopathic, 218
    avoidant personality disorder, 218
    borderline personality disorder, 218
    dependent personality disorder, 218
    narcissistic personality disorder, 218
    obsessive-compulsive personality disorder,
        218–19
    paranoid personality disorder, 218
    schizoid personality disorder, 218
    schizotypal personality disorder, 218
    research evidence for treatment effectiveness, 219
pet therapy, 226, 529–30
pharmocodynamics, 315
pharmokinetics
    definition, 306
phobia, 215–16
Piaget, J., 149–51
placebo effect, 601–2
play therapy, 552
poetry therapy, 553
positive reinforcement
    as fostered in the adolescent, 91–92
postrotary nystagmus, 154
posttraumatic stress disorder (PTSD), 216
praxis
    constructional, 154
    on verbal command, 153
    oral, 154
    postural, 154
    sequencing, 154
prayer
    as a form of alternative medicine, 520–21

preferred provider organizations (PPOs), 588
Professional Standard Review Organizations
    (PSRO), 561–62
Profile of Mood State (POMS), 284
private payment insurance systems, 587–88
psychiatry
    forensic, 70
    goals of, 28–32
    landmarks in the 20th century, 29
psychiatric rehabilitation program, 31
psychoanalysis (')
    application to occupational therapy, 128–29
    critical analysis of, 128–29
    impact on occupational therapy, 127–28
    key concepts in, 116–28
psychodrama, 552–53
psychodynamic frame of reference, 129–33
psychodynamic theoretical model, 112–29
    assumptions, 112–14
    definition, 112
psychoeducational model, 433
psychological development
    adolescence (12 to 20 years), 207–10
    childhood (3 to 11 years), 203–7
    infancy (0 to 2 years), 203
    middle adulthood (36 to 65 years), 222
    old age (over 65), 223–27
    prenatal and perinatal, 203
    stages of, 202–27
    young adulthood (21 to 35 years), 210–22
psychosexual stages of development, 119
psychosocial assessment
    suggested test battery for, 253–94
psychosocial dysfunction
    evaluation and assessment of individuals with,
        241–94
    process of, 2–3
psychosocial occupational therapy, 9–18
    applied versus basic research in, 592–3
    applying the group process to, 359–84
        activity groups, 360–61
        behavioral groups, 364
        cognitive dysfunction groups, 365–66
        cognitive-behavioral groups, 371–73
        developmental groups, 363–64
        directive group therapy, 370–71
        human occupation groups, 364–65

integrative group therapy, 369–70
    reality-oriented groups, 362
    role-oriented groups, 363
    self-awareness groups, 361
  concepts of positive mental health for, 227–32
  creative and expressive arts and their application
    to, 539–54
  critique of clinical research studies in, 597
  future of, 12
  generating research in, 593–96
  model for a therapeutic group in, 373–81
  research on therapeutic groups in, 381–84
  short- and long-term treatment goals in, 227
  teaching the creative arts versus creative expres-
    sion, 541
  theoretical models underlying, 109–75
  treatment model, 142–43
psychosocial practice
  holistic approach in, 1–23
psychosocial stages of development, 119
psychotherapy, "the talking cure," 115
psychostimulants, 324
"psychotic art," 545
puppetry
  as used in therapy, 553

Qi gong, 520
quality assurance
  and the need for documentation, 566–79
  assessment of quality in health care, 565–66
  credentialing and, 563–65
  definition, 560, 562–63
  historical notes on, 560–62
  in mental health care, 559–85

range of motion (ROM) dance, 550
Reilly's Work-Play frame of reference, 170–73
reinforcement, 137
relaxation response, 452
relaxation therapy, 520
  as alternative treatment, 530–31
reminiscence groups, 226
research
  on therapeutic groups, 381–84
  protection of subjects in, 604
residential treatment center (RTC), 86
Role Activity Performance Scale (RAPS), 285

Role Checklist, 286
rolfing, 520
Rosenfield, J., 497
rural mental health, 76

safety margin, 314
schizophrenia, 14, 16, 122–23
  art of individuals with, 545–48
  comprehensive treatment planning for, 209
  definition, 207
  diagnosis, 208–9
  patient with chronic, 84–85
  precipitating factors, 208
  presumed causes and predisposing factors of, 208
  prevalence of, 14
  subdiagnostic groups (types of schizophrenia),
    209
schizoid personality disorder, 218
schizotypal personality disorder, 218
self
  as treatment agent, 56
  in healthy individuals, 227–32
self-actualization, 230
self-care activities, 471
  and skills necessary for independent living, 472
  apartment and home maintenance, 473
  communication aids, 472–73
  definition, 471
  medical management, 473
  money management, 473
  health maintenance, 473–74
  teaching, 471
  transportation, 473
  validation of the individual's competencies in,
    474
    standardized tests, 475
    in vivo observations, 475
self-confidence, 229
self-regulation, 12, 487
Selye, H., 417
sense of identity, 207
Sensory Integration and Praxis Tests (SIPT), 153
sensory integration treatment modalities, 155–58
sensory integrative therapy frame of reference,
    151–62
  assumptions, 152
  clinical research studies of, 159–62

definition, 151–52
  theoretical concepts of, 152–53
sensory stimulation, 226
Short-Form McGill Pain Questionnaire (SF-MPQ), 275
Short Portable Mental Status Questionnaire (SPMSQ), 276
single-subject research, 597–98
  proposal for, 604–8
sleep hygiene, 438
social dysfunction
  process of, 3
social phobia, 216
social skills
  assertiveness training and, 488
  assessment of, 482
  definition, 478
  effectiveness of training in (recent studies), 489
  initiating a program in, 482, 489
    assessment, 483–84
  teaching methods, 484–85
  training, 478–81
  need for, 481–82
Soranus, 32
Southern California Sensory Integration Tests (SCSIT), 153
space visualization, 153
  contralateral use, 154
  preferred hand use, 154
spiritual healing, 520–21
standing and walking balance, 154
State-Trait Anxiety Inventory (STAI), 287
stimulus, 137
Street Survival Skills Questionnaire (SSSQ), 288
stress
  and its relationship to mental illness, 418–23
  as a precipitating factor in mental illness, 421
  assessment of, 423–25
  causes of, 420
  definition, 418–20
    resistance to, 230–31
  symptoms of, 421–23
Stress Audit Questionnaire, 289
stress management program, 417–57
  application of, 425
  as a critical life skill, 436–37
  compliance with, 441–44

  designing, 431–33
Stress Management Questionnaire (SMQ), 290
  components of, 424
  conceptual definition of stress as defined by the, 423–24
  conceptual development of the, 424–25
  test instrument, 426–30
Strong-Campbell Interest Inventory (SCII), 291
structured environments
  for adolescents, 92
substance abuse
  alcohol use, 220
  etiology, 220
  illicit drug use, 219–20
  occupational therapy treatment for, 222
  treatment objectives for, 220–22
substance-related disorders, 16, 216
superego, 119
Support Network (Madison, WI), 81–85

Tai Ch'i, 521
tactile defensiveness, 152
test battery for psychological assessment, 254–94
Three Frames of Reference, 132–33
theory (ies)
  as clustered into theoretical models, 111–12
  characteristics of, 111–12
  definition, 111
theoretical model(s), 111–29
  behavioral, 134–43
  developmental, 149–50
  psychodynamic, 112–29
therapeutic guided imagery, 521
therapeutic social clubs, 74
therapeutic touch, 521
threshold dosage level, 313
tonic labyrinth reflex, 154
Trager® approach, 521
treatment
  evaluation of, 598–99
  outcome, 598–99
tripartite mind (id, ego, superego), 116–19

unconditional stimulus, 137

Valpar (Valpar Corp.), 292
vestibular system function, 155

visualization exercise, 456–57
vocational assessment tools, 400
vocational rehabilitation, 391–413
    affirmative businesses, 398
    cooperatives, 397–98
    delivery of services for, 396–97
    home employment for, 398–99
    principles of work for, 394–95
    process, 404–11
    sheltered work, 397
    theories of career development for, 393–94
    volunteer work, 397
    work as treatment in, 395–96
Wilson, Louise, 202–22

West, W. L., 559
work
    adjustment training, 401
    definition, 464
    hardening, 401
Worker Role Interview (WRI), 293

youth at risk
    and community care model, 86–88
    community residential treatment center for, 89
    therapeutic goals for, 86–88

Zung Self-Rating Depression Scale (ZSRDS), 294